Timothy R. Deer
Editor-in-chief

Michael S. Leong
Associate Editor-in-chief

Albert L. Ray
Associate Editor

Treatment of Chronic Pain by Integrative Approaches

the AMERICAN ACADEMY *of* PAIN MEDICINE
Textbook on Patient Management

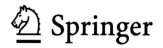 Springer

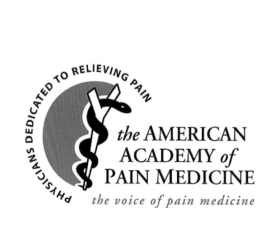

the AMERICAN
ACADEMY *of*
PAIN MEDICINE
the voice of pain medicine

Editor-in-chief
Timothy R. Deer, M.D.
President and CEO
The Center for Pain Relief
Clinical Professor of Anesthesiology
West Virginia University School of Medicine
Charleston, WV, USA

Associate Editor
Albert L. Ray, M.D.
Medical Director
The LITE Center
South Miami, FL, USA

Clinical Associate Professor
University of Miami Miller School of Medicine
Miami, FL, USA

Associate Editor-in-chief
Michael S. Leong, M.D.
Clinic Chief
Stanford Pain Medicine Center
Redwood City, CA, USA

Clinical Associate Professor
Department of Anesthesiology
Stanford University School of Medicine
Stanford, CA, USA

ISBN 978-1-4939-1820-1   ISBN 978-1-4939-1821-8 (eBook)
DOI 10.1007/978-1-4939-1821-8
Springer New York Heidelberg Dordrecht London

Library of Congress Control Number: 2014953009

Springer is part of Springer Science+Business Media (www.springer.com)

To my wonderful wife, Missy, and the blessings I have been given in my children Morgan, Taylor, Reed, and Bailie.
I also want to thank my team for their awesome, continued support:
Chris Kim, Rick Bowman, Doug Stewart, Matt Ranson, Jeff Peterson, Michelle Miller, Wil Tolentino, and Brian Yee.

Timothy R. Deer, M.D.

To all of my mentors, colleagues, and patients who have taught me about pain medicine. I would also like to acknowledge the patience and love of my family, particularly my children, Isabelle and Adam, as well as Brad, PFP, and little Mia. I have discovered more about myself during my short career than I thought possible and hope to help many more people cope with pain in the exciting future.

Michael S. Leong, M.D.

To my family and The LITE Center team, who have been patient and allowed me time to do this work.

Albert L. Ray, M.D.

Foreword to *Comprehensive Treatment of Chronic Pain by Medical, Interventional, and Integrative Approaches*

A brand new textbook is a testament to many things—an editor's vision, many authors' individual and collective expertise, the publisher's commitment, and all told, thousands of hours of hard work. This book encapsulates all of this, and with its compendium of up-to-date information covering the full spectrum of the field of pain medicine, it stands as an authoritative and highly practical reference for specialists and primary care clinicians alike. These attributes would be ample, in and of themselves, yet this important addition to the growing pain medicine library represents a rather novel attribute. It is a tangible embodiment of a professional medical society's fidelity to its avowed mission. With its commission of this text, under the editorial stewardship of highly dedicated and seasoned pain medicine specialists, the American Academy of Pain Medicine has made an important incremental step forward to realizing its ambitious mission, "to optimize the health of patients in pain and eliminate the major public health problem of pain by advancing the practice and specialty of pain medicine."

This last year, the Institute of Medicine (IOM) of the National Academies undertook the first comprehensive evaluation of the state of pain care in the United States. This seminal work culminated in a report and recommendations entitled "Relieving Pain in America: A Blueprint for Transforming Prevention, Care, Education, and Research." Clearly, as a nation, we have much work to do in order to meet the extraordinary public health needs revealed by the IOM committee. This comprehensive textbook is both timely and relevant as a resource for clinicians, educators, and researchers to ensure that the converging goals of the American Academy of Pain Medicine and the Institute of Medicine are realized. This book has been written; it is now all of ours to read and implement. Godspeed!

Salt Lake City, UT, USA   Perry G. Fine, M.D.

Foreword to *Comprehensive Treatment of Chronic Pain by Medical, Interventional, and Integrative Approaches*

The maturation of a medical specialty rests on both its ability to project its values, science, and mission into the medical academy and the salience of its mission to the public health. The arrival of the American Academy of Pain Medicine (AAPM)'s *Comprehensive Treatment of Chronic Pain by Medical, Interventional, and Integrative Approaches: the American Academy of Pain Medicine Textbook on Patient Management* is another accomplishment that signals AAPM's emergence as the premier medical organization solely dedicated to the development of pain medicine as a specialty in the service of patients in pain and the public health.

Allow me the privilege of brief comment on our progress leading to this accomplishment. The problem of pain as both a neurophysiological event and as human suffering has been a core dialectic of the physician-healer experience over the millennia, driving scientific and religious inquiry in all cultures and civilizations. The sentinel concepts and historical developments in pain medicine science and practice are well outlined in this and other volumes. Our history, like all of medicine's, is replete with examples of sociopolitical forces fostering environments in which individuals with vision and character initiated major advances in medical care. Thus the challenge of managing chronic pain and suffering born of injuries to troops in WWII galvanized John Bonica and other pioneers, representing several specialties, into action. They refused to consider that their duty to these soldiers, and by extension their brethren in chronic pain of all causes, was finished once pain was controlled after an acute injury or during a surgical procedure. They and other clinicians joined scientists in forming the IASP (International Association for the Study of Pain) in 1974, and the APS (American Pain Society) was ratified as its American chapter in 1978. Shortly thereafter, APS physicians with a primary interest in the development of pain management as a distinct medical practice began discussing the need for an organizational home for physicians dedicated to pain treatment; in 1984, they formally chartered AAPM. We soon obtained a seat in the AMA (American Medical Association). Since then, we have provided over two decades of leadership to the "House of Medicine," culminating in leadership of the AMA's Pain and Palliative Medicine Specialty Section Council that sponsored and conducted the first Pain Medicine Summit in 2009. The summit, whose participants represented all specialties caring for pain, made specific recommendations to improve pain education for all medical students and pain medicine training of residents in all specialties and to lengthen and strengthen the training of pain medicine specialists who would assume responsibility for the standards of pain education and care and help guide research.

Other organizational accomplishments have also marked our maturation as a specialty. AAPM developed a code of ethics for practice, delineated training and certification requirements, and formed a certifying body (American Board of Pain Medicine, ABPM) whose examination was based on the science and practice of our several parent specialties coalesced into one. We applied for specialty recognition in ABMS (American Board of Medical Specialties), and we continue to pursue this goal in coordination with other specialty organizations to assure the public and our medical colleagues of adequate training for pain medicine specialists. We have become a recognized and effective voice in medical policy. The AAPM, APS, and AHA (American Hospital Association) established the Pain Care Coalition (PCC), recently joined by the ASA (American Society of Anesthesiologists). Once again, by garnering sociopolitical support galvanized by concern for the care of our wounded warriors, the PCC was able to partner with the American Pain Foundation (APF) and other organizations to pass three new laws requiring the Veterans Administration and the military to report yearly on advances in pain management, training, and research and requiring the NIH (National Institute of Health) to examine its pain research portfolio and undertake the recently completed IOM report on pain.

AAPM has developed a robust scientific presence in medicine. We publish our own journal, *Pain Medicine*, which has grown from a small quarterly journal to a respected monthly publication that represents the full scope of pain medicine science and practice. Annually, we conduct the only medical conference that is dedicated to coverage of the full scope of pain medicine science and practice and present a robust and scientific poster session that represents our latest progress. Yet, year to year, we lament that the incredible clinical wisdom displayed at this conference, born out of years of specialty practice in our field, is lost between meetings. Now comes a remedy, our textbook—*Comprehensive Treatment of Chronic Pain by Medical, Interventional, and Integrative Approaches*.

Several years ago, Editor Tim Deer, who co-chaired an Annual Meeting Program Committee with Todd Sitzman, recognized the special nature of our annual conference and proposed that the AAPM engages the considerable expertise of our membership in producing a textbook specifically focused on the concepts and practice of our specialty. Under the visionary and vigorous leadership of Tim as Editor-in-Chief and his editorial group, *Comprehensive Treatment of Chronic Pain by Medical, Interventional, and Integrative Approaches* has arrived. Kudos to Tim, his Associate Editor-in-Chief Michael Leong, Associate Editors Asokumar Buvanendran, Vitaly Gordin, Philip Kim, Sunil Panchal, and Albert Ray for guiding our busy authors to the finish line. The expertise herein represents the best of our specialty and its practice. And finally, a specialty organization of physician volunteers needs a steady and resourceful professional staff to successfully complete its projects in the service of its mission. Ms. Susie Flynn, AAPM's Director of Education, worked behind-the-scenes with our capable Springer publishers and Tim and his editors to assure our book's timely publication. Truly, this many-faceted effort signals that the academy has achieved yet another developmental milestone as a medical organization inexorably destined to achieve specialty status in the American medical pantheon.

Philadelphia, PA, USA   Rollin M. Gallagher, M.D., M.P.H.

Preface to *Treatment of Chronic Pain by Integrative Approaches*

We are grateful for the positive reception of *Comprehensive Treatment of Chronic Pain by Medical, Interventional, and Integrative Approaches:* **The AMERICAN ACADEMY OF PAIN MEDICINE *Textbook on Patient Management*** following its publication last year. The book was conceived as an all-encompassing clinical reference covering the entire spectrum of approaches to pain management: medical, interventional, and integrative. Discussions with pain medicine physicians and health professionals since then have persuaded us that the book could serve even more readers if sections on each of the major approaches were made available as individual volumes – while some readers want a comprehensive resource, others may need only a certain slice. We are pleased that these "spin-off" volumes are now available. I would like to take this opportunity to acknowledge once more the outstanding efforts and hard work of the Associate Editors responsible for the sections:

Treatment of Chronic Pain by Medical Approaches:
The American Academy of Pain Medicine *Textbook on Patient Management*
Associate Editor: Vitaly Gordin, MD

Treatment of Chronic Pain by Interventional Approaches:
The American Academy of Pain Medicine *Textbook on Patient Management*
Associate Editors: Asokumar Buvanendran, MD, Sunil J. Panchal, MD, Philip S. Kim, MD

Treatment of Chronic Pain by Integrative Approaches:
The American Academy of Pain Medicine *Textbook on Patient Management*
Associate Editor: Albert L. Ray, MD

We greatly appreciate the feedback of our readers and strive to continue to improve our educational materials as we educate each othcr. Please send me your input and thoughts to improve future volumes.

Our main goal is to improve patient safety and outcomes. We are hopeful that the content of these materials accomplishes this mission for you and for the patients to whom you offer care and compassion.

Charleston, WV, USA   Timothy R. Deer, M.D.

Preface to *Comprehensive Treatment of Chronic Pain by Medical, Interventional, and Integrative Approaches*

In recent years, I have found that the need for guidance in treating those suffering from chronic pain has increased, as the burden for those patients has become a very difficult issue in daily life. Our task has been overwhelming at times, when we consider the lack of knowledge that many of us found when considering issues that are not part of our personal repertoire and training. We must be mentors of others and elevate our practice, while at the same time maintain our patient-centric target. Not only do we need to train and nurture the medical student, but also those in postgraduate training and those in private and academic practice who are long separated from their training. We are burdened with complex issues such as the cost of chronic pain, loss of functional individuals to society, abuse, addiction, and diversion of controlled substances, complicated and high-risk spinal procedures, the increase in successful but expensive technology, and the humanistic morose that are part of the heavy load that we must strive to summit.

In this maze of difficulties, we find ourselves branded as "interventionalist" and "non-interventionalist." In shaping this book, it was my goal to overcome these labels and give a diverse overview of the specialty. Separated into five sections, the contents of this book give balance to the disciplines that make up our field. There is a very complete overview of interventions, medication management, and the important areas of rehabilitation, psychological support, and the personal side of suffering. We have tried to give a thorough overview while striving to make this book practical for the physician who needs insight into the daily care of pain patients. This book was created as one of the many tools from the American Academy of Pain Medicine to shape the proper practice of those who strive to do the right things for the chronic pain patient focusing on ethics and medical necessity issues in each section. You will find that the authors, Associate Editor-in-chief, Associate Editors, and I have given rise to a project that will be all encompassing in its goals.

With this text, the American Academy of Pain Medicine has set down the gauntlet for the mission of educating our members, friends, and concerned parties regarding the intricacies of our specialty. I wish you the best as you read this material and offer you my grandest hope that it will change the lives of your patients for the better.

We must remember that chronic pain treatment, like that of diabetes and hypertension, needs ongoing effort and ongoing innovation to defeat the limits of our current abilities. These thoughts are critical when you consider the long standing words of Emily Dickinson…

"Pain has an element of blank; it cannot recollect when it began, or if there were a day when it was not. It has no future but itself, its infinite realms contain its past, enlightened to perceive new periods of pain."

Best of luck as we fight our battles together.

Charleston, WV, USA

Timothy R. Deer, M.D.

Contents

Contributors

Hakan Alfredson, M.D., Ph.D. Sports Medicine Unit, University of Umea, Umea, Sweden

John F. Barnes, P.T., L.M.T., N.C.T.M.P. Myofascial Release Treatment Centers and Seminars, Paoli, PA, USA

Cheryl D. Bernstein, M.D. University of Pittsburgh School of Medicine, Pittsburgh, PA, USA

Cady Block, M.S. Department of Psychology, University of Alabama at Birmingham, Birmingham, AL, USA

Christopher R. Brigham, M.D. Improvement Resources LLC, San Diego, CA, USA
American Board of Independent Medical Examiners, San Diego, CA, USA
AMA Guides Newsletter and Guides to Casebook, San Diego, CA, USA

Daniel Bruns, Psy.D. Health Psychology Associates, Greeley, CO, USA

Marsha Campbell-Yeo, R.N., M.N., Ph.D. Candidate IWK Health Care, Maternal Newborn Program, Halifax, NS, Canada

Christopher J. Centeno, M.D. Physical Medicine and Rehabilitation, Pain Medicine, and Regenerative Medicine, Centeno-Schultz Clinic, Broomfield, CO, USA

Leanne R. Cianfrini, Ph.D. Pain and Rehabilitation Institute, Birmingham, AL, USA

David Crane, M.D. Regenerative Medicine, Crane Clinic Sports Medicine, Chesterfield, MO, USA

Geralyn Datz, Ph.D. Forrest General Pain Management Program, Hattiesburg, MS, USA

Timothy R. Deer, M.D. President and CEO, The Center for Pain Relief, Clinical Professor of Anesthesiology, West Virginia University School of Medicine, Charleston, WV, USA

John Mark Disorbio, Ed.D. Integrated Therapies, LLC, Lakewood, CO, USA

Daniel M. Doleys, Ph.D. Pain and Rehabilitation Institute, Birmingham, AL, USA

Allen R. Dyer, M.D., Ph.D. International Medical Corps, Washington, DC, USA

Rachel Feinberg, P.T., D.P.T. Feinberg Medical Group, Palo Alto, CA, USA

Steven D. Feinberg, M.D. Feinberg Medical Group, Palo Alto, CA, USA
Stanford University School of Medicine, Stanford, CA, USA
American Pain Solutions, San Diego, CA, USA

Ananda Fernandes, M.S.N., Ph.D. Candidate Coimbra School of Nursing, Coimbra, Lisbon, Portugal

Michael C. Francis, M.D. St. Jude Medical, New Orleans, LA, USA
Integrative Pain Medicine Center, New Orleans, LA, USA

Rollin M. Gallagher, M.D., M.P.H. Department of Psychiatry, Anesthesiology and Critical Care, University of Pennsylvania Perelman School of Medicine, Philadelphia, PA, USA

Pain Policy Research and Primary Care, Penn Pain Medicine Center, Philadelphia, PA, USA

Pain Management, Philadelphia Veterans Health System, Philadelphia, PA, USA

Robert J. Gatchell, Ph.D., A.B.P.P. Department of Psychology, College of Science, The University of Texas at Arlington, Arlington, TX, USA

Stuart Gitlow, M.D., M.P.H., M.B.A. Department of Psychiatry, Mount Sinai School of Medicine, New York, NY, USA

Claire E. Goodchild, B.Sc., M.Sc., Ph.D. Department of Psychology, Clinical Institute of Psychiatry, King's College London, London, UK

J. David Haddox, D.D.S., M.D., D.A.B.P.M., M.R.O. Tufts University School of Medicine, Boston, MA, USA

Department of Health Policy, Purdue Pharma L.P., Stanford, CT, USA

Julia Hallisy, D.D.S. San Francisco, CA, USA

Ji-Sheng Han, M.D. Neuroscience Research Institute, Peking University, Beijing, China

Valerie Johnson-Montieth, M.A., Ph.D. Candidate Department of Psychology, University of Texas at Arlington, Arlington, TX, USA

Celeste Johnston, R.N., D.Ed. School of Nursing, McGill University, Montreal, QC, Canada

Jordan F. Karp, M.D. University of Pittsburg School of Medicine, Pittsburgh, PA, USA

Department of Psychiatry, University of Pittsburgh Medical Center, Pittsburgh, PA, USA

Barry Kerner, M.D., D.A.B.P.M. Silver Hill Hospital, New Canaan, CT, USA

Kenneth L. Kirsh, Ph.D. Department of Behavioral Medicine, The Pain Treatment Center of the Bluegrass, Lexington, KY, USA

Michael S. Leong, M.D. Clinic Chief, Stanford Pain Medicine Center, Redwood City, CA, USA

Clinical Associate Professor, Department of Anesthesiology, Stanford University School of Medicine, Stanford, CA, USA

Felix S. Linetsky, M.D. Department of Osteopathic Principles and Practice, Nova Southeastern University of Osteopathic Medicine, Clearwater, FL, USA

Norman Marcus, M.D. Division of Muscle Pain Research, Departments of Anesthesiology and Psychiatry, New York University Langone School of Medicine, New York, NY, USA

Natalia E. Morone, M.D., M.S. University of Pittsburgh School of Medicine, Pittsburgh, PA, USA

Geriatric Research Education and Clinical Center, VA Pittsburgh Healthcare System, Pittsburgh, PA, USA

Jason Ough, M.D. Department of Pain Management/Anesthesiology, New York University Langone Medical Center, New York, NY, USA

Steven D. Passik, Ph.D. Professor of Psychiatry and Anesthesiology, Vanderbilt University Medical Center, Psychosomatic Medicine, Nashville, TN, USA

Manon Ranger, R.N., Ph.D. Candidate School of Nursing, McGill University, Montreal, QC, Canada

Albert L. Ray, M.D. Medical Director, The LITE Center, South Miami, FL, USA

Clinical Associate Professor, University of Miami Miller School of Medicine, Miami, FL, USA

Ben A. Rich, J.D., Ph.D. Department of Bioethics, University of California, Davis School of Medicine, Sacramento, CA, USA

William Rowe, M.A. American Pain Foundation, Baltimore, MD, USA

David Spiegel, M.D. Department of Psychiatry and Behavioral Sciences, Stanford University School of Medicine, Stanford, CA, USA

Steven Stanos, D.O. Department of Physical Medicine and Rehabilitation, Center for Pain Management, Rehabilitation Institute of Chicago, Chicago, IL, USA
Northwestern University Medical School, Feinberg School of Medicine, Chicago, IL, USA

Richard L. Stieg, M.D., M.H.S. Denver, CO, USA

Heidi J. Stokes Minneapolis, MN, USA

Nicole K.Y. Tang, D. Phil. (Oxon) Department of Primary Care Sciences, Arthritis Research UK Primary Care Centre, Keele University, Staffordshire, UK

Rhonwyn Ullmann, M.S. The LITE Center, South Miami, FL, USA

Lynn R. Webster, M.D. Lifetree Clinical Research and Pain Clinic, Salt Lake City, UT, USA

Debra K. Weiner, M.D. University of Pittsburgh College of Medicine, Pittsburgh, PA, USA
Geriatric Research Education and Clinical Center, VA Pittsburgh Healthcare System, Pittsburgh, PA, USA

September Williams, M.D. Ninth Month Productions, San Francisco, CA, USA

Pain as a Perceptual Experience

Albert L. Ray, Rhonwyn Ullmann, and Michael C. Francis

Key Points
- Human perception
- Pain perception
- Physical contribution, including nervous system and fascial network
- Cognitive contribution
- Memory contribution
- Emotional contribution
- Mind contribution

Definitions

Hologram: A three-dimensional image created by intersecting two or more laser beams of light. The more laser beams intersecting, the richer the image.

Pain hologram: A perceptual experience likened to a hologram comprised of "laser beam" inputs from physical nervous system and fascia,

cognitions, emotions, memory, and mindful contributions, differing in intensity from person to person, thereby creating the uniqueness to each person's pain experience.

Neuroplasticity: The ability of the nervous system to change itself throughout the entire life cycle. The operating system by which the nervous system develops its patterns of functioning in both states of health and illness and by which it maintains the balance between sensory and motor function.

Sensitization: A process by which the neuroplastic nature of the nervous system alters normal transmission into an abnormal state. This can occur in pain states and result in pain as a disease state (maldynia), rather than as a normal occurrence (eudynia). It can also happen in other sensory states, as well, such as auditory, visual, olfactory, and tactile sensations.

Eudynia: Normal nociceptive pain; warning pain; pain as a symptom; has value to the person.

Maldynia: Abnormal pain; pain as a disease state and not a symptom; has no value to the person.

Persistent pain: A state of unremitting maldynia, with or without the additional input of eudynia.

TANS: Tonically active neurons; an area in the caudate that modulates cognitive input with emotional input, interacting with memory and having output to the thalamus and basal ganglia and eventually to the motor cortex. TANS are also responsive to auditory or visual stimuli that are linked to reward.

A.L. Ray, M.D. (✉)
Medical Director, The LITE Center, 5901 SW 74 St, Suite 201, South Miami, FL 33143, USA

Clinical Associate Professor, University of Miami Miller School of Medicine, Miami, FL, USA
e-mail: aray@thelitecenter.org

R. Ullmann, B.S., M.S.
The LITE Center, 5901 SW 74 St, Suite 201, South Miami, FL 33143, USA
e-mail: bearrab@aol.com

M.C. Francis, M.D.
St. Jude Medical, New Orleans, LA, USA

Integrative Pain Medicine Center, New Orleans, LA, USA
e-mail: integrativepmc@gmail.com

T.R. Deer et al. (eds.), *Treatment of Chronic Pain by Integrative Approaches: the AMERICAN ACADEMY of PAIN MEDICINE Textbook on Patient Management*, DOI 10.1007/978-1-4939-1821-8_1,
© American Academy of Pain Medicine 2015

Tensegrity: A term derived from a contraction of "tensional integrity"; a term to describe a structural relationship that allows for a system to yield without breaking; a term used to describe how the fascial system maintains its integrity while allowing movement of its encapsulated structures, such as muscle; a term that allows for an understanding of why the fascial system could stand on its own, if the bones and muscles were removed from the body.

Price's Two Dimensions of All Pains

Sensory-discriminative: Highly localized; discrete; signal transmitted from dorsal horn via spinothalamic tract to thalamus and contralateral sensory cortex; we call it the "ouch" portion of pain.

Affective-motivational: Vague; not localized; signal transmitted from dorsal horn via parabrachial tract to limbic system, ACC, insula and prefrontal cortex and distributed bilaterally throughout brain; we call it the "yuck" portion of pain.

Introduction

"The mind creates the brain." J. Schwartz, MD, PhD: The Mind and the Brain

Human perception has been likened to a hologram [1]. A hologram exists by converging two or more laser beams together, producing a three-dimensional vision that is very real, but does not really exist. You can put your hand right through a hologram, yet it is quite visible and not disturbed by your hand. The more laser beams we add to the hologram, the richer the vision. This analogy is often used to address human perception [1–3].What our brain creates as a perception and how we project these perceptions onto the outside world are called qualia [4]. The qualia we call our conscious experience of pain cannot be fully explained by neurophysiological events only [5, 6]. Some qualia, or perceptions, can be up to 90 % memory [7]. Thus, our qualia are produced by a dynamic interaction between mind and brain and most likely through the mechanics of quantum physics [6, 8].

In this chapter, we will look at what component "laser beams" comprise our "holographic" perception of pain, and we will understand why each person's pain perception is unique to them. Even with the addition of *f*MRIs, which can demonstrate confluence of multiple brain areas utilized during pain perception [9], the experience on the part of the person in pain remains unique to them [10]. The goal of our treatment of pain, then, is to deconstruct as much of the pain hologram as possible, by reducing or eliminating as many laser beams as possible. The weakening of the hologram can come about by reducing laser beams from any number of perspectives, as we will see below, and this accounts for why interdisciplinary/multidisciplinary treatment is so often the best choice.

Doidge said, "When we wish to prefect our senses, neuroplasticity is a blessing; when it works in the service of pain, plasticity can be a curse" [11]. We now understand how sensitization, through neuroplastic reorganization, can also influence and change perceptions [12, 13]. In abnormal pain states, these neuroplastic changes cause a sensitization which enhances pain perceptions in a negative way, by increasing either the sensory-discriminative dimension or the affective-motivational dimension of pain, or both. In the previous chapter, we have reviewed the issue of neuroplasticity, "for better or for worse," and its role in the production of abnormal pain perception. However, to understand the ultimate perceptual experience of abnormal pain, we must look beyond just the physical neuroplastic sensitization of the nervous system and incorporate the role of the mind and its effect on the physical system. What we will see is that mindful will and attentional focus also can actually change the neuroplastic structure of the brain [6].

Pain Perception

Price has identified two dimensions to all pain [14, 15]: the sensory-discriminative and the affective-motivational dimensions, and these have been further discussed by others [12, 16, 17]. The sensory-discriminative dimension is perceived as a highly localized sensation and is processed via the spinothalamic tract through the thalamus and up to the contralateral somatosensory cortex. This part of the pain experience we refer to as the "ouch" portion of pain. The affective-motivational dimension contributes the vague coloration to pain and is processed via the spinoparabrachial tract to the amygdala, hippocampus, prefrontal cortex, insula anterior cingulate gyrus (ACC), etc., and is distributed bilaterally throughout the brain. This part of the pain experience we refer to as the "yuck" portion of pain. Obviously, these two separate dimensions of pain are perceived as one final integrated perception [18–21]. In our experience, the affective-motivational dimension of pain is the most difficult for people to tolerate. In other words, the "suffering" component of pain is harder to live with than the "ouch" portion [22, 23].

Price's concepts are applicable to all pain, whether it be eudynia (acute nociceptive warning pain) or maldynia (pain as a disease process unto itself which is not useful to the person)

[13, 24–27]; Rome and Rome [28] have previously described LAPS (limbically augmented pain syndrome) in terms of sensitization of the nervous system through neuroplastic reorganization resulting in a condition in which the pain perception is "out of proportion" to physical findings. Previously, these pain sufferers have been labeled as hysterics, "crocks," and even malingerers. However, we now understand that the intensity of their pain perception is quite genuine and real.

In addition, we do know that the brain is similarly activated by actual events or by imagined events within one person [29–31], and this brain activation function has also been demonstrated between two different persons who are highly sympathetic with each other [32]. "Performing" an activity in our mind's eye causes brain function to occur as if we were actually doing that same activity [6, 29]. The development of new neuroplastic patterns in the brain or the arousal of previously established patterns can be excited by imagination. This is a well-documented happening with musicians and athletes, who "practice" at times even when they are away from their actual activity. Brain activity on fMRIs is identical whether visualizing or actually playing. In terms of pain perception, this concept was very nicely demonstrated by Krämer et al. in a rather enlightening experiment with imagined allodynia in subjects who had a history of allodynia, but no current allodynia. fMRIs done while touching the subjects' hands demonstrated excitation of S_1 and S_2 somatosensory cortices bilaterally. However, when the subjects imagined their allodynia while having their hand touched, their simultaneous fMRIs indicated activity of brain areas congruent with those of someone experiencing "real" allodynia [29].

Turning to the pain hologram produced by the neuromatrix network and the mind, besides the "physical" laser beam input from the peripheral and/or central nervous system to the brain or via the fascial network [2], there are multiple other major laser beam inputs which have a significant influence on the ultimate perception of "I hurt." These inputs can include, but are not limited to, emotional, cognitive, memory, and mindful contributions, and these other inputs can frequently be of greater significance to our pain hologram [4, 12, 20]. We will now discuss the components of a hypothetical painful hologram (Table 1.1).

Table 1.1 Contributions to a pain hologram

Physical neuromatrix, including peripheral and central nervous systems plus fascial network:
• Emotional
• Cognitive
• Memory
• Mind

Physical Laser Beams

We live with and through a dynamically fluctuating nervous system, one which has a marvelously complex functioning in terms of pain transmission [13, 18, 19]. To briefly review, eudynia starts with stimulation of chemical, mechanical, or temperature nociceptors in the periphery [33, 34]. Via transduction, an action potential is created, and this electrical signal is conducted to the spinal dorsal horn (Fig. 1.1). Here, a complex series of interactions occur, with Aδ and C fibers working to enhance the signal strength, while Aβ fibers and descending inhibitory fibers work to inhibit the signal, and all of this interaction receives an additional excitatory influence from the glial cells [35, 36] within the dorsal horn. Once the dorsal horn interactions reach a final summation of factors, the remaining signal is then transmitted via the spinothalamic and spinoparabrachial tracts to the brain (Fig. 1.2). The spinothalamic transmission is delivered to the thalamus and is processed on to the contralateral somatosensory cortex. The spinoparabrachial transmission is processed through the hippocampus, amygdala, and onward to the prefrontal cortex, ACC, and other areas of the brain bilaterally (Fig. 1.3) [13, 26, 27, 37–40].

Intensification of the laser beam being generated by the periphery or spinal cord can occur via sensitization of the peripheral nociceptors, which increases the intensity of the signal reaching the spinal cord [12]. At the spinal level, we can experience recruitment of new nociceptive inputs or even non-nociceptive fibers (as with Aβ fibers) when the signals are strong enough. When enough stimulation has occurred via root input or dorsal horn sensitization, the spinal cord can go into "automatic" mode, where it no longer needs peripheral input to fire. Thus, we can wind up with very strong and enduring laser beams from the physical generators below the brain [13, 38, 39, 41].

Within the brain, adding further to this complex process which happened in the dorsal horn, an area of the caudate contains TANS (tonically active neurons). It is in this area of the brain where a confluence of signals from the hippocampus (memory), our emotions (amygdala), and our cognitions are processed, with the resultant signals being sent to the globus pallidus and up to the motor cortex. Thus, messages that come from areas of our brain that are overlapping and interacting with pain signals can incorporate cognitive, emotional, and memory inputs that have a direct effect on our motor system as well as our sensory system [6]. This provides an understanding to the concept that our brain processing is geared to result in "action" and is responsive to our sensory perceptions such as pain. We do not experience sensory perceptions for the sake of experiencing alone [61422, 42, 43].

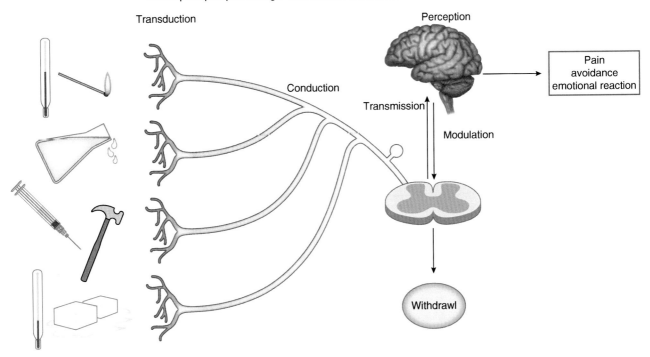

Nociceptive pain processing*: Transduction to perception

Transduction

Perception

Conduction

Transmission

Modulation

Pain avoidance emotional reaction

Withdrawl

*The stimulus is well localized; its duration, intensity, and quality are clear

Fig. 1.1 Nociceptive pain processing. Transduction to perception

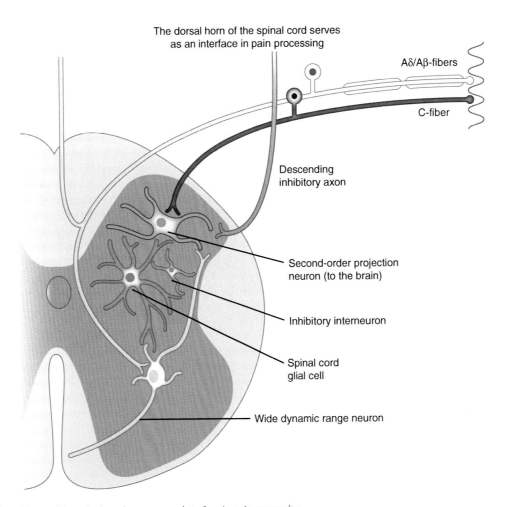

The dorsal horn of the spinal cord serves as an interface in pain processing

Aδ/Aβ-fibers

C-fiber

Descending inhibitory axon

Second-order projection neuron (to the brain)

Inhibitory interneuron

Spinal cord glial cell

Wide dynamic range neuron

Fig. 1.2 The dorsal horn of the spinal cord serves as an interface in pain processing

Fig. 1.3 Processing of pain in the brain occurs in several regions

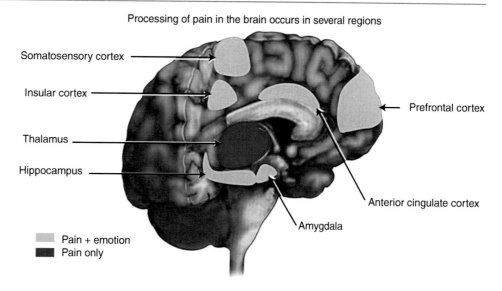

Processing of pain in the brain occurs in several regions

Somatosensory cortex

Insular cortex

Thalamus

Hippocampus

Prefrontal cortex

Anterior cingulate cortex

Amygdala

Pain + emotion
Pain only

In addition to the neural network, physical input to our pain hologram can be strongly influenced by the fascial system, described as the organ system of stability and mechano-regulation [44], and wherein lies ten times more sensory nerve endings than in muscle [45, 46]. Fascia lines all body parts, as John Barnes puts it: "fascia is a tough connective tissue that spreads throughout the body in a three-dimensional web from head to foot functionally, without interruption" [2]. The purpose of fascia is to maintain body shape and keep organs in their proper positions, as well as resist mechanical stresses from any source such as trauma and inflammation [47]. This function of fascia is best understood through the construct of tensegrity, a concept that explains the relationship between skeleton, tensional forces of the fascia, contractility of muscle, and hydrostatic pressure of fascial compartments [48]. Restrictions of the fascia have been found to cause limitations in movement and pain which can have non-dermatomal referral patterns [49, 50], thus demonstrating that the physical input to our pain hologram from fascia is not by activation of peripheral nociceptors. While often ignored in evaluating a person's pain perception, fascial contribution to pain has been demonstrated in such diverse problems as Achilles tendinopathy [51], plantar fasciitis [52], systemic lupus erythematosus [53], and acute compartment syndrome of the upper extremity [54].

Researchers have demonstrated an energy transmission system throughout fascial planes. This energy wave is faster than neural transmission and is very nicely visually demonstrated by Guimberteau [55]. Body memory of past events or trauma (physical, emotional, or sexual) [3] can be stored in the fascia, similarly to neural storage, and this stored memory can interrupt the smooth flow of energy via the fascial system [2, 55–57]. We do know that traumatic events are processed by the person immediately after they happen. However, what is not totally processed at that time is stored in cellular body memory traces that become like a three-dimensional photo (although the storage is in energy units and not pictures) and incorporates all contingencies of that event, placing them in "storage" at an unconscious level. Barnes has found that a part of these stored memory traces in the fascial network are positionally dependent [2]. Through Barnes' unwinding technique, bodily positions that can replicate the same body part position at the time of the trauma can release and make conscious the stored unconscious memories and allow the person to finish working through that event [2].

Other therapeutic applications that take advantage of this fascial network input to pain are being used for surgical anesthesia and post-op pain control. Fascial iliaca compartment block has been used in fractured neck of femur [58], hip arthroplasty [59], and this same block has been shown to reduce emergence agitation in children having thigh surgery [60]. One study cited has replaced epidural anesthesia with fascial anesthesia in prostatectomies [61]. Although the fascial network is not processed via the peripheral nociceptors, there is some recent animal research to indicate some dorsal horn activity via the fascial network in addition to fascial activation itself, and this article concludes that fascial input is a significant contributing force to painful syndromes [62].

Emotional Laser Beams

We are all familiar with the fact that people with persistent pain frequently have complaints of anger, anxiety, depression, and sometimes fear attached to their pain experience. These reactions have been categorized into phasic, acute, and chronic by Craig, with phasic and acute representing anticipatory fear and relief, while chronic represents depression, fear, anger, disgust, social distress, guilt, subservience, resignation, and abandonment [63]. The question then arises as to whether these emotional complaints are representative of primary psychological illnesses or are they part and parcel of normal and/or dysfunctional brain activity relative to pain perception? Do people living with maldynia have multiple illnesses or was Osler correct to have us think of "one person, one disease"?

Perhaps we can make more sense of this question by looking at brain function. Brain areas significantly involved in emotion in the brain include the amygdala, hippocampus, lateral hypothalamus, caudate, anterior cingulate cortex (ACC), supraorbital cortex, and prefrontal cortex [13, 37]. These same areas have been well documented in depression, anxiety, obsessive-compulsive disorder, and fear among others [4, 6, 11]. Interestingly, if we look at the affective dimension of pain, according to Price and the Rome article, these same brain areas are the ones involved [14, 15, 28]. Thus, what we are beginning to identify is that pain perception and emotional problems share some of the same "brain railroad tracks." The brain doesn't "know" what it is doing, it just does. Therefore, if the brain is utilizing the same tracks for two different types of perception, it cannot tell which train is riding that track at any given time, nor does it care. In fact, two trains can use the same tracks at the same time, and by so doing, they can signal a "go" to each other. This mixed signaling helps us understand why people in pain, especially those with maldynia, will report that stressful or depressing events can exacerbate their pain. In our holographic analogy, this would be equivalent to adding strength to some of the laser beams making up our pain hologram, by non-painful inputs. This could be likened to "recruitment" in the spinal cord, where we intensify a pain signal through recruitment of non-nociceptive fibers. (Spinal recruitment is a lower level route to add strength to the "physical" pain laser beam being fed into our hologram.)

The medical literature supports the reverse concepts to also be a frequent occurrence; that is, psychiatric patients with affective disorders often have pain as a symptom of their affective disorder. Phillips and Hunter identified an increased prevalence and intensity in tension-type headaches in a psychiatric population compared to the general population [64]. Melzack and Katz have discussed that stressful events have been associated with angina pectoris, ulcers, rheumatoid arthritis, painful menses, ulcerative colitis, and regional enteritis [20].

In addition, some psychiatrists have taken the position that pain is no more than a symptom of psychiatric disease and is not a disease unto itself. We believe the distinction is better conceived by understanding perception rather than disease states. For example, Romano and Turner have written that approximately 50 % of all patients with pain and depression develop the two "disorders" simultaneously [65]. In view of brain imaging studies and our current understanding of overlapping brain areas in pain and depression, it makes

sense that some patients may experience pain and depression simultaneously, while others may feel one or the other first. If both perceptions are utilizing the same brain areas and reinforcing each other, then it becomes easier to understand why depression could stimulate a pain perception, pain could stimulate depression, or both could start together. Remember, the brain is the only part of the body that can "perceive," and since the brain only "does," without understanding, then any combination of perceptions can take place if the same areas of the brain are being utilized for them.

Cognitive Laser Beams

Marcus Aurelius [66] once said:

> If you are distressed by anything external, the pain is not due to the thing itself, but to your estimate of it. THIS you have the power to revoke at any time.

Our brain is structured such that the most primitive areas, in terms of development, are lower in location. Our cortex has been described as having evolved to be sitting on top of the older brain. Thus, the areas that are so highly integrated into the affective dimension of pain, as well as much of the pain areas associated with maldynia, are for the most part sub/lower cortical. As mentioned above, the TANS is the location where the cognitive areas meet the emotional areas, which have had input already from memory. Like so many of our sensory perceptions, the lower brain takes charge rather than the logical inputs we are capable of. It is often said that in most any issue between emotions and logic, the emotions will win out, that is, we will default to the "heart." This is another way of saying that decisions and responses, unless consciously influenced, will include "unconscious" influences that are more emotionally driven. Perlmutter and Villodo discuss the role of prefrontal cortex in reasoning and creative thinking and how changes in prefrontal functioning can lead to a "dysregulation" of the balance necessary for optimum brain function [67].

This "default" system can often lead us into difficulty. For example, when a person takes a medication for pain relief, the feeling of relief ("feels good") can easily lead us into the behavior of "if one feels good, then two or three must be even better." And hence, we can wind up with a patient developing significant adverse medication reactions by their instinctual (unconscious) desire to be pain free. Too much NSAID, acetaminophen, antidepressant, antiepileptic, etc., can produce physical harm to the body. Too much controlled substance can produce adverse bodily reactions and/or behaviors that result in legal trouble as well. The ultimate expression of this "action without thinking" response can be the development of pseudoaddiction, where the perception of pain relief is the desired goal, and our behaviors can mimic those of someone with a true addictive disorder. One person's actions are driven by the desire to relieve pain, while the person with an addictive disorder demonstrates behavior driven by the need to get high and, further into the disease, by the need to avoid crashing and experiencing withdrawal. The behaviors may be very similar on the part of those two different people, with lack of demonstrable control in following prescription directions, drug seeking behaviors, actually placing themselves in harm's way at times, lying to those around them in order to obtain more medications, etc. (see Chap. 6 on Addictive Disorders and Pain). What we experience in situations where the lower brain centers are controlling our responses are cognitive rationalizations, that is, "if one pill works, two is better" as a way to justify our desire to have less pain. This kind of cognitive laser beam is one in which the cognition follows the affective dimension rather than lead it.

Various issues regarding the cognitive input to pain perception have been described [4]. These contributions have looked at such issues as the roles of language descriptors [68], emotion and attitudes [69], culture and attention [70], ethnicity [71], gender differences [72], and age differences (see Chap. 19, Pain in the Elderly Population) [73]. The literature also supports the significance of the affective dimension through the cognitive inputs [23]. These contributions from mind and cognition support Schwartz's description of processing the affective, memory, and cognitive processes through the TANs, described earlier.

Conversely, when cognitive-behavioral therapies are utilized in treating pain or other problems such as depression or OCD, the success of the patient depends on their ability, through much practice, to have the cognitive abilities of the higher cortex take charge and present alternative "thinking" to the patient. This change allows for a reframing of thoughts and a refocusing of attention as well as the consequent behaviors away from the "painful" thoughts, that is, "I hurt," "I am suffering," "I will never be able to enjoy family picnics again," etc [4, 74]. These examples are of our cognitive system in a passive mode (default system). The alternatives, through cognitive-behavioral approaches, would be to assertively place into consciousness such concepts as "this pain has no beneficial meaning to me, therefore, I will focus on the love I have for antique cars and review some pictures of old convertibles now," or "since this pain is meaningless to me, I choose to breathe deep ten times and allow my body to feel the flow of positive energy course through me," etc. Utilizing our higher cortical powers assertively, then, allows us to change the "default" system by building in new neuroplastic patterns. We literally can control our lives by creating the new set of railroad tracks we want our train to utilize and set up the switching mechanisms by practicing, until the new track becomes our "default." This becomes active mode for our cognitive inputs [6].

Thus, the cognitive contribution to pain lasers can be positive or negative and can be minimal when in passive mode (old default), or when in active mode, the cognitive input has the potential, in many instances, to become the most powerful influence to overcome adverse emotional reactions [23]. As we will see below, the cognitive force from our mind through our cortical thinking brain can become a valuable source of positive neuroplastic retraining of our brain. Cognitive-behavioral processes have been shown to be the most effective in helping people with maldynia to restore their functional status and maximize their abilities to take charge of their lives again [4, 74]. Our developmentally highest level of brain function is often needed to help us deal with our most significant life problems, when our lower brain levels that normally run on automatic default fail us. The paradox is that it so often requires professional help to teach us how to utilize these higher level approaches to alter our life experiences, which are our perceptions (see Chap. 7).

Another example of how we can utilize our higher cognitive power to defeat pain is through hypnosis. Rainville et al. have demonstrated that if we use hypnosis to alter the affective-motivational dimension of pain first, there is often a reduction in the sensory-discriminative pain dimension that follows it [75]. However, this approach makes changes in brain function through the lower centers which mediate the affective dimension of pain and does not involve the somatosensory cortex. On the other hand, the reverse is not true. If we utilize hypnosis to alter the sensory-discriminative dimension of pain first, the process does involve the somatosensory cortex, but even if we alter the pain intensity, the affective dimension (the "yuck") doesn't change [75]. Thus, how we build our new railroad tracks and which "switchers" we utilize can have a rather dramatic effect on the "retraining" process of the brain (see Chap. 9).

Memory Laser Beams

Memory in humans is a complex process, which involves multiple inputs to go from immediate memory to long-term memory. Memory is made in the body cells [7, 56] as well as in the brain, but it is not made in pictures. It is made in mnemonics, with different memory storage for each part of the memory. For example, the memory for a traumatic event (painful or not) will have memory traces for the event itself, the place it happened, the smells involved, the sounds heard, the sights seen, the emotions perceived, the thoughts associated with the event, our judgment of what has happened, etc. The memory is made and stored according to events and patterns. The memory may or may not remain in our conscious awareness, but long-term memory is permanent [76, 77].

Brain areas involved in memory involve left prefrontal, temporal, and parahippocampal cortices. The level of activation of these areas predicts which memory becomes long term or not [78, 79]. The hippocampus and amygdala relate to emotional memory (remember the TANS) via NMDA and dopamine, and long-term potentiation in the hippocampus may underlie learning and memory [76, 77, 80]. Prefrontal cortex is involved with object identity, spatial locations, memory and coding, and analysis of the meaning of items [81–83]. Prefrontal cortical involvement increases as the semantic complexity rises [78, 79]. Thus, we can begin to see how memory becomes entwined with the confluence of brain patterning involved in pain perception. Through the TANS, the feed-in of memory, emotions, and meaning all meld together. When the input is of sufficient intensity, memory will be made [83].

When we want to actively recall a memory, such as "what did I eat for lunch today," our brain must activate these brain areas, pull up the mnemonic for each part of that hologram for "lunch," and converge them all to produce the three-dimensional holographic picture in my mind's eye of lunch today. This will include all my senses, including taste, color, food presentation, sounds in the room where lunch was eaten, the conversation that took place, who was there, the temperature of the food and room, how much comfort or discomfort was involved both physically and emotionally, etc.

Thus, memory is made in parallel for the events and for the emotional and other components [15, 28]. Hence, when we have to converge multiple mnemonics to produce our pain perception hologram, the mnemonic for any portion of the pain (sensory-discriminative, affective, memory, or both) can be overloaded by previous memory mnemonics for that particular quality of the pain [4, 84]. If the affective component is overloaded, we can see the limbically augmented pain syndrome (LAPS) described by Rome and Rome. Thus, memory, and sensitization of the memory system, can result in augmentation of the pain perception. This accounts for why sufferers of persistent pain often have a more frequent history of trauma compared to the general population.

Returning to our great Roman emperor, Marcus Aurelius [66], we can again quote him:

> As for pain, a pain that is unbearable carries us off; but that which lasts a long time is bearable; the mind retires into itself, and the ruling faculty is not injured. As for the parts which are hurt by the pain, let them, if they can, give their opinion of it.

If we view this memory system through the lenses of the brain areas involved, and realize those same brain areas are involved with the physical, emotional, cognitive, and meaningfulness of any perception, including pain, we can see the genius behind Marcus Aurelius' two observations about pain perception. He demonstrated a far-reaching wisdom about pain perception, without any scientific knowledge of how accurate his statements have turned out to be in terms of modern investigations into brain functioning.

Mind Control and Mind Laser Beams

Building on the foundation that our mind is something different from our brain, even though it operates through the brain, we can add some very powerful laser beams and control over the entire system through mindfulness.

As Schwartz has described, "quantum theory creates a causal opening for the mind, a point of entry by which mind can affect matter, a mechanism by which mind can shape brain. That opening arises because quantum theory allows intention, and attention, to exert real, physical effects on the brain…" [6].

This same author has brought together the work of many neuroscientists, such as William James, Henry Stapp, and Benjamin Libet in order to demonstrate how the mind can physically affect the brain. It has been demonstrated that a wave of "readiness" energy appears in the brain about 350–550 ms before a motor movement occurs. In addition, the sense of will occurs 150–200 ms prior to a movement. This free will offers an opportunity to make the movement a "go" or "not go" [6]. Stowell has previously described a similar time delay in pain perception [85], and the impact of psychosocial feedback has been investigated in the timing of events by Lee and colleagues [42].

Hence, the understanding of free will becomes a process by which the brain "bubbles up" unconscious thoughts that could lead to action; but free will, as a conscious system, provides an opportunity to screen these bubbling ideas and exert control over which ones are a go or not. It has been proposed that the initiatives that bubble up in the brain are based on the person's past memories, experiences, values inculcated from society, and present circumstances. Interestingly, studies of brain function in relationship to free will demonstrate that the prefrontal cortex is activated as a primary area. Disorders such as schizophrenia, which is marked by autistic behavior and inactivity, and clinical depression, one symptom of which is lack of initiative, demonstrate a consistently low level of activity in the prefrontal cortex [6].

Additionally, studies cited by Schwartz have demonstrated activation of brain regions which affect perception, such as auditory-language association cortices in the temporal lobe without any associated activity of the auditory cortex in schizophrenic patients who are having active auditory hallucinations. In fact, the hippocampus (retrieving contextual information), ventral striatum (integrating emotional experience with perception), and thalamus (maintaining conscious awareness) were also involved in these patients, but the frontal cortex remained quiet. Another example of a patient with amyotrophic lateral sclerosis (ALS) showed that by implanting electrodes into his motor cortex, he was able to will his brain to activate his motor cortex by imagining his finger moving.

This enabled him to be able to move a cursor on his computer through brain activation via his imagination [6]. We have previously discussed in this chapter how imagination also activates brain function consistent with allodynia, in people without any current allodynia, but only a history of same.

It has been shown that long-standing pain can interrupt time perception, causing a disorganization of the patient's being in the world [86]. Spatial additivity and attention also had impact on the mind-pain relationship [87]. One of the most powerful demonstrations of mindfulness "power" is presented by Fitzgibbon and colleagues, in which "synesthesia" is used to explain how, if we experience another person's pain, similar brain areas that are activated in the pain person are activated in the sympathetic person as well [32]. Rainville et al. [75]. have shown the brain activation associated with hypnosis, and Krämer's group has shown brain activation through imagination, another mindful activity [29].

Our spiritual perspectives also contribute to our mindful contributions to our pain lasers. Perlmutter and Villoldo describe nicely the relationship between our spiritual beliefs and brain function (see also Chap. 14, for a more comprehensive discussion of this important input to our pain hologram) [67].

Another area that deserves discussion in terms of mind laser beam input to our pain hologram is that of post-traumatic stress disorder (PTSD). We have long known of an association between PTSD, either military or civilian, and pain perception. The trauma, which can be due to physical calamity, emotional abuse, sexual abuse, or combinations of these, results in neuroplastic changes causing a sensitization in brain regions overlapping with some of those involved in pain perception [88–92]. The limbic system, especially amygdala, demonstrates hypersensitivity, while the medial frontal cortex fails to exert governance [93]. For example, loud noise results in a more severe and exaggerated effect in people with PTSD [94]. Other clinical symptoms, such as intrusive rethinking of the traumatic event, intrusive dreaming of same, diminished interests, constriction of affective responses, as well as heightened responses to events that arouse recollections of the trauma, are all congruent with the dysfunction of the limbic and prefrontal cortex areas seen in chronic pain sufferers. As we discuss in this chapter, the more attention we pay to things that activate similar areas of the brain, the more intensely those brain areas react to less intense stimuli or even imagined stimuli. Thus, we can see why trauma and maldynia so frequently coexist and how two seemingly different happenings can serve to reinforce each other. Treatments directed at one, can conversely, reduce the intensity of the perceptual experience of the other. Perception within PTSD victims has been described as "you can never feel just a little bit: it is all or nothing" [95]. This is very similar to the heightened pain perceptions in such painful conditions as limbically augmented pain syndrome (LAPS) [28], phantom pain [11, 96, 97],

irritable bowel syndrome (IBS) [98, 99], chronic daily headache [100, 101], chronic depression [102, 103], and fibromyalgia [104–106]. Dohrenbusch et al. have also demonstrated the heightened sensory system in general in patients with fibromyalgia [106]. Hence, in all of these conditions, our mindful perception is increased secondary to the neuroplastic sensitization of the brain.

Finally, Schwartz has discussed how volitional attention is the key to inducing neuroplastic changes through mindfulness. Attention determines brain activity, through the selection process discussed earlier. "Attention can do more than enhance the responses of selected neurons. It can also turn down the volume in competing regions" [6]. "When it comes to determining what the brain will process, the mind (through the mechanism of selective attention) is at least as strong as the novelty or relevance of the stimulus itself" [6]. This attention seems to originate in the frontal and parietal lobes, but like other functions, imaging studies show that there is no attention center in the brain. Rather, we see similar patterns as those associated with pain perception, that is, prefrontal cortex and anterior cingulate. In addition, parietal cortex, basal ganglia, and cerebellum are involved. Furthermore, studies have shown that when you pay attention to something, the brain parts involved in processing that something become more active. "Attention, then, is not some fuzzy, ethereal concept. It acts back on the physical structure and activity of the brain" [6]. Indeed, hypnosis, one of our potentially powerful treatment tools, is best understood as focused awareness (highly selective attention) with a resulting reduction in peripheral awareness (see Chap. 9, Hypnosis and Pain Control) [107]. Tai Chi, another mindfulness system, also incorporates attentional focus to utilize slow movements that promote balance, agility, flexibility, and strength to develop synergy of mind and body [108].

In creating neuroplastic changes to aid control over pain holograms, repeatedly utilizing patterns of attention will actually result in changes in patterns of sensory processing, and this remapping of sensory cortex has been demonstrated. Animal studies that have documented these neuroplastic changes in primary auditory cortex, somatosensory cortex, and motor cortex support the position that it is the attentional state of the animal which is crucial to make the change, not the sensory input itself. "Every stimulus from the world outside impinges on a consciousness that is predisposed to accept it, or to ignore it. We can therefore go further: not only do mental states matter to the physical activity of the brain, but they can contribute to the final perception even more powerfully than the stimulus itself" [6]. In fact, it has been shown that when stimuli identical to those inducing neuroplastic changes in an attending brain are delivered to a non-attending brain, there is no induction of neuroplastic cortical change [6]. Hence, "the willful focusing of attention is not only a psychological intervention. It is also a biological one" [6].

Schwartz nicely summarizes the contribution of mind via quantum brain functioning in the following quote [6]:

> Our will, our volition, our karma, constitutes the essential core of the active part of mental experience. It is the most important, if not the only important, active part of consciousness. We generally think of will as being expressed in the behaviors we exhibit: whether we choose this path or that one, whether we make this decision or that. Even when will is viewed introspectively, we often conceptualize it in terms of an externally pursued goal. But I think the truly important manifestation of will, the one from which our decisions and behaviors flow, is the choice we make about the quality and direction of attentional focus. Mindful, or unmindful, wise or unwise--- no choice we make is more basic, or important, than this one.

Pain Holograms

We have looked at how perception is analogous to holograms. When we want to evaluate a person's pain, we need to just look at what laser beam is part of the pain hologram. Is there a contribution to their pain perception from physical inputs, emotional inputs, cognitive inputs, mindful inputs, memory inputs, or multiple sources linked together by brain function? Only by understanding their entire hologram can we then begin to devise the appropriate treatments to deconstruct as much of their hologram as possible.

The importance of evaluating and treating a person's pain by identifying what laser beams may be contributing to their pain hologram is critically important to our success in finding them relief. For example, a 34-year-old female migraine sufferer had been averaging 2–3 headaches/month, relieved by an injection at local emergency rooms, for years. One evening, she suffered a severe headache, went to an emergency room for treatment, and was told "you're having a migraine; go home and go to bed." The patient, who sought treatment at a different hospital, was found to have a ruptured brain aneurysm, which was successfully surgically repaired. However, she began to experience a daily headache from that time forward. She had been to several headache clinics and neurologists, all of whom treated her for "transformed migraine" for over 2 years with multiple classes of migraine pharmacological treatments, biofeedback, acupuncture, and meditation without success. She was referred to our clinic for treatment of the PTSD from the night of the ruptured aneurysm, as she clearly thought she was going to die that night. Processing the PTSD with eye movement desensitization and reprocessing (EMDR), a psychological treatment that seems to "delink" linked memories and possibly reverse the long-term potentiation associated with this memory storage, was successful in alleviating her PTSD symptoms completely. However, her headache continued. EMDR was then used to target the daily headache itself, and after six sessions, her daily headache was resolved and has not returned in over 8+ years.

She does continue with her 2–3 migraines/month. Her daily headache hologram appears to have been a "phantom headache." EMDR is a useful treatment for phantom pain and can resolve it permanently, as it did in this case, unless the person is re-traumatized [109]. Thus, only by continuing to search for what laser beams may have been underlying her pain hologram were we able to identify and treat her with a treatment that allowed deconstruction of that hologram and resolution of her daily headache.

John Barnes has said that, "prior to seeing any patient that day, if we believe we know what we are going to do based on their diagnosis, then we don't know what we are doing." This is not only an observation, but we consider it to be a medical principle [2, 3]. Our patients' pain holograms are dynamic, not static, just like our physical nervous system. Thus, we owe it to ourselves and our patients to find out what that pain hologram is comprised of and the importance of each contributing factor on any given day in order to properly plan treatment. This approach allows us to treat people, not body parts. Pain holograms are three-dimensional, just like any other hologram, and we can be more successful with pain sufferers if we approach pain perception through those lenses.

Summary

In this chapter, we have explored human perception and pain as a perceptual experience. We have looked at how individual parts of pain perception are processed in the brain, with overlapping of multiple different inputs within brain regions resulting in the enabling, enhancement, sensitization, and altered perceptions which can result from this. This perspective allows a better understanding of why pain has so many comorbid psychological consequences, as well as altered motor behaviors.

By utilizing an analogy to holograms, we have discussed how various sources of input into a pain hologram can come from physical inputs, including the nervous system and fascial tissue energy, and/or from emotional, cognitive, memory, as well as mindful sources. These different inputs, which operate via the brain, are best explained through both traditional and quantum physics. Traditional physics can help us understand some of the hard-wiring nervous system (peripheral, spinal, and brain) functions. However, it is only through a "quantum brain" perspective that we can make sense out of the perspectives of mind, thoughts, fascial energies, memory, and our cognitions which include our social, cultural, familial, spiritual, and personal values. Through these traditional and quantum brain approaches, we can understand why each person's pain hologram is unique to them, regardless of the type of pain. If five people all suffered a tibial fracture in an auto accident, there would be five different holograms created, and those five individuals' experiences with "tibial fracture pain" would all be different from each other.

Our ultimate formula for successful treatment is to restore a sense of balance to the system [110]. An example of this is seen in intracranial electrical stimulation for chronic depression and pain control. Here, the stimulation, which reduces brain activity, is applied to the motor cortex and not the sensory cortex, thus reestablishing a better balance within the brain [111]. The results are immediate.

Through comprehensive exploration of our patients' pain holograms, we are better able to identify appropriate treatments [21]. Patients who don't respond "as expected" may well have laser beams that we have not yet found or perhaps undervalued. If we keep in mind our old adage that the patient is always "right," it can lead us to unexplored paths to seeing their pain hologram differently and allow us newer approaches to those "difficult" cases. It can help us to keep in our consciousness, as pain treaters, the opening thought to this chapter: *the mind creates the brain.*

References

1. Talbot M. The holographic universe. New York: HarperCollins; 1991.
2. Barnes J. Myofascial release: the missing link in traditional treatment. In: Davis C, editor. Complementary therapies in rehabilitation, evidence for efficacy in treatment, prevention, and wellness. 3rd ed. Thorofare: Slack In; 2009. p. 89–112.
3. Barnes JF. Myofascial release: the search for excellence-A comprehensive evaluatory and treatment approach. Paoli: Rehabilitation Services Inc; 1990.
4. Ray A, Zbik A. Cognitive behavioral therapies and beyond. In: Tollison CD, editor. Practical pain management. 3rd ed. Philadelphia: Lippincott Williams and Wilkins; 2002. p. 189–208.
5. Benini A. Pain as a biological phenomenon of consciousness. Praxis. 1998;87(7):224–8.
6. Schwartz J, Begley S. The mind and the brain neuroplasticity and the power of mental force. New York: Harper Perennial; 2002. p. 372–7.
7. Gregory R. Brainy mind. BMJ. 1999;317:1693–5.
8. Satinover J. The quantum brain. New York: Wiley; 2001.
9. Schweinhardt P, Lee M, Tracey I. Imaging pain in patients: is it meaningful? Curr Opin Neurol. 2006;19:392–400.
10. Songer D. Psychotherapeutic approaches in the treatment of pain. Psychiatry. 2005;2(5):19–24.
11. Doidge N. The brain that changes itself. New York: Penguin Books; 2007.
12. Stohler C, Kowalski C. Spatial and temporal summation of sensory and affective dimensions of deep somatic pain. Pain. 1999;79(2–3):165–73.
13. Apkarian A, Bushnell M, Treede R-D, Zubieta J. Human brain mechanisms of pain perception and regulation in health and disease. Eur J Pain. 2005;9:463–84.
14. Price D. Psychological mechanisms of pain and analgesia. Seattle: IASP Press; 1999.
15. Price D, Harkins S. The affective-motivational dimension of pain: a two-stage model. APS J. 1992;1:229–39.
16. Auvray M, Myin E, Spence C. The sensory-discriminative and affective-motivational aspects of pain. Neurosci Biobehav Rev. 2010;34(2):214–23.
17. Gracely R. Affective dimensions of pain: how many and how measured? APS J. 1992;1:243–7.
18. Melzack R. Evolution of the neuromatrix theory of pain: the Prithvi Raj Lecture. Presented at the third world congress of World Institute of pain, Barcelona, Spain, 2004. Pain Pract. 2005;5(2):85–94.
19. Melzack R. Pain – an overview. Acta Anaesthesiol Scand. 1999;43(9):880–4.
20. Melzack R, Katz J. Pain assessment in adult patients. In: McMahon S, Koltzenburg M, editors. Wall and Melzack's textbook of pain. 5th ed. Oxford: Elsevier Churchill Livingstone; 2006. p. 291–304.
21. Pesut B, McDonald H. Connecting philosophy and practice: implications of two philosophic approaches to pain for nurses' expert clinical decision making. Nurs Philos. 2007;8(4):256–63.
22. Sitges C, Garcia-Herrera M, Pericas M, et al. Abnormal brain processing of affective and sensory pain descriptors in chronic pain patients. J Affect Disord. 2007;104(1–3):73–82.
23. Mialet J. From back pain to life-discontent: a holistic view of psychopathological contributions to pain. Ann Med Interne (Paris). 2003;154(4):219–26.
24. Bonica J. Neurophysiologic and pathologic aspects of acute and chronic pain. Arch Surg. 1977;112(6):750–61.
25. Lippe P. An apologia in defense of pain medicine. Clin J Pain. 1998;14:189–90.
26. Casey K, Tran T. Cortical mechanisms mediating acute and chronic pain in humans. In: Cervero F, Jensen T, editors. Handbook of clinical neurology. Boston: Elsevier; 2006. p. 159–77.
27. Voscopoulos C, Lema M. When does acute pain become chronic? Br J Anaesth. 2010;105 Suppl 1:i69–85.
28. Rome H, Rome J. Limbically augmented pain syndrome (LAPS): kindling, corticolimbic sensitization, and convergence of affective and sensory systems in chronic pain disorders. Pain Med. 2000;1:7–23.
29. Krämer H, Stenner C, Seddigh S, et al. Illusion of pain: preexisting knowledge determines brain activation of 'imagined allodynia. J Pain. 2008;9(6):543–51.
30. Fontani G, Migliorini S, Benocci R, et al. Effect of mental imagery on the development of skilled motor actions. Percept Mot Skills. 2007;105(3 Pt 1):803–26.
31. Sanders CW, Sadoski M, Bramson R, et al. Comparing the effects of physical practice and mental imagery rehearsal on learning basic surgical skills by medical students. Am J Obstet Gynecol. 2004;191(5):1811–4.
32. Fitzgibbon B, Giumarra M, Georgiou-Karistianis N, et al. Shared pain: from empathy to synaesthesia. Neurosci Biobehav Rev. 2010;34(4):500–12.
33. Meyer R, Ringkamp M, Campbell J, Raja S. Peripheral mechanisms of cutaneous nociception. In: McMahon S, Koltzenburg M, editors. Wall and Melzack's textbook of pain. 5th ed. London: Elsevier; 2006. p. 3–34.
34. Julius D, McCloskey E. Cellular and molecular properties of primary afferent neurons. In: McMahon S, Koltzenburg M, editors. Wall and Melzack's textbook of pain. 5th ed. London: Elsevier; 2006. p. 35–48.
35. Ji R, Kawasaki Y, Wen Y, Decostrel I. Possible role of spinal astrocytes in maintaining chronic pain sensitization: review of current evidence with focus on bFGF/JNK pathway. Neuron Glia Biol. 2006;2:259–69.
36. Hertz L, Hansson E. Roles of astrocytes an microglia in pain memory. In: DeLeo J, Sorkin L, Watkins L, editors. Immune and glial regulation of pain. Seattle: IASP Press; 2007. p. 21–41.
37. Woolf C. Pain: moving from symptom control toward mechanism specific pharmacological management. Ann Intern Med. 2004;140:441–51.
38. Baron R. Mechanisms of disease: neuropathic pain – a clinical perspective. Nat Clin Pract Neurol. 2006;2(2):95–106.
39. Basbaum A, Jessell T. The perception of pain. In: Kandel E et al., editors. Principles of neural science. 4th ed. New York: Oxford University Press; 2000. p. 472–91.

40. Fields H, Heinricher M, Mason P. Neurotransmitters in nociceptive modulating circuits. Annu Rev Neurosci. 1991;14:219–45.

41. Kuner R. Central mechanisms of pathological pain. Nat Med. 2010;16(11):1258–66.

42. Lee M, Mouraux A, Iannetti G. Characterizing the cortical activity through which pain emerges from nociception. J Neurosci. 2009;29(24):7909–16.

43. Nicolelis M, Katz D, Krupa D. Potential circuit mechanisms underlying concurrent thalamic and cortical plasticity. Rev Neurosci. 1998;9(3):213–24.

44. Varela F, Frenk S. The organ of form. J Soc Biol Struct. 1987;10(1):1073–83.

45. Myers T. Fascial fitness: training in the neuromyofascial web. Fitness J. 2011:36–43.

46. Myers T. Anatomy trains: myofascial meridians for manual and movement therapists. New York: Churchill Livingstone; 2009.

47. Scott J. Molecules that keep you in shape. New Sci. 1986;111:49–53.

48. Juhan D. Job's body. Barrytown: Station Hill Press; 1987.

49. Travell J. Myofascia pain and dysfunction. Baltimore: Williams and Wilkins; 1983.

50. Hackett G, Hemwall G, Montgomery G. Ligament and tendon relaxation treated by prolotherapy. 5th ed. Oak Park: Beulah Land Press; 2002.

51. van Sterkenburg M, et al. The plantaris tendon and a potential role in mid-portion Achilles tendinopathy: an observational anatomical study. J Anat. 2011;218(3):336–41.

52. Sahin N, Oztürk A, Atici T. Foot mobility and plantar fascia elasticity with plantar fasciitis. Acta Orthop Traumatol Turc. 2010;44(5):385–91.

53. Ball T. Structural integration-based fascial release efficacy in systemic lupus erythematosus (SLE): two case studies. J Bodyw Mov Ther. 2011;15(2):217–25.

54. Prasarn ML, Oullette EA. Acute compartment syndrome of the upper extremity. J Am Acad Orthop Surg. 2011;19(1):49–58.

55. Guimberteau J. Strolling under the skin. New York: Elsevier SAS; 2004.

56. Pert C. The molecules of emotion. New York: Touchstone; 1999.

57. Oschman J. Energy medicine: the scientific basis. New York: Churchill Livingstone; 2000.

58. Elkhodair S, et al. Single fascia iliaca compartment block for pain relief in patients with fractured neck of femur in the emergency department: a pilot study. Eur J Emerg Med. 2011;18:340–3.

59. Kearns R, et al. Intrathecal opioid versus ultrasound guided fascia iliaca plane block for analgesia after primary hip arthroplasty: study protocol for a randomized, blinded, noninferiority controlled trial. Trials. 2011;21:12–51.

60. Kim HS, et al. Fascia iliaca compartment block reduces emergence agitation by providing effective analgesic properties in children. J Clin Anesth. 2011;23(2):119–23.

61. Boström P, Karjalainen V. Epidural or fascial anesthesia for postoperative pain? Duodecim. 2011;127(3):281–3.

62. Hoheisel U, Taguchi T, Treede RD, Mense S. Nociceptive input from the rat thoracolumbar fascia to lumbar dorsal horn neurones. Eur J Pain. 2011;15(8):810–5. Epub 2011 Feb 16.

63. Craig K. Emotions and psychobiology. In: McMahon S, Koltzenburg M, editors. Wall and Melzack's textbook of pain. 5th ed. Philadelphia: Elsevier Churchill Livingstone; 2006. p. 231–9.

64. Phillips HC, Hunter M. Headache in a psychophysical population. J Nerv Ment Dis. 1982;170:1–12.

65. Romano J, Turner J. Chronic pain and depression: does the evidence support a relationship? Psychol Bull. 1985;97:18–34.

66. Aurelius M. The meditations of Marcus Aurelius. In: Eliot C, editor. Plato, Epictetus, Marcus Aurelius the Harvard Classics. New York: Collier & Son; 1937. p. 245–61.

67. Perlmutter D, Villoldo A. Power up your brain the neuroscience of enlightenment. Carlsbad: Hay House; 2011. p. 26–31.

68. Kusumi T, Nakamoto K, Koyasu M. Perceptual and cognitive characteristics of metaphorical pain language. Shinrigaku Kenkyu. 2010;80(6):467–75.

69. Moroni C, Laurent B. Pain and cognition. Psychol Neuropsychiatr Vieil. 2006;4(1):21–30.

70. Kirmayer L. Culture and the metaphoric mediation of pain. Transcult Psychiatry. 2008;45(2):318–38.

71. Campbell C, France C, Robinson M, et al. Ethnic differences in the nociceptive flexion reflex (NFR). Pain. 2008;134(1–2):91–6.

72. Fillingham R. Sex differences in analgesic responses: evidence from experimental pain models. Eur J Anaesthesiol. 2002; 26(suppl):16–24.

73. Gibson S, Farrell M. A review of age difference in the neurophysiology of nociception and the perceptual experience of pain. Clin J Pain. 2004;20(4):227–39.

74. Turk D, Flor H. The cognitive-behavioral approach to pain management. In: McMahon S, Koltzenburg M, editors. Wall and Melzack's textbook of pain. 5th ed. New York: Elsevier Churchill Livingstone; 2006. p. 339–48.

75. Rainville P, Hofbauer RK, Paus T, et al. Cerebral mechanisms of hypnotic induction and suggestion. J Cogn Neurosci. 1999;11(1): 110–25.

76. Malenka R, Nicoll R. Long-term potentiation – a decade of progress. Science. 1999;285:1870–4.

77. Engert F, Bonhoeffer T. Dendritic spine changes associated with hippocampal long-term synaptic plasticity. Nature. 1999;399:66–70.

78. Wagner A, Schacter D, Rotte M, et al. Building memories: remembering and forgetting of verbal experiences as predicted by brain activity. Science. 1998;281:1188–91.

79. Brewer J. Making memories: brain activity that predicts how well visual experience will be remembered. Science. 1998;281:1185–7.

80. Shi S, Hayashi Y, Petralia R, et al. Rapid spine delivery and redistribution of AMPA receptors after synaptic NMDA receptor activation. Science. 1999;284:1811–6.

81. Damasio A. On some functions of the human prefrontal cortex. Ann N Y Acad Sci. 1995;769:241–51.

82. Owen A, Herrod N, Menon D, et al. Redefining the functional organization of working memory processes with human lateral prefrontal cortex. Eur J Neurosci. 1999;11:567–74.

83. D'Esposito M, Detre J, Alsop D, et al. The neural basis of the central executive system of working memory. Nature. 1995; 378:279–81.

84. Shapiro F. Eye movement desensitization and reprocessing. New York: Guilford Press; 1995.

85. Stowell H. Event related brain potentials and human pain: a first objective overview. Int J Psychophysiol. 1884;1(2):137–51.

86. Hellström C, Carlsson S. The long-lasting now: disorganization in subjective time in long-standing pain. Scand J Psychol. 1996;37(4):416–23.

87. Lautenbacher S, Prager M, Rollman G. Pain additivity, diffuse noxious inhibitory controls, and attention: a functional measurement analysis. Somatosens Mot Res. 2007;24(4):189–201.

88. van der Kolk B. The psychobiology of posttraumatic stress disorder. J Clin Psychiatry. 1997;58 Suppl 9:16–24.

89. van der Kolk B, Fisler R. Childhood abuse and neglect and loss of self-regulation. Bull Menninger Clin. 1994;58(2):145–68.

90. van der Kolk B, Greenberg M, Boyd H, et al. Inescapable shock, neurotransmitters, and addiction to trauma: toward a psychobiology of post-traumatic stress. Biol Psychiatry. 1985;20(3):314–25.

91. van der Kolk B, Greenberg M, Orr S, et al. Endogenous opioids, stress induced analgesia, and posttraumatic stress disorder. Psychopharmacol Bull. 1989;25(3):417–21.

92. van der Kolk B, Pelcovitz D, Roth S, et al. Dissociation, somatization, and affect dysregulation: the complexity of adaptation of trauma. Am J Psychiatry. 1996;153(7 Suppl):83–93.

93. Rauch S. Neuroimaging and the neuroanatomy of PTSD. CNS Spectr. 1998;3 Suppl 2:31–3.

94. Shalev A, Peri T, Brandes D, Freedman S, Orr SP, Pitman RK. Auditory startle response in trauma survivors with PTSD: a prospective study. Am J Psychiatry. 2000;157:255–61.

95. van der Kolk B. Psychological trauma. Washington: American Psychiatric Press; 1987.

96. Ramachandran V, Rogers-Ramachandran D. Phantom limbs and neural plasticity. Arch Neurol. 2000;57(3):317–20.

97. Wade N. Beyond body experiences: phantom limbs, pain and the locus of sensation. Cortex. 2009;45(2):243–55.

98. Kwan C, Diamant N, Mikula K, Davis K. Characteristics of rectal perception are altered in irritable bowel syndrome. Pain. 2005;113(1–2):160–71.

99. Pain Giamberardino M, et al. Referred muscle pain and hyperalgesia from viscera. J Musculoskeletal Pain. 1999;7(1–2):61–9.

100. Silberstein S, et al. Neuropsychiatric aspects of primary headache disorders. In: Yudofsky S, Hales R, editors. Textbook of neuropsychiatry. 3rd ed. Washington: American Psychiatric Press; 1997. p. 381–412.

101. Burstein R, Strassman A. Peripheral and central sensitization during migraine. In: Devor M et al., editors. Proceedings of the 9th world congress on pain. Seattle: IASP Press; 2000. p. 589–602.

102. Post R, Weiss S, Smith M. Sensitization and kindling: implications for the evolving neural substrates of post-traumatic stress disorder. In: Friedman M, Charney D, Deutch A, editors. Neurobiological and clinical consequences of stress: from normal adaptation to post-traumatic stress disorder. Philadelphia: Lippincott-Raven; 1995. p. 203–24.

103. Weiss S, Post R. Caveats in the use of the kindling model of affective disorders. Toxicol Ind Health. 1994;10:421–7.

104. Vecchiet L, Giamberardino M. Muscle pain, myofascial pain, and fibromyalgia: recent advances. J Musculoskeletal Pain. 1999;7(1–2).

105. Graven-Nielson T. Central hyperexcitability in fibromyalgia. J Musculoskeletal Pain. 1999;7(1–2):261–72.

106. Dohrenbusch R, Sodhi H, Lamprecht J, Genth E. Fibromyalgia as a disorder of perceptual organization? An analysis of acoustic stimulus processing in patients with widespread pain. Z Rheumatol. 1997;56(6):334–41.

107. Spiegel H, Spiegel D. Trance and treatment: clinical uses of hypnosis. 2nd ed. Washington: American Psychiatric Publishing Inc; 2004.

108. Francis M. Mindfulness exercises may help chronic pain patients. In: Pain medicine network. Spring; 2011: p. 6–7.

109. Schneider J, Hofmann A, Rost C, Shapiro F. EMDR in the treatment of chronic phantom limb pain. Pain Med. 2008;9(1):76–82.

110. Sumatani M, Miyachi S, Uematsu H, et al. Phantom limb pain originates from dysfunction of the primary motor cortex. Masui. 2010;59(11):1364–9.

111. Levy R, Deer T, Henderson J. Intracranial neurostimulation for pain control: a review. Pain Physician. 2010;13(2):157–65.

Neuroplasticity, Sensitization, and Pain

Albert L. Ray

> **Key Points**
> - Neuroplasticity is the "operating system" for the nervous system.
> - Eudynia: "the good"; acute nociceptive pain; a symptom; useful; warning pain
> - Maldynia: "the bad"; sensitized system at peripheral nerves, cord, and/or brain; no benefits to the person; pain becomes the disease process itself
> - Persistent pain: "the ugly"; continual maldynia; LAPS, CRPS, phantom pain, myofascial pain, IBS, fibromyalgia, chronic headaches, chronic mood changes

Introduction

Neuroplasticity is a term that is used quite frequently these days in pain-related literature, and in many ways, it has come to be a term especially associated with maldynia [1, 2]. However, neuroplasticity is a term that more accurately delineates the way our nervous system operates, peripherally and centrally, and it should have no intrinsic judgment placed upon it. It simply is what it is.

Neuroplasticity implies a mechanism whereby the physical anatomy and physiological workings of our nervous systems happen, both in normal and pathological conditions. It is the operating system for our nervous system "computer." It is like a combined hardware and software program. It is programmable, and when neuroplastic changes occur, they cause both physical changes, that is, anatomical changes to neurons, and physiological changes in the neurological patterns of operation. In many ways, these changes are analogous to laying down a set of railroad tracks. Once the tracks are in place, a train has no options but to follow the tracks, unless a switcher makes a change in the track and sends the train onto another set of tracks. In a similar way, once neuroplastic changes occur, our nervous system has no option but to follow these tracks, unless something causes a switch onto new tracks. However, the old tracks remain available indefinitely, and certain circumstances can switch our neurological train back onto the old track again.

In normal conditions, we foster the utilization of neuroplastic development to not only develop "railroad tracks" but also to polish them. For example, we develop the ability to walk from about 1 year of age, and hence, we lay down some early tracks for mobilization. As we age, and as we utilize walking in our everyday life, we polish those tracks till we become adept at walking. Eventually, we finely polish the system to allow for balance, mobility at low speed (walking) or high speed (running), and we develop variations on the mobility theme, such as skipping and hopping. With practice, we become better and better at it, adding more and more polished tracks as we develop. Later, we utilize neuroplasticity to accomplish more sophisticated tasks, such as developing the ability to play musical instruments, develop craft skills, or become athletes. In these situations, we merrily go our way without paying much attention to the fact that we are building new neurons devoted to the task at hand, and then, we are polishing and fine-tuning how the neurons work together in patterns that allow us to become proficient and efficient at what our task is. These neuroplastic changes are what allows us to become very accomplished at "within-self" activities, such as practicing at a musical instrument until the finger movements become "automatic," thus allowing the musician to concentrate on how they want the music to sound rather than on how to move fingers to produce the desired sound. But practicing also allows for neuroplastic changes to affect social activities with others, for example,

A.L. Ray, M.D. (✉)
Medical Director, The LITE Center, 5901 SW 74 St, Suite 201, South Miami, FL 33143, USA

Clinical Associate Professor, University of Miami Miller School of Medicine, Miami, FL, USA
e-mail: aray@thelitecenter.org

T.R. Deer et al. (eds.), *Treatment of Chronic Pain by Integrative Approaches: the AMERICAN ACADEMY of PAIN MEDICINE Textbook on Patient Management*, DOI 10.1007/978-1-4939-1821-8_2,
© American Academy of Pain Medicine 2015

when linemen members of a football team describe the state of being where they "know" what their teammates will do without having to verbally communicate during plays. This happens from concentrated practice until the neuroplastic tracks for working together are highly polished.

Certain principles have been attributed to neuroplastic development and functioning [3–5]:

1. Our brain is constantly changing, based on our current experiences.
2. Cells that fire together, wire together, and, through practice, stay together.
3. "Use it or lose it" works for brain activity and numbers of neurons.
4. Our brain works best when the system is "balanced."
5. The left and right hemispheres work together within this balance, under normal conditions, as a whole and not separately.
6. The corpus callosum is the bridge between hemispheres, and it is denser in females than in males, making the female brain more symmetrical and women more intuitive.
7. Male brains have an asymmetrical torque, with a right frontal lobe larger than the left and the left occiput larger than the right.
8. Right hemispheres process visual and spatial information related to the big picture and is more active while we are learning something new, while left hemispheres are more adept at details, categories, and linearly arranged information such as language, and the left hemisphere becomes more involved once something is "overlearned" and is now routine.
9. Right brain makes more connections with centers below the cortex and hence has more to do with emotional things.
10. Women have a greater density of neurons in the temporal lobe, which specializes in language, and in developing language skills; they activate the left hippocampus (related to memory) more than men do, while men generally have greater visual and spatial skills, because they show greater activity in the right hippocampus.
11. Prefrontal cortex provides our most complex cognitive, behavioral, and emotional capacities. The dorsolateral prefrontal cortex is involved in higher-order thinking, attention, and short-term memory, while the orbital frontal cortex processes emotions via connections through the amygdala and is involved in social issues. Right prefrontal cortex develops foresight and "gets the gist of it," allowing us to stay on course to our goals and understand metaphor, whereas left prefrontal cortex focuses on details of individual events.
12. The major neurotransmitters function in coordination with each other according to the following general understandings:

(a) Gamma-aminobutyric acid (GABA) is inhibitory and quiets the brain, while glutamate is excitatory and stirs it up. These neurotransmitters account for about 80 % of brain signaling.
(b) Serotonin, norepinephrine, and dopamine act more as neuromodulators, alter sensitivity of receptors, make transmission more efficient, and instruct neurons to make more glutamate. They also have other modulating duties: serotonin helps the system stay in control, norepinephrine activates attention and amplifies signals for perception, arousal, and motivation, and both serotonin and norepinephrine are associated with mood. Dopamine sharpens and focuses attention and is involved with reward, movement, learning, and pleasure.

13. Neuroplastic development and changes occur via long-term potentiation (LTP). This happens through electrochemical changes. Glutamate in presynaptic cells builds up, while the postsynaptic cell increases receptivity of receptor sites, increasing the voltage to attract more glutamate. If the increased firing continues, the genes within neurons turn on and build more infrastructures to enhance the system. This occurs via brain-derived neurotrophic factor (BDNF). BDNF increases gene activation, voltage, serotonin, and even more of itself. It also regulates apoptosis.

Under normal conditions, the system described above works in harmony within the brain to regulate our learning, emotions, thinking, and controls through a marvelous balance of a feedback system of neurophysiology. Through the development of neuroplastic brain anatomy and physiology, we function in a state of health.

However, when we are dealing with neuroplastic changes that have negative consequences for our lives, we tend to place a "black cloud" value onto them. For example, the neuroplastic changes that account for fibromyalgia, complex regional pain syndrome, and neuropathic pain are all understood through negative lenses. In these painful conditions, we focus our understandings on how neuroplastic changes produce such ravaging conditions that account for so much human suffering.

Neuroplasticity, then, can account for "the good, the bad, and the ugly" of pain perception. In the remainder of this chapter, we will focus on how neuroplasticity can result in the normal transmission of pain and how sensitization of the nervous system, peripherally and centrally, can alter a rather magnificent "pain system" and place the pain train on different tracks. Through the remainder of this chapter, we will describe what happens in terms of normal pain transmission and the neuroplastic changes of the nervous system in the disease of pain and principles of treatment applications designed to retrain the brain for health, by taking advantage of the principles listed above.

Neuroplasticity in Pain

Eudynia: The "Good"

In our normal development, our nervous system becomes wired and develops the ability to transmit pain as a warning symptom. For example, if we fall down and break a bone, the warning pain says "something is wrong; fix it and I will go away." This transmission of a warning signal comes about through what we consider the "normal" development of our nervous system, but this is accomplished via our neuroplastic system of development. That system is a most complex and wonderful system that helps protect us.

It begins with transduction from nociceptors in the skin. These nociceptors respond to mechanical, chemical, and temperature extremes of hot or cold. They turn their response into an electrical/chemical signal that conducts information to the dorsal horn of the spinal cord (see Fig. 1.1).

At the dorsal horn, multiple inputs can have an effect on that information signal, some acting to enhance and some acting to diminish it. Once these influences occur, a final summated signal is then sent up to the brain, where it is further processed (see Fig. 1.2). Some of the signal passes up the spinothalamic tract, through the thalamus, and on to the contralateral somatosensory cortex, while some of it passes via the parabrachial tract to be distributed to multiple brain regions including the limbic system, the anterior cerebral cortex (ACC), the prefrontal cortex, the amygdala, and the striatum and on to the somatosensory cortex and also the motor cortex via the basal ganglia. The first part accounts for Price's sensory-discriminative dimension (the ouch) of pain, while the latter accounts for Price's affective-motivational dimension (the yuck) of pain (see Fig. 1.3) [6–9].

Overall, this system of eudynia offers us the security and protection against many threats, including injury, infection, and tumors, by alerting us to the pain associated with these threats. (The details of normal pain transmission are covered elsewhere in this book.) Hence, our system, through helpful neuroplastic development, will continue to serve us well indefinitely, unless something goes awry.

Sensitization of the System

Maldynia: The "Bad"

Negative changes in the transmission of pain tend to occur through a process of sensitization. The nervous system can become sensitized at peripheral sites as well as centrally at dorsal horn and/or brain. Hence, a system that once worked to protect us can transform into one that produces ongoing pain [10]. Long-term potentiation (LTP) is the cellular model for sensitization [2, 11], whereas long-term depression (LTD) inhibits pain [12].

For example, peripheral sensitization is known to happen at trigger point sites in muscle. Trigger points have been described as consisting of sensory (sensitive locus) and motor (active locus) combinations with sensitized nociceptors [13]. Allodynic and hyperalgesic areas have been found in trigger points secondary to peripheral sensitization in chronic muscle pain [14, 15], tension-type headaches [16], and postmastectomy pain [17]. Both nociceptor and nonnociceptor sensitization secondary to ischemia due to sustained contraction have been identified in trigger points [18]. The peripheral sensitization of trigger points feeds into the dorsal horn and contributes to the beginning of central sensitization. However, this peripheral sensitization resolves with treatment of the trigger points, whereas the central sensitization appears to continue if LTP has occurred.

Likewise, plastic changes have been noted in peripheral nerve injuries, and these injuries also contribute to spinal and brain sensitizations [19]. The plasticity of the peripheral system is not quite as well identified as that of the central system.

Central sensitization is more studied, especially at the spinal dorsal horn level and, more recently, brain level, which has been undervalued in the past. "Central sensitization represents an enhancement in the function of neurons and circuits on nociceptive pathways caused by the increases in membrane excitability and synaptic efficacy as well as to reduced inhibition and is a manifestation of the remarkable plasticity of the somatosensory nervous system in response to activity, inflammation, and neural injury" (Fig. 2.1) [20].

At the cord level, many interactions can lead to sensitization, both in terms of functional and structural changes [21]. Voltage-gated calcium channels (VGCC) [22, 23], transient receptor potential vanilloid type 1 (TRPV1) receptors [24, 25], glutamate [7, 26–29], protein kinases [30, 31], serotonin, and N-methyl-D-aspartate (NMDA) [32] have all been described in functional roles within both the spinal cord and brain for sensitization (Figs. 2.1 and 2.2).

Structural and functional changes also occur in the spinal cord level regarding astrogliosis, and this effect seems to be mediated through secretion of diffusible transmitters, such as interleukins, ATP, and nitric oxide. The glial cells, via glutamate release, are thought to sensitize second-order neurons. However, they may also have a direct effect via the astrocytic networks that can transduce signals intrinsically [33, 34]. Additionally, animal studies have demonstrated an increase in the number of synapses within the dorsal horn in neuropathic pain [35].

Within the brain, reduced opioid neurotransmission has been noted in animal studies of spinal LTP, especially in brain areas associated with pain modulation and affective-emotional response [36]. LTP in the hippocampus is also

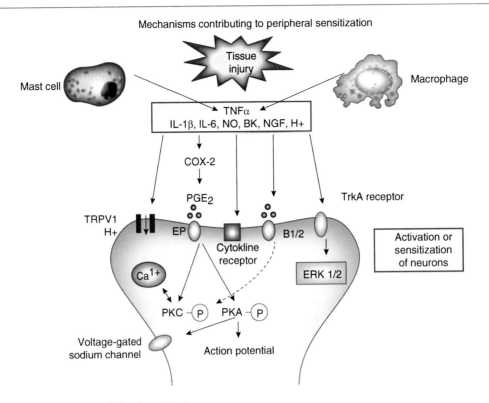

Fig. 2.1 Mechanisms contributing to peripheral sensitization

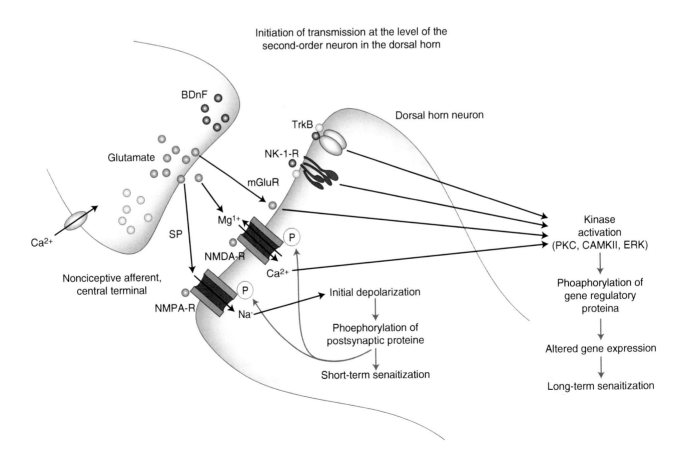

Fig. 2.2 Initiation of transmission at the level of the second-order neuron in the dorsal horn

involved with memory [37] and fear changes [38]. Spatiotemporal hippocampal changes have been observed in response to persistent nociception [39]. Tetanic stimulation of the ACC increased neurons in the central lateral nucleus of the medial thalamus [40]. fMRI, magnetoencephalography (MEG), positron emission tomography (PET), and voxel-based morphometry (VBM) studies in neuropathic pain have also shown reorganization of cortical somatotropic maps in sensory and motor areas, increased activity in nociceptive areas, recruitment of new cortical areas usually not activated by nociceptive stimuli, aberrant brain behavior normally involved with descending inhibitory pathways, changes in excitatory and inhibitory transmitter systems, and significant structural changes of neurodegeneration (use it or lose it) [41, 42]. These changes have been noted in phantom pain, chronic back pain, irritable bowel syndrome (IBS), fibromyalgia (FM), and two types of headaches. The alterations were different for each pain syndrome but overlapped in the cingulated cortex, the orbitofrontal cortex, the insula, and the dorsal pons [43]. These recent studies support an earlier proposition that the syndromes of chronic daily headache, chronic depression, IBS, and FM may all be different "phenotypes" of one "genotype" secondary to central sensitization [44]. Also, in post-spinal cord injury-related neuropathic pain, VBM studies have shown anatomical changes in pain-related and classic reward circuitry, including the nucleus accumbens, orbitofrontal, dorsolateral prefrontal, and posterior parietal cortices, and the right posterior parietal cortex projected to most of these affected areas [45]. Emotional-affective and cognitive dimensions of pain seem to also demonstrate structural and functional changes in maldynia, especially amygdala and prefrontal cortical areas [46, 47]. In fact, animal models for the amygdala-medial prefrontal cortex-driven pain-related cognitive deficits, including decision making, demonstrated that the cortical deactivation resulted from a shift of balance between excitatory and inhibitory transmission [47]. Hormones may have a role in neuroplasticity as well. Changes in neuroactive steroids during the estrous cycle have been shown to affect GABA-A receptor expression in female rats, resulting in an upregulation of GABA-A receptors late diestrus causing an increased excitability of output neurons in the periaqueductal gray (PAG) and clinically resulting in hyperalgesia [48].

Hence, we now have seen a neuroplastic transformation within the nervous system from a marvelous eudynic pain transmission model to one which demonstrates anatomic cellular changes, chemical transmitter and neuromodulator changes, and physiological functional changes via the process of sensitization. Indeed, our pain train now has different numbers of cars, different speeds at which to travel, changes in the stations along the way, and different tracks upon which it must now travel. It is what it has become!

Neuroplastically Remodeled Pain System

Persistent Pain: The "Ugly"

We will now turn more toward the clinical side of neuroplasticity and look at some specific pain problems. Ultimately, we will look at what can be done about them to ease our patient's suffering.

Limbically Augmented Pain Syndrome (LAPS) [49]

LAPS was described in a seminal pain paper to account for people who demonstrate more pain and pain behaviors than would be expected based solely on physical findings. These patients had previously been labeled as "hysterics," "crocks," and malingerers. Their presentation was usually affectively colorful, intense, and consisted of dramatic levels of dysfunction based on what previously looked like very little wrong physically. Through a very extensive comparison of clinical symptoms to sensitization research work, this paper clarified the role of central sensitization in both the traditional pain pathways and non-pain pathways regarding the affective-motivational and cognitive dimensions to pain perception. LAPS provides a foundational understanding of how sensitization presents clinically and why the primary pain and secondary non-pain complaints make sense. This includes many maldynia-accompanying complaints such as memory problems, slower thinking, non-restful sleep, decreased energy, lack of drive, decreased mental concentration and focus, anxiety, depression, anger, irritability, social isolation, a marked change in self-perception, and other frequent complaints we hear from our patients. The neuroplastic changes secondary to sensitization which account for decreased pain threshold, increased pain perception, recruitment, amplification of pain signaling within the central nervous system, and the intertwined role of pain- and non-pain-related inputs to pain have all been borne out and clarified through the research that has progressed since LAPS was identified, primarily due to improved technologies, but based on the core principles presented in the LAPS paper.

Through the LAPS foundation, we can make more sense out of the two dimensions of pain: the sensory-discriminative and affective-motivational dimensions described by Price [8]. Understanding these two dimensions and the overlapping brain functions involved with both helps unify our understanding of a person's pain perception, again reminding us of Osler's decree: one person, one disease. Rather than separate the two dimensions of pain and their respectively related symptoms, we can now focus on one person with all those complaints related to alterations in neuroplastic changes of the brain.

Fibromyalgia

Clinical aspects of neuroplastic changes in fibromyalgia are easily delineated, including many of those identified by the LAPS paper. However, peripheral evidence of change is basically lacking, in spite of much research on the peripheral tissues and peripheral pain transmissions. Within the central nervous system, however, much has been demonstrated. Fibromyalgia sufferers demonstrate hyperalgesia and allodynia, and this seems to result from an abnormal temporal summation of pain [50]. Changes in both sensory and motor brain have been found. One MRI and VBM study showed decreases in gray matter in the right superior temporal gyrus and left posterior thalamus, with increased gray matter in the left orbitofrontal cortex, left cerebellum, and striatum [51]. Another study found increased levels of serum BDNF in 30 female fibromyalgia patients, with no correlation to age, disease duration, pain score, number of pain tender points, or depression rating scores (HAM-D) [52].

Some of the treatments for fibromyalgia include pharmacological approaches designed to lower the level of pain transmission secondary to the neuroplastic sensitization by "calming down" the system at spinal and brain levels (see Part I. Medical Approaches). Other treatments include mind-body paradigms, as well as physical modalities. One study demonstrated benefit with a mind-body treatment utilizing psychosocial genomic postulates coupled with ideodynamic hand movements [53]. One study is being planned to utilize virtual exercise for those fibromyalgia patients who tend to avoid exercise as part of a catastrophizing style [54]. Moderate exercise for 24 weeks has been shown to have benefit for those able to tolerate it, resulting in improved health status and quality of life [55]. A separate 10-week exercise study demonstrated reduction in anxiety, improved sleep, and improved quality of life [56]. However, a group who had demonstrated improved daily step count by 54 %, improved functioning by 18 %, and reduced pain by 54 % in a 12-week trial found poor sustainability at 12-month follow-up, at which time the patients did not differ from controls on pain, physical activity, tenderness, fatigue, depression, the 6-min walk test, or self-reported functioning [57]. These findings would raise question as to what could be done to maintain the home treatment strategies long enough, or what could be added to them, in order to establish positive neuroplastic changes (i.e., what fires together wires together and what fires apart, wires apart).

Phantom Pain

Phantom limb sensations and pain have become more prominent in the literature since the incidence of amputation has increased as a result of the recent wars throughout the world [58]. The most recent successful treatments for phantom pain have also been based on what can change the brain LTP, hence, utilizing neuroplasticity to understand the pathophysiology of phantom pain and also to reverse it.

Studies have shown changes in the cortical representation of the affected limb and a correlation between these changes and the phantom pain. Mechanisms for the phantom pain are thought to relate to a loss of gamma-amino-butyric acid (GABA)-ergic inhibition, glutamate-mediated LTP changes, and structural changes such as axonal sprouting, and furthermore, these changes and consequent pain seem to be more extensive if chronic pain precedes the amputation [59].

One proposal suggests the imbalance of the system to be part of the problem. Specifically, the motor cortical body-representation cells involute, while the sensory cortical body-representation cells remain, the resulting imbalance producing the phantom pain. Reconciliation of this imbalance produces relief [60]. In fact, one treatment protocol utilizing imagined amputated limb movement coupled with existing counterpart limb movement resulted in fMRI evidence of elimination of the cortical reorganization and a reduction in constant pain and exacerbation pain [61]. Eye movement desensitization and reprocessing (EMDR) has also been shown to virtually eliminate phantom pain, without return barring further trauma to the body, through a similar process of alternating sensory input coupled with mental processing of the phantom pain [62, 63].

Complex Regional Pain Syndrome (CRPS)

CRPS is currently understood to be a complex of altered somatosensory, motor, autonomic, and inflammatory systems. But the central feature is both peripheral and central sensitization. Especially important to this sensitization is the neuroplastic alterations in the dorsal horn of postsynaptic NMDA receptors via chronic C-fiber input, among other changes. Motor changes are effected by calcitonin gene-related peptide (CGRP), substance P, and pro-inflammatory cytokines involved in the inflammatory process. Recent evidence implicates sensitization of adrenergic receptors in the sympathetic system having an influence on the C-fibers [64]. In animal studies, chronic peripheral inflammation has been shown to increase AMPA receptor-mediated glutamergic transmission in the ACC, which then increases the central excitatory transmission [65].

Visceral Pain

Visceral pain drives many doctor visits by patients, and it is one of the most common complaints in primary care offices. Visceral afferents have been found to play a role in tissue homeostasis by monitoring the viscera and contributing efferent functions via the release of small molecules such as CGRP that can drive inflammation. These afferents are highly plastic and are responsive to their cellular environment. They are quite susceptible to long-term changes associated with irritable bowel syndrome (IBS), pancreatitis, and visceral cancers [66]. In fact, recent work on chronic pancreatitis links sensitization to this syndrome, with descriptions of temporal and spatial alterations of intrapancreatic nerves and central neuroplastic consequences [67]. This process in chronic pancreatitis, then, seems to involve peripheral nociception, peripheral pancreatic neuropathy and neuroplasticity, and central neuroplastic changes as follows: sustained sensitization of pancreatic peripheral nociceptors by neurotransmitters and neurotrophic factors following neural damage, resulting in intrapancreatic autonomic "neural remodeling," which in turn causes our familiar hyperexcitability of second-order dorsal horn neurons, followed by viscerosensory cortical spatial reorganization [68].

Headache

Much work has been done regarding sensitization involving headache [69]. Recent understanding of sensitization in migraine considers peripheral sensitization leading to intracranial hypersensitivity (worsening the headache with cough and activity) and sensitized neurons becoming hyperresponsive to normally innocuous and unperceived fluctuations in intracranial pressure changes from arterial pulsation, resulting in the throbbing sensation. Central sensitization results in hyperexcitability of second-order neurons in the trigeminocervical complex, again a result of increased glutamate sensitivity of NMDA receptors and neuronal nitric oxide synthase activity. Clinically, this is manifested by facial and scalp allodynia along with neck stiffness [70].

Additionally, in chronic posttraumatic headache, a VBM study found spatial cortical reorganization to include decreased gray matter in the ACC and dorsolateral prefrontal cortex after 3 months. After resolution of the headache, at 1-year follow-up, patients who had developed the chronic headaches also showed an increase in gray matter in antinociceptive brainstem centers, thalamus, and cerebellum [71].

Postsurgical Pain

Chronic postoperative pain is becoming more prominently recognized. It is again thought to follow sensitization of the peripheral and central system by persistent acute postoperative pain. In most patients, it resembles neuropathic pain and occasionally follows continuous post-op inflammation [72]. This problem is estimated at between 10 and 80 %, and increased risk is associated with the existence of preoperative pain, the intensity and duration of post-op pain, and the type of surgery (high-risk surgeries) such as thoracotomy, breast, inguinal herniorrhaphy, and amputations [73]. The use of perioperative regional anesthesia has been shown to reduce the incidence, compared with intravenous morphine [74].

What to Do About It: Retraining the Brain

Multiple treatment approaches have been investigated for persistent pain, some designed to reduce the pain, others to improve functional status, and still others to reestablish a sense of contentment with life. The main theme behind all treatments is to try to establish a reversal of the neuroplastic sensitization or find ways to diminish its significance [75, 76].

Low back pain has been improved utilizing a training program model of delayed postural activation of the deep abdominal muscle, the transverse abdominis (TrA). Motor skill training induced an anterior and medial shift in motor cortical representation of the TrA, more closely resembling that of healthy persons. This training reversed the neuroplastic reorganization associated with chronic low back pain [77]. Other paradigms for chronic musculoskeletal pain also identify the need for motor learning as an important component for success, secondary to their ability at cortical reorganization [78]. One example is the use of peripheral electrical stimulation, which has been shown to develop rapid plastic change in the motor cortex, with parameters of variation in intensity of stimulation and longer periods of stimulation having the most sustained effects [79]. A fMRI study involving low-frequency electrical stimulation of cutaneous afferents in healthy volunteers resulted in pain relief and increased activity in the ACC, anterior insula, striatum, and frontal and temporal cortices, demonstrating long-term depression (LTD) of pain-related cerebral activation involving sensory, affective, cognitive, and attentional processes [80].

Acupuncture (see Chap. 10 for a detailed analysis of the approach) and massage have also been found to be peripheral stimulations which can cause central reorganizations. This has been described in terms of changing the neuroplastic adaptations associated with pain and addictive disorders [81].

Other therapeutic approaches include training of perceptual abilities, motor function, direct cortical stimulation, and behavioral approaches. Treatments that combine several modalities, such as imagery, mirror treatment, and prostheses, have been shown to have benefit [82]. For example, mirror therapy has been utilized for phantom pain, hemiparesis from stroke, and CPRS [83]. A somatosensory evoked potential (SEP) study involving chiropractic manipulation of the neck in subjects without current pain, but a history of chronic cervical pain, suggested alteration of the cortical integration of dual somatosensory input [84]. Paired associative stimulation in which peripheral nerve stimulation is followed by transcranial magnetic stimulation resulted in increased volleys of the descending inhibitory pathways [85], resulting in apparent LTD [86]. Even such techniques such as caloric restriction, via reduced intake of calories or intermittent fasting, have been shown to stimulate neurogenesis, enhance plasticity affecting pain sensation, cognitive function, and possibly resist brain aging. This is felt to occur through neurotrophic factors, neurotransmitter receptors, protein chaperones, and mitochondrial biosynthesis regulators which contribute to stimulation of the neuronal plasticity and resistance to oxidative metabolic insults [87]. Interestingly, one of the three worldwide characteristics of people who live the longest is eating 25 % less than the rest of their community members (caloric restriction) [4]. Cognitive-behavioral approaches have included somatosensory amplification associated with training in affect differentiation and the interaction of somatoform pain and interpersonal relationships [88].

It has been the clinical experience of the current author that the most effective treatment for maldynia or maldynia-eudynia combinations is a comprehensive approach designed to *retrain the brain*. This includes the utilization of some/all of the below modalities, individualized for each patient, such as myofascial release, unwinding, movement, electrical stimulations, muscle and ligament injections, exercising, postural training, guided imagery, body manipulations, visualization, meditation, spiritual healing, energy work, hypnosis, use of appropriate medications, inappropriate medication reductions, low-glycemic load nutritional approaches, nutritional supplements, bioidentical hormones, aroma therapy, graduated functional increases, massage and therapeutic touch, acupuncture, cognitive-behavioral treatment, Eye Movement Desensitization and Reprogramming (EMDR), NeuroEmotional Technique (NET), music therapy, family therapy and education, and patient education including neuroplasticity and brain function and how they are affecting their lives. The author of this chapter also utilizes written materials, some self-created and some published. Patients are referred to such items such as the American Pain Foundation (APF) website, the American Chronic Pain Association (ACPA) website, The Brain That Changes Itself [5], Rewire Your Brain [3], The Mind and the Brain [4], You Can Heal Your Life [89], The Quantum Brain [90], Power versus Force [91], and Healing and Recovery [92], among others.

These various therapies, educational materials, and philosophical approaches are often delivered individually, but sometimes simultaneously in a dual stimulatory approach through co-treatment (i.e., two therapists utilizing different treatments simultaneously, often incorporating two different senses/physical modalities at the same time). Treatments such as EMDR and NET incorporate two types of brain activity within one treatment approach. Some of these modalities take time and ritualistic practice in order to make neuroplastic changes (LTD, depotentiation of the LTP that occurred, or new LTD which is positive), while others, such as EMDR and NET, can have a rapid and lasting response, implying a neuroplastic reorganization that is immediate. Most of the therapeutic approaches mentioned above, however, must be done extensively and relatively frequently to make cortical changes permanently. We view ALL of these possible treatment modalities to have the same ultimate goal: RETRAINING THE BRAIN!

Summary

In this chapter, we have discussed the concept of neuroplasticity as the operating system of our nervous system computer. Without judgment, neuroplasticity can be of extreme usefulness, or it can produce, via sensitization, an "altered computer program" with devastating life effects of pain and suffering.

We have looked at the normal neuroplastic pain system for eudynia and what can go awry to result in maldynia, a disease. We have seen how neuroplasticity and sensitization can account for the good, the bad, and the ugly for pain transmission.

Although the mechanisms involved with neuroplastic sensitization of peripheral and central nervous components have been studied and continue to be researched, we still do not know which is the chicken or the egg. Exactly why this sensitization occurs, and who are the vulnerable people, is still a mystery. We do know that the brain can undergo neuroplastic reorganization from lower level (peripheral and spinal) changes or from higher level (mind) inputs. The system remains plastic throughout time and is responsive to inputs from any level.

However, successful treatment approaches all seem to be explained in terms of their effect on the neuroplastic changes (i.e., LTP that have happened). Successful treatments either seem to cause LTD, dampen the sensitized transmission of the disordered system, or cause new LTP that results in positive change rather than negative change.

Ultimately, however, the most significant changes appear to be related to those that occur in the brain. The brain has the ability to respond to the mind inputs and/or peripheral and spinal inputs. This input from above and below the brain can result in devastating negative changes in pain and suffering perception. However, effective treatment modalities seem to be those that can take advantage of the plastic nature of the brain to utilize those same higher and lower inputs to the brain to resolve and lessen pain and increase joy in life (see Chap. 1 on Pain as a Perceptual Experience for an extension of this topic).

References

1. Lippe P. An apologia in defense of pain medicine. Clin J Pain. 1998;14:189–90.
2. AMA Council on Science and Public Health Report 5. Maldynia: pathophysiology and non-pharmacologic treatment. 2010.
3. Arden J. Rewire your brain. New York: Wiley; 2010.
4. Schwartz J, Begley S. The mind and the brain: neuroplasticity and the power of mental force. New York: Harper Collins; 2002.
5. Doidge N. The brain that changes itself. New York: Penguin Group; 2007.

6. Voscopoulos C, Lema M. When does acute pain become chronic? Br J Anaesth. 2010;105 Suppl 1:169–85.

7. Apkarian A, Bushnell M, Treede R-D, Zubieta J. Human brain mechanisms of pain perception and regulation in health and disease. Eur J Pain. 2005;9:463–84.

8. Price D, Harkins S. The affective-motivational dimension of pain: a two-stage model. APS J. 1992;1:229–39.

9. Reichling DB, Levine JD. Critical role of nociceptor plasticity in chronic pain. Trends Neurosci. 2009;32(12):611–8.

10. Basbaum AI, Bautista DM, Scherrer G, Julius D. Cellular and molecular mechanisms of pain. Cell. 2009;139(2):267–84.

11. Descalzi G, Kim S, Zhuo M. Presynaptic and postsynaptic cortical mechanisms of chronic pain. Mol Neurobiol. 2009;40(3):253–9.

12. Treede RD. Highly localized inhibition of pain via long-term depression (LTD). Clin Neurophysiol. 2008;119(8):1703–4.

13. Hong CZ. New trends in myofascial pain syndrome. Zhonghua Yi Xue Za Zhi (Taipei). 2002;65(11):501–12.

14. Nielsen LA, Henriksson KG. Pathophysiological mechanisms in chronic musculoskeletal pain (fibromyalgia): the role of central and peripheral sensitization and pain disinhibition. Best Pract Res Clin Rheumatol. 2007;21(3):465–80.

15. Henrikssen KG. Hypersensitivity in muscle pain syndromes. Curr Pain Headache Rep. 2003;7(6):426–32.

16. Bendtsen L, Fernández-de-la-Peñas C. The role of muscles in tension-type headache. Curr Pain Headache Rep. 2011;15(6):451–8.

17. Fernández-Lao C, Cantarero-Villanueva I, Fernández-de-la-Peñas C, et al. Myofascial trigger points in neck and shoulder muscles and widespread pressure pain hypersensitivity in patients with postmastectomy pain: evidence of peripheral and central sensitization. Clin J Pain. 2010;26(9):798–806.

18. Ge HY, Fernández-de-la-Peñas C, Yue SW. Myofascial trigger points: spontaneous electrical activity and its consequences for pain induction and propagation. Chin Med. 2011;6:3.

19. Navarro X. Neural plasticity after nerve injury and regeneration. Int Rev Neurobiol. 2009;87:483–505.

20. Latremoliere A, Woolf CJ. Central sensitization: a generator of pain hypersensitivity by central neural plasticity. J Pain. 2009;10(9):895–926.

21. Kuner R. Central mechanisms of pathological pain. Nat Med. 2010;16(11):1258–66.

22. Park J, Luo ZD. Calcium channel functions in pain processing. Channels (Austin). 2010;4(6):510–7.

23. Tuchman M, Barrett JA, Donevan S, et al. Central sensitization and Ca(V)α₂δ ligands in chronic pain syndromes: pathologic processes and pharmacologic effect. J Pain. 2010;11(12):1241–9.

24. Palazzo E, Luongo L, de Novellis V, et al. Moving towards supraspinal TRPV1 receptors for chronic pain relief. Mol Pain. 2010;6:66.

25. Alter BJ, Gereau RW. Hotheaded: TRPV1 as mediator of hippocampal synaptic plasticity. Neuron. 2008;57(5):629–31.

26. Adedoyin MO, Vicini S, Neale JH. Endogenous N-acetylaspartylglutamate (NAAG) inhibits synaptic plasticity/transmission in the amygdala in a mouse inflammatory pain model. Mol Pain. 2010;6:60.

27. Larsson M, Broman J. Synaptic plasticity and pain: role of ionotropic glutamate receptors. Neuroscientist. 2011;17(3):256–73. Epub 2010 Apr 1. Review.

28. Zhou HY, Chen SR, Chen H, Pan HL. Functional plasticity of group II metabotropic glutamate receptors in regulation spinal excitatory and inhibitory synaptic input in neuropathic pain. J Pharmacol Exp Ther. 2011;336(1):254–64.

29. Liu XJ, Salter MW. Glutamate receptor phosphorylation and trafficking in pain plasticity in spinal cord dorsal horn. Eur J Neurosci. 2010;32(2):278–89.

30. Sanderson JL, Dell'Acqua ML. AKAP signaling complexes in regulation of excitatory synaptic plasticity. Neuroscientist. 2011;17(3):321–36. Epub 2011 Apr 15.

31. Li XY, Ko HG, Chen T, et al. Alleviating neuropathic pain hypersensitivity by inhibiting PKMzeta in the anterior cingulated cortex. Science. 2010;330(6009):1400–4.

32. Maneepak M, le Grand S, Srikiatkhachorn A. Serotonin depletion increases nociception-evoked trigeminal NMDA receptor phosphorylation. Headache. 2009;49(3):375–82.

33. Hald A. Spinal astrogliosis in pain models: cause and effects. Cell Mol Neurobiol. 2009;29(5):609–19.

34. Gwak YS, Hulsebosch CE. GABA and central neuropathic pain following spinal cord injury. Neuropharmacology. 2011;60(5):799–808.

35. Peng B, Lin JY, Shang Y, et al. Plasticity in the synaptic number associated with neuropathic pain in the rat spinal dorsal horn: a stereological study. Neurosci Lett. 2010;486(1):24–8.

36. Hjornevik T, Schoultz BW, Marton J, et al. Spinal long-term potentiation is associated with reduced opioid neurotransmission in the rat brain. Clin Physiol Funct Imaging. 2010;30(4):285–93.

37. Blanchard J, Chohan MO, Li B, et al. Beneficial effect of a CNTF tetrapeptide on adult hippocampal neurogenesis, neuronal plasticity, and spatial memory in mice. J Alzheimers Dis. 2010;21(4):1185–95.

38. Zhuo M. A synaptic model for pain: long-term potentiation in the anterior cingulate cortex. Mol Cells. 2007;23(3):259–71. Review.

39. Zhao XY, Liu MG, Yuan DL, et al. Nociception-induced spatial and temporal plasticity of synaptic connection and function in the hippocampal formation of rats: a multi-electrode array recording. Mol Pain. 2009;5:55.

40. Zhang L, Zhao ZQ. Plasticity changes of neuronal activities on central lateral nucleus by stimulation of the anterior cingulate cortex in rat. Brain Res Bull. 2010;81(6):574–8.

41. Maihöfner C. Neuropathic pain and neuroplasticity in functional imaging studies. Schmerz. 2010;24(2):137–45.

42. Teutsch S, Herken W, Bingel U, et al. Changes in brain gray matter due to repetitive painful stimulation. Neuroimage. 2008;42(2):845–9.

43. May A. Chronic pain may change the structure of the brain. Pain. 2008;137(1):7–15.

44. Ray A, Zbik A. Cognitive therapies and beyond. In: Tollison CD, editor. Practical pain management. 3rd ed. Philadelphia: Lippincott Williams and Wilkins; 2002. p. 189–208.

45. Gustin SM, Wrigley PJ, Siddall PJ, Henderson LA. Brain anatomy changes associated with persistent neuropathic pain following spinal cord injury. Cereb Cortex. 2010;20(6):1409–19.

46. Neugebauer V, Galhardo V, Maione S, Mackey SC. Forebrain pain mechanisms. Brain Res Rev. 2009;60(1):226–42.

47. Ji G, Sun H, Fu Y, et al. Cognitive impairment in pain through amygdala-driven prefrontal cortical deactivation. J Neurosci. 2010;30(15):5451–64.

48. Lovick TA, Devall AJ. Progesterone withdrawal-evoked plasticity of neural function in the female periaqueductal grey matter. Neural Plast. 2009;2009. doi:10.1155/2009/730902;730902. Epub 2008 Dec 2. Review.

49. Rome H, Rome J. Limbically augmented pain syndrome (LAPS): kindling, corticolimbic sensitization, and convergence of affective and sensory symptoms in chronic pain disorders. Pain Med. 2000;1(1):7–23.

50. Staud R, Spaeth M. Psychophysical and neurochemical abnormalities of pain processing in fibromyalgia. CNS Spectr. 2008;13 (3 Suppl):12–7.

51. Schmidt-Wilcke T, Luerding R, Weigand T, et al. Striatal grey matter increase in patients suffering from fibromyalgia- – a voxel-based morphometry study. Pain. 2007;132 Suppl 1:s109–16.

52. Haas L, Portela LV, Böhmer AE, et al. Increased plasma levels of brain derived neurotrophic factor (BDNF) in patients with fibromyalgia. Neurochem Res. 2010;35(5):830–4.

53. Cuadros J, Vargas M. A new mind-body approach for a total healing of fibromyalgia: a case report. Am J Clin Hypn. 2009;52(1):3–12.

54. Morris LD, Grimmer-Somers KA, Spottiswoode B, Louw QA. Virtual reality exposure therapy as a treatment for pain catastrophizing in fibromyalgia patients: proof-of-concept study (study protocol). BMC Musculoskelet Disord. 2011;12(1):85.

55. Sañudo B, Galliano D, Carrasco L, et al. Effects of prolonged exercise program on key health outcomes in women with fibromyalgia: a randomized controlled trial. J Rehabil Med. 2011;43(6):521–6.

56. Arcos-Carmona IM, Castro-Sánchez AM, Matarán-Peñarrocha GA, Gutiérrez-Rubio AB, Ramos-González E, Moreno-Lorenzo C. Effects of aerobic exercise program and relaxation techniques on anxiety, quality of sleep, depression, and quality of life in patients with fibromyalgia: a randomized controlled trial. Med Clin (Barc). 2011; 137(9):398–401. doi:10.1016/j.medcli.2010.09.045.Epub 2011 Feb 22 [Article in Spanish].

57. Fontaine KR, Conn L, Clauw DJ. Effects of lifestyle physical activity in adults with fibromyalgia: results at follow-up. J Clin Rheumatol. 2011;17(2):64–8.

58. Weeks SR, Anderson-Barnes VC, Tsao JW. Phantom limb pain: theories and therapies. Neurologist. 2010;16(5):277–86.

59. Flor H. Maladaptive plasticity, memory for pain and phantom limb pain: review and suggestions for new therapies. Expert Rev Neurother. 2008;8(5):809–18.

60. Sumitani M, Miyauchi S, Uematsu H, et al. Phantom limb pain originates from dysfunction of the primary motor cortex. Masui. 2010;59(11):1364–9.

61. MacIver K, Lloyd DM, Kelly S, et al. Phantom limb pain, cortical reorganization and the therapeutic effect of mental imagery. Brain. 2008;131(Pt 8):2181–91.

62. Shapiro F. Eye movement desensitization and reprocessing. New York: Guilford; 1995.

63. Schneider J, Hofmann A, Rost C, Shapiro F. EMDR in the treatment of chronic phantom limb pain. Pain Med. 2008;9(1):76–82.

64. Nickel FT, Maihöfner C. Current concepts in pathophysiology of CRPS I. Handchir Mikrochir Plast Chir. 2010;42(1):8–14.

65. Bie B, Brown DL, Naguib M. Increased synaptic Glur1 subunits in the anterior cingulated cortex of rats with peripheral inflammation. Eur J Pharmacol. 2011;653(1–3):26–31.

66. Christianson JA, Bielefeldt K, Altier C, et al. Development, plasticity and modulations of visceral afferents. Brain Res Rev. 2009; 60(1):171–86.

67. Ceyhan GO, Demir IE, Maak M, Friess H. Fate of nerves in chronic pancreatitis: neural remodeling and pancreatic neuropathy. Best Pract Res Clin Gastroenterol. 2010;24(3):311–22.

68. Demir IE, Tieftrunk E, Maak M, et al. Pain mechanisms in chronic pancreatitis: of a master and his fire. Langenbecks Arch Surg. 2011;396(2):151–60.

69. Silberstein S, et al. Neuropsychiatric aspects of primary headache disorders. In: Yudofsky S, Hales R, editors. Textbook of neuropsychiatry. 3rd ed. Washington DC: Amer Psychiatric Press; 1997. p. 381–412.

70. Tajti J, Vécsei L. The mechanism of peripheral and central sensitization in migraine. A literature revie. Neuropsychopharmacol Hung. 2009;11(1):15–21.

71. Obermann M, Nebel K, Schumann C, et al. Gray matter changes related to chronic posttraumatic headache. Neurology. 2009;73(12): 978–83.

72. Nau C. Pathophysiology of chronic postoperative pain. Anasthesiol Intensivmed Notfallmed Schmerzther. 2010;45(7–8):480–6.

73. Schnabel A, Pogatzki-Zahn E. Predictors of chronic pain following surgery. What do we know? Schmerz. 2010;24(5):517–31.

74. Chauvin M. Chronic pain after surgery. Presse Med. 2009;38(11): 1613–20.

75. Berger JV, Knaepen L, Janssen SP, et al. Cellular and molecular insights into neuropathy-induced pain hypersensitivity for mechanism-based treatment approaches. Brain Res Rev. 2011; 67(1-2):282–310.

76. Engineer ND, Riley JR, Seale JD, et al. Reversing pathological neural activity using targeted plasticity. Nature. 2011;470(7332): 101–4.

77. Tsao H, Galea MO, Hodges PW. Driving plasticity on the motor cortex in recurrent low back pain. Eur J Pain. 2010;14(8): 832–9.

78. Boudreu SA, Farina D, Falla D. The role of motor learning and neuroplasticity in designing rehabilitation approaches for musculoskeletal pain disorders. Man Ther. 2010;15(5):410–4.

79. Chipchase LS, Schabrun SM, Hodges PW. Peripheral electrical stimulation to induce cortical plasticity: as systematic review of stimulus parameters. Clin Neurophysiol. 2011;122(3):456–63.

80. Rottmann S, Jung K, Vohn R, Ellrich J. Long-term depression of pain-related cerebral activation in healthy man: an fMRI study. Eur J Pain. 2010;14(6):615–24.

81. Zhao HY, Mu P, Dong Y. The pathological neural plasticity and its applications in acupuncture. Zhen Ci Yan Jiu. 2008;33(1):41–6.

82. Flor H, Diers M. Sensorimotor training and cortical reorganization. NeuroRehabilitation. 2009;25(1):19–27.

83. Ramachandran VS, Altschuler EL. The use of visual feedback, in particular mirror visual feedback, in restoring brain function. Brain. 2009;132(Pt 7):1693–710.

84. Taylor HH, Murphy B. Altered central integration of dual somatosensory input after cervical spine manipulation. J Manipulative Physiol Ther. 2010;33(3):178–88.

85. Di Lazzaro V, Dileone M, Profice P, et al. Associative motor cortex plasticity: direct evidence in humans. Cereb Cortex. 2009;19(10): 2326–30.

86. Di Lazzaro V, Dileone M, Profice P, et al. LTD-like plasticity induced by paired associative stimulation: direct evidence in humans. Exp Brain Res. 2009;194(4):661–4.

87. Fontán-Lozano A, López-Lluch G, Delgado-Garcia JM, et al. Molecular bases of caloric restriction regulation of neuronal synaptic plasticity. Mol Neurobiol. 2008;38(2):167–77.

88. Lahmann C, Henningsen P, Noll-Hussong M. Somatoform pain disorder-overview. Psychiatr Danub. 2010;22(3):453–8.

89. Hay L. You can heal your life. Carlsbad: Hay House; 1999.

90. Satinover J. The quantum brain. New York: Wiley; 2001.

91. Hawkins D. Power vs Force. New York: Hay House; 2002.

92. Hawkins D. Healing and recovery. Sedona: Veritas Publishing; 2009.

Muscle Pain Treatment

Norman Marcus and Jason Ough

Key Points

- Muscle pain: history and nomenclature
- Assessment of the community standard of care for muscle pain
- Epidemiology
- Pathophysiology: muscle nociceptors, clinical mediators
- Peripheral and central sensitization and conditioned pain modulation—the mechanisms of chronicity and referred pain patterns
- Trigger points
- History, physical examination, and treatments
- Atypical muscle pain presentations
- Future directions

The greatest enemy of knowledge is not ignorance…it is the illusion of knowledge

—Stephen Hawking

Introduction

Muscles represent approximately 40 to 50 % of the body by weight yet are generally absent from our evaluation and treatment protocols for common pain syndromes. This chapter will provide a brief background on the history of the understanding of muscle pain, its epidemiology and patho-

physiology, problems in implementing a universally accepted approach to its diagnosis and treatment, and a suggested protocol for the inclusion of muscle evaluation and treatment in all instances of subacute and chronic pain presentations.

Background and Historical Perspectives

Muscle pain and tenderness interfering with physical function has been observed for centuries. However, its etiology has been elusive. The understanding of pain mechanisms in general has been helped from experiments on cutaneous pain fibers and our understanding of obvious neuronal pathways. For example, we know that damage to skin will start a cascade of neurochemical events that results in stimulation of cells in the dorsal horn of the spinal cord and possibly goes on to be consciously experienced as a generally unpleasant sensation. Likewise, we recognize that compression of a spinal nerve can produce pain in the distribution of that nerve. However, medical training has generally not shown us how mechanisms in muscles can generate local pain, which in turn may refer pain to adjacent and distant regions. Muscle nociceptors actually excite spinal cord neurons more than cutaneous nociceptors [1].

A review of comprehensive pain treatment textbooks [2–5] finds no chapters dealing with muscle pain aside from sections on "myofascial pain syndrome" discussing "trigger points" as the defining characteristic of syndromes with painful muscles.

A fundamental problem in discussing and understanding clinical muscle pain is the lack of agreed terminology to describe clinical findings. To better appreciate this obstacle, the history of muscle pain should be reviewed.

The same confusion encountered today is found as early as the sixteenth century when Guillaume de Baillou first referred to a clinical entity, *muscular rheumatism*, while describing diffuse soft tissue pain [6]. Other clinicians subsequently offered their explanations, inventing new terms along the way. In the nineteenth century, many believed that

N. Marcus, M.D. (✉)
Division of Muscle Pain Research, Departments of Anesthesiology and Psychiatry, New York University Langone School of Medicine, 30 East 40th Street, New York 10016, NY, USA
e-mail: njm@nmpi.com

J. Ough, M.D.
Department of Pain Management/Anesthesiology, New York University Langone Medical Center, 317 E. 34th Street, Suite 902, New York 10016, NY, USA
e-mail: jkough@gmail.com

T.R. Deer et al. (eds.), *Treatment of Chronic Pain by Integrative Approaches: the AMERICAN ACADEMY of PAIN MEDICINE Textbook on Patient Management*, DOI 10.1007/978-1-4939-1821-8_3,
© American Academy of Pain Medicine 2015

muscle pains were a disease of the muscle itself (a "serous exudative process") [7]. Tender nodules were thought to be a clinical manifestation of this disease and were first reported during this period. In 1919, Schade also observed muscle nodules and coined the term *myogelosen* (muscle gelling), and in 1921, Max Lange used the term *muskelhärten*, meaning hardened muscle [8]. Various other authors referred to some type of muscular or fibrous inflammation and used terms such as *fibrositis* and *myofibrositis*, but with the absence of clear signs of inflammation, these terms eventually lost favor. The debate on the importance of tender nodules in muscles, which began at the turn of the last century [7], continues [9], with some authors denying their importance and observing their presence in patients who are otherwise without pain complaints [10].

Muscle Pain Referral Patterns

A distinct aspect of painful muscles is the referring of pain to adjacent and distant muscles. Pioneering work regarding muscle pain and referral patterns was conducted in the 1930s when Jonas Kellgren, a student in the laboratory of Sir Thomas Lewis, performed experiments on approximately 1,000 patients over a 3-year period [11–13]. Kellgren's initial groundbreaking observations showed that muscle can refer pain to another region, and preclinical studies since the 1970s have demonstrated that the mechanisms of referred pain and windup are related to peripheral sensitization of muscle nociceptors and central sensitization of spinal cord neurons [14, 15].

The term "trigger points" was introduced in the literature as early as 1921 [16], elaborated on by Lange in 1931 [17], and in 1940, first used by Steindler [18] to describe tender areas in muscles that referred pain to other muscles. It was Janet Travell (and later, with David Simons), however, who popularized its use when she published papers describing the treatment of trigger points with injection of local anesthetic [19] and in the 1950s also popularized the term myofascial pain syndrome [20]. Travell and Simons played an important role in teaching colleagues about the presence of trigger points and typical patterns of referred pain from specific muscles [21]. Although myofascial pain syndrome (MPS) refers generically to pain from muscle and connective tissue, it is frequently used to infer that the muscle pain is the result of trigger points (TrPs) and tender points, contributing to the conceptual distortion that all muscle pain is from TrPs or tender points. A noteworthy episode in the muscle pain saga is the contrasting treatment approaches of Janet Travell and Hans Kraus who both treated President John F. Kennedy [22] for his low back pain. When Kennedy had been unable to walk without pain for months, trigger point injections were ineffective. Providing exercises addressing his weakness, stiffness, and tension resulted in pain reduction and restoration of function. Dr. Kraus shared with the senior author (NM) (1995) that JFK was planning to establish a national back pain institute so that his own experience of success and failure with various interventions could be studied. Following the death of Kennedy, two phenomena would interfere with the acceptance of muscles as a legitimate area of interest for pain-treating clinicians: (1) muscle pain treatment overemphasizing TrPs became the world community standard rather than a comprehensive muscle evaluation and treatment approach, thus laying the foundation for the overemphasis of trigger points as the sole area of interest in clinical muscle pain, and (2) the introduction of sophisticated imaging (e.g., CT scans, MRI) allowed clinicians to believe that the source of pain could be visualized, minimizing the importance of the physical examination [22] and relegating it frequently to a perfunctory ritual.

Chronic Widespread Pain (CWP) and Fibromyalgia Syndrome (FMS)

A subset of patients with muscle pain has diffuse pain and tenderness. The cause of widespread pains has been debated. Is the origin in the soft tissues in the periphery or in the central nervous system? Smythe and Moldofsky reintroduced the term fibrositis to describe patients with widespread pain and later renamed it fibromyalgia syndrome (FMS), when they described a collection of symptoms that included persistent widespread pain, fatigue, nonrestorative sleep, and multiple tender points at specific locations in the body [23, 24]. FMS was originally thought to be related to peripheral muscle pain generators [25], but research suggesting central dysregulation [26] as the cause has moved the entire field toward the concept that FMS is a CNS phenomenon typified by lowered thresholds to painful stimuli, accounting for the muscle pain. Peripheral pain generators have been recently reintroduced as important causes of FMS [27–30].

Psychogenic Muscle Pain

The debate over central versus peripheral origins of muscle pain includes the concept that in patients with widespread regional pain, the underlying problem may be psychiatric (*psychogenic rheumatism*) [31]. The concept of psychiatric/psychological etiologies of muscle-related pain may not properly distinguish neurophysiological effects of emotion on brain function from psychodynamic aspects of pain initiation and perpetuation. Chronic pain patients will frequently report that their pain is increased when they experience stressful events or feelings. Psychological factors producing specific physiological changes, including muscle tension patterns, have been described [32–34]. Denial or repression of uncomfortable feelings appears to be an important aspect in perpetuating pain in some patients with chronic pain syndromes [35]. Kasamatsu showed how CNS adaptation to interrupting stimuli could easily block out (deny) the presence of the stimulus in novices but not in seasoned meditaters, and Asendorpf demonstrated the deleterious physiological effects of denial of affect [36, 37]. The effectiveness of various psychological interventions associated with enhancing the patient's capacity to tolerate uncomfortable thoughts and feelings may operate in part by reducing or eliminating sustained muscle tension patterns, relieving discomfort in chronic muscular-related pain syndromes [38–43]. The reduction in pain will produce decreased emotional discomfort; decreased emotional discomfort will decrease the perception of pain [44, 45].

Present Terminology

The term myofascial pain syndrome is used in lieu of muscle pain in most articles and textbooks on chronic pain, and multiple theories have been offered to explain myofascial pain syndromes [46–56]. The resultant confusion in the literature prevents the creation of universally accepted approaches to study painful muscles.

Review of Muscle Pain in the Literature

According to the core curriculum of the International Association for the Study of Pain, myofascial pain is defined as pain emanating from muscle and connective tissue that causes pain in common clinical regional pain syndromes and "lacks reliable means [for physicians] to identify, categorize, and treat such pain" [57, 58]. Studies of clinicians attempting to identify painful muscles demonstrate poor inter-rater reliability in the identification of myofascial trigger points [59–64]. Clinicians will frequently and mistakenly use the terms "myofascial trigger point" and "myofascial pain" interchangeably. Myofascial trigger points are only one possible source of myofascial pain. Muscle and other soft tissue pain are thought to be responsible for most of acute back pain [91] and yet muscle pain evaluation and treatment are absent in low back treatment guidelines [66]. Failure to agree on nomenclature and methods of evaluation and treatment and the absence of valid RCTs to provide evidence of effectiveness of specific treatment approaches, has contributed to the rejection of trigger point injections (TPIs) and sclerosant injections as recommended treatment options for low back pain [67]. Ignoring muscle facilitates an overemphasis on structural abnormalities demonstrated on imaging and not necessarily identifying the true source of the patient's pain. Subsequent inappropriate

treatments contribute to the $86 billion spent in 2005 on neck and back pain in the United States [68].

Possible Etiologies of Myofascial Pain Are Not Fully Recognized by Clinicians

Myofascial pain can be caused by various etiologies. However, the current community standard of establishing the diagnosis is limited to palpating the putative muscle causing regional pain and identifying any TrPs. The standard treatment is to give TPIs to the putative muscle, injecting into a discrete area that includes only the TrPs and associated taut bands. The evaluation of TrPs without a complete assessment of muscle conditioning contributes to unexplainable variability in treatment outcomes because diagnoses are confounded when clinicians fail to consider weakness, stiffness, spasm, or tension as a primary source of pain [69]. Therefore, even if the putative muscle is correctly identified and injection is effective, failure to acknowledge and/or appropriately treat pain from these other causes of myofascial pain may leave the patient with persistent discomfort, and clinically unchanged.

Limits of Palpation as a Diagnostic Tool

Palpation alone used to detect areas of muscle pain introduces two confounding variables. First, varying amounts of pressure may be applied, diminishing the reliability of the examination. Pressure-recording devices have been introduced to determine more accurately the amount of applied pressure necessary to elicit discomfort in the patient [70, 71]. However, the accuracy of these devices is compromised because examiner preconceptions have been reported to influence the assessment [72]. Second, palpation to elicit a subjective experience of pain is often performed in a sedentary muscle. Most functional muscle pain is experienced with muscle activity versus rest. Therefore, an examination of a resting muscle is likely to be less accurate in determining the source of the muscle pain, frequently identifying a referred pain pattern, compared with an examination utilizing movement of discrete muscles [73, 74].

Two technologies to image muscles thought to harbor taut bands and TrPs have been suggested as possible means to more objectively identify the presence of pain-generating structures. Magnetic resonance elastography (MRE) allows visualization and identification of tissues with varied elasticity and has been shown to be reliable than palpation in identifying taut bands [75]. Visualization of TrPs is more elusive, but recent studies have demonstrated the use of ultrasound in identifying TrPs [76, 77]. Both of these techniques may help to objectify the identification of taut bands and TrPs but have not yet been clinically tested to determine if they will improve the effectiveness of treatment for muscle pain.

Injection Techniques

The description of TPIs and the assessment of their effectiveness in the literature has great variability. At least one published study used the return of 75 % of the pre-injection pain as a measure of success in studying TPIs using different injectates [78], and other studies have commented on the need to reinject TrPs [79, 80].

Other studies address the specific number of trigger points in a muscle [81], the importance of eliciting a "twitch response" [79] or of thoroughly injecting the "taut band" [82]. We suggest an approach modeled on that of Kraus who had originally thought that injecting TrPs when present could successfully diminish or eliminate muscle pain. Kraus observed that many of his patients treated with TPIs would frequently return with the need for reinjection in the same muscle. He speculated that as the muscle-tendon and bone-tendon attachments had the least blood supply versus the muscle tissue, these areas might also be the source of the recurrent pain pattern, and therefore modified his injection technique so that it always included the origin and the insertion of the identified painful muscle. Gibson et al. [83] has reported that the tendon-bone junction is more sensitive and susceptible to sensitization by hypertonic saline than muscle tissue. This observation would support our clinical impression of the importance of the tendon-bone junction in the course of muscle needling [84].

Exercise

Exercise is defined as a "series of movements to promote good physical health." Therefore almost any activity can be defined as an exercise protocol, thus accounting for the wide variety of outcomes achieved through "exercise" [85]. The existing protocols for MPS (and for diagnoses of regional pain that are relied upon to support the use of prolotherapy) usually include some general prescription for "exercise." The utility of exercise in the treatment paradigm makes sense, and a systematic review has concluded that a variety of non-specific exercises has produced long-term results in NSLBP patients [86, 87]. A problem in the exercise literature is the general absence of subgroups of patients [88] based on psychosocial variables and specific assessments for level of conditioning (strength and flexibility). Trigger point injection therapy and prolotherapy protocols suggest the generic use of exercise following injections [89]. Idiosyncratic provision of exercise protocols without patient subclassification may confound outcome data and eliminate the possibility of valid systematic review or meta-analysis.

Statistically significant effects of exercise in pain populations may not reflect clinical significance. Van Tulder et al. [85] found that of 43 Cochrane-reviewed trials on exercise for the treatment of low back pain, 18 of the trials reported a positive response, but only four showed any statistically significant reduction of pain. We believe that the absence of specific goals based in part on the results of specific muscle testing which could provide subclassification of patients, along with the nonspecific nature of the exercise protocols administered in conjunction with muscle injections, contributes to the inconsistent outcomes, even when apparently similar injection techniques are used.

Epidemiology

Difficulty in Obtaining Accurate Survey Data

The search for the incidence of muscular pain leads to a confusing array of concepts. Musculoskeletal pain is an umbrella term that describes pain originating in bones, joints, and muscles. Low back, neck, and shoulder pains are frequently thought to be caused by soft tissue [90]. Chronic widespread pain and fibromyalgia may have peripheral muscle pain generators contributing to the pain presentation.

Therefore, the interpretation of incidence and prevalence data for muscle-related pain is confounded. In addition, patients diagnosed with other comorbidities may indeed have muscles as the source of their pain but may be excluded from survey data. Indeed, it is the premise of this chapter that muscles are an overlooked contributing etiology of many common pain syndromes which are incorrectly attributed to only nonmuscular causes.

Low back pain is an example of the difficulty encountered. The most frequent diagnosis for low back pain in an ambulatory setting is nonspecific or idiopathic low back pain, generally referred to as sprains or strains of soft tissue, and represents 70–80 % of patients seen in large-scale studies [91], yet soft tissue-/muscle-generated pain is a small percentage (which has been diminishing over time) of all causes in a large national study [68].

Prevalence and Incidence of Musculoskeletal Low Back and Shoulder Pain

Adolescent Data

Musculoskeletal pain is frequently experienced in adolescence. Multinational surveys report lifetime prevalence rates of approximately 50 % when patients are queried on their past experience of low back pain, chronic widespread pain (CWP), fibromyalgia, shoulder or musculoskeletal pain with similar rates for prospective studies lasting 1–5 years [92]. When pain occurs at more than one site and at least once a week, there is a significant reduction in health-related quality of life scores [93]. A 2009 European study reported a 1-month period prevalence of LBP of nearly 40 % in adolescents [94].

Adult Data

According to the 2008 National Health Interview Survey report, 27 % of adults reported low back pain in the preceding 3 months and 14 % reported neck pain [95]. A 2009 study demonstrated a rising prevalence of chronic LBP across all age groups over a 14-year period [96]. The lifetime prevalence of chronic LBP in the UK general population is estimated to be 6.3–11.1 % [97].

In 2008, The Bone and Joint Decade 2000–2010 Task Force on Neck Pain and Its Associated Disorders reported the 12-month prevalence of neck pain was 30–50 % [98]. The 1-month period prevalence of shoulder pain is between 20 and 33 % [99].

Data for CWP (US and UK) shows 10–11 % point prevalence with females affected 1.5 times more often than males [100–102]. The same data shows 0.5–4 % point prevalence for FMS, with females affected 10 times more often than males. Lawrence et al. in 2008 estimated that approximately five million American adults over 18 years of age have primary fibromyalgia (this data was extrapolated from Wolfe's Wichita survey in 1993 and another from London, Ontario) [103]. Another study in 2009 reported that chronic widespread pain had a lifetime prevalence of 5–10 % of the general population [104].

Data also show that patients with FMS may have a history of work-related neck and shoulder pain, whiplash, low back pain, and muscle tension [105, 106], and therefore, the authors believe that many of these patients have undetected and potentially treatable muscles as a source of pain.

No matter how the data is analyzed, muscles appear to be a significant source of pain in a wide range of diagnoses and age groups.

Pain in Cancer Patients

Ten percent of patients diagnosed with cancer have pain unrelated to their disease, and it is generally related to muscles and connective tissue [107] and often overlooked in practice [108].

Pathophysiology and Scientific Foundations

Much of the preclinical data in the literature on the pathophysiology of muscle pain is based on animal studies, and therefore much of our knowledge in humans is extrapolative. This section can only provide a limited introduction to the existence of known mechanisms that account for the presence of pain originating in muscles. Therefore, the reader is encouraged to refer directly to source material on muscle pain and at least review the 2009 IASP textbook, *Fundamentals of Musculoskeletal Pain*, edited by Arendt-

Nielsen, Graven-Nielsen, and Mense, and *Muscle Pain: Understanding the Mechanisms* edited by Mense and Gerwin.

Neurologic Mechanisms of Pain Originating in Muscle

Morphology of Muscle Nociceptors

The structure typically mediating muscle pain is free nerve endings that have a high mechanical threshold in the noxious range/and or respond to pain producing chemicals [109]. Whereas cutaneous pain is localized to an injury site, muscle pain tends to be diffuse, based on the fact that muscle nociceptors have a larger receptor field and lower innervation densities [14].

Neuropeptide Content of Nociceptors

Dorsal root ganglion cells projecting into muscle contain substance P, calcitonin gene-related peptide, and somatostatin, which may be released when nociceptors are sensitized, causing further stimulation of the nociceptor.

Functional Types of Muscle Nociceptors

There are three types of muscle nociceptors:
1. High-threshold mechanoreceptors, activated by tissue-threatening mechanical stimuli, which allow the organism to respond to threats of damage as well as actual damage.
2. Chemonociceptors which respond to algesic substances but not to mechanical stimuli. For example, a receptor would respond to ischemic contraction of the muscle but not normal contraction.
3. Polymodal nociceptors which respond to both mechanical and chemical stimuli.

Nociceptors Are Equipped with Specific Molecular Receptors for Various Ligands

Inflammatory Chemical Mediators
These particular nociceptors may respond to a variety of chemical mediators, including inflammatory mediators released by damaged muscle tissue (bradykinin, serotonin, and prostaglandin E2).

Proton Receptors
These receptors respond to lowered pH (e.g., due to exhausting muscle work), which excites acid-sensing ion channels. With aggressive work or exercise, the pH may be less than

5.0 and in extreme conditions as low as 4.0 with resultant severe pain [110].

Vanilloid receptors are specific for capsaicin and are also sensitive to protons and heat.

Purinergic receptors bind ATP and its metabolites.

Excitatory amino acid receptors bind glutamate.

Nerve growth factor (NGF) exclusively excites high-threshold mechanoreceptors. Mense cautions that since multiple mediators are present at the same time, it is not possible to determine which are key mediators since there are important synergies among them [111].

Pathophysiological Mechanisms That Produce Spread of Muscle Pain

Nerve Growth Factor (NGF)

Experimental evidence suggests that NGF may be important in the production of certain chronic muscle pain syndromes, such as work-related musculoskeletal pain. NGF, released by a repetitively used inflamed muscle, may painlessly sensitize spinal neurons and ultimately lead to chronic muscle pain [110, 112, 113].

Peripheral Sensitization

Nociceptors in muscles become sensitized following a variety of events such as repetitive strain (overuse), direct trauma, and ischemia. These events all produce sensitization of type III and IV nerve fibers through stimulation of the aforementioned receptors, which lowers the stimulation threshold for pain, with resultant tenderness (hyperalgesia) and pain with movement (muscle allodynia) [114]. Axonal reflexes will then excite previously uninvolved branches of the same nerve (that were not directly stimulated by the tissue damage), with a spread of sensitization so that adjacent areas will also be experienced as tender.

Central Sensitization

Central sensitization may also result in muscle allodynia and hyperalgesia. Mense and his colleagues have shown that experimental inflammation in the leg muscles of rats produced three observable changes in the excitability of dorsal horn neurons [115]:

1. An increase in the spontaneous activity of the dorsal horn neurons.

2. An increase in the response of neurons in spinal segments L4 and L5 (the segments to which gastrocnemius/soleus (GS) muscle afferents travel for the rat; in human L5–S1) to mechanical stimulation of the GS. If there is persistent stimulation of the GS, neuroplastic changes will occur in the dorsal horn.

3. Excitation of adjacent spinal segments that are not usually stimulated by the GS.

Previously ineffective connections that become effective in pathological conditions may become opened, leading to a larger number of neurons being excited in response to an input which was previously nonexciting. The clinical significance of these changes is seen in the development of pain with movement of a sensitized muscle (muscle allodynia) and exaggerated pain (hyperalgesia) with painful stimuli. In addition, the opening of previously unaffected channels connected to adjacent spinal segments may be another mechanism of referred pain often seen in muscle pain syndromes. Central sensitization should not be confused with windup—although they have similarities in transmitters and neuronal pathways responsible for the heightened responsiveness to stimuli, they are not identical. Windup does not persist for a long time after stimulation unlike central sensitization, which can be long lasting [15].

Clinical Significance of Conditioned Pain Modulation (CPM) - formerly known as Diffuse Noxious Inhibitory Control, in the Treatment of Muscle Pain Syndromes and in the Relationship of FMS to Regional Muscle Pain

Central sensitization is known to be a normal event in acute pain [116], but it becomes pathologic when it is long standing or permanent. There is now ample evidence for central sensitization in fibromyalgia [117]. However, there have been differing schools of thought on the role peripheral generators play in the maintenance and development of central sensitization in a chronic pain syndrome such as fibromyalgia. While some scholars focus on the lack of direct evidence of peripheral input as proof that there is no true muscular pathology in FMS, others believe that peripheral generators should be considered the primary cause of pain in FMS unless proven otherwise [25, 116]. In a 2006 review article, Vierck offers several examples of possible muscle pathology supporting a peripheral generator theory, including red, ragged fibers on muscle biopsy, constricting band-like structures, mitochondrial abnormalities, metabolic changes, and vascular effects [25]. In further support of the idea that FMS can develop from a local or peripheral source, Arendt Nielsen points out that most patients diagnosed with fibromyalgia initially present with localized or regional pain, which subsequently leads to chronic, widespread pain [116].

It is already understood that in certain diseases, continuous peripheral input maintains central sensitization, resulting in painful conditions such as hyperalgesia and allodynia [118]. Studies have been done which continue to support the idea of peripheral generators playing a significant role in central sensitization in fibromyalgia. A randomized, double-blind, placebo-controlled study by Staud and others in 2009 showed that lidocaine injections into the trapezius muscle increased local pain thresholds and, in cases of FM, decreased remote secondary heat hyperalgesia [118]. Ignoring potential primary afferent mechanisms may lead to the mistaken impression that all FMS patients have a chronic intractable condition and deprive those with treatable peripheral pain generators the chance to eliminate an actual pain source and avoid the prolonged administration of serotonin/norepinephrine reuptake inhibitors or anticonvulsants.

Loss of centrally mediated inhibitory pain modulation is a proposed mechanism of pain in fibromyalgia. Two mechanisms have been discussed: (1) Fields and Basbaum described a tonic descending inhibitory mechanism that when impaired decreases pain thresholds and may be associated with the pain seen in FMS [119]. (2) In experiments performed on healthy controls, normally functioning central pain inhibitory mechanisms were demonstrated when a secondary tonic stimulation reduced brief episodes of experimentally induced pain. This pain modulation, referred to as diffuse noxious inhibitory control (DNIC) and recently renamed conditioned pain modulation (CPM) [120], was not observed in patients with FMS, and there is evidence suggesting that this mechanism is impaired or deficient in a chronic pain state such as FMS [121, 122]. The functional role of CPM is still unclear, but it is possible that lack of CPM may play a role in central sensitization itself and may further be involved in the transformation of acute pain to chronic pain [122].

Observations by the senior author (NM) suggest that both central sensitization and CPM may be evident in the course of treatment of patients with multiple painful muscles requiring needling. Approximately 20 % of muscles identified in the initial consultation of patients with pain duration of more than 1 year and with more than five muscles identified as sources of regional pain were found not to be present in the course of ongoing muscle injections [57]. Conversely, muscles that did not test positive on the initial consultation sometimes would become painful over the course of injections, reflecting the belief of NM that this may be a function of CPM, i.e., when the most painful area is eliminated, a less painful area can be identified. Based on these observations, after the first muscle is injected, a reevaluation should be performed prior to each additional muscle injection.

Prolonged inactivity results in weakness and stiffness and diminished endurance, all contributing to the overall pain experience in FMS. A recent Cochrane review of exercise in FMS concluded that exercise was effective as related in part to improved muscle conditioning rather than decreased pain or tender points [123]. Another small study by E. Ortega et al. [124] suggests that exercise reduces inflammation as measured by inflammatory markers in FMS.

Trigger Points (TrPs) or Myofascial Trigger Points

Trigger points are tender nodular spots in muscles that are frequently associated with a taut band of muscle fibers and when palpated will frequently radiate pain to a distant site. Laboratory studies have found evidence of dysfunctional neuromuscular end plates [55], and recent studies have reported alteration in the biochemical milieu of the TrPs [125]. Although numerous articles have been written on the evaluation and treatment of trigger points, there is diminishing interest in their importance and even disbelief in the construct [9] based in part on the inconsistency of evaluation and treatment methodology and relative transient relief of pain following injection of TrPs. It does appear that TrPs are important sources of localized and diffuse [126, 127] muscle pain [10], but the lack of agreed nomenclature and treatment approaches has rendered the available clinical literature unusable for meta-analyses, systematic reviews, and inclusion as a validated approach [128] in published guidelines for common pain syndromes such as low back pain [129]. Altered muscle tissue is not only present in TrPs in the belly of the muscle but has been noted by Simons et al. [130] as occurring in the muscle attachments as well. The typical examination using palpation will frequently miss these areas of tenderness especially in deep muscles. NM has used electrical stimulation to contract discreet muscles. When a muscle is painful to stimulation, in contrast to surrounding muscles that are non-painful to stimulation, it is considered a putative source of pain in that region of the body. An important aspect of the examination is the production of pain along the entire course of a suspected muscle, from origin to insertion, in order to unambiguously identify that muscle as a source of pain.

Peripheral Nerve Entrapments

Muscle spasm, either in the entirety of the muscle or in a small region, may result in compression of an adjacent nerve (e.g., the piriformis muscle compressing the sciatic nerve). Kopell and Thompson [131] report on the "fall from grace" of the diagnosis of the "piriformis syndrome," which had been an important explanation for sciatic pain in the mid-twentieth century, because surgical sectioning of the muscle to release the sciatic nerve was often unsuccessful, but the practice of sectioning the piriformis muscle persists [132, 133]. The piriformis syndrome is an important consideration in the differential diagnosis of apparent lumbosacral radicular pains, and proper identification and nonsurgical treatment of a painful piriformis muscle may result in sciatic pain relief. Other referral patterns of pain associated with peripheral entrapment neuropathies are reported [131] and in the author's opinion are important sources of apparent "radicular" patterns of pain.

Impediments to Creating a Reliable, Valid Muscle Pain Protocol

General absence of education in medical school and postgraduate training of the published basic science mechanisms of muscle pain has lead to the perpetuation of the belief that muscle pain is only a response to problems in the spine or the CNS [9]. Functional muscle pain from tension, weakness, stiffness, and spasm should be part of the standard assessment leading to specific diagnosis-driven treatments of patients presenting with regional pain syndromes. Absence of these functional pain categories leads to overdiagnosis and treatment of trigger points and the ensuing suboptimal results.

The Need for a Protocol That Recognizes and Incorporates Muscle Pain and Physical Function into the Evaluation and Treatment of Common Pain Syndromes

We have an obligation to come together as a discipline and attempt to formulate testable protocols that could facilitate reasonably equivalent data collection. This could lead to valid meta-analyses and systematic reviews of the evaluation and treatment of muscles as a source of pain in a variety of chronic pain syndromes. In this spirit, the authors present the following protocol for consideration as a comprehensive model of evaluation and treatment for all persistent pain presentations to facilitate the study of muscle as a putative source of pain.

History

When taking a patient's history, clinicians should always inquire about the presence and duration of any muscle tenderness. Pre- and posttreatment use of a self-administered test instrument for assessment of pain and its effect on daily

function, such as the Brief Pain Inventory [134], is encouraged. The history should gather appropriate data to establish possible habits, postures, and activities that could contribute to and perpetuate muscle dysfunction and pain. For example, patients can be asked if pain is worsened with prolonged positioning (such as sitting or standing in one place for too long), or if movements such as walking diminish pain, which suggests that a muscle pain component is present. For headaches or pain in the upper body, neck or shoulder, some common habits may contribute to the perpetuation and exacerbation of pain: (A) reading or watching TV in bed (causing a stiffening isometric contraction of the muscles of the shoulder and neck), (B) typing with a keyboard placed too high (causing a nonergonomic elbow bend of less than 90°), (C) not positioning a computer monitor straight ahead and at eye level or slightly below and not using a telephone head set to avoid isometric contraction of the neck and shoulder muscles.

Physical Exam

The physical examination should contain a method to establish whether or not the patient has an acceptable minimal level of strength and flexibility in the upper and/or lower body. The Kraus-Weber (KW) (see Fig. 3.1) test is proposed for key trunk muscle strength and flexibility. An examination for neck and shoulder range of movement, a neurological examination, and palpation for muscle tenderness and resilience are all suggested evaluation tools. If available, an evaluation with an electrical instrument to stimulate specific muscles (NM uses the MPDD [SPOC, Inc. Stamford, CT]) to locate those producing pain is also recommended. The MPDD is thought to work by contracting a specific muscle, which stimulates nociceptors in (1) the muscle attachments and (2) in the muscle belly in trigger points when deformed by the muscle contraction. In the practice of NM, palpation for tenderness and resilience is performed to identify presumptive sources of muscle pain, but the diagnosis of muscle pain amenable to injection (MPAI) is only made with the MPDD. For MPAI to be diagnosed in a muscle, the entire course of the muscle from origin to insertion must be experienced as painful (tender, aching, or sore) during the stimulation. Sustained pain produced by MPDD in only a portion of the muscle suggests that another muscle is the true source of the pain.

In the absence of an electrical device to identify the muscular source of pain, manual palpation can sometimes correctly identify the muscle where the tenderness originates versus a referred muscle pain. To maximize the accuracy of the manual examination, an instrument that facilitates the application of a standard amount of pressure is suggested [135–137].

Fig. 3.1 KW test for strength and flexibility of key postural muscles; failure—inability to perform any of the tasks (Courtesy of the Norman Marcus Pain Institute)

Six Basic Muscle Tests

These six standardized tests of musular function may help to "pinpoint" deficiencies of strength or flexibility (Test 6). They are done as slowly and smoothly as possible. Avoid jerky movements. Do not strain. Stop and rest briefly after each test.

Test 1. Lie on your back, hands behind your neck, legs straight. Keeping your legs straight, raise both feet 10 inches off the floor and hold for 10 seconds. This is a test of your hip-flexing muscles.

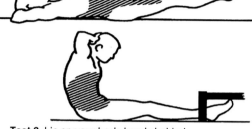

Test 2. Lie on your back, hands behind your neck, feet under a heavy object which will not topple over. Try to "roll" up to a sitting position.This tests your hip-flexing and abdominal muscles.

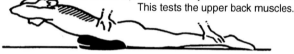

Test 3. Lie on your back, hands behind your neck, knees flexed, feet under a heavy object which will not topple over. Again try to "roll" up to a sitting position. This is a test of your abdominal muscles.

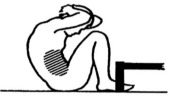

Test 4. Lie on your stomach with a pillow under your abdomen, hands behind your neck. With someone holding your feet and hips down, raise your trunk and hold for 10 s. This tests the upper back muscles.

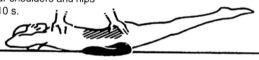

Test 5. Taking the same position as that used for Test 4, but this time having someone holding your shoulders and hips down, try to raise your legs and hold for 10 s. This test the muscles of the lower back.

Test 6. Stand erect with shoes off, feet together, knees stiff, hands at sides. Try to touch the floor withe your fingertips. If you can not, try it again. Relax, drop your head forward, and try to let your torso "hang" from your hips. Keep your knees stiff. Chances are you'll do better the second time.This is a test of muscle tension or flexibility.

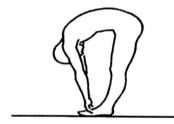

Treatment Protocols

Patients who are diagnosed with muscle pain that does not lend itself to injection should receive treatment appropriate to the diagnosis. Therefore, patients who have stiffness, but not weakness, should not be given strengthening exercises since this will only further stiffen their muscles. The current nostrum (following the fads of low-impact aerobics [138–140] and then closed-chain exercises [141, 142]) using core strengthening for back pain without any test of strength and flexibility is ill-founded [143].

Injection Technique

When muscle involvement is suggested and the evaluation protocol finds that injections are indicated, the authors suggest the use of the term Muscle Pain Amenable to Injection (MPAI), as opposed to "trigger point pain." Suggested treatment consists of muscle-tendon injections (MTIs) instead of only TrP injections (TPIs), in order to include the regions (the entheses) with possibly the greatest density of sensitized nociceptors, followed by a structured physical therapy protocol which includes a validated set of exercises [144].

Patients should not be injected if they have a concurrent physical diagnosis (including morbid obesity, profound weakness and/or stiffness, Parkinson's disease, severe peripheral neuropathy, or significant psychological comorbidities) that discourages aggressive treatment of the diagnosed muscle pain until the underlying problem is adequately addressed.

We suggest that only one muscle is injected during a given injection treatment. A needle that is long enough to reach the bony attachment of the muscle (between 25 gauge × 5/8 in. and 20 gauge × 3½ in.) is used, depending on the size and depth of the identified muscle. The treatment is the needle disrupting the muscle tissue with particular attention to the origin and insertion. NM refers to the injection as a muscle-tendon injection (MTI) because of the significant difference in location of the injections versus TPIs. An entire muscle, and not just a "point or taut band," is injected.

The patient will typically first receive an intravenous analgesic. After seeing ketamine used for minor procedures at Walter Reed Army Medical Center, NM routinely uses it at a dose of <1 mg/kg, with total doses between 15 and 50 mg maximum, along with Midazolam 1–2 mg IV, with patients experiencing no pain from the procedure. Patients are counseled prior to the use of ketamine that they will have an unusual experience but that they will be able and are encouraged to keep discussing with me what they are feeling and thinking. Most patients elect to have ketamine on subsequent injections. The few that do not because of discomfort from the psychological effects of the ketamine, or lack of available recovery time, will be given a low-dose opioid, determined by the patient's past response to opioids.

The area to be injected is swabbed with iodine. Next, up to 10 ml of 0.5 % lidocaine is injected into the subcutis overlying the indexed muscle (5 ml for muscles in the neck and above). After 5–8 min, the muscle is needled from its origin to its insertion point (including the muscle belly) with an additional 10 ml of 0.5 % lidocaine (5 ml for muscles in the neck and above) for comfort, down to the bony attachment. With such doses of lidocaine, NM has never produced a systemic lidocaine reaction.

To illustrate the treatment technique, consider the example of giving an MTI to the infraspinatus (see Figs. 3.1 and 3.2). After instilling subcutaneous lidocaine, the muscle is injected at the vertex of the scapula with a 22-gauge × 1½-in. needle, and with the needle still inserted, it is moved along the medial and lateral borders of the scapula, withdrawing and reinserting the needle as one proceeds up toward the spine of the scapula and the rotator cuff. Ice is applied for 4 min after the injection. The area is cleansed, and when all bleeding stops, the stable patient is released.

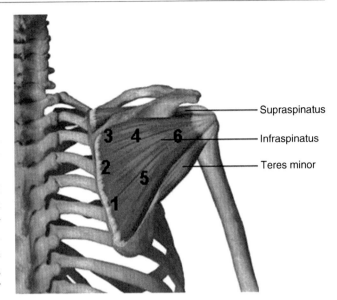

Fig. 3.2 The numbers represent the suggested sequence of muscle-tendon injections into the infraspinatus muscle down to the periosteum (With permission from the University of Washington)

Postinjection Physical Therapy

The MTI procedure causes some degree of pain both during and after the procedure. In order to facilitate additional injections and subsequent mobilization, the patient receives physical therapy on the day following the MTI. The physical therapy lasts for three consecutive days postinjection and consists of the patient receiving neuromuscular sine-wave stimulation (with ice) to a visible contraction, 2 seconds on and 2 seconds off, for a total of 15–20 min. This is followed by the first seven Kraus exercises for the lower body or the eight exercises for the upper body (see Figs. 3.3 and 3.4). Treatment always commences on a Monday to allow more than one muscle to be injected per week and to allow time for the three required post-MTI physical therapy sessions to be completed for each MTI. Therefore, treatment is considered complete on the final day of the post-MTI physical therapy session, of the last week that injections are given. Patients are given further instructions on the final day of physical therapy for the remaining 14 additional lower body exercises.

Summary of Suggestions for the Inclusion of Muscle Assessment in All Patients with Persistent Pain

1. Any patients with persistent pain should undergo a thorough examination of all muscles that could possibly contribute to the pain complaint.

Fig. 3.3 Kraus-Marcus level 1 exercises for the relaxation and limbering of the lower body musculature (Courtesy of the Norman Marcus Pain Institute)

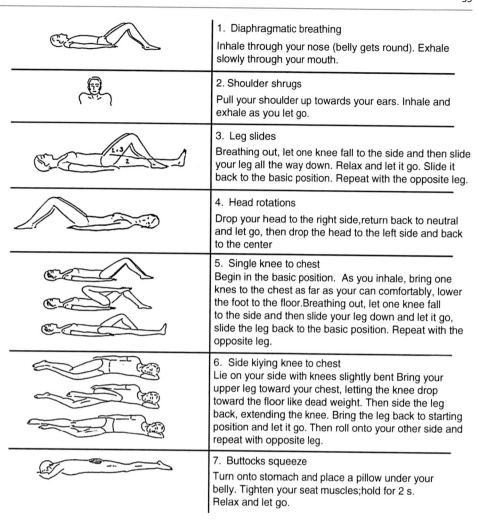

	1. Diaphragmatic breathing Inhale through your nose (belly gets round). Exhale slowly through your mouth.
	2. Shoulder shrugs Pull your shoulder up towards your ears. Inhale and exhale as you let go.
	3. Leg slides Breathing out, let one knee fall to the side and then slide your leg all the way down. Relax and let it go. Slide it back to the basic position. Repeat with the opposite leg.
	4. Head rotations Drop your head to the right side,return back to neutral and let go, then drop the head to the left side and back to the center
	5. Single knee to chest Begin in the basic position. As you inhale, bring one knes to the chest as far as your can comfortably, lower the foot to the floor.Breathing out, let one knee fall to the side and then slide your leg down and let it go, slide the leg back to the basic position. Repeat with the opposite leg.
	6. Side kiying knee to chest Lie on your side with knees slightly bent Bring your upper leg toward your chest, letting the knee drop toward the floor like dead weight. Then side the leg back, extending the knee. Bring the leg back to starting position and let it go. Then roll onto your other side and repeat with opposite leg.
	7. Buttocks squeeze Turn onto stomach and place a pillow under your belly. Tighten your seat muscles;hold for 2 s. Relax and let go.

2. Distinguish injectable muscle pain from pain related to tension, deficiency (weakness and/or stiffness), and spasm. We suggest the Kraus-Weber test for strength and flexibility of key postural muscles for low back and lower extremity pain. We suggest standard tests of upper body strength along with assessment of forward elevation and abduction of the arm and functional internal and external rotation of the shoulder (scapulohumeral and scapulothoracic motion) to find asymmetries of motion in the shoulder girdles which may suggest which muscle(s) may be involved.

3. Attempt to identify primary versus referred muscle pain. (Identification through muscle stimulation appears to be more accurate than palpation.)

4. Utilize a standardized exercise program to correct muscle deficiencies. We recommend the Kraus exercises: 8 for the upper body and 21 for the lower body.

5. When injecting a specific muscle, pay particular attention to the entheses of the identified muscle rather than just TrPs and taut bands. Consider injecting only one muscle at a given injection session.

6. If you use an injection procedure that targets the entire muscle, we recommend following up with 3 days of a postinjection physical therapy protocol to minimize postinjection soreness and stiffness.

7. If more than one MPAI is identified and multiple treatments are planned, reassess the patient for continued presence of MPAI prior to injecting the next planned muscle. It is possible that changes may have taken place as a result of successful injection. These changes may be related to central sensitization (the next muscle is no longer painful to manual or electrical stimulation) or CPM (a new muscle is painful after the previous; most severely painful muscle was successfully treated).

In future editions of this textbook, we hope to be able to publish head-to-head comparisons of other proposed and published comprehensive protocols.

Fig. 3.4 Kraus upper quadrant exercises for flexibility of the neck and shoulder girdle (Courtesy of the Norman Marcus Pain Institute)

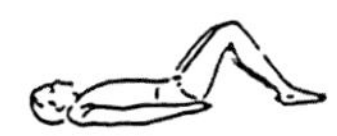	**1. Diaphragmatic breathing** Inhale through your nose (belly gets round). Exhale slowly through your mouth.
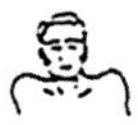	**2. Shoulder shrugs** As you inhaling pull your shoulders up towards your ears, exhale and let go.
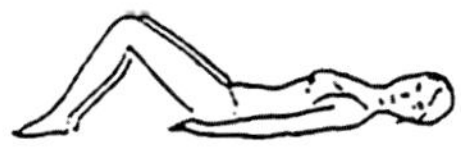	**3. Head rotations** Drop your head to the right side as you inhale, return back to neutral on the exhale and let go, then drop the head to the left side and back to center.
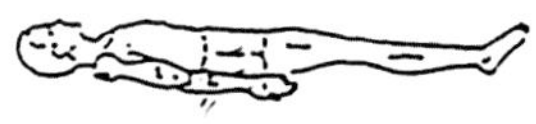	**4. Elbow bend** As you are inhaling close fists and bend elbows, as you are exhaling-let go.
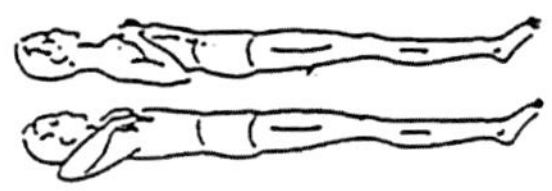	**5. "Chicken wings"** Basic position with hands on the chest. Inhale first. slide the arms out to the sides as you are exhaling and bring them back as you continue to exhale.
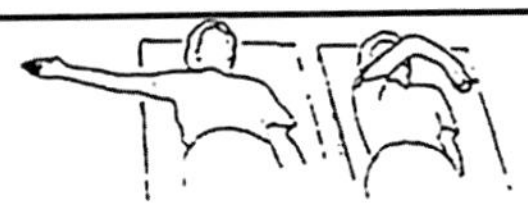	**6. Horizontal abduction–adduction** Bring the arm across the chest and bring it back (out to the side.)
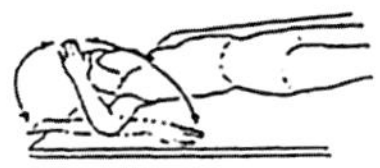	**7. Shoulder rotation** Abduct the arm with elbow flexed. Make sure to maintain a 90° angle as you rotate in and out.
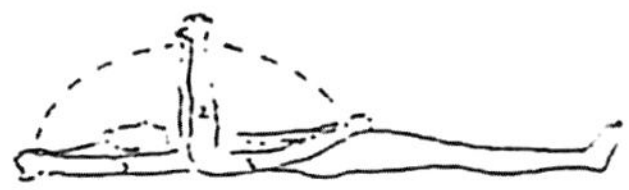	**8. Shoulder bend** Clasp your hands together and straighten your arms as you inhale. Exhale as you elevate your arms. Return back to basic position as you continue to exhale. If it is too diffcult or painful, lower both hands and let the strong/less painful, side assist with raising and lowering the arms.

Unusual Clinical Presentations in Which Muscles Played a Role

The following extraordinary case examples are presented not as a suggestion that all patients with the initial putative diagnoses below have muscle pain, but rather that we do not know whether any of our patients with persistent pain complaints have an overlooked, treatable muscle pain because we are not routinely and systematically looking at their muscles as a possible source of pain. Ignoring muscles in patients with chronic pain may lead to unnecessary treatment failures and, in some cases, exacerbation rather than elimination of the pain complaint.

Complex Regional Pain Syndrome (CRPS)

A 50-year-old woman suffered a right-sided tibia/fibula fracture requiring open reduction and internal fixation and postoperatively developed complex regional pain syndrome in her foot and lower leg with discoloration, swelling, restricted range of motion, allodynia, and decreased temperature. Her initial diagnosis was made at a prominent New York City hospital. She received ketamine infusions, spinal cord stimulation, and a variety of traditional medications utilized for CRPS. She was unable to wear a sock or a closed-toe shoe. She was severely depressed. She was seen for assessment five and a half years after the onset of her symptoms. Examination revealed pain emanating from the bilateral quadratus lumborum, left piriformis, left peroneus, left tibialis posterior, left soleus, left extensor hallucis longus, and left extensor digitorum longus muscles. The muscles were treated in the fashion previously described. She was pain free for approximately 4 months after her last treatment, with no restrictions and no medication, wearing a normal shoe and playing golf.

Her pain then returned, coincident with failed rotator cuff surgery and cessation of her prescribed lower body exercises, as well as the onset of wintry weather. Interestingly, only the dysesthetic pain and allodynia at the surgical scar site returned and not the skin color, temperature, and sweat changes. She was found to have MPAI in the following muscles: right quadratus lumborum (pain reduced 50 % after injection), piriformis (pain reduced 30 % after injection), extensor digitorum longus (pain reduced 10 % after injection), and extensor hallucis longus (complete relief of pain after injection). At the time of this writing, the patient has been essentially pain free for more than two years.

Failed Back Surgery Syndrome (FBSS)/ Spinal Stenosis

A 65-year-old entrepreneur with a 15-year history of back and leg pain was diagnosed with spinal stenosis and underwent two failed lumbar spine fusions at a prominent surgically oriented hospital. He was told that his only option for his persistent pain, which prevented him from leaving his home and socializing with friends and family, was a spinal cord stimulator or an epidural morphine pump. He was on round-the-clock opioid analgesia. In November 2005, he was evaluated for the presence of muscles as a source of his now persistent bilateral anterior thigh pain. Three muscles were identified—the right gluteus maximus and the left tensor fascia lata and vastus lateralis—and injected. One month after, he was essentially pain free and ambulating normally and remains pain free 5 years after his last injection. He has been able to travel to Vietnam and China and reports no impairments secondary to back or proximal leg pain.

FBSS is generally considered to be only amenable to palliative interventions such as spinal cord stimulation and/or lifelong delivery of potent analgesics, orally or parenterally. We have previously reported on a series of patients with FBSS successfully treated for muscle pain in the same fashion [145].

Fibromyalgia/Disk Protrusion

A 42-year-old woman with a 2-year history of neck, head, back, and lower extremity pain following an auto accident (causing her to spend days and weeks in bed with severe pain) was evaluated by multiple physicians and diagnosed with fibromyalgia. It was suggested that she undergoes cervical/lumbar spinal fusion as well. She was evaluated for the presence of muscle pain, and 13 muscles were identified— in the upper body, bilateral frontalis, infraspinatus, pectoralis minor, and left anterior/medial scalenes; and in the lower body, bilateral quadratus lumborum, gluteus medius, and right gluteus maximus, and piriformis. Since the most intense and disabling pain was in her head and neck, this region was treated first. After five muscles had been injected in her upper body (bilateral infraspinatus, frontalis, and left pectoralis minor), she reported that nearly all of the upper and lower

body pain was eliminated. No other muscle injections needed to be done. She is now without any pain-related impairment, 1 year after her last treatment.

Patients with imaging studies suggesting clinically meaningful spinal pathology may also present with diffuse pain diagnosed as FMS. Spinal fusion may be suggested. Some of these patients may have treatable muscle pain.

Rotator Cuff Tear

A 60-year-old medical assistant with a 2-year history of severe right shoulder pain and markedly restricted of range of motion was found to have a full-thickness buttonhole tear of the supraspinatus tendon on MRI. He was scheduled for rotator cuff surgery repair but was evaluated prior to surgery for muscle-based pain and found to have tenderness in six muscles of his shoulder girdle—coracobrachialis, trapezius, levator scapula, posterior para-cervicals, biceps brachii, and pectoralis major—which were successfully injected with elimination of all pain and total restoration of his range of motion (and subsequent cancellation of his surgery). He remained without pain or restriction for the 1 year he was followed.

Shoulder pain is inconsistently evaluated and treated [146–148]. Including the routine examination for specific shoulder muscle pain and dysfunction could decrease unnecessary surgeries and long-term use of analgesics.

Future Directions

The addition of a muscle protocol into the standard pain treatment paradigm should be supported by adequate RCTs to establish the validity of any intervention. In the realm of injection techniques to treat NSCLB, such a formidable task has uniquely been done by Francisco Kovacs.

Neuroreflexotherapy (NRT)

Neuroreflexotherapy (NRT) consists of the temporary implantation of a number of epidermal devices (surgical staples and small "burins" implanted subcutaneously) in trigger points in the back at the site of dermatomes and at the referred tender points located in the ear. The purpose is to "deactivate" neurons assumed to be involved in the persistence of pain, neurogenic inflammation, muscle dysfunction, and contracture.

As recognized by the Cochrane Back Review Group, NRT is one of the few technologies which has shown to be effective through high-quality, randomized, controlled trials and to provide "unusually positive" results [149]. This technology is currently implemented in Spain through the Spanish National Health System [150], and its evaluation in other countries is warranted.

Fascial Pain

Muscles do not function in a vacuum, and the relationship of muscle to its adjacent fascia and ligaments has not been systematically explored. As obscure as the data on muscle pain may be, fascial pain is even more so. The dynamic structure and function of fascia has not been appreciated. Fascia appears to have contractile properties that make it integral to efficient muscle contraction [151], as well as mechanosensitive properties which provide important information to surrounding muscles. Fascia has been shown to refer pain to different structures [152]. Therefore, damaged fascia may play an important role in chronic and recurrent low back pain [153, 154].

Stretching of injured muscle and tendon appears to inhibit scarring, which may be related to the production of transforming growth factor (TGF) beta 1 by damaged fascia [155]. In surgical procedures where fascia is resected, one should at least consider preservation of functional integrity whenever possible.

Regional Nonspecific Neck Pain

Regional pain such as neck pain is loosely defined [156], and although muscles are acknowledged as one of the pain-producing structures, little data exist on their importance. Andersen et al. [157] demonstrated that when pain was predominantly from the trapezius muscle (i.e., trapezius myalgia), strength training of the trapezius and surrounding muscles resulted in large decreases in pain that were sustained months after cessation of the study. Vuillerme and Pinsault [158] demonstrated the importance of intact non-painful neck muscles in maintaining normal balance. In using manual palpation to identify muscle-related neck pain, facet arthropathy may be confused with pain associated with muscle attachments on the cervical spine [159]. Multifaceted treatment remains the norm for generic neck pain. In a systematic review, Chow found low-level laser therapy (LLLT) to be effective for acute- and moderate-duration neck pain [160], although a recent Cochrane review found that LLLT appeared to be ineffective [161].

Summary

Muscle and other soft tissue may be a primary source of common pain complaints and, if consistently acknowledged in our evaluation and treatment protocols, could result in improved treatment outcomes.

References

1. Wall PD, Woolf CJ. Muscle but not cutaneous C-afferent input produces prolonged increases in the excitability of the flexion reflex in the rat. J Physiol. 1984;356:443–58.
2. Fishman SM, Ballantyne JC, Rathmell JP, editors. Bonica's management of pain. 4th ed. Philadelphia: Lippincott Williams & Wilkins; 2009.
3. McMahon SB, Koltzenburg M, editors. Wall and Melzack's textbook of pain. 5th ed. Philadelphia: Elsevier/Churchill Livingstone; 2005.
4. Aronoff GM. Evaluation and treatment of chronic pain. 3rd ed. Baltimore: Lippincott Williams & Wilkins; 1999.
5. Benzon H, Rathmell J, Wu C, Turk D, Argoff C, editors. Raj's practical management of pain. 4th ed. St. Louis: Mosby; 2008.
6. Wallace DJ. The history of fibromyalgia. In: Wallace DJ, Clauw DJ, editors. Fibromyalgia and other central pain syndromes. 1st ed. Philadelphia: Lippincott Williams & Wilkins; 2005. p. 1–5.
7. Reynolds MD. The development of the concept of fibrositis. J Hist Med Allied Sci. 1983;38(1):5–35.
8. Inanici F, Yunus MB. History of fibromyalgia: past to present. Curr Pain Headache Rep. 2004;8:369–78.
9. Cohen M, Quintner J. The horse is dead: let myofascial pain syndrome rest in peace [letter]. Pain Med. 2008;9(4):464–5.
10. Marcus N. Response to letter to the editor by Dr. Cohen and Dr. Quintner [letter]. Pain Med. 2008;9(4):466–8.
11. Kellgren JH. Observations on referred pain arising from muscle. Clin Sci. 1938;3:174–90.
12. Kellgren JH. On distribution of pain arising from deep somatic structures with charts of segmental pain areas. Clin Sci. 1939;4:35–6.
13. Lewis T, Kellgren JH. Observations relating to referred pain, visceromotor reflexes and other associated phenomena. Clin Sci. 1939;4:47–71.
14. Mense S, Hoheisel U. Central hyperexcitability and muscle nociception. In: Graven-Nielsen T, Arendt-Nielsen L, Mense S, editors. Fundamentals of musculoskeletal pain. 1st ed. Seattle: IASP; 2008. p. 61–73.
15. Arendt-Nielsen L, Graven-Nielsen T. Translational aspects of musculoskeletal pain. In: Graven-Nielsen T, Arendt-Nielsen L, Mense S, editors. Fundamentals of musculoskeletal pain. 1st ed. Seattle: IASP; 2008. p. 347–66.
16. Schade H. Untersuchungen in der Erkaltungsfrage. III: Ueber den rheumatismus, insbesondere den muskelrheumatismus (myogelose). Munch Med Wschr. 1921;68:418–20.
17. Lange M. Die Muskelhärten (Myogelosen): Ihre Entstehung und Heilung. Munich: Lehmann; 1931.
18. Steindler A. The interpretation of sciatic radiation and the syndrome of low-back pain. J Bone Joint Surg Am. 1940;22:28–34.
19. Travell JG, Rinzler SH, Herman M. Pain and disability of the shoulder and arm: treatment by intramuscular infiltration with procaine hydrochloride. JAMA. 1942;120:417–22.
20. Travell JG, Rinzler SH. The myofascial genesis of pain. Postgrad Med. 1952;11:425–34.
21. Simons DG, Travell JG. Myofascial origins of low back pain. 1. Principles of diagnosis and treatment. Postgrad Med. 1983;73(2):66–73.
22. Reeves R. President Kennedy: profile of power. New York: Simon and Schuster; 1993. p. 15, 82–85, 120, 242–3.
23. Smythe H. Tender points: the evolution of concepts of the fibrositis/fibromyalgia syndrome. Am J Med. 1986;81(3A):2–6.

24. Moldofsky H, Scarisbrick P, England R, Smythe H. Musculoskeletal symptoms and non-REM sleep disturbance in patients with "fibrositis syndrome" and healthy subjects. Psychosom Med. 1975;37: 341–51.

25. Vierck CJ. Mechanisms underlying development of spatially distributed chronic pain (fibromyalgia). Pain. 2006;124(3):242–63.

26. Mease PJ. Fibromyalgia syndrome: review of clinical presentation, pathogenesis, outcome measures, and treatment. J Rheumatol Suppl. 2005;75:6–21.

27. Borg-Stein J. Management of peripheral pain generators in fibromyalgia. Rheum Dis Clin North Am. 2002;28(2):305–17.

28. Ge HY, Nie H, Madeline P, Danneskiold-Samsøe B, Graven-Nielsen T, Arendt-Nielsen L. Contribution of the local and referred pain from active myofascial trigger points in fibromyalgia syndrome. Pain. 2009;147(1–3):233–40.

29. Stein C, Clark JD, Oh U, et al. Peripheral mechanisms of pain and analgesia. Brain Res Rev. 2009;60(1):90–113.

30. Staud R. The role of peripheral input for chronic pain syndromes like fibromyalgia syndrome. J Musculoskelet Pain. 2008;16(1–2):67–74.

31. Ellman P, Shaw D. The "chronic rheumatic" and his pains; psychosomatic aspects of chronic non-articular rheumatism. Ann Rheum Dis. 1950;9(4):341–57.

32. Sarno JE. Etiology of neck and back pain. An automatic myoneuralgia? J Nerv Ment Dis. 1981;169(1):55–9.

33. Burns JW. Arousal of negative emotions and symptom-specific reactivity in chronic low back pain patients. Emotion. 2006;6(2):309–19.

34. Cathcart S, Petkov J, Winefield AH, Lushington K, Rolan P. Central mechanisms of stress-induced headache. Cephalalgia. 2010;30(3):285–95.

35. Asendorpf JB, Scherer KR. The discrepant repressor: differentiation between low anxiety, high anxiety, and repression of anxiety by autonomic-facial-verbal patterns of behavior. J Pers Soc Psychol. 1983;45(6):1334–46.

36. Kasamatsu A, Hirai T. An electroencephalographic study on the zen meditation (Zazen). Folia Psychiatr Neurol Jpn. 1966;20(4):315–36.

37. Weinberger DA, Schwartz GE, Davidson RJ. Low-anxious, high-anxious, and repressive coping styles: psychometric patterns and behavioral and physiological responses to stress. J Abnorm Psychol. 1979;88(4):369–80.

38. Budzynski TH, Stoyva JM, Adler CS. EMG biofeedback and tension headache: a controlled outcome study. Psychosom Med. 1973;35(6):484–96.

39. Jacobson E. The technique of progressive relaxation. J Nerv Ment Dis. 1924;60(6):568–78.

40. Luthe W. Autogenic training: method, research and application in medicine. Am J Psychother. 1963;17:174–95.

41. Holroyd KA, Andrasik F, Westbrook T. Cognitive control of tension headache. Cogn Ther Res. 1977;1(2):121–33.

42. Stenn PG, Mothersill KJ, Brooke RI. Biofeedback and a cognitive behavioral approach to treatment of myofascial pain dysfunction syndrome. Behav Ther. 1979;10(1):29–36.

43. Kabat-Zinn J, Lipworth L, Burney R. The clinical use of mindfulness meditation for the self-regulation of chronic pain. J Behav Med. 1985;8(2):163–90.

44. Campbell C, Edwards R. Mind-body interactions in pain: the neurophysiology of anxious and catastrophic pain-related thoughts. Transl Res. 2009;153(3):97–101.

45. Martenson M, Cetas J, Heinricher M. A possible neural basis for stress-induced hyperalgesia. Pain. 2009;142(3):236–44.

46. Gunn CC. Radiculopathic pain: diagnosis and treatment of segmental irritation or sensitization. J Musculoskelet Pain. 1997;5(4): 119–43.

47. Gunn CC. Reply to Chang-Zern Hong [letter]. J Musculoskelet Pain. 2000;8(3):137–42.

48. Gunn CC, Milbrandt WE, Little AS, Mason KE. Dry needling of muscle motor points for chronic low-back pain: a randomized clinical trial with long-term follow-up. Spine. 1980;5(3):279–91.

49. Hong CZ. Comment on Gunn's radiculopathy model of myofascial trigger points [letter]. J Musculoskelet Pain. 2000;8(3):133–5.

50. Hong CZ. Treatment of myofascial pain syndrome. Curr Pain Headache Rep. 2006;10(5):345–9.

51. Hopwood MB, Abram SE. Factors associated with failure of trigger point injections. Clin J Pain. 1994;10(3):227–34.

52. Kraus H, Fischer AA. Diagnosis and treatment of myofascial pain. Mt Sinai J Med. 1991;58(3):235–9.

53. Marcus N, Kraus H. Letter to the editor in response to article by Hopwood and Abram [letter]. Clin J Pain. 1995;11(1):84.

54. Rachlin E, Rachlin I. Myofascial pain and fibromyalgia. St. Louis: Mosby; 2002. p. 234–44.

55. Simons DG, Travell J. Myofascial pain and dysfunction (the trigger point manual). 2nd ed. Baltimore: Lippincott Williams & Wilkins; 1999.

56. Tough EA, White AR, Richards S, Campbell J. Variability of criteria used to diagnose myofascial trigger point pain syndrome – evidence from a review of the literature. Clin J Pain. 2007;23(3):278–86.

57. Marcus NJ, Gracely EJ, Keefe KO. A comprehensive protocol to diagnose and treat pain of muscular origin may successfully and reliably decrease or eliminate pain in a chronic pain population. Pain Med. 2010;11(1):25–34.

58. International Association for the Study of Pain (IASP). Core curriculum. 3rd ed. Seattle: IASP; 2005.

59. Christensen HW, Vach W, Manniche C, et al. Palpation for muscular tenderness in the anterior chest wall: an observer reliability study. J Manipulative Physiol Ther. 2003;26(8):469–75.

60. Levoska S. Manual palpation and pain threshold in female office employees with and without neck-shoulder symptoms. Clin J Pain. 1993;9(4):236–41.

61. Maher C, Adams R. Reliability of pain and stiffness assessments in clinical manual lumbar spine examination. Phys Ther. 1994;74(9):801–9; discussion 9–11.

62. Marcus N, Kraus H, Rachlin E. Comments on K.H. Njoo and E. Van der Does, pain 58 (1994) 317–323 [letter]. Pain. 1995; 61(1):159.

63. Njoo KH, Van der Does E. The occurrence and inter-rater reliability of myofascial trigger points in the quadratus lumborum and gluteus medius: a prospective study in non-specific low back pain patients and controls in general practice. Pain. 1994;58(3):317–23.

64. Wolfe F. Stop using the American College of Rheumatology criteria in the clinic. J Rheumatol. 2003;30(8):1671–2.

65. Kraus H. Diagnosis and treatment of muscle pain. Chicago: Quintessence Books; 1988. p. 11–37.

66. Chou R, Qaseem A, Snow V, et al. Diagnosis and treatment of low back pain: a joint clinical practice guideline from the American College of Physicians and the American Pain Society. Ann Intern Med. 2007;147(7):478–91.

67. Van Tulder MW, Koes B, Seitsalo S, Malmivaara A. Outcome of invasive treatment modalities on back pain and sciatica: an evidence-based review. Eur Spine J. 2006;15 suppl 1:S82–92.

68. Martin BI, Deyo RA, Mirza SK, et al. Expenditures and health status among adults with back and neck problems. JAMA. 2008;299(6):656–64.

69. Rachlin E, Rachlin I. Myofascial pain and fibromyalgia. 2nd ed. St. Louis: Mosby; 2002. p. 438.

70. Fischer AA. Documentation of myofascial trigger points. Arch Phys Med Rehabil. 1988;69(4):286–91.

71. Jensen K, Andersen HO, Olesen J, Lindblom U. Pressure-pain threshold in human temporal region. Evaluation of a new pressure algometer. Pain. 1986;25(3):313–23.

72. Orbach R, Crow H. Examiner expectancy effects in the measurement of pressure pain thresholds. Pain. 1988;74:163–70.

73. Hunter C, Dubois M, Zou S, Oswald W, Coakley K, Shehebar M, Conlon AM. A new muscle pain detection device to diagnose muscles as a source of back and/or neck pain. Pain Med. 2010;11(1):35–43.

74. Simons D, Travell J. Myofascial pain and dysfunction (the trigger point manual). 2nd ed. Baltimore: Lippincott Williams & Wilkins; 1999. p. 166.

75. Chen Q, Basford J, An K-N. Ability of magnetic resonance elastography to assess taut bands. Clin Biomech. 2008;23(5):623–9.

76. Sikdar S, Shah JP, Gebreab T, et al. Novel applications of ultrasound technology to visualize and characterize myofascial trigger points and surrounding soft tissue. Arch Phys Med Rehabil. 2009;90(11):1829–38.

77. Park G-YMDP, Kwon DRMDP. Application of real-time sonoelastography in musculoskeletal diseases related to physical medicine and rehabilitation. Am J Phys Med Rehabil. 2011;90(11): 875–86.

78. Graboski CL, Gray DS, Burnham RS. Botulinum toxin a versus bupivacaine trigger point injections for the treatment of myofascial pain syndrome: a randomized double blind crossover study. Pain. 2005;118(1–2):170–5.

79. Hong CZ. Lidocaine injection versus dry needling to myofascial trigger point. The importance of the local twitch response. Am J Phys Med Rehabil. 1994;73(4):256–63.

80. Hong CZ. Consideration and recommendation of myofascial trigger point injections. J Musculoskelet Pain. 1994;2:29–59.

81. Kamanli A, Kaya A, Ardicoglu O, et al. Comparison of lidocaine injection, botulinum toxin injection, and dry needling to trigger points in myofascial pain syndrome. Rheumatol Int. 2005;25(8):604–11.

82. Fischer AA. New injection techniques for treatment of musculoskeletal pain. Philadelphia: Mosby; 2002.

83. Gibson W, Arendt-Nielsen L, Graven-Nielsen T. Referred pain and hyperalgesia in human tendon and muscle belly tissue. Pain. 2006;120(1–2):113–23.

84. Starr M. Theory and practice of myofascial pain as both practicing clinician and patient. J Back Musculoskelet Rehabil. 1997;8(2): 173–6.

85. Van Tulder M, Malmivaara A, Hayden J, Koes B. Statistical significance versus clinical importance: trials on exercise therapy for chronic low back pain as example. Spine. 2007;32(16):1785–90.

86. Hayden JA, van Tulder MW, Malmivaara A, Koes BW. Exercise therapy for treatment of non-specific low back pain. Cochrane Database Syst Rev. 2005;(3):CD000335.

87. Abenhaim L, Rossignol M, Valat JP, et al. The role of activity in the therapeutic management of back pain. Report of the International Paris Task Force on Back Pain. Spine. 2000;25 suppl 4:1S–33.

88. Fersum KV, Dankaerts W, O'Sullivan PB, Maes J, Slcouen JS, Bjordal JM, Kvale A. Integration of sub-classification strategies in RCTs evaluating manual therapy treatment and exercise therapy for non-specific chronic low back pain (NSLBP): a systematic review Br J Sports Med. 2010;44(14):1054–62.

89. Van Tulder M, Malmivaara A, Esmail R, Koes B. Exercise therapy for low back pain. Spine. 2000;25(21):2784–96.

90. Natvig B, Picavet HS. The epidemiology of soft tissue rheumatism. Best Pract Res Clin Rheumatol. 2002;16(5):777–93.

91. Deyo RA, Weinstein JN. Low back pain. N Engl J Med. 2001;344(5):363–70.

92. McBeth J, Jones K. Epidemiology of chronic musculoskeletal pain. Best Pract Res Clin Rheumatol. 2007;21(3):403–25.

93. Petersen S, Hägglöf BL, Bergström EI. Impaired health-related quality of life in children with recurrent pain. Pediatrics. 2009;124(4):e759–67.

94. Pellisé F, Balagué F, Rajmil L, et al. Prevalence of low back pain and its effect on health-related quality of life in adolescents. Arch Pediatr Adolesc Med. 2009;163(1):65–71.

95. Pleis JR, Lucas JW, Ward BW. Summary health statistics for U.S. adults: National Health Interview Survey, 2008. National Center for Health Statistics. Vital Health Stat. 2009;10(242):6–7.

96. Freburger JK, Holmes GM, Agans RP, et al. The rising prevalence of chronic low back pain. Arch Intern Med. 2009;169(3):251–8.

97. Juniper M, Le TK, Mladsi D. The epidemiology, economic burden, and pharmacological treatment of chronic low back pain in France, Germany, Italy, Spain and the UK: a literature-based review. Expert Opin Pharmacother. 2009;10(16):2581–92.

98. Hogg-Johnson S, van der Velde G, Carroll LJ, et al. The burden and determinants of neck pain in the general population: results of the bone and joint decade 2000–2010 task force on neck pain and its associated disorders. Spine. 2008;33(4 Suppl):S39–51.

99. Pope DP, Croft PR, Pritchard CM, Silman AJ. Prevalence of shoulder pain in the community: the influence of case definition. Ann Rheum Dis. 1997;56(5):308–12.

100. Croft P, Rigby AS, Boswell R, Schollum J, Silman A. The prevalence of chronic widespread pain in the general population. J Rheumatol. 1993;20(4):710–3.

101. Wolfe F, Ross K, Anderson J, Russell IJ, Hebert L. The prevalence and characteristics of fibromyalgia in the general population. Arthritis Rheum. 1995;38(1):19–28.

102. Weir PT, Harlan GA, Nkoy FL, et al. The incidence of fibromyalgia and its associated comorbidities: a population-based retrospective cohort study based on international classification of diseases, 9th revision codes. J Clin Rheumatol. 2006;12(3):124–8.

103. Lawrence RC, Felson DT, Helmick CG, et al. Estimates of the prevalence of arthritis and other rheumatic conditions in the United States. Part II. Arthritis Rheum. 2008;58(1):26–35.

104. Staud R. Chronic widespread pain and fibromyalgia: two sides of the same coin? Curr Rheumatol Rep. 2009;11(6):433–6.

105. Buskila D, Neumann L. The development of widespread pain after injuries. J Musculoskelet Pain. 2002;10:261–7.

106. Littlejohn G. Regional pain syndrome: clinical characteristics, mechanisms and management. Nat Clin Pract Rheumatol. 2007; 3(9):504–11.

107. Marcus N. Pain in cancer patients unrelated to the cancer or treatment. Cancer Invest. 2005;23(1):84–93.

108. Marcus N. Treating nonacute pain in the cancer population [letter]. Pain Med. 2007;8(6):539.

109. Stacey M. Free nerve endings in skeletal muscle of the cat. J Anat. 1969;105:231–254.

110. Mense S. Algesic agents exciting muscle nociceptors. Exp Brain Res. 2009;196(1):89–100.

111. Mense S, Hoheisel U. Morphology and functional types of nociceptors. In: Graven-Nielsen T, Arendt-Nielsen L, Mense S, editors. Fundamentals of musculoskeletal pain. 1st ed. Seattle: IASP; 2008. p. 14–5.

112. Svensson P, Wang K, Arendt-Nielsen L, Cairns BE. Effects of NGF-induced muscle sensitization on proprioception and nociception. Exp Brain Res. 2008;189(1):1–10.

113. Nie H, Madeleine P, Arendt-Nielsen L, Graven-Nielsen T. Temporal summation of pressure pain during muscle hyperalgesia evoked by nerve growth factor and eccentric contractions. Eur J Pain. 2009;13(7):704–10.

114. Mense S. Muscle pain: mechanisms and clinical significance. Dtsch Arztebl Int. 2008;105(12):214–9.

115. Mense S, Simons DG, Hoheisel U, Quenzer B. Lesions of rat skeletal muscle after local block of acetylcholinesterase and neuromuscular stimulation. J Appl Physiol. 2003;94(6):2494–501.

116. Nielsen LA, Henriksson KG. Pathophysiological mechanisms in chronic musculoskeletal pain (fibromyalgia): the role of central and peripheral sensitization and pain disinhibition. Best Pract Res Clin Rheumatol. 2007;21(3):465–80.

117. Yunus MB. Role of central sensitization in symptoms beyond muscle pain, and the evaluation of a patient with widespread pain. Best Pract Res Clin Rheumatol. 2007;21(3):481–97.

118. Staud R, Nagel S, Robinson ME, Price DD. Enhanced central pain processing of fibromyalgia patients is maintained by muscle afferent input: a randomized, double-blind, placebo-controlled study. Pain. 2009;145(1–2):96–104.

119. Fields HL, Basbaum AI. Central nervous system mechanisms of pain modulation. In: Wall PD, Melzack R, editors. Textbook of pain. Edinburgh: Churchill Livingstone; 1999. p. 309–29.

120. Moont R, Pud D, Sprecher E, Sharvit G, Yarnitsky D. 'Pain inhibits pain' mechanisms: is pain modulation simply due to distraction? Pain. 2010;150(1):113–20.

121. Lautenbacher S, Rollman GB. Possible deficiencies of pain modulation in fibromyalgia. Clin J Pain. 1997;13(3):189–96.

122. Staud R, Robinson ME, Vierck CJ, Price DD. Diffuse noxious inhibitory controls (DNIC) attenuate temporal summation of second pain in normal males but not in normal females or fibromyalgia patients. Pain. 2003;101(1–2):167–74.

123. Busch AJ, Barber KA, Overend TJ, Peloso PM, Schachter CL. Exercise for treating fibromyalgia syndrome. Cochrane Database Syst. Rev. 2007;(4):CD003786.

124. Ortega E, García JJ, Bote ME, Martín-Cordero L, Escalante Y, Saavedra JM, Northoff H, Giraldo E. Exercise in fibromyalgia and related inflammatory disorders: known effects and unknown chances. Exerc Immunol Rev. 2009;15:42–65.

125. Shah JP, Gilliams EA. Uncovering the biochemical milieu of myofascial trigger points using in vivo microdialysis: an application of muscle pain concepts to myofascial pain syndrome. J Bodyw Mov Ther. 2008;12(4):371–84.

126. Ge H, Nie H, Madeleine P, Danneskiold-Samsøe B, Graven-Nielsen T, Arendt-Nielsen L. Contribution of the local and referred pain from active myofascial trigger points in fibromyalgia syndrome. Pain. 2009;147(1–3):233–40.

127. Staud R. Are tender point injections beneficial: the role of tonic nociception in fibromyalgia. Curr Pharm Des. 2006;12(1):23–7.

128. Scott NA, Guo B, Barton PM, Gerwin RD. Trigger point injections for chronic non-malignant musculoskeletal pain: a systematic review. Pain Med. 2009;10(1):54–69.

129. Chou R, Qaseem A, Snow V, et al. Diagnosis and treatment of low back pain: a joint clinical practice guideline from the American College of Physicians and the American Pain Society. Ann Int Med. 2007;147(7):478–91.

130. Simons D, Travell J, Simons L. Myofascial pain and dysfunction: the trigger point manual. 2nd ed. Baltimore: Williams & Wilkins; 1999. p. 122.

131. Kopell HP, Thompson WA. Peripheral entrapment neuropathies of the lower extremity. N Engl J Med. 1960;262:56–60.

132. Byrd JW. Piriformis syndrome. Oper Tech Sports Med. 2005;13(1):71–9.

133. Fishman LM, Dombi GW, Michaelsen C, et al. Piriformis syndrome: diagnosis, treatment, and outcome – a 10-year study. Arch Phys Med Rehabil. 2002;83(3):295–301.

134. Tan G, Jensen MP, Thornby JI, Shanti BF. Validation of the brief pain inventory for chronic nonmalignant pain. J Pain. 2004;5(2):133–7.

135. Fischer AA. Pressure algometry over normal muscles. Standard values, validity and reproducibility of pressure threshold. Pain. 1987;30(1):115–26.

136. Kinser AM, Sands WA, Stone MH. Reliability and validity of a pressure algometer. J Strength Cond Res. 2009;23(1):312–4.

137. Bendtsen L, Jensen R, Jensen NK, Olesen J. Pressure-controlled palpation: a new technique which increases the reliability of manual palpation. Cephalalgia. 1995;15(3):205–10.

138. Neuberger GB, Press AN, Lindsley HB, et al. Effects of exercise on fatigue, aerobic fitness, and disease activity measures in persons with rheumatoid arthritis. Res Nurs Health. 1997;20(3):195–204.

139. Liemohn W. Exercise and arthritis. Exercise and the back. Rheum Dis Clin North Am. 1990;16(4):945–70.

140. Mannion AF, Müntener M, Taimela S, Dvorak J. A randomized clinical trial of three active therapies for chronic low back pain. Spine. 1999;24(23):2435–48.

141. Graham VL, Gehlsen GM, Edwards JA. Electromyographic evaluation of closed and open kinetic chain knee rehabilitation exercises. J Athl Train. 1993;28(1):23–30.

142. Kibler WB. Closed kinetic chain rehabilitation for sports injuries. Phys Med Rehabil Clin North Am. 2000;11(2):369–84.

143. Lederman E. The myth of core stability. J Bodyw Mov Ther. 2010;14(1):84–98.

144. Kraus H, Nagler W, Melleby A. Evaluation of an exercise program for back pain. Am Fam Physician. 1983;28(3):153–8.

145. Hunter C, Marcus N, Shehebar M. Muscles as a treatable pain source in patients with failed back surgery syndrome. Poster session presented at: American Academy of Pain Medicine (AAPM) 25th Annual Meeting; 2009 Jan 28 – 31; Honolulu, HI.

146. Bamji A. Interventions to treat shoulder pain. Lack of concordance between rheumatologists may render multicentre studies invalid. BMJ. 1998;316(7145):1676–7.

147. Szebenyi B, Dieppe P. Interventions to treat shoulder pain. Review was overly negative. BMJ. 1998;316(7145):1676; author reply 1677.

148. Green S, Buchbinder R, Glazier R, Forbes A. Systematic review of randomized controlled trials of interventions for painful shoulder: selection criteria, outcome assessment, and efficacy. BMJ. 1998;316(7128):354–60.

149. Urrútia G, Burton AK, Morral Fernández A, Bonfill Cosp X, Zanoli G. Neuroreflexotherapy for non-specific low-back pain. Cochrane Database of Syst Rev. 2009;(2):CD003009.

150. Corcoll J, Orfila J, Tobajas P, Alegre L. Implementation of neuroreflexotherapy for subacute and chronic neck and back pain within the Spanish public health system: audit results after one year. Health Policy. 2006;79:345–57.

151. Schleip R, Klingler W, Lehmann-Horn F. Active fascial contractility: fascia may be able to contract in a smooth muscle-like manner and thereby influence musculoskeletal dynamics. Med Hypotheses. 2005;65(2):273–7.

152. Hackett GS, Hemwall GA, Montgomery GA. Ligament and tendon relaxation treated by prolotherapy. Oak Park: Beulah Land Press; 2002.

153. Langevin HM, Sherman KJ. Pathophysiological model for chronic low back pain integrating connective tissue and nervous system mechanisms. Med Hypotheses. 2007;68(1):74–80.

154. Langevin HM. Potential role of fascia in chronic musculoskeletal pain. In: Audette JF, Bailey A, editors. Integrative pain medicine: the science and practice of complementary and alternative medicine in pain management. Totowa: Humana; 2008. p. 123–32.

155. Bouffard NA, Cutroneo KR, Badger GJ, et al. Tissue stretch decreases soluble TGF-beta1 and type-1 procollagen in mouse subcutaneous connective tissue: evidence from ex vivo and in vivo models. J Cell Physiol. 2008;214(2):389–95.

156. Ariëns GAM, Borghouts JAJ, Koes BW. Neck pain. In: Crombie IK, Croft PR, Linton SJ, LeReseche L, Von Korff M, editors. Epidemiology of pain. London: IASP; 1999.

157. Andersen LL, Kjaer M, Søgaard K, Hansen L, Kryger AI, Sjøgaard G. Effect of two contrasting types of physical exercise on chronic neck muscle pain. Arthritis Rheum. 2008;59(1):84–91.

158. Vuillerme N, Pinsault N. Experimental neck muscle pain impairs standing balance in humans. Exp Brain Res. 2009;192(4):723–9.

159. Bogduk N, Simons DG. Neck pain: joint pain or trigger points? Pain Res Clin Manag. 1993;6:267–73.

160. Chow RT, Johnson MI, Lopes-Martins RA, Bjordal JM. Efficacy of low-level laser therapy in the management of neck pain: a systematic review and meta-analysis of randomised placebo or active-treatment controlled trials. Lancet. 2009;374(9705):1897–908.

161. Gross AR, Aker PD, Goldsmith CH, Peloso P. Physical medicine modalities for mechanical neck disorders. Cochrane Database Syst Rev. 2000;(2):CD000961.

Addictive Disorders and Pain

Lynn R. Webster and Stuart Gitlow

Key Points

- Patients with chronic pain occupy a subset of the general population as do patients with addictive disorders. The two subsets sometimes overlap, an occurrence that cannot be judged solely by the quantity of opioid consumption.
- Addiction requires genetic vulnerability, conducive environmental conditions, and exposure to a chemical that triggers expression of the disorder, which itself results in a compromised reward system.
- Problematic drug-related behaviors and medication-induced side effects do not necessarily indicate addiction. Substance-induced disorders and substance-related symptoms may, therefore, arise in the absence of addictive disease and require a different treatment approach.
- Components of effective opioid therapy include screening patients for drug-related risks and psychiatric comorbidities and monitoring patients for regimen adherence, pain control, and stressors that could compromise treatment.
- Patients with histories of substance-use disorders may benefit from strong support systems, including 12-step groups.
- Patients who exhibit continued nonadherence to medical direction and inadequate analgesia may be humanely tapered from opioids.

L.R. Webster, M.D. (✉)
Lifetree Clinical Research and Pain Clinic, 3838 South 700 East, Suite 200, Salt Lake City, UT 84106, USA
e-mail: lynnw@lifetreepain.com

S. Gitlow, M.D., M.P.H., M.B.A.
Department of Psychiatry, Mount Sinai School of Medicine, New York, NY, USA
e-mail: drgitlow@aol.com

Introduction

People consume opioids for many reasons, some medically beneficial and others harmful to themselves and to society. It is difficult to conclude that opioid use is harmful by evaluating consumption alone. Consider Fig. 4.1, in which we first have a population of individuals none of whom have been exposed to opioid use. Within that population are those who do not have addictive disease involving opioids; these individuals will not demonstrate signs and symptoms of addiction whether exposed to opioids or not. A smaller group within the population, shown in red and blue, has addictive disease. Those shown in blue do not know they have addictive disease simply because they have never been exposed to opioids. Phenotypically, then, they do not have addiction despite the underlying physiology. The group of individuals depicted in red, however, will show signs of addiction, resulting from medical or nonmedical use of opioids.

The two populations can be subdivided differently. Users of any substance, for medical or nonmedical reasons, do so with a range of frequency and quantity (addicted people have a further non-correlated range of disease severity). People with addictive disease might actually use less of the substance less frequently than those without addictive disease, particularly when those without addiction use the substance because they have been prescribed it. It is equally critical to realize that patients with addictive disease and with pain might use opioids precisely as prescribed with close monitoring and that in such cases the signs and symptoms of addiction may be absent despite the development of physiologic dependence.

Clinical evaluation and treatment are complicated when pain and addiction coexist. When addiction is present without the added component of pain, the focus is not on dissecting what a patient means by terms such as "occasional" or "experimental" use but on why the patient has used at all. When pain is added to the equation, that signal is valueless,

T.R. Deer et al. (eds.), *Treatment of Chronic Pain by Integrative Approaches: the AMERICAN ACADEMY of PAIN MEDICINE Textbook on Patient Management*, DOI 10.1007/978-1-4939-1821-8_4,
© American Academy of Pain Medicine 2015

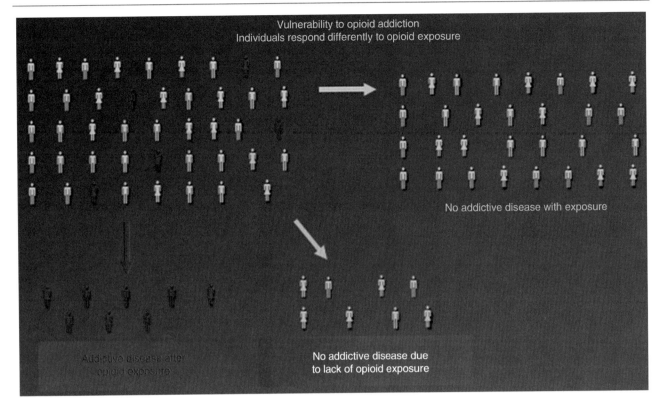

Fig. 4.1 First, we have a population of individuals none of whom have been exposed to opioid use. Within that population are those who do not have addictive disease involving opioids; these individuals will not demonstrate signs and symptoms of addiction whether exposed to opioids or not. A smaller group within the population, shown in *red* and *blue*, has addictive disease. Those shown in *blue* do not know they have addictive disease simply because they have never been exposed to opioids. Phenotypically, then, they do not have addiction despite the underlying physiology. The group of individuals depicted in *red*, however, will show signs of addiction, resulting from medical or nonmedical use of opioids

because the patient has been prescribed the substance and is expected to use it. Furthermore, because denial is inherent to addictive illness, one always questions subjectively provided information when a patient is being treated for addiction but not pain. When pain is added, detective work is needed to determine whether the patient has taken the amount prescribed; whether he has doctor shopped to gain access to additional medication; whether he is taking the opioid only to avoid withdrawal; whether objective data exist to support the subjective report of pain; and many other factors.

Background

A subset of patients who are prescribed opioids for pain will eventually use their medication in ways not intended by their prescribing clinicians. Addiction is one reason why. Addiction prevalence among opioid-treated pain patients has been reported between 2 and 5 % [1, 2]; however, the prevalence of problematic opioid use is far higher. A prospective cohort study showed that 62 of 196 (32 %) patients enrolled in a chronic pain disease management program had at least one episode of opioid misuse after 1 year [3].

Patients who engage in multiple, repeated, or egregious aberrant drug-related behaviors are in danger of self-harm and are nearly certain to realize poor outcomes from pain therapy. Many problematic drug-related behaviors can be handled by screening opioid candidates, stratifying patients by risk category, monitoring them closely, and treating them for comorbid depression, anxiety, and other mental conditions. Patients with strong risk factors for problematic opioid use, such as a family history of addiction or a personal history of addictive disease, present a special challenge because the potential for triggering or reactivating a substance-use disorder is real. Another reality is the frequent overlap of pain and addiction. In a study of patients receiving methadone for chemical dependency, 37 % experienced chronic, severe pain [4]. In a separate study, an association between chronic pain and self-reported prescription drug abuse was confirmed in veterans referred for a behavioral health evaluation [5]. Given the subjective nature of pain, these studies suggest the possibility that those with addictive disease are either more aware of painful stimuli or more susceptible to a subjective experience of pain than those without addictive illness when exposed to identical stimuli. This is consistent with Hennecke's findings with respect to stimulus augmentation in children of alcoholic fathers [6].

Failure to treat pain is poor medical practice as is failure to treat addiction, including opioid use disorders. Physicians, however, often receive little medical training on addiction or clinical pain treatment [7]. The treatment plan for chronic nonmalignant pain may include opioids, even for patients with substance-abuse histories or strong risk factors, if accompanied by careful screening, medication selection, and monitoring. However, some patients cannot be managed with opioid therapy, because their nonadherence or lack of analgesic response renders opioid therapy more harmful than helpful. In such cases, compassionate discontinuation of opioids can improve outcomes. The key is to personalize the treatment plan and to adjust when needed.

Scientific Foundation of Addiction

Definitions

The field of addictive disease suffers from a plethora of terminology, much of which has been defined and redefined over the years by different groups of specialists. Use, abuse, misuse, heavy use, dependence, and addiction: these terms are all in general use. Dependence carries a specific meaning to the pain physician as it refers to a physiologic neuroadaptation of the central nervous system to the effects of a given substance, in which an individual will experience objective physiologic symptoms of withdrawal should the substance use be terminated without tapering. Dependence has a different meaning to the reader of *DSM-IV-TR* where it refers to the medical disorder in which an individual repetitively uses an addictive substance despite that person's best interest. This latter definition is more widely applied to the class of disease known as addiction, with the acknowledgment that consensus among experts regarding terminology is not complete. Table 4.1 contains suggested definitions to clarify opioid use and misuse [8, 9].

The critical point is that, whatever terminology you choose, addictive disease is an illness or class of illnesses of the brain in which one marker is that of repetitive substance use; this approach simplifies the concept of pre-addiction, in which an individual is predisposed to the development of observable symptoms but has not yet developed them as a result of not having been exposed to the drug.

Neurobiology of Addiction

As addiction develops, changes occur within neuroanatomic structures, communication pathways, and neurochemical processes of the nervous system. Drugs of abuse impact the mesolimbic dopaminergic system, the region of the brain linked to basic emotions, by activating the ventral tegmental area and releasing dopamine into the nucleus accumbens,

Table 4.1 Definitions associated with opioid use and misuse [8, 9]

Misuse	Use of a medication for a medical purpose other than as directed or as indicated, whether willful or unintentional and whether harm results or not
Abuse	Any use of an illegal drug; the intentional self-administration of a medication for a nonmedical purpose such as altering one's state of consciousness (e.g., getting high)
Addiction	A primary, chronic neurobiologic disease influenced by genetic, psychosocial, and environmental factors. It is characterized by impaired control over drug use, compulsive use, continued use despite harm, and craving
Tolerance	A physiologic state resulting from the regular use of an opioid where increased doses are needed to maintain the same effects. In *analgesic tolerance*, increased opioid doses are needed to maintain pain relief
Physical dependence	A physiologic state characterized by abstinence syndrome (withdrawal) if an opioid is stopped or decreased abruptly or if an opioid antagonist is administered. It is an expected result of opioid therapy and does not, by itself, equal addiction

amygdala, prefrontal cortex, and ventral palladium [10]. Dopamine has been called the master molecule of addiction, but glutamate and gamma-amino butyric acid (GABA) also play key roles [10]. Opioids and other drugs decrease GABA activity in the ventral tegmental area, causing an increase in glutamate release in the nucleus accumbens which increases dopamine release. The release of dopamine in the nucleus accumbens appears to reinforce memories of pleasant drug experiences, boosting craving.

The amygdala mediates anxiety and other strong emotions. Not only does it help to regulate craving and relapse in addicted people, but amygdala stimulation may partially explain why certain chronic pain patients overuse opioids or anxiolytics, looking for relief from the stress and fear associated with chronic pain.

The activation of the reward pathway from the ventral tegmental area to the nucleus accumbens is crucial to the formation of addiction but is not in itself sufficient to cause addiction. Changes, which are both structural and functional, create in the vulnerable individual a behavioral compulsion to use drugs. With repeated use, the brain experiences neuroadaptive changes that can include tolerance, necessitating larger quantities of the substance to achieve the desired effects, and sensitization or heightened reward. Chronic drug abuse results in neuroplastic learning and altered brain systems with results that are observable in behavior. The brain becomes unable to distinguish between stimuli to engage in behaviors related to survival, such as eating, and the reward incentive delivered by addictive drugs. The result is a compromised reward system, and the changes are long term.

Observing the addicted brain is easier than understanding how it got that way, and the reason why some people become addicted while others do not must remain the subject of ongoing inquiry. Genetic and environmental vulnerabilities exist for the individual, who, in order to trigger the underlying neurobiologic mechanisms that lead to addiction, must be exposed to a drug of abuse. According to the National Institute on Drug Abuse, changes in frontal activity that accompany loss of control and compulsive drug intake are observable in addicted people during brain imaging studies [11]. What is still unclear is whether the changes preceded or followed drug use. Young people, whose central nervous systems are still developing, appear to be at particular risk for sustaining changes to the prefrontal cortex that could lead to compulsive drug behaviors when drug use is initiated early [12]. A study conducted by researchers at Rockefeller University in New York City found that adolescent mice allowed to self-administer oxycodone took less of the drug than adult mice did; however, when reexposed as adults, they exhibited increased striatal dopamine levels at the lowest dose [13]. Neither effect was found in the adult mice studied, and investigators concluded that both effects suggest greater sensitivity to oxycodone's effects in younger mice [13].

Disorders such as posttraumatic stress disorder, depression, and anxiety disorders also frequently coincide with substance abuse [12]. Whether psychiatric disorders confer vulnerability to addiction or vice versa – or whether both proceed from a common genetic vulnerability – is a question still to be answered.

Clinical Practice

Screening Opioid-Treated Patients for Risk of Abuse or Addiction

The universal precautions of opioid prescribing include initial screening and ongoing assessment for the presence of substance-use disorders [14]. High-risk patients, those likely to fit in the right-hand circle of Fig. 4.1, generally display risk factors such as personal or family history of substance abuse [2, 5], younger age [2, 5], history of preadolescent sexual abuse [2], mental disease [2, 5], social patterns of drug use [15], psychological stress [15], lack of a 12-step program [16], polysubstance abuse [16], poor social support [16], cigarette dependency [5, 17], and repeated drug or alcohol rehabilitations [17]. Conversely, low-risk patients, those likely to fit in the left-hand circle of Fig. 4.1, are those with fewer risk factors. Perhaps, they have completed a regimen of opioids in the past without difficulty or evidence of addiction.

Several tools are available to screen for the risk of opioid abuse. Opioid guidelines jointly released by the American Pain Society (APS) and the American Academy of Pain Medicine (AAPM) [18] endorse the Opioid Risk Tool (ORT) [2], the Screener and Opioid Assessment for Patients with Pain (SOAPP) [19], and the Diagnosis, Intractability, Risk, Efficacy (DIRE) [20]. Unlike the ORT and the SOAPP, which guide risk stratification, the DIRE purports to identify who would not be a suitable candidate. Other opioid-specific tools include the Screening Instrument for Substance Abuse Potential (SISAP) [21] and the Pain Medication Questionnaire (PMQ) [22].

A comparison study of the SOAPP, the ORT, and the DIRE found the SOAPP to be the most sensitive, followed by the ORT and then the DIRE [23]. Little data exist to differentiate the validity of self-administered vs. clinician-administered tools, although face-to-face interviews may give the clinician opportunity to gauge the patient's reactions and facial cues. However, self-administered tools are more practical for most clinical environments, and the choice is likely to be influenced by the time available.

The possibility of deception always exists when a patient is asked to share sensitive information. It is important to build trust and rapport during the assessment process to encourage honesty. The validity of the information provided is enhanced when [10]:

- Confidentiality is observed.
- Patients fear no negative consequences from disclosing information.
- The information disclosed has a likelihood of subsequent verification.
- The clinician is nonjudgmental and matter of fact.
- The clinician treats substance-use questions as an important, routine component of the medical history, no different than data on diet, exercise, and smoking.

Management of High-Risk, Opioid-Treated Patients

Screening can help clinicians to stratify and monitor patients by risk level – usually high, moderate, or low risk. There is a triage associated with chronic pain treatment [14]. The highest-risk patients who also experience moderate-to-severe chronic pain should be treated only by physicians trained to care for this complex population. In moderate-to-high-risk patients, care may be coordinated with appropriate specialists in addiction, pain, and mental health. Low-risk patients typically may be treated by primary care physicians.

All patients should receive at least the routine level of monitoring with monitoring measures intensifying as the level of risk rises (Table 4.2) [10]. Patients with histories of substance-use disorders require the strictest monitoring measures. In addition to cooperation with the high-risk measures listed in Table 4.2, patients with addiction histories should provide proof of continuing involvement with substance-related treatment, including 12-step programs or some equivalent.

Table 4.2 Monitoring methods according to patient risk for drug abuse [10]

Low-risk (routine)	Pain assessment
	Substance-abuse assessment
	Informed consent
	Signed treatment agreement
	Regular follow-up visits, prescriptions
	Initial prescription database check
	Medical reports
	Initial UDT
	No specialist consult required
	Med type, unrestricted
	Document 4A's
	Document patient/physician interactions
Moderate risk	Biweekly visits
	Biweekly prescriptions
	Regular prescription database check
	Verification via family members/friends
	Random UDT
	Question comorbid disease
	Consider psychiatry/pain specialist evaluation
	Consider medication counts
	Consider limiting RO analgesics
High risk	Weekly visits
	Weekly prescriptions (on attendance)
	Quarterly prescription database check
	Friend/family member controls medication
	UDT: scheduled and random
	Consider blood screens
	Psychiatry/addiction specialist evaluation
	Consider pain specialist evaluation
	Limit RO analgesics
	Consider limiting SAO

RO rapid onset, *SAO* short-acting opioids, *UDT* urine drug testing, *4A's* analgesia, activities, adverse events, and aberrant drug taking

Ongoing monitoring of the patient and clear documentation of the treatment process must take place at every clinic visit. Useful clinical monitoring tools include the Pain Assessment and Documentation Tool (PADT) [24] and the Current Opioid Misuse Measure (COMM) [25]. Urine drug screens (administered according to risk as shown in Table 4.2) and opioid treatment agreements that spell out the terms of treatment and the consequences for failure to comply are particularly valuable for patients at high risk for nonadherence. Agreements clarify expectations and also provide for early intervention if a high-risk patient exhibits problems managing opioid use. Prescription monitoring programs (PMPs), in the states where they are available, enable clinicians to ascertain whether patients are obtaining unauthorized prescriptions from more than one provider.

Any patient being considered for chronic opioid treatment should be screened for the history and presence of psychiatric comorbidities, and care should be coordinated with experts in mental-health fields when indicated. Recently, investigators have concluded that mental disorders among pain patients place them at special risk for abusing their medications [26]. A history of substance-use disorders is a red flag for potential abuse of prescription medications [10]. Patients with a trio diagnosis of chronic pain, addictive disorder, and psychiatric comorbidity should be treated for all three problems simultaneously. Agreement should be reached on the medications to be prescribed by each provider. It is vital to know what is being prescribed and by whom in order to manage medication use as safely and effectively as possible. Whenever possible, one physician should prescribe all medications with additional specialists to contribute consultations and recommendations as needed. Bipartite or tripartite management requires clear, timely, and complete communication for maximum success.

Deviations from the treatment program should result in a tightening of monitoring measures such as increased clinic visit frequency, reduced prescription quantities, and the involvement of a third party to control the dispensing. Patients with psychiatric comorbidities should receive treatment in tandem with addiction and pain treatment as these can worsen addiction-related behaviors involving opioids.

Choice of pain therapy is influenced by substance-related risk and pain condition. In high-risk patients with chronic pain, rapid-onset and short-acting opioids possess the potential to produce more rapid effects, including the potential for a reward that could prove reinforcing. If the pain severity allows, non-opioid therapies should be tried first. Medications with properties similar to drugs abused in the past should be avoided. Clinical decisions must be reached based on the individual patient; however, slow-release opioids that are difficult to alter or manipulate are preferred for high-risk patients with pain.

Support Systems

Addictive disease, as with many disease states, has two components that must be addressed: the genetic and the environmental. We can look at the genetic component as being phenotypically expressed in terms of a patient's heightened level of discomfort with life. We can look at the environmental expression as the patient's failure to learn a coping mechanism that does not involve self-medication for dealing with the discomfort.

Twelve-step programs and equivalent self-help groups are methods of providing patients with new coping mechanisms. This fresh approach to dealing with discomfort, which should not be confused with treatment, provides a helpful adjunct at every stage of addiction therapy. Indeed, patients who attend 12-step meetings achieve rates of abstinence that are nearly double that of patients who do not attend such meetings [27]. Furthermore, higher levels of attendance are related to higher rates of abstinence [27]. Given the significant improvement in addiction treatment efficacy provided by attendance at 12-step meetings, an important area of focus for treating clinicians is to facilitate meeting attendance. It has been demonstrated that it is possible to increase such involvement and that this increase directly leads to reduced use [28].

Narcotics Anonymous (NA), started in 1947, has since become international just as Alcoholics Anonymous (AA) has. NA is open to users of any drug regardless of whether the drug is a narcotic. NA promotes a spiritual awakening; some think of this as a religious experience, while others disregard any religious overtones. While NA started in part due to concern about drugs other than sedatives within AA, nearly all of the NA traditions, steps, and policies are based upon those of AA. The groups have a history of cooperating with one another.

Patients should be encouraged to build support systems in all areas of their lives. Factors that can contribute to first-time abuse or relapse include unrelieved pain, family difficulties, unemployment, and financial strain. Patients should be counseled to avoid social and family contacts that could influence them to misuse opioids or any other substance. Encourage the patient to seek help if stressors tempt him or her to overuse medication or lead to drug cravings. Facilitation of involvement with 12-step programs can be helpful here as well.

Discontinuation

A patient with an addictive disorder may be successfully treated with opioids given strict monitoring by the treating clinician and the patient's commitment to adherence. A poor candidate for opioid therapy is one whose physical functioning and quality of life continues to deteriorate and whose adherence to the treatment regimen cannot be established despite stringent measures. Clinical indications that it may be time to consider cessation of opioid therapy include the following [29]:

- Lack of benefit despite dose adjustment, side effect management, and/or opioid rotation
- Poor tolerance at analgesic dose
- Persistent adherence problems
- Presence of a comorbid condition that makes opioid therapy more likely to harm than help (e.g., sleep apnea, addiction)

Tapering from opioids is performed to prevent a physically dependent patient from going through withdrawal and to allow the clinician to observe the effect of tapering on pain level. Table 4.3 contains a suggested exit strategy [10].

Table 4.3 Exit strategy to discontinue opioid therapy [10]

Meet with the patient and review exit criteria agreed on in treatment agreement
Clarify that exit is for the patient's benefit
Clarify that exiting opioid therapy is not synonymous with abandoning pain management
Consider tapering opioids gradually over 1 month
Implement non-opioid pain strategies, including:
Psychiatric/behavioral therapies
Physical therapy
Non-opioid analgesics
Treatment for insomnia, anxiety, or depression
Consideration of interventional procedures
If patient does not cooperate with outpatient taper:
Do not provide additional opioids.
Refer to inpatient program or comprehensive outpatient program for opioid discontinuation as available.
Provide non-opioid medical maintenance until admission.
If addiction is the problem, refer for addiction management or comanagement.

Future Directions

No one argues that opioids are a panacea, certainly not doctors who frequently treat chronic pain. Medical research is currently focused on finding less abusable opioid formulations and testing alternatives to opioids. Much exciting research is being done in the field of genetics as it impacts pain perception and response to analgesic medication. Individuals demonstrate wide variations in responses to morphine and other opioids, and research implicates slight variations in DNA sequencing as a reason [30]. Opioids produce very effective pain control for some people and not for others. Science is moving in the direction of creating drugs that are tailored for individual genetic makeup.

Buprenorphine, a partial mu-receptor agonist, is being considered as an alternative to full mu agonists for certain types of pain [31]. Although buprenorphine has long been available, increased interest in its use has resulted from the possibility it could control pain while posing a reduced risk for addiction. Its value in addressing perioperative pain has also been broadly recognized [32]. Buprenorphine is available as a sublingual agent combined with naloxone. In this formulation, when used as directed, the naloxone has little-to-no direct effect. As a result, this combination drug works as one would expect buprenorphine to work while further reducing the potential misuse of the agent. Specific studies looking at the combination drug as a method of treating chronic pain have found it to be efficacious [33]. However, as a partial mu agonist, buprenorphine has limited analgesic potency. Used alone, it may not provide adequate analgesia for many patients with moderate-to-severe pain.

Summary

The overlap of pain and addiction presents special challenges to the clinical treatment of both disorders. Some patients with histories of substance-use disorders or other risk factors for addiction who also suffer moderate-to-severe pain may be successfully managed using opioids when alternative treatments would be ineffective. For other patients, opioids may be ineffective, retrigger abuse, and clearly be the wrong treatment for the individual patient. Every clinician who provides opioids should be familiar with risk factors for opioid addiction and screen patients for possible addictive disorders, remembering that the spectrum of aberrant behaviors ranges from misuse to the disease of addiction. Effective ongoing management requires an understanding of the motivations underlying drug-related behaviors and a recognition that not all substance use is addiction. Ongoing management is then tailored by setting the level of clinical monitoring appropriate to the degree of risk, reassessing the patient frequently, and being prepared to humanely taper the patient from opioids if necessary.

Acknowledgment Technical writing and manuscript review are provided by Beth Dove of Medical Communications, Salt Lake City, Utah.

References

1. Fleming MF, Balousek SL, Klessig CL, Mundt MP, Brown DD. Substance use disorders in a primary care sample receiving daily opioid therapy. J Pain. 2007;8(7):573–82.
2. Webster LR, Webster RM. Predicting aberrant behaviors in opioid-treated patients: preliminary validation of the opioid risk tool. Pain Med. 2005;6(6):432–42.
3. Ives TJ, Chelminski PR, Hammett-Stabler CA, et al. Predictors of opioid misuse in patients with chronic pain: a prospective cohort study. BMC Health Serv Res. 2006;6:46.
4. Rosenblum A, Joseph H, Fong C, Kipnis S, Cleland C, Portenoy RK. Prevalence and characteristics of chronic pain among chemically dependent patients in methadone maintenance and residential treatment facilities. JAMA. 2003;289(18):2370–8.
5. Becker WC, Fiellin DA, Gallagher RM, Barth KS, Ross JT, Oslin DW. The association between chronic pain and prescription drug abuse in veterans. Pain Med. 2009;10(3):531–6.
6. Hennecke L. Stimulus augmenting and field dependence in children of alcoholic fathers. J Stud Alcohol Drugs. 1984;45(6):486–92.
7. Public policy statement on the rights and responsibilities of healthcare professionals in the use of opioids for the treatment of pain: a consensus document from the American Academy of Pain Medicine, the American Pain Society, and the American Society of Addiction Medicine. Adopted 2004. Available at http://www.ampainsoc.org/advocacy/pdf/rights.pdf. Accessed 7 Jan 2010.
8. Katz NP, Adams EH, Chilcoat H, et al. Challenges in the development of prescription opioid abuse-deterrent formulations. Clin J Pain. 2007;23(8):648–60.
9. Federation of State Medical Boards of the United States, Inc. Model policy for the use of controlled substances for the treatment of pain. 2004. Available at: http://www.fsmb.org/pdf/2004_grpol_Controlled_Substances.pdf. Accessed 7 Jan 2010.
10. Webster LR, Dove B. Avoiding opioid abuse while managing pain: a guide for practitioners. 1st ed. North Branch: Sunrise River Press; 2007. p. 145.
11. National Institutes of Health, U.S. Department of Health and Human Services. Drugs, brains, and behavior: the science of addiction. NIH Pub No. 07–5605. Printed Apr 2007.
12. National Institutes of Health, U.S. Department of Health and Human Services. Research report series. Comorbidity: addiction and other mental illnesses. NIH Pub No. 08–5771. Printed Dec 2008.
13. Zhang Y, Picetti R, Butelman ER, Schlussman SD, Ho A, Kreek MJ. Behavioral and neurochemical changes induced by oxycodone differ between adolescent and adult mice. Neuropsychopharmacology. 2009;34(4):912–22.
14. Gourlay DL, Heit HA, Almahrezi A. Universal precautions in pain medicine: a rational approach to the treatment of chronic pain. Pain Med. 2005;6(2):107–12.
15. Savage SR. Assessment for addiction in pain-treatment settings. Clin J Pain. 2002;18(4 Suppl):S28–38.
16. Dunbar SA, Katz NP. Chronic opioid therapy for nonmalignant pain in patients with a history of substance abuse: report of 20 cases. J Pain Symptom Manage. 1996;11(3):163–71.
17. Friedman R, Li V, Mehrotra D. Treating pain patients at risk: evaluation of a screening tool in opioid-treated pain patients with and without addiction. Pain Med. 2003;4(2):182–5.
18. Chou R, Fanciullo GJ, Fine PG, et al. Clinical guidelines for the use of chronic opioid therapy in chronic noncancer pain. J Pain. 2009;10(2):113–230.
19. Butler SF, Budman SH, Fernandez K, Jamison RN. Validation of a screener and opioid assessment measure for patients with chronic pain. Pain. 2004;112(1–2):65–75.
20. Belgrade MJ, Schamber CD, Lindgren BR. The DIRE score: predicting outcomes of opioid prescribing for chronic pain. J Pain. 2006;7(9):671–81.
21. Coambs RB, Jarry JL. The SISAP; a new screening instrument for identifying potential opioid abusers in the management of chronic nonmalignant pain in general medical practice. Pain Res Manag. 1996;1(3):155–62.
22. Adams LL, Gatchel RJ, Robinson RC, et al. Development of a self-report screening instrument for assessing potential opioid medication misuse in chronic pain patients. J Pain Symptom Manage. 2004;27:440–59.
23. Moore TM, Jones T, Browder JH, Daffron S, Passik SD. A comparison of common screening methods for predicting aberrant drug-related behavior among patients receiving opioids for chronic pain management. Pain Med. 2009;10(8):1426–33.
24. Passik SD, Kirsh KL, Whitcomb L, et al. A new tool to assess and document pain outcomes in chronic pain patients receiving opioid therapy. Clin Ther. 2004;26(4):552–61.
25. Butler SF, Budman SH, Fernandez KC, et al. Development and validation of the current opioid misuse measure. Pain. 2007; 130(1–2):144–56.
26. Wasan AD, Butler SF, Budman SH, Benoit C, Fernandez K, Jamison RN. Psychiatric history and psychologic adjustment as risk factors for aberrant drug-related behavior among patients with chronic pain. Clin J Pain. 2007;23(4):307–15.
27. Kaskutas LA. Alcoholics anonymous effectiveness: faith meets science. J Addict Dis. 2009;28(2):145–57.
28. Donovan DM, Floyd AS. Facilitating involvement in twelve-step programs. Recent Dev Alcohol. 2008;18:303–20.
29. Katz N. Patient level opioid risk management: a supplement to the PainEDU.org manual. Newton: Inflexxion, Inc; 2007.
30. Webster LR. Pharmacogenetics in pain management: the clinical need. Clin Lab Med. 2008;28(4):569–79.
31. Induru RR, Davis MP. Buprenorphine for neuropathic pain: targeting hyperalgesia. Am J Hosp Palliat Care. 2009;26(6):470–3.
32. Vadivelu N, Hines RL. Buprenorphine: a unique opioid with broad clinical applications. J Opioid Manag. 2007;3(1):49–58.
33. Malinoff HL, Barkin RL, Wilson G. Sublingual buprenorphine is effective in the treatment of chronic pain syndrome. Am J Ther. 2005;12(5):379–84.

The "Five-Minute" Mental Status Examination of Persons with Pain

J. David Haddox and Barry Kerner

Key Points
- Mental status findings are common in patients with pain.
- Many medicines employed in pain care can induce or worsen underlying psychiatric problems.
- Examining the mental status in routine pain care requires little additional work.
- Pain physicians should understand the well-defined terms to describe mental status findings.

Introduction

The mental status examination (MSE) is just that – a set of processes that systematically examine various aspects of a person's mental functioning – in essence, a physical examination of the mind. A complete MSE constitutes a distinct portion of a complete psychiatric assessment. In practice, whether in psychiatry or other specialties, the MSE can be less comprehensive than a complete MSE, according to the clinical setting. MSEs can be partial – focusing only a particular aspect, such as mood or intelligence, or can be exhaustive. Abbreviated MSEs can range anywhere from keen observations of people, to structured interviews (e.g., Structured Clinical Interview for DSM-IV (SCID)), to the use of validated instruments for the assessment of a specific aspect of the mental status (e.g., Profile of Mood States, Wechsler Adult Intelligence Test, Minnesota Multiphasic Personality Inventory, State-Trait Anxiety Inventory), and to multi-hour assessments of specific

J.D. Haddox, DDS, M.D., DAPBM, MRO (✉)
Tufts University School of Medicine, Boston, MA, USA

Department of Health Policy, Purdue Pharma L.P.,
One Stanford Forum, Stanford, CA 06901, USA
e-mail: dr.j.david.haddox@pharma.com

B. Kerner, M.D., DABPM
Silver Hill Hospital, 208 Valley Road, New Canaan, CT 06840, USA
e-mail: bkerner@silverhillhospital.org

functions (e.g., Halstead-Reitan Neuropsychological Test Battery) [1]. MSEs can involve standardized clinical assessment techniques (e.g., "serial sevens" or copying a figure) or can be less formal. Incorporating certain aspects of the MSE into clinical pain assessment and care is important because persons in pain may present with mental status findings that (a) predate the onset of pain (e.g., the presence of generalized anxiety disorder long before a cancer diagnosis), (b) date to the onset of pain (e.g., posttraumatic stress disorder initiated by the same motor vehicle accident that caused the spinal fracture that gave rise to the pain for which they are being evaluated or treated), (c) follow the onset of, but are related to, the pain syndrome (e.g., depression or anxiety due in part or in whole to chronic, unremitting pain), or (d) are related to treatment (e.g., cognitive impairment due to medications prescribed). Because virtually all medications used to treat pain have the potential for significant effects on various aspects of a patient's mental status, it is important to assess the mental status at baseline and note any changes over time. The thorough way to do this is to learn how to observe patients in clinical interactions while keeping the potential MSE findings in mind, to record the findings using precise, unambiguous, and proper terms, and to interpret these findings in the assessment and plan.

An abbreviated MSE in pain practice does not necessarily have to take a lot of time, or even be a separate part of the initial or ongoing evaluation of patients undergoing treatment for pain. Certain aspects of mental function can have significant influences on the course of treatment and potential treatment outcomes. Documenting important aspects of the patient's mental status can be very helpful in the overall assessment by affording a chronology of the presence, absence, improvement, or worsening of specific symptoms and signs from visit to visit. The inclusion or absence of documentation of important MSE findings can have significant medical/legal consequences as well.

Fortunately, once the physician has learned the principles of an abbreviated MSE, most information needed to document MSE findings can be readily obtained as part of the normal conversation and observation that occurs during a typical clinical encounter. Just as a pain physician begins their observation of pain behaviors immediately upon seeing the patient and ends it as the patient leaves their sight (e.g., walking down the hall to schedule an appointment), the abbreviated MSE becomes part of the entire interaction, to be separately described and interpreted in the health record.

The "Five-Minute Mental Status Examination for Persons in Pain" (5-MSEPP) is a distillation of some salient aspects of the MSE that the authors have found useful from decades of direct clinical care of persons in pain and is specifically aimed at assisting the nonpsychiatrist in routine care of their patients (see Table 5.1). There will, of course, be cases in which a more structured, formal MSE is indicated, but these should be done by a psychiatrist or psychologist, rather than the pain physician without such qualification.

In this chapter, the authors will review the various aspects of the mental status that can be assessed during the provision of clinical pain care, provide precise terminology and definitions for the phenomena commonly encountered, suggest some methods for mental status assessment that can easily be incorporated into clinical routines, and provide a framework for how to document such findings in the health care record.

The MSE includes assessment and interpretation of both subjective and objective aspects of the person's mental function. The subjective aspects are called *symptoms* and represent experiences, beliefs, thoughts, feelings, etc., which are *reported* by the patient. The objective findings are referred to as *signs* and are those phenomena and behaviors that are directly *observed* by the practitioner. Just as during the physical examination a physician would note and record the speed and amplitude of the biceps tendon reflex objectively (e.g., "3+, normal recovery, no clonus"), so, too, should the findings of the MSE be recorded objectively, leaving the interpretation of the constellation of history, MSE, physical examination, and laboratory findings to the assessment section of consultation, initial visit, or progress note.

As will be clear from the information that follows, the traditional separation of "mental status" from "neurological" findings is somewhat arbitrary and may be of questionable clinical relevance, since both are ways of assessing the function and abnormalities of the same nervous system. For example, if a person with dementia (a "neurological" diagnosis) presents with psychosis (a "psychiatric" diagnosis), both need addressing, whether by a psychiatrist, a neurologist, a geriatrician, or a family physician.

Background Concepts and Terms

There are well-defined aspects of an abbreviated MSE that can be readily assessed in the provision of pain care. The following are the various domains assessed as part of a typical

Table 5.1 5-MMSEPP – key points to observe and describe

Appearance
Development
Nutritional status – including change over time
Dress/grooming
Level of consciousness – alert, somnolent, lethargic, obtunded, stuporous, comatose
Orientation – person, place, time, situation
Motor activity
Quantity – hypoactive, normoactive, hyperactivity, agitation
Quality – altered gait (antalgic, ataxic, festinating, etc.)
Fluidity – tremors
Spontaneity
Speed
Abnormal signs – cogwheel rigidity, tics, stereotypies, chorea, athetosis
Affect and mood – range, amplitude, stability, appropriateness, relation to examiner
Suicidality – ideation, plans, intent, threats, gestures, attempts
Homicidality – ideation, plans, intent, threats, attempts, duty to protect intended victim
Thought process
Speech – spontaneity, rate, amount, rhythm, articulation, idiosyncrasies
Associations – fragmentation, derailment, non sequiturs, flight of ideas, circumlocution, tangential
Thought content – delusions, hallucinations (sensory modality), illusions
Memory – registration, short-term, long-term, confabulation
Judgment and insight

MSE: appearance, level of consciousness, orientation, motor activity, affect and mood, thought content and processes, intellect, memory, and judgment.

Appearance

The first thing typically noticed is the patient's *appearance*. Aspects of appearance that warrant observation and characterization include the apparent degree of development (i.e., the patient is well developed or, if not, describes what aspects of development deviate from normal), the nutritional status (i.e., well nourished, overweight, cachectic, emaciated, etc.), and the degree of grooming/dress/hygiene (i.e., well groomed, appropriately dressed, disheveled, poor hygiene, etc.). Because various drugs encountered in pain care can directly or indirectly cause either weight gain (increased body mass from antidepressants or fluid retention from corticosteroid injections) or weight loss (stimulant use/abuse, cocaine abuse, opioid abuse), note should be made of changes in appearance over time.

Eye contact can be revealing, but like many signs, whether a patient makes good eye contact with the examiner can have different meanings. For example, it is common, in Western cultures, to infer that someone not making good eye contact is being evasive. However, this behavior must be interpreted carefully because in certain cultures, looking at an authority figure, such as a physician, directly in the eye is considered disrespectful or sexually provocative [2, 3].

Overall comments about the nature of the interaction deserve documentation, such as the patient's demeanor, courtesy, and cooperativeness. The term *guarded* is used to describe a person who appears to be *inappropriately* cautious or reserved about the interaction or reluctant to provide information.

Level of Consciousness

This aspect of a patient's presentation is virtually always perceived by the clinician, but is often not reported. The normal level of consciousness in a clinical situation is, of course, is *alert* (which implies that the person being evaluated is also awake). Other descriptors commonly employed included *somnolent* (i.e., drowsy, or sleepy), *lethargic* (i.e., very sleepy, in which the person can be verbally or physically aroused to a level of communication, but when unprovoked, will drift back to sleep), *obtunded* (i.e., more sleepy than lethargic), *stuporous* (i.e., repeated, vigorous stimuli can arouse the person, but ceasing the stimuli results in immediate return to sleep), and *comatose* (i.e., unresponsive to any stimulus mode – auditory, tactile, etc.) [4]. Degree of attention or engagement is important to observe and report. For example, an alert patient can be disengaged from the interaction (e.g., a person with drug-induced hallucinations may be alert, but completely or intermittently disengaged with the clinician because they are attending to the hallucinations).

Orientation

Orientation is typically assessed and described in four domains: orientation to *person, place, time*, and *situation*. A patient who is oriented to person knows who they are and who others they should know are. Orientation to place is the ability to indicate where they are. With organic brain syndromes, whether degenerative, metabolic, traumatic, infectious, or drug-induced, orientation to time can be an especially sensitive indicator. In a rapidly changing organic brain syndrome (e.g., a person who is admitted to hospital for an overdose of a tricyclic antidepressant), incremental improvement in orientation to time can be a useful adjunct to monitoring progress, as the toxicity resolves, in that the person may initially be disoriented with respect to time, then may know what year it is, but still be disoriented to season or month and will gradually regain orientation to month and

date. Orientation to situation is sometimes referred to as situational insight and is used to describe the person who demonstrates an understanding of the context of what is happening at that time.

Motor Activity

The *quantity, quality, fluidity, spontaneity*, and *speed* of motor activity should be described, as should the presence of any *abnormal motor signs*. The terms used to quantify activity include normoactive, hypoactive (less spontaneous or responsive activity than normally observed, as might be seen in a patient with drug-induced Parkinsonian syndrome or a person with chronic benzodiazepine toxicity), and hyperactive. *Hyperactivity* specifically describes an excess amount of *goal-directed* activity, such as might be seen in a child with attention deficit hyperactivity disorder, in which the clinical presentation may include the child hopping out of their chair, opening and closing the examining room door or drawers in the cabinetry, taking off their shoes, etc.

Excess, purposeless, voluntary motor activity is referred to as *agitation*. Agitation is often associated with alteration in affect or mood. Pacing, frequently switching positions, hand wringing, finger drumming, or pulling on one's hair are all examples of agitation. Purposeless, involuntary motor activity, such as *tremors*, should be described. Tremors can be characterized with regard to their *location* (e.g., finger, arm), *amplitude* (small or large), *frequency* (low or high), whether they are *resting* or *intention* (intention tremors appear when an action is attempted, such as reaching for a pencil), and whether they *diminish* or *disappear* with distraction. A well-described tremor of note is the *pill-rolling tremor*, which describes a low-amplitude, high-frequency resting tremor involving the thumb and index finger (with possible involvement of other digits, as well), that is named because it is reminiscent of the rolling of medicinal compounds into round pills by early apothecaries (the dominant technique of creating oral formulations before tableting presses were invented). Another tremor equivalent is that of constant or nearly constant head bobbing or low-amplitude shaking (as if one was repeatedly signaling "no") that is referred to as *titubation*. This is seen in a variety of neurodegenerative diseases and drug-induced neurological syndromes.

Drugs may induce several disorders of motor activity, including agitation (e.g., cocaine, stimulants), cogwheel rigidity, tics, and stereotypies. *Cogwheel rigidity* is the term used to describe a ratchet-like quality of the muscles when flexing and extending a joint. This can be visually observed in some cases, with the hand moving through the flexion-extension arc in a jerky or "start-and-stop" fashion, but often is detectable only by placing the examiner's thumb over, for example, the biceps tendon and asking the patient to allow the examiner to smoothly, but relatively quickly, flex and extend the elbow (passive flexion and extension). It results in a subtle "bumping" or "ratcheting" feeling of the tendon under the thumb, likened by some to feeling as though a string of pearls is being pulled subcutaneously under the examiner's thumb. Cogwheel rigidity is an *extrapyramidal* phenomenon (i.e., it is mediated via neural pathways that are *outside* of the corticospinal tracts – most of which cross the midline in the medulla oblongata at the pyramidal decussation). *Drug-induced* extrapyramidal side effects (EPSE) result from dopamine antagonism. Extrapyramidal findings can also occur with disease processes that cause the loss of dopaminergic neurons in the basal ganglia, such as Parkinson's disease. In general, the corticospinal tracts mediate coarse motor activity and the extrapyramidal paths mediate fluidity and "fine-tuning" of movement. A person with basal ganglia dysfunction may be able to reach for a glass of water, but the movement will be so coarse that they will overshoot the target or knock the glass over. Other features of the Parkinsonian syndrome, whether drug-induced or naturally occurring, include gait abnormalities (see below), masklike facies (i.e., far less activity in the muscles of facial expression than is normal – which can also be seen in chronic depression resulting in so-called *pseudodementia* and myotonic dystrophy), general hypoactivity, and difficulty initiating an activity or initiating a change in activity. For example, a person with Parkinsonian syndrome may appear to sit comfortably in an examination room chair, but at the conclusion of the visit demonstrate significant difficulty rising from the chair. This difficulty initiating or changing movement is often reported to the physician as difficulty rising from the toilet, or going up stairs (which requires initiation of change of activity with every step). Another characteristic presentation that can be induced by administration of dopamine antagonists is *tardive dyskinesia* (Fr, *tardif*, late, as in *tardy*, + Gk, *dys* + *kinesia*, movement). Tardive dyskinesia usually affects the muscles of the head, causing involuntary lip pursing or tongue protrusion, but can affect other muscle groups, as well, even creating restrictive pulmonary compromise.

Drug-induced EPSE can also occur acutely, following the administration of dopamine antagonists used as antiemetics (e.g., droperidol, promethazine), and can manifest as an overwhelming urge to move, or restlessness, called *akathisia* (Gk, *a* + *kathízein*, to sit). This phenomenon can typically be treated with the administration of a drug with antimuscarinic properties, such as diphenhydramine or benztropine. It is important to remember that akathisia refers to the *urge* to move, not to the movement itself, which may take the form of agitation or hyperactivity. Administration of dopamine antagonists (e.g., some antiemetics or antipsychotics) rarely results in *acute dystonias*, or sudden increased tone of certain muscles, but not their antagonist muscles, such that the person presents, for example, with their head painfully rotated to one side, and is unable to voluntarily rotate it to a neutral, forward-looking position. The most dramatic of the drug-induced acute dystonias is opisthotonos (Gk, *opistho*, behind + *tonos*, tension) in which the extensor muscles of the axial spine and extremities are acutely contracted such that the only contact with the floor is the occiput and the heels – a bridging or arching posture.

Tic (Fr, from It, *ticchio*) is the term used to describe a rapid, involuntary, repetitive movement of small muscles, such as it can involve the muscles of facial expression. Common tics are throat clearing, blinking, and nose twitching. Tics often disappear during sleep, and can be exacerbated in frequency with anxiety. It is common for persons with tics to describe increasing emotional discomfort the longer they consciously suppress a tic, which discomfort is relieved when they allow the tic to reemerge.

Complex, repetitive, voluntary movements of larger muscle groups are referred to as *stereotypies* (pronounced "stereo-TIP-eez") (Gk, *stereos*, hard or fixed + type). Stereotypies can involve many muscle groups, including muscles involved in speech. They can appear almost mechanical in their repetition and can be difficult for a patient to consciously suppress. A stereotypy can take the form of assuming a particular posture, movements that appear almost purposeful (crossing and uncrossing legs, periodic rubbing a body part not due to pain, rocking, arm flapping), or utterances as one might observe in Tourette's syndrome. Abusers of methamphetamine or amphetamines may engage in stereotypies that involve picking at their skin, excessive grooming, and disassembling and reassembling or plucking at things. These stereotypies are sometimes referred to in the addiction community as *tweaking* or *punding*. Tweaking may also occur in patients treated for Parkinson's disease with L-DOPA.

Chorea, or choreia, (Gk, *choreia*, a circle dance) is used to describe brief, irregular contractions that are not repetitive or rhythmic, but appear to flow from one muscle to the next [5]. Chorea is common in Huntington's disease, but can also occur following infection with group A beta-hemolytic streptococci (GABHS) which cause rheumatic fever; some cases of which can present with *Sydenham chorea*, which is characterized by rapid, irregular, and aimless involuntary movements of the arms and legs, trunk, and facial muscles, affecting females more often and typically occurring between the ages of 5 and 15 years. The etiology is likely via an autoimmune reaction from infection-induced antibodies that attack neurons [6]. Chorea can also present in Wilson's disease, can be drug-induced (dopamine agonists and antagonists, and anticonvulsants), or can be due to cerebrovascular accidents.

Not infrequently, chorea is accompanied by *athetosis* (Gk, *a* + *thetos*, not placed), which is the term used to describe writhing, twisting movements involving multiple muscle groups. When chorea is accompanied by athetosis, the term *choreoathetosis* is used.

One aspect of a patient's motor behavior typically observed by pain physicians is gait. A normal gait includes a reasonable stride length, a fluid shift from leg to leg, a moderate arm swing, and an upright or nearly upright posture. A common gait abnormality encountered in care of persons with pain is referred to as *antalgic* (literally, "against pain," in clinical use, "pain avoiding") gait which is characterized by limping, guarding, one lower extremity consistently moving more rapidly than the contralateral extremity to reduce the amount of time weight is borne on the painful side, or significant flexion of the lumbar spine or hips, any of which is done to avoid or minimize pain on ambulation. Ankylosing spondylitis resulting in a fused vertebral column presents with the so-called *simian* ("apelike") gait in which there is prominent, fixed flexion of the spine, which pitches the upper body well forward of the feet. A simian gait, because of the forward position of the torso, is also characterized by arms dangling in front of the feet. A person with a simian gait who is wearing a coat or jacket may not be able to see their feet because the forward position of the torso causes the jacket to drape in front of the person and obscures their view of their feet. This can, of course, make the person prone to trips and falls, especially when descending stairs.

An *ataxic* gait is an unsteady or uncoordinated manner of walking that often includes a *broad-based* gait (i.e., the lateral distance between the feet is greater than normal and often exceeds the shoulder-to-shoulder width). Ataxic gaits can result from inherited or acquired neurodegenerative conditions (e.g., Friedreich's ataxia, cerebellar ataxia from inhalant toxicity), acute or chronic drug exposure (e.g., ethanol, benzodiazepines), may be due to conditions affecting the vestibular system (e.g., Meniere's disease, drug-induced vertigo from calcium antagonists, orthostatic hypotension), or may be due to cerebrovascular disease.

A *festinating* gait is characterized by short, staccato, accelerating steps in an effort to move forward, almost as if the person is falling forward in order to move and they are having trouble making their feet keep pace with their body. It is often seen in Parkinsonian conditions, as well as other neurological syndromes.

Fortunately, neurologic complications from *syphilis* infection are currently rare in the USA, but its prevalence is rising. Persons who have *tabes dorsalis* (peripheral neuropathy, ataxia, autonomic dysfunction) have a characteristic gait due to dorsal column disease causing them to lose proprioception. The tabetic gait is characterized by several distinct components – an inordinate degree of hip flexion, resulting in a high lift of the knee (to ensure that the foot clears the floor, since the lack of proprioception prevents the person from sensing if their ankle is flexed or extended), followed by a forceful "slapping" of the foot on the floor wherein the entire plantar surface contacts the floor at or nearly at once (instead of a normal gait, wherein the heel strikes the floor and the rest of the sole "rolls" down to the floor as weight is shifted). The forceful slapping, in addition to accommodating for a partial or complete foot drop, also provides a supranormal amount of proprioception, so that the person perceives some feedback with regard to position in space, even though dorsal columnar function is impaired. Dorsal spinal space tumors, hematomas, and infection can cause a tabetic-like presentation. Persons with unilateral foot drop, due to tibial nerve injury or early amyotrophic lateral sclerosis, may exhibit features of a tabetic-like gait only in the affected extremity.

A *hemiplegic* gait, as might be seen following a cerebrovascular accident, is typified by lower extremity circumduction (swinging it laterally as it is brought forward) and exaggerated hip flexion, both of which combine to ensure the foot clears the floor. A *spastic* gait is that in which the lower extremities are stiff and do not flex normally, causing a "stiff-legged" walking pattern.

Affect and Mood

Surprisingly, there is some disagreement over the precise constructs referred to as *affect* and *mood*. Some authors consider mood to be a parameter of affect (e.g., "affect is the emotional tone underlying all behaviors" and "mood is only one facet of affect") [7]. Other authors prefer the convention of affect being the immediately observable expression of emotion which typically changes during a conversation, while mood is the prevailing or underlying emotional state. In other words, affect is to weather as mood is to climate. For example, a person could be in a bad mood, yet still respond with an affective change to something they found very humorous [8]. Others would describe them by analogy, as mood being the channel a person is watching on television, while affect is the color saturation of the image (Ray A, 2011, personal communication).

The parameters of affect that are typically described include the range, amplitude, stability, appropriateness, and ability to relate to the examiner (which is inferred from the affect observed).

Range of affect refers to the person's emotional repertoire. A person who does not react much to various emotionally laden comments during a clinical encounter would be described as having a *constricted* range, whereas a *full* range of affect is the societal norm. With a full range of affect, the person exhibits transient changes in the immediate emotional state the course of an interaction (e.g., frowning when describing the intensity and impact of their pain, furrowing their brow while listening intently to counseling instructions, and smiling at the conclusion of the visit as they are leaving the office and saying their goodbyes).

Amplitude, or intensity, is the degree to which a particular affective vector is expressed. The difference between a chuckle and guffaw is a difference in range along the same vector, as is the difference between indicating annoyance with a scowling expression and screaming at someone, which is an affective vector of a very different nature than laughing. Affect may be of normal amplitude, exaggerated (e.g., in mania or intoxication with certain substances), diminished, blunted, or *flat* (e.g., schizophrenics, when their psychotic symptoms are not prominent, exhibit a marked and characteristic reduction in affective amplitude).

Stability refers to the rapidity with which the affect changes during a clinical encounter. If the person is doing well, with their pain under good control, it is likely that their affect will be relatively stable. If, on the other hand, a person is laughing or smiling one moment, crying the next, and appears irritable the next, their affect is described as *labile*. Labile affect can be observed in drug-induced conditions (e.g., steroid use, intoxication) or in idiopathic or reactive mental diagnoses, such as depression, mania, or dementia.

Appropriateness refers to the degree of correlation of affect to the content of conversation or situation. Usually, what is appropriate for the examiner is appropriate for the patient. Therefore, if the patient describes getting into a serious automobile accident in which they and others were injured and is smiling during the description, the patient's affect would be described as *inappropriate*.

The *ability to relate* to the examiner refers to the patient's ability to express emotional warmth, establish rapport, and interact with the examiner. When a patient does this, they are described *relating well*. When a patient remains cold or unfeeling and no rapport is apparent, they are described as exhibiting *relating poorly*. Due to the flat affect that characterizes schizophrenia, examiners typically describe a poor ability to relate. Historically, this was referred to as the *praecox feeling*, a reference to an obsolete term once used to describe schizophrenia, *dementia praecox* (premature dementia, i.e., "dementia" occurring in a young person, when schizophrenia typically manifests) [9].

Mood is the prevailing or underlying emotional state being experienced by the patient. Mood generally falls into one of these classifications: sad, happy, angry, anxious, or apathetic. A person who has what is considered a normal mood is described as *euthymic* (Gk, *eu*, true or normal + *thymia*, mood; ancient practitioners believed the function of the thymus gland was to control mood). Mood on the depressed side of normal is designated as *dysthymic*. Excessive mood on the happy side of euthymia is referred to as *hypomania* (Gk, *hypo*, beneath or under + via L, *mania*, loss of reason, from Gk, *mainesthai*, to rage).

Anger is a common concomitant of chronic, unrelenting pain [10]. It is strongly related to self-reported assessments of pain intensity, pain behaviors, and perceived pain interference in activities of daily living. In the person with chronic pain, anger is often diffuse and nondirected, such that they lash out at the examiner for asking a simple question. This is often followed by guilt, which can then contribute to sadness.

Anxiety often occurs in patients with acute or chronic pain [11]. As noted at the beginning of the chapter, it may antedate, co-occur, or follow the onset of a chronic pain condition.

Depression and depressive spectrum disorders (pervasive sad mood, loss of interest in social interactions, etc., but not to the degree as is seen in clinically diagnosable depression) frequently accompany persistent pain [11].

Suicidality should be regularly assessed as part of the mental status examination of persons with persistent pain [12–18]. Depression is prevalent among this population, and it, coupled with the loss of hope that so commonly occurs as a result of repeated treatment failures, can cause patients with chronic pain to have thoughts of killing themselves. Treatments used for certain chronic or recurrent conditions (e.g., β-adrenergic antagonists for migraine prophylaxis) can also cause depression through alteration of the brain neurochemistry, as can antidepressants, themselves, as noted in the boxed warning most antidepressants now carry. The motivation for suicidal thoughts can range from ideas of stopping suffering once and for all, to simply giving up ("I just don't have the energy to go on."), to getting even with someone who the person feels has wronged them ("I'll show them!"). The assessment of suicidality is often overlooked or avoided by practitioners not trained in the behavioral sciences. Inquiring about suicide does not increase the risk of suicidal thoughts [19]. Since the best predictor of future risk of successful suicide is a history of suicide attempts, it is important to assess this in providing clinical pain care. When assessing and characterizing suicidal thoughts and behaviors, one should document *suicidal ideation* (i.e., *thoughts* of suicide), *suicidal plans* (the more detailed and thought-out the plan, the greater the risk of completion), *suicidal intent* (a person could have thought about suicide and formulated a plan, but have no intent to carry it out), *suicidal threats* (i.e., communication to others of the intent to commit suicide – sometimes used to manipulate, sometimes a serious plea for help), *suicidal gestures* (i.e., actions without lethal intent that are intended to appear lethal – which may also be manipulation or a genuine call for help), or *suicidal attempts* (i.e., actions with sincere intent to end one's life). The process of suicidal thoughts represents a psychiatric emergency and should be referred immediately to a psychiatrist/hospital emergency department for further assessment.

Similarly, *homicidal* ideation or plans should be assessed [20]. Unfortunately, a not uncommon occurrence is the plan of a desperate person to "take out" someone they hold responsible for harm or wrong, followed by taking their own life or, in some cases, "suicide by police" (constructing a situation in which there is a high probability that the police will use lethal force to protect the public or themselves).

Case law has established an affirmative duty to protect the intended victim when the examiner believes the homicidal threat is credible [21].

Thought Processes and Content

The content of a patient's thoughts and their thought processes are inferred largely from their speech, although some other behaviors may provide clues to thought content or process (e.g., a person suffering from paranoid delusions may present as electively mute, anxious, and hypervigilant with an exaggerated startle response). Thought processes refer to how the patient is thinking; what the patient is thinking (talking) about is called content.

Speech qualities that can be characterized include *spontaneity, rate, amount, rhythm, articulation, idiosyncratic* word usage, and the tightness and form of *associations*.

Spontaneous speech is typical in a normal clinical interaction; however, the lack of spontaneity, as with all mental status signs, must be interpreted in the totality of the presentation. As with eye contact, in some cultures, a sign of deference to an authority figure is to "speak only when spoken to." Thus, the lack of spontaneous speech in a person from such a culture, in the absence of other findings, may be of no clinical significance from the standpoint of assessing their mental state.

The *rate* of speech can be described as normal, slow, or rapid. *Pressured speech* refers to the behavior which results from an apparent drive to keep talking. A person with pressured speech is difficult to interrupt. Persons with pressured speech often "do all the talking" (i.e., in addition to the rate and uninterruptability of speech, the *amount* of speech is also abnormal) or appear that their thoughts are coming faster than their mouth can get them out. In the latter presentation, the presence of *racing thoughts* can be inferred. Racing thoughts are common in mania, whether endogenous (e.g., bipolar disorder) or drug-induced (e.g., methamphetamine abuse). Abnormally slow or labored speech can be a feature of benzodiazepine or opioid toxicity [22].

Most patients speak with a *normal rhythm*; however, certain clinical conditions exhibit unusual rhythm of speech. *Scanning speech*, where certain words or syllables are stressed, producing a slow, sliding cadence is observed in multiple sclerosis. *Hesitant speech* can accompany Huntington's disease. Persons with early Huntington's disease or other incipient dementias can appear normal until exposed to drugs with antimuscarinic properties, after which the disease will become manifest. *Staccato speech*, which is abrupt and clipped, can be present in temporal lobe epilepsy. *Stuttering or stammering speech* can be a persistent problem for some persons. The acute onset of stammering during a procedure, however, may be an indication of systemic toxicity of a local anesthetic.

Articulation, or the accuracy with which syllables and words are pronounced, can be affected by numerous diseases and drugs. Acute intoxication with ethanol, sedative-hypnotics, or marijuana can induce *slurring of speech* (a form of *dysarthria*). Cerebrovascular accidents in different parts of the brain can affect most speech in various ways, including the ability to articulate words.

Some patients may use words or word-like sounds in idiosyncratic ways. A person who repeatedly uses approximations of or substitution of correct words is described as having *paraphasia* (Gk, *para*, to one side of + *phrasein*, to utter). In *verbal* or *semantic paraphasia*, there is a complete word substitution (e.g., the person says "dog" when referring to a photograph of a cat). *Literal* or *phonemic paraphasia* is characterized by substitution or addition of syllables ("phonemes") or letters (e.g., the use of "rice" instead of "nice" or "shoots" to mean "shoes"). The term *neologism* is used to describe a new word created by the patient. Neologisms often sound-like words or are composed of parts of existing words. The apparent meaning of a neologism may vary during a conversation. Anomia (Gk, *a* + L, *nom*, name), or nominal aphasia, refers to the inability to find the right word for an object. A person with expressive anomia when asked, "Can you tell me what this is?" (with the examiner pointing to their watch), may answer, "Oh, it's … you know … it's …, it's a time-telling thing." Paraphasic speech often indicates an organic brain lesion, such as a cerebrovascular accident, but can also be observed in some primary mental disorders. When caused by the former, the type of dysfluency of speech can facilitate anatomic localization of the lesion. *Complete aphasia* is the apparent inability to speak despite an effort to do so (as contrasted with *elective mutism*, where the examiner has reason to believe the person can speak, but is choosing not to). Complete aphasia is most commonly due to cerebrovascular accidents.

The *tightness and form of associations* refer to the way in which ideas or concepts are linked together. Normal speech manifests tight associational linkages, that is, each element of speech is logically linked to the previous ones and the thought behind the speech is goal-directed. In some conditions, there is a disruption of the tightness of association, which is referred to as *loose association*. The form of thought disorder can be partially determined by where the loosening of the association occurs. In the most severe form, called *word salad*, sometimes called *gibberish*, or *jargon* (old Fr, *jargoun*, gibberish) speech, the loosening of associations occurs between words, such that consecutive words seem to have no relationship (e.g., "red up tolerable cloud fine want"). *Fragmentation* is defined as a loosening of associations that occurs between clauses or sentences. In fragmentation, a person begins to relate a thought in a sequential, coherent manner, but winds up changing the content within a sentence or a paragraph. *Derailment* refers to a sudden switch from one line of thinking to a new parallel line of thought. A *non sequitur* (L, "it does not follow") refers to a totally unrelated response. *Flight of ideas* is characterized by rapid switching of the line of thought which may be somewhat understandable but is often interpreted as reflecting the patient's distraction by external or internal stimuli. *Circumstantial speech*, also called *circumlocution* (L, *circum*, around + *locutio*, speech), has tightly linked associations, but contains extraneous, nonessential material that is interspersed throughout before ultimately reaching its goal. *Tangential speech* refers a series of tightly linked associations which never reach a goal.

Thought content can be inferred by listening to and probing the drive behind speech content. A patient's thought content may indicate preoccupation with a particular issue, paranoia, guilt, shame, etc. A *delusion* is a fixed, false belief, which is held by the person despite evidence to the contrary. The presence of delusions is considered to represent a *psychotic* state (i.e., an inability to relate to reality). Delusions are described by their content, for example, *delusions of guilt*, *persecutory delusions*, *religious delusions*, etc. *Perceptual disorders* are those in which there is an abnormality manifesting as a report of alteration of or interference with one of the senses. A hallucination is a perception in any sensory modality in the absence of a stimulus. When a patient reports having a hallucination while fully awake with a clear *sensorium* (consciousness and connectedness to the environment), he or she is said to have reported a psychotic symptom. Hallucinations can be *visual* (most commonly encountered with intoxication (e.g., antimuscarinic toxicity), withdrawal (e.g., ethanol), or diffuse Lewy body disease, which typically presents with the triad of dementia, Parkinson's syndrome, and psychosis, involving delusions and hallucinations, especially visual ones), *auditory* (the most prevalent type of hallucination in idiopathic psychotic disorders, such as schizophrenia), *olfactory*, *gustatory* (reports of which can also be due to *candidiasis*, vitamin or mineral deficiency (e.g., zinc), medications, or pyorrhea), or *tactile*, or *haptic*, a particular form of which *formication* (L, *formica*, ant), is association with abuse of certain substances ("*coke* (or *crack*) *bugs*," or ethanol withdrawal) and is so named because the person reports the sensation of ants or other insects crawling on or underneath their skin [23]. With the so-called phenomenon of coke bugs, rarely does the individual report actually seeing the insects (which would be a visual hallucination) or report believing that there are bugs crawling beneath the skin (which would be a delusion). When a hallucination is present, it is important to explore it further to determine its form; for example, an olfactory hallucination of the smell of sulfur or burning rubber may indicate the presence of a temporal lobe lesion. Also, hearing voices telling the patient to kill himself or somebody else clearly has important implications in terms of intervention.

Auditory hallucinations that are ordering a person to do something are referred to as *command hallucinations*. Most people have experienced at some time a specific kind of hallucination usually during the transition period between sleep and wakefulness. A hallucination while falling asleep is called a *hypnagogic* (Gk, *hypno*, sleep + *agogos*, leading) hallucination, and a hallucination that occurs while awakening is called *hypnopompic* (Gk, *hypno*, sleep + *pompe*, sending forth) hallucination. These can emerge or become more prevalent when a person is taking medicines that alter sleep architecture, especially those that cause REM sleep rebound, such as tricyclic antidepressants.

Because so many drugs have significant antimuscarinic properties, especially in situations of multiple medications or overdoses, the pain clinician should be aware of the presentations of persons so affected [24, 25]. Drugs with antimuscarinic properties include some antidepressants (e.g., tricyclic antidepressants), skeletal muscle relaxants (e.g., cyclobenzaprine), medicines used for urinary incontinence (e.g., oxybutynin), antidiarrheals (e.g., diphenoxylate + atropine), antiemetics (e.g., promethazine, transdermal scopolamine), antipsychotics (e.g., chlorpromazine), drugs used to treat dopamine antagonist-induced movement disorders or Parkinson's disease (e.g., benztropine), cardiovascular drugs (e.g., nifedipine), antispasmodics (e.g., dicyclomine), antiulcer drugs (e.g., cimetidine), and antihistamines (both prescription and over-the-counter). The features of the antimuscarinic syndrome can include tachycardia; blurred vision (especially difficulty with accommodation); worsening of narrow-angle glaucoma; larger than normal pupils; visual hallucinations or other psychotic symptoms and signs; delirium; impaired memory; ataxia; hyperthermia; urinary retention; constipation; xerostomia; fever; and warm, red, and dry skin. All these effects are mediated by blockade of the actions of acetylcholine upon muscarinic receptors.

If a person misperceives a real sensory stimulus, the reported perception is called an *illusion*. For this same reason, magicians who do coin tricks, etc., are referred to as illusionists because adults know the coin has not, in fact, disappeared, but our eyes tell us it did. An illusion is often associated with an intense affective state (e.g., when walking past a cemetery at midnight, one may perceive shadows to be objects).

Assessment of *intellect* can be initially done during the general conversation with the patient. Noted are whether the patient's vocabulary is consistent with their educational background. The ability to think abstractly and form concepts by the use of words, numbers, and other symbols is also assessed. Subtraction of serial sevens from 100 to 75 is a way to assess the patient's ability to concentrate. If the person has difficulty with the arithmetic, one can assess concentration by asking them to add 3 to 20, and then keep adding 3 to the resultant sum. A useful clinical tool is the mini-mental state exam, which is a brief, structured, valid procedure to assess cognitive function, when impairment is suspected from the clinical encounter [26]. The MMSE is sensitive to changes in cognitive function, such as might occur when a person is recovering from a concussion or drug-induced cognitive decrements.

Memory is typically assessed conversationally by paying attention to the person's ability to recall for recent and remote events. If impairment of memory is suspected during the interview, a more formal assessment of memory can easily be performed in the clinical setting. Memory functions are generally divided into *registration, immediate recall,* and *long-term recall.* The ability to register information can be tested by naming three unrelated objects and asking the patient to repeat them as soon as you finish. Once that has occurred, ask the patient to remember those three objects while you continue the interview. The continuation of the interview serves as a distraction, preventing them from simply repeating the names of the objects to themselves repeatedly. About three minutes later, ask the patient to repeat those objects named earlier, which assesses *immediate recall.* Long-term memory can be assessed by asking them to recall the last three US presidents or some similar well-known but sequential information that spans several years. People with organic causes for memory gaps will sometimes fill in those gaps with so-called false memories, which they believe to be real. This is referred to as *confabulation* [27–29].

Fibromyalgia syndrome and chronic fatigue syndrome are both associated with a particular, but vaguely defined, cluster of cognitive deficits known among patients as "brain fog" [30]. Interestingly, neuropsychological testing does not always confirm the degree of memory dysfunction reported by patients. Recent research suggests that short-term memory is worsened by distraction in persons with fibromyalgia syndrome, which may explain common complaints in this population, such as, "I walk from the kitchen to the living room to get something and then can't remember what I went to get" [31].

Judgment refers to the ability to evaluate various situations and information and reach an effective conclusion. Decisions about the patient's real-life situations are the best way to evaluate judgment. Asking the patient, "What are you going to tell your boss about this?" or "What are your plans for dealing with this problem?" assists in evaluating the patient's judgment. Judgment is described as good, fair, or poor. Some choose to describe judgment as intact or impaired and modify how impaired it is, for example, mildly impaired, moderately impaired, or severely impaired.

Performing the 5-MSEPP

As can be inferred from the information presented in this chapter, much of the 5-MSEPP is accomplished merely by being attuned to the patient's presentation during the clinical encounter and using precise terminology to document it.

In actual practice, observing and describing various aspects of mental functioning do not add much time to a typical interaction. Yet, doing so can have important ramifications for clinical care, as well as in the medicolegal realm.

Documentation of findings is relatively simple and can constitute one additional paragraph in the progress note. For example, during asking how a person is doing since the last visit, one can make many observations. It is human nature to only recall or document those observations which catch one's attention. However, it is just as important in a clinical practice dealing with persons in pain to document normal findings, instead of believing that someone else reading a progress note in which normal findings were not documents will assume they were observed and interpreted as within normal limits. Thus, for an uncomplicated visit in a patient with low back pain and unilateral, chronic lumbar radiculopathy who is stable on a medication regimen, a typical 5-MMSEPP comment would be:

> The patient is alert and oriented in all spheres (or: oriented × 4, which refers to person, place, time, and situation). They are well-nourished, well-developed, dressed appropriately, and well-groomed. The patient relates well, and affect is slightly constricted, stable, and appropriate. Mood is slightly depressed. Speech is fluid, articulate, and reveals no indication of disorder of thought process or content. Memory appears intact × 3 (referring to registration, immediate recall, and long-term recall). Judgment appears unimpaired. Other than an antalgic gait, favoring the affected side, there is no evidence of abnormal motor activity. The patient denies suicidal and homicidal ideation at this time.

Conclusion

The astute pain practitioner unwittingly performs aspects of a mental status examination as part of everyday clinical encounters. Learning the material presented in this chapter and incorporating a conscious assessment of these parameters into routine pain care will translate to better diagnoses, improved documentation, more precise and thorough documentation, and enhanced care for patients presenting with pain.

References

1. Pull CB, Cloos J-M, Pull-Erpelding M-C. Clinical assessment instruments in psychiatry. In: Maj M, Gaebel W, López-Ibor JJ, Sartorius N, editors. Psychiatric diagnosis and classification. Chichester: Wiley; 2002.
2. Galanti G-A. Caring for patients from different cultures. Philadelphia: University of Pennsylvania Press; 2004. p. 33–4. http://books.google.com/books?id=nVgeOxUL3cYC&pg=PA34#v=onepage&q&f=false. Accessed 2 Oct 2011.
3. Teal CR, Street RL. Critical elements of culturally competent communication in the medical encounter: a review and model. Soc Sci Med. 2009;68:533–43.

4. Tindall SC. Level of consciousness. In: Walker HK, Hall WD, Hurst JW, editors. Clinical methods: the history, physical, and laboratory examinations. 3rd ed. Boston: Butterworths; 1990. p. 296–9. http://www.ncbi.nlm.nih.gov/books/NBK380/#A1732. Accessed 2 Oct 2011.

5. NINDS. Chorea information page. http://www.ninds.nih.gov/disorders/chorea/chorea.htm. Accessed 2 Oct 2011.

6. NINDS. Sydenham chorea information page. http://www.ninds.nih.gov/disorders/sydenham/sydenham.htm. Accessed 2 Oct 2011.

7. Taylor MA. The neuropsychiatric mental status examination. New York: SP Medical & Scientific Books; 1981. p. 36–8.

8. Sadock BJ, Sadock VA, Ruiz P. Kaplan & Sadock's comprehensive textbook of psychiatry. 9th ed. Philadelphia: Lippincott Williams & Wilkins; 2009. 1083p.

9. Ungvaria GS, Xianga Y-T, Hong Y, et al. Diagnosis of schizophrenia: reliability of an operationalized approach to 'praecox-feeling'. Psychopathology. 2010;43:292–9.

10. Bruehl S, Burns JW, Chung OY, Chont M. Pain-related effects of trait anger expression: neural substrates and the role of endogenous opioid mechanisms. Neurosci Biobehav Rev. 2009;33:475–91.

11. Tsang A, von Korff M, Lee S, et al. Common chronic pain conditions in developed and developing countries: gender and age differences and comorbidity with depression-anxiety disorders. J Pain. 2008;9(10):883–91.

12. Fishbain DA. The association of chronic pain and suicide. Semin Clin Neuropsychiatry. 1999;4(3):221–7.

13. Cheatle MD. Depression, chronic pain, and suicide by overdose: on the edge. Pain Med. 2011;12:S43–8.

14. Edwards RR, Smith MT, Kudel I, Haythornthwaite J. Pain-related catastrophizing as a risk factor for suicidal ideation in chronic pain. Pain. 2006;126:272–9.

15. Ilgen MA, Zivin K, McCammon RJ, Valenstein M. Pain and suicidal thoughts, plans and attempts in the United States. Gen Hosp Psychiatry. 2008;30:521–7.

16. Braden JB, Sullivan MD. Suicidal thoughts and behavior among adults with self-reported pain conditions in the National Comorbidity Survey Replication. J Pain. 2008;9(12):1106–15.

17. Smith MT, Edwards RR, Robinson RC, Dworkin RH. Suicidal ideation, plans, and attempts in chronic pain patients: factors associated with increased risk. Pain. 2004;111:201–8.

18. Tang NKY, Crane C. Suicidality in chronic pain: a review of the prevalence, risk factors and psychological links. Psychol Med. 2006;36:575–86.

19. Gould MS, Frank A, Marrocco FA, Kleinman M, et al. Evaluating iatrogenic risk of youth suicide screening programs: a randomized controlled trial. JAMA. 2005;293(13):1635–43.

20. Fishbain DA, Bruns D, Lewis JE, et al. Predictors of homicide – suicide affirmation in acute and chronic pain patients. Pain Med. 2011;12:127–37.

21. Tarasoff v. Regents of the University of California, 17 Cal. 3d 425, 551 P.2d 334, 131 Cal. Rptr. 14 (Cal. 1976).

22. Mokhlesi B, Leiken JB, Murray P, Corbridge TC. General approach to the intoxicated patient. Part I. Chest. 2003;123:577–92.

23. Crack Cocaine. http://www.cesar.umd.edu/cesar/drugs/crack.asp. Accessed 2 Oct 2011.

24. Mokhlesi B, Leiken JB, Murray P, Corbridge TC. General approach to the intoxicated patient. Part II. Chest. 2003;123:897–922.

25. Examples of medications with anticholinergic properties. In: Center for Medicare and Medicaid Services. State operations manual, appendix PP – Guidance to surveyors for long term care facilities. p. 410–412. https://cms.gov/manuals/Downloads/som107ap_pp_guidelines_ltcf.pdf. Accessed 2 Oct 2011.

26. Folstein MF, Folstein SE, McHugh PR. Mini-mental state. A practical method for grading the cognitive state of patients for the clinician. J Psychiatr Res. 1975;12(3):189–98.

27. DeLuca J, Cicerone KD. Confabulation following aneurysm of the anterior communicating artery. Cortex. 1991;27(3):417–23.

28. Gundogar D, Demirci S. Multiple sclerosis presenting with fantastic confabulation. Gen Hosp Psychiatry. 2006;28(5):448–51.

29. Schnider A. Spontaneous confabulation, reality monitoring, and the limbic system – a review. Brain Res Rev. 2001;36:150–60.

30. Jason LA, Boulton A, Porter NS, et al. Classification of myalgic encephalomyelitis/chronic fatigue syndrome by types of fatigue. Behav Med. 2010;36(1):24–31.

31. Leavitt F, Katz RS. Distraction as a key determinant of impaired memory in patients with fibromyalgia. J Rheumatol. 2006;33(1):127–32.

The Psychological Assessment of Patients with Chronic Pain

Daniel Bruns and John Mark Disorbio

6

Key Points

- There is strong evidence that the biopsychosocial model does not apply only to dysfunctional patients with chronic pain, but rather represents the inherent nature of pain.
- There is strong evidence that psychological tests are scientifically as valid and reliable as medical tests with regard to diagnostics and predicting a patient's response to treatments for pain.
- As many payors and guidelines require psychological evaluations prior to authorizing certain treatments for pain, pain clinics increasingly use some form of psychological assessment.
- While there are a large number of psychometric questionnaires used to assess patients with chronic pain, only a few have undergone the rigorous process required to become standardized tests, and these are reviewed.
- Both evidence and opinion are converging on a set of psychosocial variables that should be assessed when treating patients with chronic pain, and these can all be organized within a biopsychosocial "vortex" paradigm.
- A standardized method of psychological assessment can identify patients who are at low, moderate, and high risk, and this is illustrated with three case vignettes.

D. Bruns, PsyD (✉)
Health Psychology Associates, 1610 29th Avenue Place, Suite 200, Greeley, CO 80634, USA
e-mail: daniel.bruns@healthpsych.com

J.M. Disorbio, EdD
Independent Practice, 225 Union Blvd. Suite 150, Lakewood, CO 80228, USA
e-mail: jmdisorbio@earthlink.net

Introduction

There is strong evidence that the biopsychosocial model does not apply only to dysfunctional patients with chronic pain, but rather represents the inherent nature of pain. Research has determined that psychological tests are scientifically as valid and reliable as medical tests with regard to diagnostics and predicting a patient's response to treatments for pain. As many payers and guidelines now require psychological evaluations prior to authorizing certain treatments for pain, pain clinics increasingly use some form of psychological assessment. While there are a large number of psychometric questionnaires used to assess patients with chronic pain, only a few have undergone the rigorous process required to become standardized tests, and these are reviewed. Both evidence and opinion are converging on a set of psychosocial variables that should be assessed when treating patients with chronic pain, and these can all be organized within a biopsychosocial "vortex" paradigm. A standardized method of psychological assessment can identify patients who are at low, moderate, and high risk, and this is illustrated with three case vignettes.

A review of the research reveals strong evidence that pain is a biopsychosocial phenomena, having biological, psychological, and social components [2, 3]. In addition to biological components of pain being the product of pathophysiology, the experience and report of pain are also strongly influenced by psychosocial factors. As the IASP notes, while pain often has a physical cause, pain can also occur in the absence of any likely pathophysiological explanation. Further, since pain is a subjective, psychological state, we are dependent on the patient's report of pain to guide our treatments [1]. However, there are a variety of psychological and social variables that affect what patients say about their pain.

T.R. Deer et al. (eds.), *Treatment of Chronic Pain by Integrative Approaches: the AMERICAN ACADEMY of PAIN MEDICINE Textbook on Patient Management*, DOI 10.1007/978-1-4939-1821-8_6,
© American Academy of Pain Medicine 2015

The Natural History of Biopsychosocial Pain Disorders

The biopsychosocial model does not apply only to dysfunctional patients with chronic pain, but rather represents the inherent nature of pain [2, 3]. Over the natural history of chronic pain disorders, the biological, psychological, and social aspects of these conditions interact in complex ways. Some psychosocial factors may lead to the onset of a pain condition, while others may arise as a reaction to a pain condition. The subsequent medical treatment of chronic pain may also be complicated by interactions with preexisting psychological vulnerabilities or conflicts in the social environment. Thus, complex biopsychosocial pain disorders do not simply appear, but rather tend to evolve over the course of their natural history.

Psychosocial Factors That Lead to the Onset of Pain Conditions

A variety of psychosocial factors have been associated with the onset of a variety of medical painful conditions (Fig. 6.1). Life stress has been associated with the onset of musculoskeletal pain [4, 5] and functional gastrointestinal pain [6], and one prospective study of workers found that the variable most predictive of the future report of back pain was job dissatisfaction [7].

Psychological dysfunction can also lead to the onset of painful conditions. A systematic review of the literature determined that risk-taking is influenced by mood and personality disorder, and associated with an increased chance of injury [8], while another study determined that risk-taking is influenced by personality type [9]. One study found that half of all traumatic brain injury hospitalizations were associated with alcohol intoxication [10], while another study found that patients reporting drug or alcohol abuse were more likely to sustain violent injuries [11]. Consequently, it is not surprising that some research has found that the prevalence of substance abuse disorders in patients with chronic pain is twice as high as that observed in the normal population [12]. Another study of patients being treated in an interventional pain medicine setting explored the prevalence of substance abuse problems. Of those patients with a prior history of drug abuse, 34 % of those who were being treated with controlled substances for pain were simultaneously abusing illicit drugs [13].

Overall, a multitude of psychosocial variables may influence lifestyle, risk-taking behaviors, and health habits that can act to increase or decrease the risk of onset of a medical condition.

Psychological Reactions to a Pain Condition

Serious illness and injury are often life-altering conditions, with a profound psychosocial impact (Fig. 6.1). Not surprisingly, in a study of patients with pain-related disability, 64 % reported one or more diagnosable psychiatric disorders, compared to a prevalence of 15 % in the general population. In this sample, the prevalence of major depression was 25 times higher than that seen in the general population. This finding is especially significant as even minimal levels of depression have been associated with increased rates of service utilization [14] and poorer adherence to treatment [15]. In many cases, though, the direction of the arrow of causality is not clear. For example, while in some cases, depression could be a reaction to a severe injury, in other cases, depression that preexisted an injury may increase the risk that the pain will become chronic [16].

Pain can alternately be associated with anxiety, depression, or anger, depending upon how pain is perceived [17]. Laboratory experiments in pain perception suggest that the presence of depression tends to magnify the perception of pain [18]. Additionally, affective distress combines with pain to produce suffering, and ultimately, this suffering may be more closely associated with the patient's level of functioning than is the pain itself [19]. Research also suggests that a number of other psychological variables are associated with poor treatment outcome. These include anger [20, 21], neuroticism [22], psychological distress [23–27], relationship with spouse [28, 29], positive or negative perceptions prior to treatment [30–32], maladaptive beliefs [33, 34], and fears of reinjury [31].

Psychological Vulnerability Risk Factors

A review of the literature on psychopathology and chronic pain concluded that psychological vulnerabilities of various types could both increase the risk of onset of chronic pain, plus shape how the pain disorder was manifested. This review also concluded that the dominant emerging perspective is that preexisting but dormant vulnerabilities of the individual may be activated by the stress of an illness or injury [35]. If this proves to be true, this would mean that some patients are inherently at increased risk for disability, but this vulnerability may not appear until an environmental event precipitates it. Consequently, understanding preexisting vulnerabilities is an important part of chronic pain assessment (Fig. 6.1).

If a person who is prone to chemical dependency becomes injured, any subsequent pain could become a rationalization for excessive opioid use [36, 37]. Under such circumstances, the possibility of opioid abuse must be addressed [38]. Similarly, patients may be at increased risk for excessive opioid abuse if they are pain intolerant or feel entitled to be

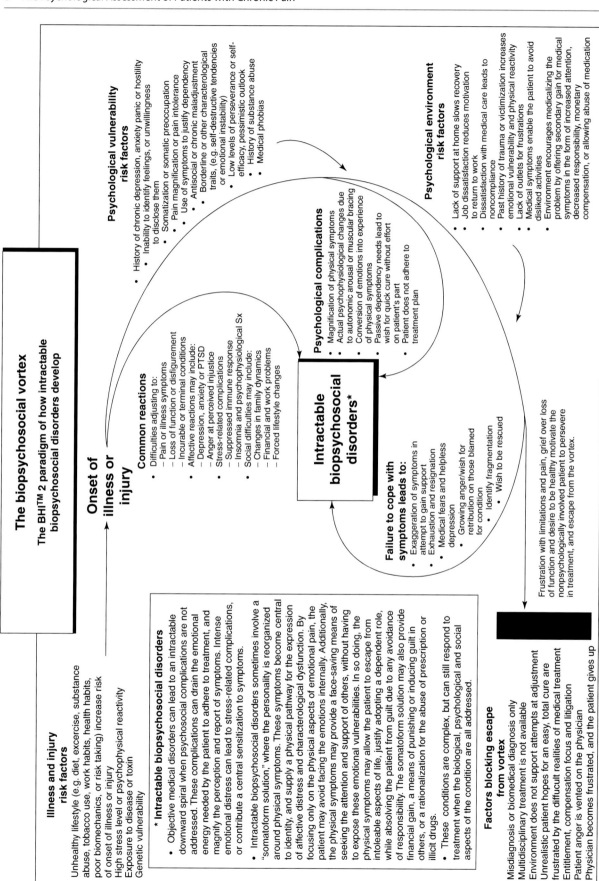

Fig. 6.1 A variety of psychosocial factors have been associated with the onset of intractable chronic pain (Biopsychosocial Vortex © 2008 by Daniel Bruns, PsyD and John Mark Disorbio, EdD. All Rights Reserved. Reprinted with permission. BHI 2 © 2003 by Pearson Assessments)

pain-free [39]. Although concerns about regulatory scrutiny can sometimes complicate the clinical decision-making process when prescribing opioids, carefully designed interdisciplinary programs can successfully treat patients at risk for addiction [38, 40]. One study found that patients with histories of substance abuse report higher levels of pain [41], and so distinguishing true pain from drug-seeking behavior becomes a matter of great importance [42]. Related to this, a review of the research determined that positive scores on substance abuse screening measures could identify patients who were at significantly higher risk for aberrant drug-related behaviors in treatment [43].

Patients with personality disorders may have an aberrant reaction to pain and may be at increased risk for chronicity. This hypothesis is supported by five studies of patients with chronic pain. These studies found the prevalence rate of personality disorders to range from 40 to 77 % [12, 16, 44–46], far higher than the estimated 5.9–13.5 % prevalence rate found in the general population [47]. However, a recent study reviewed psychological characteristics of patients with chronic pain and determined that a decrease in pain tends to produce a decrease in signs of personality disorder as well [48]. Thus, dysfunctional traits observed in patients with chronic pain may be partially attributable to the destabilizing effect of pain rather than to an enduring personality disorder. This suggests that estimates of personality disorders in patients with chronic pain could be spuriously inflated.

Non-characterological personality traits or cognitive styles can also constitute risk factors for recovery. For example, patients who are prone to catastrophizing [49, 50] have a low sense of self-efficacy [51], and who are prone to pessimism [52] are at risk for failing to make needed behavioral changes and for generally poor functioning. Conversely, positive personality traits such as perseverance have been found to be associated with favorable outcomes from pain conditions [53]. In general, a history of maladjustment [28], low educational level [54], or the presence of a personality disorder can undermine a patient's ability to cope satisfactorily with an illness or injury, increase the risk of noncompliance, and thus increase the risk of delayed recovery [47, 55]. Severe psychopathology may sometimes affect pain reports in mysterious ways. For example, patients with dissociative disorders often present with psychogenic pain symptoms [56, 57], and in patients with dissociative identity disturbance (multiple personality), each personality may manifest different pain and disability symptoms [58, 59].

Social Environment Risk Factors

Environmental stressors are known to be associated with numerous psychophysiological reactions (Fig. 6.1). A patient's social environment includes relationships with family, friends, professionals in the medical setting, and supervisors and coworkers in the workplace. The onset of a disabling condition can stress the family system [60, 61] and leads to family conflicts if the disability prevents the patient from performing expected family responsibilities [62, 63]. The problems arising from these changes can be overcome if the patient is a member of a healthy, supportive family. However, in response to disability, an overly solicitous family may reinforce patient passivity and encourage the patient to adopt a disabled role [64, 65], while a dysfunctional family may exacerbate a patient's condition.

For example, patients who have experienced adverse childhood experiences, such as childhood abuse, have been found to exhibit increased pituitary-adrenal and autonomic responses to stress compared with controls [66–71] and suppressed immunological resistance to cancer and infection [72–74]. These findings may help to explain the association between stress and poor surgical outcome [75], increased mortality [76–78], and slowed speed of wound recovery [79, 80] observed in numerous studies. Consistent with this, studies have found that psychological traumas in childhood are associated with a poor treatment outcome [75, 81].

Within the medical setting, research has found that the therapeutic alliance between the physician and the patient strongly influences the course of treatment [82, 83]. If the physician is perceived as competent and empathic, a positive relationship can develop. This can facilitate the flow of information between physician and patient and promote patient compliance. In contrast, these studies have found that a poor physician/patient relationship can complicate the recovery process and increase the risk of noncompliance. A history of physical or sexual abuse has also been found to increase the risk of delayed recovery [84, 85], as patients reporting a history of assault may feel more physically vulnerable, exhibit more stress-related symptomatology, and resist examinations that they find threatening [86].

Disability is most often considered in the context of the patient's ability to be gainfully employed. Consequently, the psychological assessment of disability needs to be especially sensitive to social aspects of the workplace that could influence disability behaviors. For example, escape from a disliked workplace environment may offer considerable secondary gain for the report of medical symptoms, and this may influence the course of recovery. In a longitudinal, prospective study of back pain, job dissatisfaction was determined to be the strongest predictor of future back pain reports [87]. This suggests that the avoidance of a disliked workplace may be a powerful negative reinforcer for both pain and disability behaviors [29].

In addition to avoidance of an aversive workplace, other types of reinforcers are also present in the social environment. Studies have shown that both litigation [88–93] and compensation play a role in treatment outcome [25, 88, 90, 92, 94–98]. In some contexts, an injury can socially empower a patient or increase the attention and support from others. Pain can cause the patient to be assigned to lighter job tasks in the workplace or avoid undesirable chores at home. However, once disability appears, the inability of the patient to function in the workplace often leads to financial distress [99] and a continuation of a downward spiral. Overall, it is not surprising that psychosocial variables have been found to be important predictors of the cost of medical treatment [100].

The lack of English proficiency can impact treatment outcome and disability [101] in a number of ways. The inability to speak English in the USA can make it much more difficult to communicate with caregivers, understand how to fill out paperwork, or in other ways access care. In the immigrant community, though, the effects of a lack of English proficiency may be confounded by a low level of education, and low education has been found to be a separate risk factor for poor medical treatment outcome [54].

Etiologically, while some biopsychosocial disorders have their origin in biology or pathophysiology, others have psychosocial origins. Thus, the assessment of biopsychosocial conditions requires not only assessing biomedical variables but also assessing the psychosocial aspects as well. These assessments are facilitated by the use of psychometric tools.

The Psychological Assessment of Patients with Pain

In a survey performed in 1996, some type of psychological screening was performed in about 70 % of surveyed pain clinics using implantable devices [102]. Since that time, multiple evidence-based medical guidelines have recommended psychological evaluation prior to SCS [103–105], and many insurers now require psychological assessment prior to implantation. More generally, multiple evidence-based medicine guidelines now recommend psychological evaluation for all patients with chronic pain [103–105]. As a result, a similar survey in 2005 found that 100 % of surveyed clinics used some type of psychological assessment for patients being considered for implantable devices for pain [106].

The reason for the increased use of psychological tests for patients with pain is the growing evidence of their utility. A recent extensive review of the literature compared the scientific merits of psychological tests to traditional medical tests [107]. After reviewing 125 meta-analyses and 800 samples, this seminal study concluded that psychological tests are scientifically as good as medical tests and can sometimes predict the outcome of medical treatment as well as medical tests. Specifically, this study of psychological tests concluded that (a) there is strong evidence for psychological test validity, (b) the evidence for psychological test validity is comparable to that of medical tests, (c) psychological test provides a unique source of information, and (d) psychological tests supply information beyond what can be obtained by an interview.

In the assessment of patients with back pain, psychological tests are sometimes stronger predictors of treatment outcome than medical tests. For example, a recent study found that psychometric assessment was better than either MRIs or discography in predicting future back pain disability [108] while another study found that psychosocial variables predicted delayed recovery from back pain correctly 91 % of the time, without using any medical diagnostic information [109]. Multiple research studies have shown that psychosocial factors can predict the results of lumbar surgery [28, 54, 75, 90, 110, 111] or spinal cord stimulation [112] correctly over 80 % of the time, and there is evidence that protocols which integrate psychological and medical assessments can provide improved care at reduced cost [196]. Beyond back pain, research sponsored by the World Health Organization found that psychopathology was a stronger contributor to disability than was disease severity [113].

Psychological Testing Concepts

Psychological tests are developed using the science of psychometrics, which is a mathematical approach to measuring intangible human abilities (such as intelligence or memory), traits (such as personality), and subjective experiences (such as sadness or pain). Bruns and Warren have noted that the science of psychometrics is less esoteric than it would first appear:

> Although psychometrics sounds mysterious, it is a science that Western society has come to rely on heavily. Perhaps the most common example of this is that on almost every edition of the news on television, the results of a poll are reported. Scientific surveys, which employ psychometric principals, have an established ability to accurately predict the sentiments of a population, with a known degree of error. In manner analogous to the way that scientific questioning of voters can assess their subjective opinions and predict voting behavior, standardized psychometric instruments can assess subjective states in patients that predict disability [114].

To use an analogy, before a medication is ready for clinical use, rigorous scientific testing is needed to show that it is safe and effective. Similarly, before a psychological test is ready for clinical use, it should be psychometrically *standardized*. While informal questionnaires may be developed without any scientific method at all, a standardized psychological test is developed using the psychometric principles outlined in a work called the *Standards for Educational and Psychological Testing* [115]. When a questionnaire has been developed to meet the criteria listed in the *Standards*, it is said to be a *standardized test*. Standardized tests offer an efficient and scientific means of gathering information about psychological, social, and medical variables.

To illustrate the impact of a lack of standardization, consider the numerical pain rating scale. Although it may have been used in over 1,000 research studies, it is not standardized, and the following clinical vignette illustrates the effect of this: Suppose a clinician asks a patient, "On a 1–10 scale, how would you rate your pain?" How should the clinician respond if the patient responds with the following questions:

1. What is a pain level of 10? My other doctor defines a pain level of 10 as pain like having a baby, but you say it is pain so bad I want to die. Which one is correct?
2. Rate my pain from 1 to 10? Does 1 mean no pain, or is that 0? Should I rate my pain from 0 to 10?
3. Do you mean my back pain, my leg pain, or my headaches? Or do you want the average of all three? Or maybe the highest?
4. Do you mean right this second while I am sitting? As soon as I stand up, it is worse.
5. My pain is a 5 – Is that high? What does the average patient say?

Since the numerical pain rating scale is not standardized, there is no test manual to supply the correct answer to the above questions. Consequently, the clinician could respond to the questions in any number of ways, and this would significantly influence which number the patient chooses to describe the pain. As a result, it has been noted that without a more rigorous method, scores returned by measures such as informal pain rating scales are essentially meaningless [116]. In contrast, with a standardized measure of pain like the BBHI 2, all of the above questions would have a definitive answer [117]. This illustrates the advantage of standardized tests. By imposing a carefully standardized method of asking questions, scoring the responses in a standardized way, and having a norm group to which the scores can be compared, a much more meaningful result is obtained.

Characteristics of a Standardized Test

The characteristics of standardized tests are defined in the *Standards for Educational and Psychological Testing*, which states that standardized psychological tests are characterized by having a number of features:

1. Standardized tests are developed to be used for a defined purpose and may have less applicability outside of that purpose.
2. A standardized test reduces error by having standardized testing materials, standardized administration procedures, standardized instructions, and standardized scoring and interpretation methods, and may even require a standardized type of writing instrument, such as a #2 pencil.
3. A standardized test must have evidence of validity, demonstrating that the test measures what it intends to measure (e.g., the report of medication side effects such as fatigue and weight gain can cause false-positive findings for depression on some psychological tests).

4. A standardized test must have evidence of reliability, demonstrating that if the test is administered twice in a short time frame, the results will be very similar.
5. Standardized tests use one or more reference groups called norm groups, which make it possible to have standardized scores with percentile ranks.
6. A standardized test takes steps to eliminate gender, race, age, and other biases.
7. A standardized test has an official manual that has recorded the psychometric details of the standardization process and provides the information needed to use the test appropriately.
8. The content of standardized tests is controlled by copyright and other methods and cannot be modified by end users, as this would destroy the standardization.
9. Standardized tests are subject to test security or trade secret restrictions, keeping the details of the test confidential (e.g., if the answers on an I.Q. test were made public, a test subject could appear to be a genius by studying the answers beforehand, and this would invalidate the test).

In addition to meeting the criteria specified by the *standards*, others have suggested that a standardized psychological test should also be peer reviewed, either by the Mental Measurements Yearbook [105, 118] or in a scientific journal [118].

What Psychosocial Variables Need to Be Assessed in Patients with Chronic Pain?

A recent review proposed what it termed the "convergent model" of biopsychosocial assessment. The term "convergent model" was intended to reflect that while at this time the field has yet to achieve any final determinations about how to perform biopsychosocial assessments, evidence and opinion are beginning to converge [119]. This review identified both cautionary risk factors or "yellow flags" (Table 6.1) and exclusionary risk factors or "red flags" (Table 6.2), and these risk factors were organized within the framework of a biopsychosocial paradigm (Fig. 6.1). Exclusionary risk factors were defined as extreme concerns (e.g., imminent risk of suicide or homicide, active psychosis, or intoxicated at medical appointments), any one of which could be sufficient to delay or exclude a patient from elective medical treatment. In contrast, cautionary risk factors were less extreme concerns (e.g., depression, poor pain tolerance), which, in combination, could negatively impact prognosis.

The convergent model was tested using 2264 US subjects obtained from 106 sites, and the demographics of the norm groups approximated US census data for gender, race, education, and age. The risk factors identified by the convergent model were assessed in a standardized manner, using the Battery for Health Improvement 2 [120] and the shorter Brief

Table 6.1 "Yellow flag" cautionary risk factors suggested by literature review

Type of risk	Potential cautionary factors	
Affective	Depression	
	Anger	
	Anxiety (fears, phobias, PTSD, etc.)	
Psychological vulnerability	History of substance abuse	
	Personality disorder	
	Cognitive disorder or low education	
	Poor coping	
	Diffuse somatic complaints	
Social	Conflict with physicians	
	Job dissatisfaction	
	Family dysfunction	
	History of being abused	
	Worker compensation	
	Compensation focus	
	Represented by attorney	
Biological	Pain and disability	Extreme pain
	Pain sensitivity	Dysfunctional pain cognitions
	Pain invariance	Diffuse pain
		Pain > 2 years
		Unexplained disability
	Exam	Degree to which patient does not meet medical criteria for procedure
		No medical necessity of procedure to preserve life or function
		Destructive/high-risk elective medical procedure
		Procedure specific risks: smoking, diet, attitude toward implant, etc.
	History	Similar procedure failed previously
		No response to any treatment
		History of nonadherence to conservative care
		No objective medical findings
	Science	Insufficient evidence that the proposed medical treatment would be effective

Adapted from Bruns and Disorbio [121]

Battery for Health Improvement 2 [117]. US national norms for the prevalence of these risk scores were generated for two groups: community members and patients with a variety of diagnoses being treated in a variety of treatment settings. The norms obtained from these samples allowed the calculation of a risk score percentile rank, which was used to establish empirical benchmarks. This made it possible to answer the question, at what point can the risk factors present be regarded as clinically elevated [119]? Using this method, standardized cautionary risk and exclusionary risk scores were shown to predict both work status and satisfaction with care for patients in multiple treatment groups (spinal surgery, upper extremity surgery, brain injury, work hardening, chronic pain, acute injury, and injured litigants). Repeat testing showed these risk scores demonstrated test-retest reliabilities ranging from 0.85 to 0.91, with no indications of race or gender bias.

Commonly Used Tests for Assessing Patients with Chronic Pain

There are a large number of psychometric tests and questionnaires commonly used to assess patients with chronic pain [121]. When determining what psychological tests to review here, a number of factors were taken into consideration. One evidence-based panel concluded that a psychological test battery for the evaluation of patients with chronic pain would include one or more tests designed for the assessment of medical patients with pain and one or more tests of personality and psychopathology [105]. With regard to selecting each of these types of tests, we would suggest the following criteria, which are that the tests (a) are standardized measures, (b) have been peer reviewed by the Burrows Institute of Mental Measures, (c) have been the subject of multiple empirical research articles in peer-reviewed journals, (d) have

Table 6.2 "Red flag" exclusionary risk factors suggested by literature review

Type of risk		Potential exclusionary factors
Affective		Active suicidal urges
		Active homicidal urges
		Severe depression
		Severe anxiety (generalized, panic, PTSD, medical phobia/death fears, etc.)
		Severe anger
		Mood elevation/mania
Other psychological risks		Psychosis/delusions/hallucinations
		Active substance abuse
		Severe somatization
		Pain-focused somatoform disorder
		Severe personality disorder
		Extremely poor coping
		Severe social isolation, family dysfunction, or current severe abuse
Social		Litigation for pain and suffering and pain-related treatment
		Intense doctor/patient conflict
Biological	Pain	Bizarre pain reports
		Dysfunctional pain cognitions
		Extreme, invariant pain
		Extreme pain sensitivity
	Exam	Medically impossible symptoms
		Gross inconsistencies between objective findings, symptom reports, and patient behavior
		Falsifying information, malingering, or factitious symptoms
		Inability to cooperate with treatment due to cognitive or other problems
	History	Same treatment failed multiple times in past
		Abuse of prescription medications, violation of opioid contracts
		History of gross noncompliance
	Science	Evidence that the proposed medical treatment would be injurious or ineffective given the circumstances

Adapted from Bruns and Disorbio [121]

been vetted by multiple evidence-based medicine panels reviewing the psychological assessment of chronic pain, (e) [if a pain-related measure] should have been designed and developed for pain assessment, and (f) [if a pain-related measure] should have standardized scores based on a norm group consisting of medical patients, and especially medical patients suffering from chronic pain. Reviews of other psychological tests for pain assessment are available elsewhere [105, 121, 122].

When you apply these criteria to measures of personality and psychopathology, four tests are identified. These are the MMPI-2, MMPI-2-RF, MCMI-III, and the PAI. If you apply these criteria to measures used for the assessment of medical patients and chronic pain, the tests identified are the BBHI 2, the BHI 2, the BSI-18, the MBMD, and the P-3.

The Three MMPIs

The three MMPI (Minnesota Multiphasic Personality Inventory) tests are arguably the most used and most researched psychological tests in existence. The original MMPI™ was published in 1943 and remained in use until the MMPI-2™ was published 1986, after which the original MMPI was phased out [123, 124]. Over the last sev-

eral decades, the MMPI (and to a lesser degree, the MMPI-2) has been used in numerous studies related to patients with chronic pain and surgical outcome. Overall, the MMPI-2 is currently the most widely used measure of psychopathology and is also a well-researched measure of malingering. With regard to the evaluation of patients with pain and injury, the MMPI/MMPI-2 have historically been the most commonly recommended tests [28, 33, 125–129].

However, the MMPI-2 (Minnesota Multiphasic Personality Inventory-2) also has a number of significant weaknesses. First of all, the MMPI-2 scales are aging and are based on archaic psychiatric constructs dating back to the 1930s, such as hysteria, psychopathic deviate, and psychasthenia. Secondly, the MMPI was developed in a time when much less was known about psychometrics and test construction. As a result, all of the clinical scales contained items that later research concluded should not have been on the scale [130].Third, it has been noted that the MMPI-2 is a lengthy test [126], sometimes prohibitively so [125], as it commonly takes up to 90 min to administer [131], and it takes considerable skill to interpret [126]. Fourth, as the MMPI-2 is not normed or designed for patients with pain, it is prone to overpathologize them [126], especially on its primary scales for assessing depression and somatization [127]. Fifth, despite the length of the MMPI-2, it does not assess many of the variables relevant to medical patients and must be combined with other measures for chronic pain assessment. To this end, Block et al. recommends that the MMPI-2 be used with three other tests [125], Burchiel et al. employed the MMPI-2 and five other tests [33], Doleys and Olson discussed the use of the MMPI-2 and seven other tests [126], Beltrutti et al. discussed the MMPI-2 and eight other tests [129], and Olson et al. employed the MMPI-2 and 10 other tests [128]. Given that the MMPI-2 is already a long test, this makes for a very lengthy test battery.

After much debate, the MMPI-2-RF™ (Minnesota Multiphasic Personality Inventory-2-Revised Form) was published in 2008 [130, 132]. This test has been called a radical departure from the MMPI-2 [133]. While most of the MMPI-2-RF scales were derived from MMPI-2 scales, none are identical, many are markedly different, while others are totally new [130, 132]. In addition to about 80 measures of psychopathology, the MMPI-2 has 15 "validity scales" used to detect exaggerating or concealing information. In contrast, the MMPI-2-RF has 50 scales including eight validity scales. The term "validity scale" is used to convey that these scales attempt to determine if the patient's test responses are valid representations of his or her true feelings or if the patient is attempting to "fake" or appear better or worse than he or she actually is by biasing the information that is presented [114]. The goal of the MMPI-2-RF development was to address the MMPI-2 shortcomings mentioned above and produce a shorter and more psychometrically sound test. Unfortunately, while there were 60 years of research on the original MMPI/MMPI-2 scales, the changed scales in the MMPI-2-RF mean that these decades of research have at best only moderate applicability to the MMPI-2-RF test.

The difference between the MMPI-2 and the MMPI-2-RF is illustrated in one study of 7,330 patients, which found that the "code type" (traditionally used to determine how the test was interpreted) agreed only 14.6 % of the time [134]. Additionally, research suggests that the MMPI-2 is substantially more likely to return a profile suggestive of psychopathology [134] or somatoform disorder [135] than the MMPI-2-RF. Overall, even though these two tests share the same name, it is probably better to think of the MMPI-2-RF as a distinctly different test. At the date of this writing, no published studies were found that utilized the MMPI-2-RF to assess patients with chronic pain. Further, it has been noted that the MMPI-2-RF Revised Clinical Scales were optimized for psychiatric assessment, and without consideration for use with medical patients or assessing somatic symptoms, possibly making them less useful for that purpose than the MMPI-2 [135]. Overall, while the relative merits of the MMPI-2 and the MMPI-2-RF tests remain the subject of ongoing debate [136, 137], both tests will likely remain popular measures of psychopathology.

The MCMI-III

The MCMI-III™ (Millon Clinical Multiaxial Inventory III) is another widely used measure of general psychopathology [138]. One of the MCMI-III's most distinctive features is that among its 25 scales are scales for the assessment of a variety of types of personality disorders, which is helpful for differential diagnosis. While the MCMI-III has the distinct advantage that its scales are keyed to DSM-IV diagnostic criteria, this will be less of an advantage once DSM-5 is released.

A feature of the MCMI-III that could be seen as either a strength or a weakness is its utilization of what are called "base rate" scores. These scales employ a psychometric method where a base rate score of above 75 suggests that some aspects of a syndrome are present, while base rates scores above 85 suggest that the full syndrome is present. While this represents an advantage in some respects, on the negative side, this psychometric method is not based on the normal curve and cannot be used to generate a percentile rank. This makes it somewhat more difficult to identify statistical outliers, but easier to identify the degree to which a particular syndrome might be present. Another feature is three validity scales and one measure random responding.

With regard to its applicability to patients with chronic pain, there is some research on the MCMI-III with regard to its use with chronic pain patients [139–141]. However, it was developed with and normed on psychiatric patients. Consequently, while the MCMI-III is a valuable measure of psychopathology, it must be remembered that like the MMPI-2 and MMPI-2-RF, its use with patients with objective physical disease or injury may lead to spuriously elevated scales scores, as patient reports of physical symptoms may inflate some of its measures of psychopathology.

The PAI

The PAI™ (Personality Assessment Inventory) is also a popular measure of general psychopathology. Psychometrically, the PAI is a carefully constructed measure, whose 22 scales assess a broad cross section of affective, characterlogical, and psychotic conditions. Like the MMPI-2, the PAI uses standardized T-scores based on community norms, which allows it to identify statistical outliers. The PAI, however, is substantially shorter than the MMPI-2, about the length of the MMPI-2-RF, but considerably longer than the MCMI-III. The PAI has four validity scales.

Some research has studied the applicability of the PAI to assess chronic pain patients [142, 143]. Like other psychological inventories designed for assessing psychiatric patients, it utilizes items about physical symptoms to diagnose depression, anxiety, and other conditions. Consequently, as with the MMPIs and the MCMI-III, it will tend to overestimate some forms of psychopathology in patients with chronic pain.

Psychological Measures for Medical Patients

As noted above, while the MMPIs, the MCMI-III, and the PAI are well-established measures of psychopathology, they are at risk for overestimating psychopathology when used with medical patients. One reason that this happens has been called the "psychological fallacy" [117], which is a problem that occurs when psychological measures intended for psychiatric patients are given to medical patients.

Most psychological tests of psychiatric conditions utilize items about physical symptoms. For example, a measure of depression might contain items about psychological symptoms (e.g., negative thoughts and sad feelings) and physical symptoms as well (e.g., fatigue, loss of libido, changes in weight). However, it has been noted that physical symptoms of this type can also be the product of injury, disease, or medication side effects. Thus, when patients report their medical symptoms on such measures, it can spuriously increase their scores on measures of psychiatric conditions. This is true not only of the MMPIs, MCMI-III, and PAI but also other common measures such as the Beck Depression Inventory [144]. In contrast, a few tests, such as the State Trait Anxiety Inventory [145] or the Battery for Health Improvement 2 [120], control this problem by avoiding the use of items containing physical symptoms to assess emotions. Another important difference in psychological measures designed for medical patients is that they are normed on medical patients, rather than psychiatric patients or community members. By comparing a patient to a group of other patients, it is much easier to identify the unusual, at risk patient [105].

The BHI 2

The BHI 2™ (Battery for Health Improvement 2) is a test designed for the biopsychosocial assessment of medical patients [120]. This test had its origins in a biopsychosocial paradigm (Fig. 6.1) and as such attempts to assess the medical, psychological, and social aspects of a patient's condition. A strength of the BHI 2 is its norms, which include both patient and community samples. Beyond this, however, the patient norms are broken down into a number of subcategories. About half of the BHI 2 patient norm group consisted of patients with acute injury or other conditions, while the other half consisted of patients with chronic conditions including patients with orthopedic injury, brain injury, headache, fibromyalgia, CRPS, and other conditions. Further, diagnosis-specific pain norms were developed for six groups, which were chronic pain, lower extremity injury, low back injury, upper extremity injury, neck injury, headache, and head injury. This allowed for many patients' pain reports to be compared to other patients in their own diagnostic category. While the BHI 2 uses pain norms for a variety of injury types, other aspects of the BHI 2 were designed to assess conditions unrelated to injury, such as somatic preoccupation

and somatization, death fears, the perception of addiction to prescription medication, the tendency to become physically tense when under stress, the perception of disability, and negative attitudes toward physicians that have been found to be associated with thoughts of litigation [146, 147] and violence [148, 149]. Additionally, in order to avoid the psychological fallacy, the BHI 2's 18 scales and 40 subscales assess the thoughts and feelings associated with depression and anxiety separately from the physical symptoms associated with depression and anxiety. Overall, since the BHI 2 was designed to assess medical patients in general and patients with chronic pain in particular, it assesses most of the risk factors identified in the literature [119]. The BHI 2 has a measure of random responding and two bidirectional validity scales, giving it two measures of exaggerating complaints and two measures of concealing information.

Weaknesses of the BHI 2 include that while it assesses some aspects of psychopathology, especially relevant to medical patients, it was not intended to assess the breadth of psychiatric conditions assessed by inventories designed for psychiatric patients. For example, it uses only critical items to assess psychosis and makes no attempt to assess mania, obsessive-compulsive disorder, and some other types of severe psychopathology. Additionally, while there is a growing body of BHI 2 research related to chronic pain [39, 119, 146–161], its research base is not as extensive as that of the MMPI/MMPI-2.

The MBMD

The MBMD™ (Millon Behavioral Medicine Diagnostic) is a psychological test designed for use with medical patients [162]. Like the BHI 2, the MBMD is theory driven, being based in part on Millon's "Evolution-based Personality Theory" [163], with the resulting coping styles being applied to the medical setting. The MBMD could be said to be the psychometric cousin of the MCMI-III, as it adapts many of the MCMI-III scales for use in a medical setting. Like the MCMI-III, the MBMD uses base rate scores. As with the MCMI-III, the strength of this approach is that it attempts to identify patients above a certain level of symptomatology, at the expense of being unable to identify statistical outliers or generate a percentile rank. The MBMD differs from the MCMI-III, however, in that while the MCMI-III attempts to assess psychopathology, the MBMD is designed to assess less extreme aspects of the same constructs that are likely to be observed in a nonpsychiatric population. For example, while the MCMI-III has a scale measuring schizoid tendencies, a similar scale on the MBMD assesses introversive tendencies.

The MBMD is a test designed for medical patients and was constructed using patients with heart disease, diabetes, HIV, and neurological problems. However, only 9 % of patients in the original patient normative group were reported to be suffering from chronic pain. More recently, bariatric and chronic pain norms for this test were also developed. The MBMD pain patient computerized interpretive report displays both the original general medical norm profile using *base rate* scores and a pain patient norm profile using *normative* scores. This produces a pain patient profile that is far less elevated than that produced by the original norm groups and adds a measure of complexity to the interpretation. Perhaps because of this, the pain patient interpretive report continues to be based on the original general medical norms. At the time of this writing, no research studies were found that applied the MBMD to patients with chronic pain.

The MBMD's 38 scales excel at describing the patient's coping style, health habits, potential for certain types of negative reactions to treatment, and factors which may potentiate the patient's distress. It also excels at the psychological assessment of medical patients who are more or less psychologically normal and is also unique in that it offers a brief assessment of spiritual resources for coping. The MBMD also has three validity measures for assessing a patient's test-taking attitude.

The BBHI 2

The BBHI 2™ (Brief Battery for Health Improvement 2) is a short (10-min) version of the BHI 2. The BBHI 2's six scales measure a number of concerns commonly seen in medical patients and especially those with chronic pain: depression, anxiety, somatization, pain, functioning, and utilization of the same norms as the BHI 2 [117]. With regard to pain, the BBHI 2 assesses pain preoccupation, pain tolerance, pain location, pain variability, and dysfunctional pain cognitions. Additionally, it uses critical items to screen for 15 other concerns such as satisfaction with care, home life problems, addiction, psychosis, sleep disorders, panic, compensation focus, and suicidality.

A strength of the BBHI 2 is that it assesses a wide variety of risk factors in a short amount of time [119] and it is the shortest psychological inventory to have validity measures for exaggerating, concealing information, and random responding, and a critical item for psychosis as well. In addition to being used diagnostically, the BBHI 2 can also be used in a serial fashion to track changes in pain, function, depression, anxiety, and somatic distress over the course of time in treatment. A weakness of the BBHI 2 is that outside of its core scales, it screens for a number of concerns using critical items, which is a less reliable method than that which can be obtained with a longer instrument.

The P-3

The P-3™ (Pain Patient Profile) is a short measure useful within pain practices [164]. The strength of the P-3 is its parsimony. The P-3 assesses three critically important variables: depression, anxiety, and somatization. Although the P-3 is tightly focused on these three scales, one strength is that

these scales have unusually high reliability. Another strength is that the P-3 utilizes both chronic pain and community norms in interpreting these scales. The appeal of the P-3 is its elegant simplicity, the strength of its norms, and its intended use with patients with chronic pain. The P-3 also has a growing base of empirical research studies pertaining to chronic pain [141, 165–173]. The primary weakness of the P-3 is that there are many risk factors it does not assess, such as coping, pain, functioning, and substance abuse.

The BSI-18

The BSI-18® (Brief Symptom Inventory 18) [174] is an 18-item version of the much longer Brief Symptom Inventory [175], which in turn was derived from the SCL-90 test [176]. Like the P-3, the BSI-18 has three scales: depression, anxiety, and somatization. Thus, it shares the P-3's parsimonious, straightforward approach, and on the surface, the BSI-18 appears identical to the P-3. However, these tests differ in three important respects. First of all, BSI-18 is much shorter than P-3, taking only about one-third of the time to complete. Secondly, while the BSI-18 scales are shorter, they also have lower reliability than the P-3 scales.

A third difference is that while the P-3 was normed on both community members and patients with chronic pain generally, the BSI-18 was normed on patients suffering from cancer-related pain. Thus, while both tests have pain norms, the two normative groups were quite different. Overall, the meaningfulness of a patient's scores on a standardized test is influenced by the degree of similarity between the patient and the norm group to which the patient is compared. Overall, the strength of the BSI-18 is assessing the psychological distress of patients with cancer [177–180].

Other Noteworthy Pain-Related Questionnaires

There are a multitude of other questionnaires pertaining to pain [121] which did not meet all of the criteria for review here, but which are nevertheless noteworthy. Three of these are the West Haven-Yale Multidimensional Pain Inventory (WHYMPI or MPI) [181], the Chronic Pain Coping Inventory (CPCI) [182], and the Survey of Pain Attitudes (SOPA) [183]. The MPI is a well-researched questionnaire that offers scales to assess attitudes about pain, the perceived attitudes of others toward the patient's pain, and the impact of pain on functioning. Weaknesses of the test include that it is not a standardized test: It does not have a formal test manual and has multiple versions [184] with alternate instructions, which have been found to significantly alter the results [185].

Conversely, the CPCI and the SOPA are both questionnaires used in research that evolved into different, standardized versions that kept the same name. Both tests are also similar in that they assess a number of variables directly related to pain. As aptly suggested by its name, the CPCI assesses a variety of strategies patients may use to cope with pain, which include three illness-focused coping strategies and six wellness-focused strategies. A weakness of this test is that it lacks a pain catastrophizing measure. The SOPA is also well researched and assesses a patient's beliefs about pain, which include two scales assessing adaptive beliefs and five scales assessing maladaptive beliefs. Both of the CPCI and the SOPA perform the important task of assessing attitudes, beliefs, and behaviors about pain. A weakness of both the CPCI and the SOPA is that their norms lack diversity in several respects, such as including less than 2 % African-American and Hispanic patients. Overall, the CPCI, SOPA, and MPI are all alike in that they all measure variables directly related to pain. However, none of these scales assess psychopathology or faking, and so they would probably best be paired with another measure.

Validity Assessment

Patients are sometimes motivated to falsely report pain or disability. Incentives range from primary gain (i.e., the individual finds some intrinsic satisfaction in being a patient, such as in being a suffering, tragic hero), secondary gain (i.e., the patient receives monetary, opiate, or other rewards for reporting pain), or tertiary gain (i.e., someone the patient cares about, often a family member, receives monetary or other rewards when the patient reports pain). Since pain is a subjective experience, reports of pain are easily faked [186], and false reports of pain are sometimes associated with malingering. An extensive review of pain-related malingering examined 68 studies and concluded that malingering was present in 1.25–10.4 % of patients with chronic pain [187]. Other more recent studies have suggested that there may be a 30–40 % incidence of malingering of pain or other symptoms in patients who were litigating or seeking benefits [188, 189] and that reports of symptoms increase when monetary compensation for them is present [190–192]. To detect these tendencies, psychometric measures called validity scales are used.

Validity measures are common features on major psychological inventories, and the MMPI-2, MMPI-2-RF, MCMI-III, PAI, BHI 2, and MBMD all have multiple validity scales. Of these, the MMPI-2 and MMPI-2-RF easily have the greatest number of and the most researched validity measures. With regard to brief psychological measures for pain, only the BBHI 2, P-3, and SOPA have validity measures. The BBHI 2 includes assessments of exaggerating, denial, random responding, and psychosis, while the P-3 has a measure of bizarre responding and the SOPA has a measure of inconsistent responding. Validity measures in general look for patterns of complaints that are so strange, improbable, or extreme as to be extraordinarily unlikely. This could involve claiming on a questionnaire to have never had a bad feeling or reporting a pattern of symptoms that is extraordinarily unlikely.

Relative Merits of the Tests Reviewed

In consideration of the relative merits of the tests above, the following observations are offered. While the MMPI-2-RF is shorter than the MMPI-2-RF and has improved psychometrics, the MMPI-2 has a far larger research base. In contrast, the MCMI-III has the advantage of being keyed to DSM-IV diagnoses and is only about 1/3 the length of the MMPI-2. When time is a factor, this is a considerable advantage. Lastly, the PAI is about the same length as the MMPI-2-RF, but about twice the length of the MCMI-III. The PAI is a well-designed measure of psychopathology and is a reasonable alternative to the other tests mentioned.

With regard to measures of chronic pain, the BHI 2 has the advantage of being intended for the assessments of patients with chronic pain. It includes standardized measures of pain, function, and most of the risk factors identified by the convergent model. The other major health psychology inventory reviewed here, the MBMD, has surprisingly little overlap with the BHI 2. While the MBMD was developed using a disease model and does not measure pain per se, it does measure some attitudes toward pain. If an assessment of how relatively normal patients cope with pain is desired, the MBMD is particularly strong. In contrast, the BHI 2 assesses a greater number of aberrant traits that may be problematic in treatment.

With regard to brief measures for medical patients, the P-3 offers a straightforward assessment of three factors known to play an important role in chronic pain in a manner that is easily understood. While the BBHI 2 is a test of similar length to the P-3, these two tests approach the assessment of pain patients differently. While the P-3 prefers the elegance of parsimony, the BBHI 2 assesses a much broader range of variables and paints a more detailed picture of the patient. Both of these tests can be used to track changes in treatment over time. The BSI-18 offers the same three scales as the P-3. However, the BSI-18 was developed and normed on patients with cancer, and so this measure has particular strengths if pain is associated with that condition.

It should be noted, however, that the final decision about tests should rest with the examiner, as unique features of a particular case or future research might indicate that a different set of tests would be warranted. At this point, however, given the current state of knowledge, the tests above meet the criteria specified.

Referral for Psychological Assessment

A multidisciplinary panel, following rules of evidence-based medicine, explored the question of when psychological assessments should be conducted in patients suffering from chronic pain [105]. The conclusion was that, given the biopsychosocial nature of pain, psychological assessment is generally indicated. Beyond this, specific indications for evaluation were also identified. These were as follows:

1. When psychological dysfunction is observed or suspected
2. When there has been inadequate recovery, as indicated by the duration of symptoms beyond the usual time, failure to benefit from all treatment, or pain complaints that cannot be explained by the patient's physical findings
3. Substance abuse and/or aberrant use of prescription medication
4. Premorbid history of major psychiatric symptoms
5. Lack of adherence to medical treatment
6. When cognitive impairment is suspected, especially if related to the medical condition or adverse effect of medications
7. When a patient has been judged to have a catastrophic medical condition
8. Prior to major surgical or invasive procedures, such as spinal cord stimulation, and prior to initiation of chronic opioid treatment

Chronic Pain Case Vignettes

For heuristic purposes, in the case vignettes below, the convergent model described above is used to assess three patients, whose biopsychosocial risk levels range from mild to extreme. It should be noted that there are other psychometric assessment protocols, and these are reviewed elsewhere [119]. However, analyzing these cases with multiple protocols would add a level of complexity that goes well beyond the vision of this chapter. In each case vignette to follow, there is both a standardized assessment of the risk factors described in Tables 6.1 and 6.2 and a clinical narrative. The first two cases assess biopsychosocial risk factors using the BBHI 2 test, while the third uses the longer BHI 2.

Case History One: Neuropathic Pain with Low Biopsychosocial Risk Level

Ms. A was a 26-year-old female college graduate and sports enthusiast, who injured her back while skiing. Initially, she had been diagnosed with a lumber strain. Later, she was determined by MRI to have bulging discs at L3-L4 and L4-L5. Ms. A wished to avoid lumbar surgery and was being evaluated for alternate treatment options. As part of a comprehensive assessment, Ms. A was administered a BBHI 2 test.

Table 6.3 summarizes the results of Ms. A's standardized testing with the BBHI 2. These results show a distribution of pain that is confined to the area near the injury, with only three body areas being involved. The pain level at testing was a four, with a high of eight and a low of two in the last month. These pain complaints were judged to be consistent with her objective medical findings. Using the convergent model to summarize Ms. A's level of risk, she had none of the extreme exclusionary risk factors and only one cautionary risk factor. This produced a cautionary risk score at the 17th percentile rank or well below average. It should be noted that these risk scores are generated solely from the testing, without any interview or chart review. Following the testing, an interview identified additional information. The overall results of the evaluation are below.

On the BBHI 2 test, Ms. A's sole cautionary risk factor was that her level of depression was higher than that seen in 88 % of a national sample of patients with pain and injury, which is significantly elevated (Table 6.3). During the interview, she reported a low mood and was very concerned that she may have to give up her active lifestyle. Additionally, her score on the functional complaints scale was in the "moderately high" range. With regard to functioning, Ms A was reporting more difficulties with functioning than was 78 % of a national sample of patients and above 98 % of a national sample of

Table 6.3 Subacute low back pain: good candidate

BBHI 2 results					
Global pain complaint		*Pain complaints areas*		*Scale ratings and percentile ranks*	
Overall pain at testing:	4	Head (headache pain):	0	Defensiveness:	Average 48 %
High pain last month:	8	Jaw or face:	0	Somatic complaints:	Average 63 %
Low pain last month:	2	Neck or shoulders:	0	Pain complaints:	Average 66 %
Peak pain:	8	Arms or hands:	0	Functional complaints:	Mod high 78 %
Pain range	6	Chest:	0	Depression:	High 88 %
Max tolerable pain	5	Abdomen or stomach:	0	Anxiety:	Average 71 %
Pain tolerance index	3	Genital area:	0	*Summary*	
Number of body areas with pain	10	Middle back:	6	Exclusionary risks = 0	
Critical concerns		Lower back:	8	Cautionary risks = 1	
Sleep disorder		Legs or feet:	3	Cautionary risk rank: 17th percentile	

Table 6.4 Subacute whiplash condition: moderate risk patient

BBHI 2 results					
Global pain complaint		*Pain complaints area*		*Scale ratings and percentile ranks*	
Overall pain at testing:	9	Head (headache pain):	8	Defensiveness:	Average 42 %
High pain last month:	10	Jaw or face:	6	Somatic complaints:	Very high 96 %
Lowest pain last month:	6	Neck or shoulders:	9	Pain complaints:	High 88 %
Peak pain:	10	Arms or hands:	4	Functional complaints:	Mod high 76 %
Pain range	8	Chest:	9	Depression:	High 90 %
Max tolerable pain	6	Abdomen or stomach:	5	Anxiety:	Very high 96 %
Pain tolerance index	−4	Genital area:	0	*Summary*	
Number of body areas with pain	6	Middle back:	0	Exclusionary risks = 0	
Clinical concerns		Lower back:	0	Cautionary risks = 5	
Panic		Legs or feet:	0	*Cautionary risk rank* = 80th percentile	
PTSD/dissociation					
Perceived disability					

persons in the community. While this is at the upper end of the average range for patients who are in rehabilitation, it is far higher than that of the average healthy person. This indicates that while a significant problem exists, it is still in the average range for patients with serious injuries. Thus, with regard to perceptions of disability and functioning, Ms. A was not an unusual patient. Additionally, Ms. A's BBHI 2 results determined that her pain, somatization, and anxiety were all in the average range. The only other significant problem reported was that the patient was having difficulty sleeping.

Importantly, the BBHI 2 Pain Tolerance Index was only −3, meaning that the patient felt that her worst pain must only be reduced by three points in order to function normally. Overall, this patient was judged to have localized back pain and a relatively low level of psychosocial complications. She was started on a trial of medications for depression and insomnia and was judged to be an excellent candidate for conservative treatment.

Case History Two: Whiplash with Moderate Biopsychosocial Risk Level

Ms. B was a 52-year-old patient who had sustained a whiplash injury in a motor vehicle accident and who had been exhibiting poor attendance in treatment. This patient complained of pain in her neck, head, and mid- to upper back, and this was judged to be consistent with the whiplash injury. In contrast, other aspects of Ms. B's pain complaints, such as the facial and jaw pain, were of uncertain etiology. It was possible that the latter pain complaints were indicative of other injuries that may have been overlooked during the acute phase or may have been attributable to dental or other conditions. Given the uncertain nature of some of her pain complaints and her lack of improvement with treatment, Ms. B was referred for psychological assessment.

Table 6.4 lists the BBHI 2 tests results of Ms. B. She had no exclusionary risk factors and five cautionary risk factors, producing a cautionary risk score at the 80th percentile rank, which is somewhat elevated. The "high" rating on the BBHI 2 pain complaints scale indicates that Ms. B's overall pain reports were substantially higher (elevated more than one standard deviation) than that seen in 88 % of patients with pain and injury. These test results also showed that Ms. B was extremely anxious, somatically preoccupied, and was reporting symptoms of panic and PTSD. This gave rise to an alternate interpretation of some of these symptoms. The interview determined that the patient was having PTSD flashbacks when driving in traffic and had also developed agoraphobia secondary to panic attacks. It was discovered that her poor attendance in treatment was not attributable to low motivation, but rather to her fear of leaving the house. Additionally, her jaw and facial pain were later determined to be associated with bruxing secondary to severe anxiety.

Ms. B's Pain Tolerance Index of −4 indicates that she felt she needed to reduce her worst pain by four points to make normal functioning possible. On the positive side, given that the patient reported that pain sometimes dropped as low as a two and a pain of six could be tolerated, it would appear that at times, the pain was quite tolerable.

In cases like this, it is important to determine the physical and psychological causes of the reported symptoms and provide appropriate treatment. If the symptoms are determined to be heavily influenced by psychosocial factors, early intervention can prevent these psychosocial complications from delaying recovery. In this case, Ms. B was referred for treatment for PTSD and agoraphobia. Later, after the PTSD and anxiety symptoms were brought under control, Ms. B no longer exhibited attendance problems. Following a two-level cervical rhizotomy, her pain symptoms decreased markedly, and she began progressing in physical therapy.

Case History Three: Chronic Low Back Pain with Extreme Biopsychosocial Risk Level

Mr. C was a 44-year-old male with failed back surgery syndrome, who was being considered for spinal cord stimulation and other treatments. Mr. C presented as a patient who had injured himself 3 years earlier while working on an oil-drilling rig. The patient reported that following the injury, there was an immediate onset of severe lumbar pain, which radiated into his left leg. A subsequent MRI revealed an L5–S1 lumbar disc herniation. Mr. C was a two to three pack a day smoker and was instructed to stop smoking prior to undergoing a lumbar fusion. He reported that he had quit, but later, after the surgery, it was discovered that he had not been honest about this. Mr. C complained that his pain after the surgery was far worse, and he increased his dose of opioid pain medications without consulting his surgeon.

Mr. C was referred for physical therapy, where he attended poorly and failed to progress. He was very pain affected, exhibited a hostile attitude, and complained that none of the treatments that had been offered to him had helped. Mr. C was offered light duty at his employer's office, which he refused. By this time, his use of opioid medication was excessive, and Mr. C became belligerent when an early refill of this medication was not allowed.

Three years postinjury, and after all other treatments had failed, Mr. C was referred to an interventional pain specialist to be evaluated for spinal cord stimulation, with hopes that this would help him decrease his opioid use. Prior to trial, Mr. C was referred for a psychological evaluation, but he regarded a referral to a psychologist as an insult, saying, "My pain is real. It is not in my head!" The physician explained that behavioral health services are a standard part of interdisciplinary care and persuaded Mr. C to attend the appointment. During the psychological evaluation, the patient was administered the BHI 2, and Table 6.5 lists Mr. C's BHI 2 results. Using the convergent model, he had 18 cautionary risk factors, producing a cautionary risk score at the 99th percentile rank, which is extremely high. Further, he also had six of the extreme exclusionary risk factors, producing an exclusionary risk score at the 99th percentile rank as well.

At the time of the psychological evaluation, Mr. C was reporting a pain of 10 in the low back, mid-back, and lower extremities, and the intensity of the pain reports was judged by his physicians to exceed what was expected. More significant perhaps was the report of pain in all seven other body areas, his report that his overall pain was a constant "10," with his pain range score of 0 indicating that he was reporting totally invariant pain over the last month. More importantly, his Pain Tolerance Index score was −10, indicating that the

Table 6.5 Chronic low back pain: high-risk candidate

BHI 2 results

Global pain complaints		Pain complaints area		Scale ratings and percentile ranks	
Overall pain at testing:	10	Headache:	10	Defensiveness:	Ext low 28 %
High pain last month:	10	Jaw/face:	6	Self-disclosure:	Mod high 80 %
Lowest pain last month:	10	Neck/shoulders:	5	Somatic complaints:	High 91 %
Peak pain:	10	Arms/hands:	2	Pain complaints:	Ext high 99 %
Pain range	0	Chest:	9	Functional complaints:	Very high 95 %
Max tolerable pain	0	Abdomen/stomach:	5	Muscular bracing	Average 58 %
Pain tolerance index	−10	Genital area:	2	Depression:	High 88 %
Number of body areas with pain	10	Middle back:	8	Anxiety:	Average 56 %
Clinical concerns		Lower back:	10	Hostility	Very high 96 %
Pain fixation		Legs or feet:	10	Borderline	Mod high 82 %
Rx addiction				Symptom dependency	Average 44 %
Violent ideation				Chronic maladjustment	Very high 95 %
Medical dissatisfaction				Substance abuse	Very high 96 %
Compensation focus				Perseverance	Average 62 %
Entitlement				Family dysfunction	Low 5 %
Cynical beliefs				Survivor of violence	Low 16 %
Aggressiveness				Doctor dissatisfaction	Ext high 99 %
Impulsiveness				Job dissatisfaction	High 84 %
Vegetative depression				Summary	
Autonomic anxiety				Exclusionary risks = 6	
Death anxiety				Cautionary risks = 18	
Sleep disorder				Exclusionary risk rank: 99th percentile	
Work disability				Cautionary risk rank: 99th percentile	

patient believed he needed to reduce the level of all his pains to 0 before he could function. Relative to this, he claimed that he had no pain at all before he was injured and he deserved to have no pain now. He stated that if spinal cord stimulation would reduce all of his pain to 0, he would have no need for medication. Overall, this patient reported more pain than did 99 % of a national sample of patients with pain and injury, including chest pain as high as 9. Given the fact that he was a heavy smoker, he was referred for coronary assessment, with negative findings. Overall, as there was no pathophysiological explanation for many of Mr. C's pain reports, therefore, psychophysiological reasons were explored.

The BHI 2 test results determined that Mr. C was at the 96th percentile rank for hostility and the 95th percentile for panic symptoms. This combination of anger and anxiety suggests extreme elevation of the fight-or-flight response, with the "fight" component being associated with anger and the "flight" component being associated with anxiety. Further, Mr. C's depression scale score was above that seen in 88 % of patients, and his depression appeared to manifest itself primarily in terms of anger and irritability. It was determined that Mr. C's reports of chest pain were associated with high levels of autonomic arousal and panic-like symptoms. Mr. C also reported a level of somatic preoccupation that was at the 91st percentile, and he was convinced that he had a severe heart condition, which his doctors were ignoring. Mr. C's BHI 2 profile also indicated that he was reporting more functional impairment than 95 % of patients, indicating that he saw himself as having a severe disability.

On the BHI 2, Mr. C also reported some violent thoughts, supported by a cynical view of others. He felt entitled to both special treatment and to financial compensation. With a level of job dissatisfaction at the 84th percentile, this patient was at odds with his employer, whom he blamed for his injury. He reported fantasies of harming his boss, "to make him feel pain the way I do." With a level of doctor dissatisfaction at the 99th percentile, he had even more negative attitudes toward physicians, who he accused of "working for the system." On the BHI 2, Mr. C reported an extensive history of substance abuse and chronic maladjustment. Overall, his BHI 2 test profile was one that has been found to be associated with thoughts of litigation [146, 147] and of assaultive behavior [148, 149, 155]. During the interview, he revealed that he had been in jail previously for domestic violence and in prison for drug-related charges.

Mr. C stated that because of his extreme pain, he needed more opioids and blamed his physicians for not increasing his dosage saying, "There is no reason why doctors couldn't cure my pain if they wanted to." Mr. C also demanded "natural" treatments, rationalizing that he should be prescribed morphine as it was a "natural treatment made from flowers." Paradoxically, though, Mr. C refused treatment with antidepressant medications out of a fear that they were "addictive" and because they were "unnatural." Similarly, he refused behavioral pain management training with a psychologist. Despite being off of work, he was often "too busy" to attend physical therapy, yet he never missed an appointment for an opioid prescription refill. Although multiple treatment referrals were offered to this patient, he did not accept them. Overall, Mr. C had unrealistic expectations of being totally cured through surgery and opioids, without effort on his own part and without changing his dysfunctional behaviors. Despite the warnings of his physicians, though, he continued to smoke heavily. It was later determined that he was combining his pain medications with methamphetamines and large amounts of alcohol. Mr. C claimed he was using both "medicinally." Mr. C did not take responsibility for his behavior, though. Instead, he blamed his orthopedic surgeon for his pain and was discussing a malpractice lawsuit.

The psychologist concluded the following:

1. Even if Mr. C did undergo spinal cord stimulation, he would almost certainly be dissatisfied with his outcome. The possibility that this patient's back pain would be reduced to 0 by spinal cord stimulation was judged to be extremely unlikely. Even if spinal cord stimulation did totally eliminate all low back and lower extremity pain, it was unlikely that it would alleviate his multitude of other pain complaints, and so the overall reported pain level would be unlikely to change.

2. Even if treatment with spinal cord stimulation was successful, it is unlikely that it would change Mr. C's demands for opioids. Spinal cord stimulation is not a treatment for addiction, which was what Mr. C was suffering from.

3. Mr. C hated his job and had no desire to return there. It was judged unlikely that spinal cord stimulation would alter Mr. C's motivation to return to work.

4. Given the fact that Mr. C was pursuing litigation, he may be reluctant to admit to any gains in treatment, as it might weaken his lawsuit against his surgeon. Additionally, since his expectation of a totally pain-free outcome was so unrealistic, Mr. C would be probably extremely unhappy with his spinal cord stimulation as well.

5. The psychologist suggested the following treatment plan for Mr. C. First of all, Mr. C should be referred to an inpatient drug rehabilitation program for polysubstance abuse. Once he had completed that, he could then benefit from an interdisciplinary treatment program for pain, which studies have shown can be effective, even for patients with personality disorders [193]. After consulting with the physician, it was decided that the interdisciplinary treatment should avoid opioids and include medical treatment as indicated, physical therapy with a focus on exercise and improving function, cognitive behavioral therapy for managing pain and emotional dysfunction, and other psychological treatments including relaxation, sleep hygiene, and mindfulness training.

After consulting with the psychologist, the pain physician felt she had a much deeper understanding of the scope of the problem and later met with Mr. C. She told Mr. C that spinal cord stimulation did not appear to be a viable treatment for him and that it was very likely that Mr. C would be unhappy with the results. The physician also said that she was committed to doing nothing to harm him and that given Mr. C's pattern of polysubstance abuse, treatment with opioids was dangerous and no longer an option. The physician said that instead, she was recommending the drug rehabilitation and interdisciplinary pain treatment program described above. The physician told Mr. C that this treatment program would not work unless he was fully invested in it and that if he faithfully adhered to it, they could continue working together. However, she also explained that if Mr. C refused this treatment, or did not adhere to it, he would be advised to seek treatment elsewhere, as this was the only treatment plan she thought was viable.

High-risk patients like Mr. C are challenging to treat. His initial injury was a serious one, but one which should have responded better to treatment. Unfortunately, Mr. C's entitled expectations, hostile attitude, noncompliance, and addictive behavior undermined the work of his treating professionals, and he suffered the consequences of his own dysfunctional tendencies.

If Mr. C followed through with the treatment plan above, one part of a 12-step treatment program for addiction would probably be a spiritual meditation commonly known as the Serenity Prayer: *God grant me the strength to change the things I am able to change, the ability to accept the things I cannot change, and the wisdom to know the difference.* Applying this approach to the treatment of pain generally, while the goal of changing physical pain is the domain of pain medicine, the emotional acceptance of having pain and coping with it is the domain of pain psychology. Knowing how to integrate these two approaches in the clinical setting requires a holistic understanding of how the patient's medical and psychological conditions interact. While events in life sometimes lead to pain, suffering comes from what you do to yourself. Thus, as the Buddha concluded, "Pain is inevitable. Suffering is optional."

Conclusions

Based on the studies reviewed here, it is evident that there is a growing consensus in the literature regarding the importance of assessing pain from a biopsychosocial perspective, which integrates both medical and psychological testing. At first glance, the specialties of pain medicine and pain psychology could seem worlds apart. Beneath the surface, though, they share a deep commonality, as both specialties focus on the assessment of subjective experiences and the attempt to alleviate painful feelings. While pain often has its origins in physical states, psychological forces can act either to alleviate or to compound the individual's suffering. Chronic pain may thus evolve into a complex biopsychosocial state, and depending upon the case, biological, psychological, or social factors may play the predominant causal role.

Given the complex nature of pain, success in treatment depends upon a full understanding of why the patient reports pain or requests opioids or other treatments. The dictum that "diagnosis precedes treatment" is nowhere more true than with the practice of pain medicine. While reports of pain are often the product of pathophysiology, they are sometimes the product of psychopathology. Consequently, when extreme pain is reported in the absence of any obvious pathophysiological explanation, tension can arise between patient and doctor. It has been said: "To have great pain is to have certainty. To hear that another has pain is to have doubt" [194]. Ultimately, successful assessment of chronic pain requires not only medical diagnostics but also a systematic investigation of the subjective world of the patient, which seeks to understand the origins of the pain reports.

From the perspective of patients, chronic pain often involves not just a loss of function but also a loss of one's future dreams and aspirations. The onset of a disabling condition may bring an abrupt end to a patient's assumptions about what the future holds, and the loss of this assumptive world can elicit profound grief [195]. Because of this, success in treatment cannot occur without addressing both medical and psychological concerns. Overall, the value of knowing one's patient, both medically and psychologically, cannot be overstated. To this end, and when integrated with medical diagnostics, psychological assessment can make an invaluable contribution to the understanding of the patient with chronic pain. In this manner, and through a determined blend of both science and humanity, more effective treatments may be identified.

References

1. International Association for the Study of Pain. Task Force on Taxonomy, Merskey H, Bogduk N. Classification of chronic pain. 2nd ed. Seattle: IASP Press; 1994.
2. Gatchel RJ, Peng YB, Peters ML, Fuchs PN, Turk DC. The biopsychosocial approach to chronic pain: scientific advances and future directions. Psychol Bull. 2007;133(4):581–624.
3. Melzack R. From the gate to the neuromatrix. Pain. 1999;Suppl 6:S121–6.
4. Joksimovic L, Starke D, v d Knesebeck O, Siegrist J. Perceived work stress, overcommitment, and self-reported musculoskeletal pain: a cross-sectional investigation. Int J Behav Med. 2002;9(2): 122–38.
5. Chen WQ, Yu IT, Wong TW. Impact of occupational stress and other psychosocial factors on musculoskeletal pain among Chinese offshore oil installation workers. Occup Environ Med. 2005;62(4):251–6.

6. Bhatia V, Tandon RK. Stress and the gastrointestinal tract. J Gastroenterol Hepatol. 2005;20(3):332–9.

7. Bigos SJ, Battie MC, Spengler DM, et al. A longitudinal, prospective study of industrial back injury reporting. Clin Orthop. 1992;279:21–34.

8. Turner C, McClure R, Pirozzo S. Injury and risk-taking behavior-a systematic review. Accid Anal Prev. 2004;36(1):93–101.

9. Levenson MR. Risk taking and personality. J Pers Soc Psychol. 1990;58(6):1073–80.

10. Corrigan JD. Substance abuse as a mediating factor in outcome from traumatic brain injury. Arch Phys Med Rehabil. 1995;76(4):302–9.

11. Drubach DA, Kelly MP, Winslow MM, Flynn JP. Substance abuse as a factor in the causality, severity, and recurrence rate of traumatic brain injury. Md Med J. 1993;42(10):989–93.

12. Dersh J, Gatchel RJ, Mayer T, Polatin P, Temple OR. Prevalence of psychiatric disorders in patients with chronic disabling occupational spinal disorders. Spine (Phila Pa 1976). 2006;31(10):1156–62.

13. Manchikanti L, Damron KS, Beyer CD, Pampati V. A comparative evaluation of illicit drug use in patients with or without controlled substance abuse in interventional pain management. Pain Physician. 2003;6(3):281–5.

14. Broadhead WE, Blazer DG, George LK, Tse CK. Depression, disability days, and days lost from work in a prospective epidemiologic survey. JAMA. 1990;264(19):2524–8.

15. Gehi A, Haas D, Pipkin S, Whooley MA. Depression and medication adherence in outpatients with coronary heart disease: findings from the Heart and Soul Study. Arch Intern Med. 2005;165(21):2508–13.

16. Polatin PB, Kinney RK, Gatchel RJ, Lillo E, Mayer TG. Psychiatric illness and chronic low-back pain. The mind and the spine – which goes first? Spine. 1993;18(1):66–71.

17. Turk DC, Monarch ES. Biopsychosocial perspective on chronic pain. In: Turk DC, Gatchel RJ, editors. Psychological approaches to pain management: a practitioner's handbook. 2nd ed. New York: The Guilford Press; 2002. xviii, 590p.

18. Carter LE, McNeil DW, Vowles KE, et al. Effects of emotion on pain reports, tolerance and physiology. Pain Res Manag. 2002;7(1):21–30.

19. Fordyce WE. Pain and suffering. A reappraisal. Am Psychol. 1988;43(4):276–83.

20. Dvorak J, Valach L, Fuhrimann P, Heim E. The outcome of surgery for lumbar disc herniation. II. A 4–17 years' follow-up with emphasis on psychosocial aspects. Spine. 1988;13(12):1423–7.

21. Herron L, Turner J, Weiner P. Does the MMPI predict chemonucleolysis outcome? Spine. 1988;13(1):84–8.

22. Hagg O, Fritzell P, Ekselius L, Nordwall A. Predictors of outcome in fusion surgery for chronic low back pain. A report from the Swedish Lumbar Spine Study. Eur Spine J. 2003;12(1):22–33.

23. Andersen T, Christensen FB, Bunger C. Evaluation of a Dallas Pain Questionnaire classification in relation to outcome in lumbar spinal fusion. Eur Spine J. 2006;10:1–15.

24. Derby R, Lettice JJ, Kula TA, Lee SH, Seo KS, Kim BJ. Single-level lumbar fusion in chronic discogenic low-back pain: psychological and emotional status as a predictor of outcome measured using the 36-item Short Form. J Neurosurg Spine. 2005;3(4):255–61.

25. Deyo RA, Mirza SK, Heagerty PJ, Turner JA, Martin BI. A prospective cohort study of surgical treatment for back pain with degenerated discs; study protocol. BMC Musculoskelet Disord. 2005;6(1):24.

26. Graver V, Haaland AK, Magnaes B, Loeb M. Seven-year clinical follow-up after lumbar disc surgery: results and predictors of outcome. Br J Neurosurg. 1999;13(2):178–84.

27. Van Susante J, Van de Schaaf D, Pavlov P. Psychological distress deteriorates the subjective outcome of lumbosacral fusion. A prospective study. Acta Orthop Belg. 1998;64(4):371–7.

28. Block AR, Ohnmeiss DD, Guyer RD, Rashbaum RF, Hochschuler SH. The use of presurgical psychological screening to predict the outcome of spine surgery. Spine J. 2001;1(4):274–82.

29. Schade V, Semmer N, Main CJ, Hora J, Boos N. The impact of clinical, morphological, psychosocial and work-related factors on the outcome of lumbar discectomy. Pain. 1999;80(1–2):239–49.

30. Cashion EL, Lynch WJ. Personality factors and results of lumbar disc surgery. Neurosurgery. 1979;4(2):141–5.

31. den Boer JJ, Oostendorp RA, Beems T, Munneke M, Evers AW. Continued disability and pain after lumbar disc surgery: the role of cognitive-behavioral factors. Pain. 2006;123(1–2):45–52.

32. Katz JN, Stucki G, Lipson SJ, Fossel AH, Grobler LJ, Weinstein JN. Predictors of surgical outcome in degenerative lumbar spinal stenosis. Spine. 1999;24(21):2229–33.

33. Burchiel KJ, Anderson VC, Wilson BJ, Denison DB, Olson KA, Shatin D. Prognostic factors of spinal cord stimulation for chronic back and leg pain. Neurosurgery. 1995;36(6):1101–10; discussion 1110–1.

34. Samwel H, Slappendel R, Crul BJ, Voerman VF. Psychological predictors of the effectiveness of radiofrequency lesioning of the cervical spinal dorsal ganglion (RF-DRG). Eur J Pain. 2000;4(2):149–55.

35. Dersh J, Polatin PB, Gatchel RJ. Chronic pain and psychopathology: research findings and theoretical considerations. Psychosom Med. 2002;64(5):773–86.

36. Spengler DM, Freeman C, Westbrook R, Miller JW. Low-back pain following multiple lumbar spine procedures. Failure of initial selection? Spine. 1980;5(4):356–60.

37. Uomoto JM, Turner JA, Herron LD. Use of the MMPI and MCMI in predicting outcome of lumbar laminectomy. J Clin Psychol. 1988;44(2):191–7.

38. Passik SD, Kirsh KL. Opioid therapy in patients with a history of substance abuse. CNS Drugs. 2004;18(1):13–25.

39. Bruns D, Disorbio JM, Bennett DB, Simon S, Shoemaker S, Portenoy RK. Degree of pain intolerance and adverse outcomes in chronic noncancer pain patients. J Pain. 2005;6(3S):s74.

40. Compton P, Athanasos P. Chronic pain, substance abuse and addiction. Nurs Clin North Am. 2003;38(3):525–37.

41. Brennan PL, Schutte KK, Moos RH. Pain and use of alcohol to manage pain: prevalence and 3-year outcomes among older problem and non-problem drinkers. Addiction. 2005;100(6):777–86.

42. Mitchell AM, Dewey CM. Chronic pain in patients with substance abuse disorder: general guidelines and an approach to treatment. Postgrad Med. 2008;120(1):75–9.

43. Chou R, Fanciullo GJ, Fine PG, Miaskowski C, Passik SD, Portenoy RK. Opioids for chronic noncancer pain: prediction and identification of aberrant drug-related behaviors: a review of the evidence for an American Pain Society and American Academy of Pain Medicine clinical practice guideline. J Pain. 2009;10(2):131–46.

44. Large RG. DSM-III diagnoses in chronic pain. Confusion or clarity? J Nerv Ment Dis. 1986;174(5):295–303.

45. Okasha A, Ismail MK, Khalil AH, el Fiki R, Soliman A, Okasha T. A psychiatric study of nonorganic chronic headache patients. Psychosomatics. 1999;40(3):233–8.

46. Fishbain DA, Goldberg M, Meagher BR, Steele R, Rosomoff H. Male and female chronic pain patients categorized by DSM-III psychiatric diagnostic criteria. Pain. 1986;26(2):181–97.

47. Dersh J, Gatchel RJ, Polatin P, Mayer T. Prevalence of psychiatric disorders in patients with chronic work-related musculoskeletal pain disability. J Occup Environ Med. 2002;44(5):459–68.

48. Fishbain DA, Cole B, Cutler RB, Lewis J, Rosomoff HL, Rosomoff RS. Chronic pain and the measurement of personality: do states influence traits? Pain Med. 2006;7(6):509–29.

49. Swinkels-Meewisse IE, Roelofs J, Oostendorp RA, Verbeek AL, Vlaeyen JW. Acute low back pain: pain-related fear and pain catastrophizing influence physical performance and perceived disability. Pain. 2006;120(1–2):36–43.

50. Smeets RJ, Vlaeyen JW, Kester AD, Knottnerus JA. Reduction of pain catastrophizing mediates the outcome of both physical and cognitive-behavioral treatment in chronic low back pain. J Pain. 2006;7(4):261–71.

51. Rapley P, Fruin DJ. Self-efficacy in chronic illness: the juxtaposition of general and regimen-specific efficacy. Int J Nurs Pract. 1999;5(4):209–15.

52. Brenes GA, Rapp SR, Rejeski WJ, Miller ME. Do optimism and pessimism predict physical functioning? J Behav Med. 2002;25(3):219–31.

53. Lin CC, Ward SE. Perceived self-efficacy and outcome expectancies in coping with chronic low back pain. Res Nurs Health. 1996;19(4):299–310.

54. den Boer JJ, Oostendorp RA, Beems T, Munneke M, Oerlemans M, Evers AW. A systematic review of bio-psychosocial risk factors for an unfavourable outcome after lumbar disc surgery. Eur Spine J. 2006;15(5):527–36.

55. Weisberg JN. Personality and personality disorders in chronic pain. Curr Rev Pain. 2000;4(1):60–70.

56. Naring GW, van Lankveld W, Geenen R. Somatoform dissociation and traumatic experiences in patients with rheumatoid arthritis and fibromyalgia. Clin Exp Rheumatol. 2007;25(6):872–7.

57. Fishbain DA, Cutler RB, Rosomoff HL, Rosomoff RS. Pain-determined dissociation episodes. Pain Med. 2001;2(3):216–24.

58. McFadden IJ, Woitalla VF. Differing reports of pain perception by different personalities in a patient with chronic pain and multiple personality disorder. Pain. 1993;55(3):379–82.

59. Packard RC, Brown F. Multiple headaches in a case of multiple personality disorder. Headache. 1986;26(2):99–102.

60. Hamberg K, Johansson E, Lindgren G, Westman G. The impact of marital relationship on the rehabilitation process in a group of women with long-term musculoskeletal disorders. Scand J Soc Med. 1997;25(1):17–25.

61. MacGregor EA, Brandes J, Eikermann A, Giammarco R. Impact of migraine on patients and their families: the Migraine And Zolmitriptan Evaluation (MAZE) survey – Phase III. Curr Med Res Opin. 2004;20(7):1143–50.

62. Kemler MA, Furnee CA. The impact of chronic pain on life in the household. J Pain Symptom Manage. 2002;23(5):433–41.

63. Harris S, Morley S, Barton SB. Role loss and emotional adjustment in chronic pain. Pain. 2003;105(1–2):363–70.

64. Kerns RD, Haythornthwaite J, Southwick S, Giller Jr EL. The role of marital interaction in chronic pain and depressive symptom severity. J Psychosom Res. 1990;34(4):401–8.

65. Block AR, Kremer EF, Gaylor M. Behavioral treatment of chronic pain: the spouse as a discriminative cue for pain behavior. Pain. 1980;9(2):243–52.

66. Heim C, Ehlert U, Hanker JP, Hellhammer DH. Abuse-related posttraumatic stress disorder and alterations of the hypothalamic-pituitary-adrenal axis in women with chronic pelvic pain. Psychosom Med. 1998;60(3):309–18.

67. Rubin RT, Phillips JJ, McCracken JT, Sadow TF. Adrenal gland volume in major depression: relationship to basal and stimulated pituitary-adrenal cortical axis function. Biol Psychiatry. 1996;40(2):89–97.

68. Heim C, Newport DJ, Bonsall R, Miller AH, Nemeroff CB. Altered pituitary-adrenal axis responses to provocative challenge tests in adult survivors of childhood abuse. Am J Psychiatry. 2001;158(4):575–81.

69. Heim C, Newport DJ, Heit S, et al. Pituitary-adrenal and autonomic responses to stress in women after sexual and physical abuse in childhood. JAMA. 2000;284(5):592–7.

70. Bremner JD, Vythilingam M, Anderson G, et al. Assessment of the hypothalamic-pituitary-adrenal axis over a 24-hour diurnal period and in response to neuroendocrine challenges in women with and without childhood sexual abuse and posttraumatic stress disorder. Biol Psychiatry. 2003;54(7):710–8.

71. De Bellis MD, Chrousos GP, Dorn LD, et al. Hypothalamic-pituitary-adrenal axis dysregulation in sexually abused girls. J Clin Endocrinol Metab. 1994;78(2):249–55.

72. Kiecolt-Glaser JK, Glaser R. Psychoneuroimmunology and cancer: fact or fiction? Eur J Cancer. 1999;35(11):1603–7.

73. Miller GE, Dopp JM, Myers HF, Stevens SY, Fahey JL. Psychosocial predictors of natural killer cell mobilization during marital conflict. Health Psychol. 1999;18(3):262–71.

74. Takahashi K, Iwase M, Yamashita K, et al. The elevation of natural killer cell activity induced by laughter in a crossover designed study. Int J Mol Med. 2001;8(6):645–50.

75. Schofferman J, Anderson D, Hines R, Smith G, White A. Childhood psychological trauma correlates with unsuccessful lumbar spine surgery. Spine. 1992;17(6 Suppl):S138–44.

76. Cossette S, Frasure-Smith N, Lesperance F. Clinical implications of a reduction in psychological distress on cardiac prognosis in patients participating in a psychosocial intervention program. Psychosom Med. 2001;63(2):257–66.

77. Donker FJ. Cardiac rehabilitation: a review of current developments. Clin Psychol Rev. 2000;20(7):923–43.

78. Frasure-Smith N, Lesperance F, Gravel G, et al. Social support, depression, and mortality during the first year after myocardial infarction. Circulation. 2000;101(16):1919–24.

79. Kiecolt-Glaser JK, McGuire L, Robles TF, Glaser R. Psychoneuroimmunology and psychosomatic medicine: back to the future. Psychosom Med. 2002;64(1):15–28.

80. Marucha PT, Kiecolt-Glaser JK, Favagehi M. Mucosal wound healing is impaired by examination stress. Psychosom Med. 1998;60(3):362–5.

81. Schofferman J, Anderson D, Hines R, Smith G, Keane G. Childhood psychological trauma and chronic refractory low-back pain. Clin J Pain. 1993;9(4):260–5.

82. Vermeire E, Hearnshaw H, Van Royen P, Denekens J. Patient adherence to treatment: three decades of research. A comprehensive review. J Clin Pharm Ther. 2001;26(5):331–42.

83. Lieberman 3rd JA. Compliance issues in primary care. J Clin Psychiatry. 1996;57 Suppl 7:76–82; discussion 83–75.

84. Green CR, Flowe-Valencia H, Rosenblum L, Tait AR. The role of childhood and adulthood abuse among women presenting for chronic pain management. Clin J Pain. 2001;17(4):359–64.

85. Winfield JB. Psychological determinants of fibromyalgia and related syndromes. Curr Rev Pain. 2000;4(4):276–86.

86. Roberts SJ. The sequelae of childhood sexual abuse: a primary care focus for adult female survivors. Nurse Pract. 1996;21(12 Pt 1):42, 45, 49–52.

87. Bigos SJ, Battie MC, Spengler DM, et al. A longitudinal, prospective study of industrial back injury reporting. Clin Orthop Relat Res. 1992;279:21–34.

88. Bernard Jr TN. Repeat lumbar spine surgery. Factors influencing outcome. Spine. 1993;18(15):2196–200.

89. DeBerard MS, Masters KS, Colledge AL, Schleusener RL, Schlegel JD. Outcomes of posterolateral lumbar fusion in Utah patients receiving workers' compensation: a retrospective cohort study. Spine. 2001;26(7):738–46; discussion 747.

90. Epker J, Block AR. Presurgical psychological screening in back pain patients: a review. Clin J Pain. 2001;17(3):200–5.

91. LaCaille RA, DeBerard MS, Masters KS, Colledge AL, Bacon W. Presurgical biopsychosocial factors predict multidimensional-patient: outcomes of interbody cage lumbar fusion. Spine J. 2005;5(1):71–8.

92. Taylor VM, Deyo RA, Ciol M, et al. Patient-oriented outcomes from low back surgery: a community-based study. Spine. 2000;25(19):2445–52.

93. Junge A, Dvorak J, Ahrens S. Predictors of bad and good outcomes of lumbar disc surgery. A prospective clinical study with recommendations for screening to avoid bad outcomes. Spine. 1995;20(4):460–8.

94. Greenough CG, Taylor LJ, Fraser RD. Anterior lumbar fusion. A comparison of noncompensation patients with compensation patients. Clin Orthop Relat Res. 1994;300:30–7.

95. Groth-Marnat G, Fletcher A. Influence of neuroticism, catastrophizing, pain duration, and receipt of compensation on short-term response to nerve block treatment for chronic back pain. J Behav Med. 2000;23(4):339–50.

96. Mannion AF, Elfering A. Predictors of surgical outcome and their assessment. Eur Spine J. 2006;15 Suppl 1:S93–108.

97. Glassman SD, Minkow RE, Dimar JR, Puno RM, Raque GH, Johnson JR. Effect of prior lumbar discectomy on outcome of lumbar fusion: a prospective analysis using the SF-36 measure. J Spinal Disord. 1998;11(5):383–8.

98. Klekamp J, McCarty E, Spengler DM. Results of elective lumbar discectomy for patients involved in the workers' compensation system. J Spinal Disord. 1998;11(4):277–82.

99. Feuerstein M, Callan-Harris S, Hickey P, Dyer D, Armbruster W, Carosella AM. Multidisciplinary rehabilitation of chronic work-related upper extremity disorders. Long-term effects. J Occup Med. 1993;35(4):396–403.

100. DeBerard MS, Masters KS, Colledge AL, Holmes EB. Presurgical biopsychosocial variables predict medical and compensation costs of lumbar fusion in Utah workers' compensation patients. Spine J. 2003;3(6):420–9.

101. Marquez de la Plata C, Hewlitt M, de Oliveira A, et al. Ethnic differences in rehabilitation placement and outcome after TBI. J Head Trauma Rehabil. 2007;22(2):113–21.

102. Nelson DV, Kennington M, Novy DM, et al. Providers' Attitudes and practices regarding psychological selection criteria for spinal cord stimulation. Seattle: International Association for the Study of Pain (IASP) Press; 1996.

103. Work Loss Data Institute. Official Disability Guidelines. Encinitas: Work Loss Data Institute; 2008.

104. Colorado Division of Worker Compensation. Chronic Pain Task Force. Rule 17, Exhibit 9: Chronic Pain Disorder Medical Treatment Guidelines: Colorado Department of Labor and Employment: Division of Worker Compensation 2007.

105. American College of Occupational and Environmental Medicine. Chronic pain treatment guidelines. In: Hegmann K, editor. Occupational medicine practice guidelines. 2nd ed. Beverly Farms: OEM Press; 2008.

106. Giordano N, Lofland K, Guay J, et al. Utilization of and beliefs about presurgical psychological screening: a national survey of anesthesiologists. J Pain. 2005;6(3 Suppl):S67.

107. Meyer GJ, Finn SE, Eyde LD, et al. Psychological testing and psychological assessment. A review of evidence and issues. Am Psychol. 2001;56(2):128–65.

108. Carragee EJ, Alamin TF, Miller JL, Carragee JM. Discographic, MRI and psychosocial determinants of low back pain disability and remission: a prospective study in subjects with benign persistent back pain. Spine J. 2005;5(1):24–35.

109. Gatchel RJ, Polatin PB, Mayer TG. The dominant role of psychosocial risk factors in the development of chronic low back pain disability. Spine. 1995;20(24):2702–9.

110. Block AR, Gatchel RJ, Deardorff WW, Guyer RD. The psychology of spine surgery. Washington, D.C.: American Psychological Association; 2003.

111. Gatchel RJ. A biopsychosocial overview of pretreatment screening of patients with pain. Clin J Pain. 2001;17(3): 192–9.

112. Giordano N, Lofland K. A literature review of psychological predictors of spinal cord stimulator outcomes. American Pain Society 24th annual scientific meeting, Boston, 2005.

113. Ormel J, VonKorff M, Ustun TB, Pini S, Korten A, Oldehinkel T. Common mental disorders and disability across cultures. Results from the WHO Collaborative Study on Psychological Problems in General Health Care. JAMA. 1994;272(22):1741–8.

114. Bruns D, Warren PA. The assessment of psychosocial contributions to disability. In: Warren PA, editor. Handbook of behavioral health disability. New York: Springer; 2010.

115. American Educational Research Association, American Psychological Association, National Council on Measurement in Education, Joint Committee on Standards for Educational and Psychological Testing (U.S.). Standards for educational and psychological testing. Washington, D.C.: American Educational Research Association; 1999.

116. Turk DC, Melzack R. Trends and future directions in human pain assessment. In: Turk DC, Melzack R, editors. Handbook of pain assessment. New York: Guilford Press; 1992. p. 473–9.

117. Disorbio JM, Bruns D. Brief battery for health improvement 2 manual. Minneapolis: Pearson; 2002.

118. Mitrushina M, Boone D, Razani J, D'Elia L. Handbook of normative data for neuropsychological assessment. 2nd ed. New York: Oxford University Press; 2005.

119. Bruns D, Disorbio JM. Assessment of biopsychosocial risk factors for medical treatment: a collaborative approach. J Clin Psychol Med Settings. 2009;16(2):127–47.

120. Bruns D, Disorbio JM. Battery for health improvement 2 manual. Minneapolis: Pearson; 2003.

121. Turk DC, Melzack R. Handbook of pain assessment. 2nd ed. New York: Guilford Press; 2001.

122. Bruns D. Psychological tests commonly used in the assessment of chronic pain patients. 2002. http://www.healthpsych.com/testing/psychtests.pdf. Accessed 7 July 2012.

123. Butcher JN, American Psychological Association. MMPI-2: a practitioner's guide. 1st ed. Washington, D.C.: American Psychological Association; 2006.

124. Butcher JN, Graham JR, Ben-Porath YS, Tellegen A, Dahlstrom WG, Kaemmer B. Minnesota Multiphasic Personality Inventory–2 (MMPI–2): manual for administration, scoring and interpretation. Rev. ed. Minneapolis: University of Minnesota Press; 2001.

125. Block A. The psychology of spine surgery. 1st ed. Washington, D.C.: American Psychological Association; 2003.

126. Doleys DM, Klapow JC, Hammer M. Psychological evaluation in spinal cord stimulation therapy. Pain Rev. 1997;4:189–207.

127. Nelson DV, Kennington M, Novy DM, Squitieri P. Psychological selection criteria for implantable spinal cord stimulators. Pain Forum. 1996;5(2):93–103.

128. Olson K, Bedder MD, Anderson VC, Burchiel KJ, Villaneuva MR. Psychological variables associated with outcome of spinal cord stimulation trials. Neuromodulation. 1998;1:6–13.

129. Beltrutti D, Lamberto A, Barolat G, et al. The psychological assessment of candidates for spinal cord stimulation for chronic pain management. Pain Pract. 2004;4(3):204–21.

130. Tellegen A, Ben-Porath YS, McNulty JL, Arbisi PA, Graham JE, Kaemmer B. The MMPI-2 restructured clinical (RC) scales. Minneapolis: Pearson Assessments; 2003.

131. Butcher JN. MMPI-2: Minnesota Multiphasic Personality Inventory-2: manual for administration, scoring, and interpretation. Rev.th ed. Minneapolis: University of Minnesota Press; 2001.

132. Ben-Porath YS, Tellegen A. MMPI-2-RF™ manual. Minneapolis: University of Minnesota; 2008.

133. Rogers R, Sewell KW. MMPI-2 at the crossroads: aging technology or radical retrofitting? J Pers Assess. 2006;87(2):175–8.

134. Rogers R, Sewell KW, Harrison KS, Jordan MJ. The MMPI-2 restructured clinical scales: a paradigmatic shift in scale development. J Pers Assess. 2006;87(2):139–47.

135. Butcher JN, Hamilton CK, Rouse SV, Cumella EJ. The deconstruction of the Hy Scale of MMPI-2: failure of RC3 in measuring somatic symptom expression. J Pers Assess. 2006;87(2):186–92.

136. Tellegen A, Ben-Porath YS, Sellbom M. Construct validity of the MMPI-2 restructured clinical (RC) scales: reply to Rouse, Greene, Butcher, Nichols, and Williams. J Pers Assess. 2009;91(3):211–21; discussion 222–6.

137. Rouse SV, Greene RL, Butcher JN, Nichols DS, Williams CL. What do the MMPI-2 restructured clinical scales reliably measure? Answers from multiple research settings. J Pers Assess. 2008;90(5):435–42.

138. Millon T, Davis R, Millon C. Millon clinical multiaxial inventory-III manual. 2nd ed. Minneapolis: Pearson Assessments; 1997.

139. Manchikanti L, Pampati V, Beyer C, Damron K. Do number of pain conditions influence emotional status? Pain Physician. 2002;5(2):200–5.

140. Manchikanti L, Fellows B, Pampati V, Beyer C, Damron K, Barnhill RC. Comparison of psychological status of chronic pain patients and the general population. Pain Physician. 2002;5(1):40–8.

141. Rivera JJ, Singh V, Fellows B, Pampati V, Damron KS, McManus CD. Reliability of psychological evaluation in chronic pain in an interventional pain management setting. Pain Physician. 2005;8(4):375–83.

142. Hopwood CJ, Creech SK, Clark TS, Meagher MW, Morey LC. Predicting the completion of an integrative and intensive outpatient chronic pain treatment with the personality assessment inventory. J Pers Assess. 2008;90(1):76–80.

143. Karlin BE, Creech SK, Grimes JS, Clark TS, Meagher MW, Morey LC. The personality assessment inventory with chronic pain patients: psychometric properties and clinical utility. J Clin Psychol. 2005;61(12):1571–85.

144. Williams AC, Richardson PH. What does the BDI measure in chronic pain? Pain. 1993;55(2):259–66.

145. Spielberger CD, Gorsuch RL, Lushene RE. Manual for the state-trait anxiety inventory. Palo Alto: Consulting Psychologists Press; 1970.

146. Fishbain DA, Bruns D, Disorbio JM, Lewis JE. What patient attributes are associated with thoughts of suing a physician? Arch Phys Med Rehabil. 2007;88(5):589–96.

147. Fishbain DA, Bruns D, Disorbio JM, Lewis JE. What are the variables that are associated with the patient's wish to sue his physician in patients with acute and chronic pain? Pain Med. 2008;9(8):1130–42.

148. Bruns D, Fishbain DA, Disorbio JM, Lewis JE. What variables are associated with an expressed wish to kill a doctor in community and injured patient samples? J Clin Psychol Med Settings. 2010;17(2):87–97.

149. Bruns D, Disorbio JM. Hostility and violent ideation: physical rehabilitation patient and community samples. Pain Med. 2000;1(2):131–9.

150. Freedenfeld RN, Bailey BE, Bruns D, Fuchs PN, Kiser RS. Prediction of interdisciplinary pain treatment outcome using the Battery for Health Improvement. Paper presented at proceedings of the 10th world congress on pain, San Francisco, 2002.

151. Bruns D, Disorbio JM, Hanks R. Chronic nonmalignant pain and violent behavior. Curr Pain Headache Rep. 2003;7(2):127–32.

152. Bruns D, Disorbio JM. Chronic pain and biopsychosocial disorders. Pract Pain Manag. 2005;5(7):52–61.

153. Disorbio JM, Bruns D, Barolat G. Assessment and treatment of chronic pain: a physician's guide to a biopsychosocial approach. Pract Pain Manag. 2006;6(2):11–27.

154. Bruns D, Disorbio JM, Hanks R. Chronic pain and violent ideation: testing a model of patient violence. Pain Med. 2007;8(3):207–15.

155. Fishbain DA, Bruns D, Disorbio JM, Lewis JE. Correlates of self-reported violent ideation against physicians in acute – and chronic-pain patients. Pain Med. 2009;10(3):573–85.

156. Fishbain DA, Bruns D, Disorbio JM, Lewis JE. Risk for five forms of suicidality in acute pain patients and chronic pain patients vs pain-free community controls. Pain Med. 2009;10(6):1095–105.

157. Fishbain DA, Bruns D, Disorbio JM, Lewis JE, Gao J. Variables associated with self-prediction of psychopharmacological treatment adherence in acute and chronic pain patients. Pain Pract. 2010;10(6):508–19.

158. Portenoy RK, Bruns D, Shoemaker B, Shoemaker SA. Breakthrough pain in community-dwelling patients with cancer pain and noncancer pain, part 2: impact on function, mood, and quality of life. J Opioid Manag. 2010;6(2):109–16.

159. Tragesser SL, Bruns D, Disorbio JM. Borderline personality disorder features and pain: the mediating role of negative affect in a pain patient sample. Clin J Pain. 2010;26(4):348–53.

160. Fishbain DA, Bruns D, Disorbio JM, Lewis JE, Gao J. Exploration of the illness uncertainty concept in acute and chronic pain patients vs community patients. Pain Med. 2010;11(5):658–69.

161. Fishbain DA, Lewis JE, Bruns D, Disorbio JM, Gao J, Meyer LJ. Exploration of anger constructs in acute and chronic pain patients vs community patients. Pain Pract. 2011;11(3):240–51.

162. Millon T, Antoni M, Millon C, Meagher S, Grossman S. Millon behavioral medicine diagnostic manual. Minnealpolis: Pearson Assessments; 2001.

163. Millon T. Toward a new personology: an evolutionary model. New York: Wiley; 1990.

164. Tollison D, Langley JC. Pain patient profile manual. Minneapolis: Pearson Assessments; 1995.

165. Willoughby SG, Hailey BJ, Wheeler LC. Pain patient profile: a scale to measure psychological distress. Arch Phys Med Rehabil. 1999;80(10):1300–2.

166. McGuire BE, Harvey AG, Shores EA. Simulated malingering in pain patients: a study with the pain patient profile. Br J Clin Psychol. 2001;40(Pt 1):71–9.

167. McGuire BE, Shores EA. Pain patient profile and the assessment of malingered pain. J Clin Psychol. 2001;57(3):401–9.

168. Manchikanti L, Pampati V, Beyer C, Damron K, Barnhill RC. Evaluation of psychological status in chronic low back pain: comparison with general population. Pain Physician. 2002;5(2):149–55.

169. Manchikanti L, Fellows B, Singh V, Pampati V. Correlates of non-physiological behavior in patients with chronic low back pain. Pain Physician. 2003;6(2):159–66.

170. Hankin HA, Killian CB. Prediction of functional outcomes in patients with chronic pain. Work. 2004;22(2):125–30.

171. Manchikanti L, Manchikanti KN, Damron KS, Pampati V. Effectiveness of cervical medial branch blocks in chronic neck pain: a prospective outcome study. Pain Physician. 2004;7(2):195–201.

172. Manchikanti L, Manchikanti KN, Manchukonda R, Pampati V, Cash KA. Evaluation of therapeutic thoracic medial branch block effectiveness in chronic thoracic pain: a prospective outcome study with minimum 1-year follow up. Pain Physician. 2006;9(2):97–105.

173. Noble J, Gomez M, Fish JS. Quality of life and return to work following electrical burns. Burns. 2006;32(2):159–64.

174. Derogatis LR. Brief symptom inventory 18 manual (BSI® 18). Minneapolis: Pearson Assessments; 2001.

175. Derogatis LR. Brief symptom inventory manual (BSI®). Minneapolis: Pearson Assessments; 2001.

176. Derogatis LR. SCL–90: Administration, scoring, and procedures manual for the revised version. Baltimore: Clinical Psychometric Research; 1983.

177. Clark KL, Loscalzo M, Trask PC, Zabora J, Philip EJ. Psychological distress in patients with pancreatic cancer-an understudied group. Psychooncology. 2010;19(12):1313–20.

178. Zeltzer LK, Recklitis C, Buchbinder D, et al. Psychological status in childhood cancer survivors: a report from the Childhood Cancer Survivor Study. J Clin Oncol. 2009;27(14):2396–404.

179. Gessler S, Low J, Daniells E, et al. Screening for distress in cancer patients: is the distress thermometer a valid measure in the UK and does it measure change over time? A prospective validation study. Psychooncology. 2008;17(6):538–47.

180. Mertens AC, Sencer S, Myers CD, et al. Complementary and alternative therapy use in adult survivors of childhood cancer: a report from the Childhood Cancer Survivor Study. Pediatr Blood Cancer. 2008;50(1):90–7.

181. Kerns RD, Turk DC, Rudy TE. The West Haven-Yale Multidimensional Pain Inventory (WHYMPI). Pain. 1985;23(4):345–56.

182. Jensen M, Turner J, Romano JM, Nielson WR. Chronic pain coping inventory manual. Lutz: Psychological Assessment Resources; 2010.

183. Jensen M, Karoly P. Survey of pain attitudes manual. Lutz: Psychological Assessment Resources; 2010.

184. Rudy TE. Multidimensional pain inventory (MPI) computer program, version 3.0. 2009. http://www.pain.pitt.edu/mpi/. Accessed 18 Sept 2010.

185. Okifuji A, Turk DC, Eveleigh DJ. Improving the rate of classification of patients with the multidimensional pain inventory (MPI): clarifying the meaning of "significant other". Clin J Pain. 1999;15(4):290–6.

186. Hall RC. Detection of malingered PTSD: an overview of clinical, psychometric, and physiological assessment: where do we stand? J Forensic Sci. 2007;52(3):717–25.

187. Fishbain DA, Cutler R, Rosomoff HL, Rosomoff RS. Chronic pain disability exaggeration/malingering and submaximal effort research. Clin J Pain. 1999;15(4):244–74.

188. Aronoff GM, Mandel S, Genovese E, et al. Evaluating malingering in contested injury or illness. Pain Pract. 2007;7(2):178–204.

189. Mittenberg W, Patton C, Canyock EM, Condit DC. Base rates of malingering and symptom exaggeration. J Clin Exp Neuropsychol. 2002;24(8):1094–102.

190. Binder LM, Rohling ML. Money matters: a meta-analytic review of the effects of financial incentives on recovery after closed-head injury. Am J Psychiatry. 1996;153(1):7–10.

191. Rohling ML, Binder LM, Langhinrichsen-Rohling J. Money matters: a meta-analytic review of the association between financial compensation and the experience and treatment of chronic pain. Health Psychol. 1995;14(6):537–47.

192. Bianchini KJ, Curtis KL, Greve KW. Compensation and malingering in traumatic brain injury: a dose–response relationship? Clin Neuropsychol. 2006;20(4):831–47.

193. Gatchel RJ, Polatin PB, Mayer TG, Garcy PD. Psychopathology and the rehabilitation of patients with chronic low back pain disability. Arch Phys Med Rehabil. 1994;75(6):666–70.

194. Scarry E. The body in pain: the making and unmaking of the world. New York: Oxford University Press; 1985.

195. Kauffman J. Loss of the assumptive world: a theory of traumatic loss. New York: Brunner-Routledge; 2002.

196. Bruns D, Mueller K, Warren PA. Biopsychosocial law, health care reform, and the control of medical inflation in Colorado. Rehabilitation psychology. 2012;57(2):81–97.

Psychological Therapies

Leanne R. Cianfrini, Cady Block, and Daniel M. Doleys

Key Points

- When we critically analyze reciprocal and plastic connections between limbic, thalamic, and sensorimotor areas of the brain, it becomes obvious that what we experience as *pain* is larger than the sum of its sensory, affective, and cognitive components.
- Acknowledging that psychological factors are involved with the pain experience does not mean that the pain is "in the patient's head."
- Cognitive behavioral therapy (CBT) is a cost-effective adjunct to medical interventions and is backed by strong empirical evidence for positive changes in health-related quality of life, coping and depression, social support, subjective pain intensity, and pain-related activity interference.
- While the cognitive techniques involve modifying pain-related maladaptive thoughts and aim to create realistic appraisals, the behavioral "conditioning" and physiological relaxation techniques can affect activity engagement, treatment adherence, overt pain behaviors, and muscle tension.
- Physicians can implement many of these basic cognitive techniques and offer potent behavioral suggestions during even the briefest of consultations; practical tips for setting appropriate expectations and encouraging self-management are suggested.
- The incremental benefit of combined treatments can address the limitations that we have seen with pain monotherapies.
- The more advanced cognitive and behavioral techniques can be secured through collaboration with mental health providers in the community or by employing a qualified therapist in the office for a seamless interdisciplinary and biopsychosocial therapeutic approach.

Introduction

Pain is a more terrible lord of mankind than even death itself.
– Albert Schweitzer, *On the Edge of the Primeval Forest*, 1914

Although the tenor of that oft-quoted sentence is dramatic, the rest of the sentiment from the humanitarian and physician reads: "We must all die. But that I can save him from days of torture, that is what I feel is my great, ever-new privilege." In the early twentieth century, Dr. Schweitzer elegantly described in three sentences the destructive nature of pain and the obligation and privilege of the physician to relieve it. He continues, "So, when the poor, moaning creature comes, I lay my hand on his head and say to him: 'Don't be afraid! In an hour's time, you shall be put to sleep, and when you wake you won't feel any more pain.'" So begins the promise of the interventionalist.

One undercurrent of this chapter is to demonstrate the *power* of such words—contained within self-reported pain descriptors and our own well-intentioned assurances—to influence pain processing and modulation. We will reveal the impact of cognitive processes (e.g., expectations, interpretations) on pain, pain-related mood issues, and behavioral responses. We will also explore the evidence-based psychological methods designed to treat unrealistic patient outcomes expectations, maladaptive pain behaviors, and the general physical and emotional consequences of chronic

L.R. Cianfrini, Ph.D. (✉) • D.M. Doleys, Ph.D.
The Doleys Clinic / Pain & Rehabilitation Center, Inc.,
2270 Valleydale Road, Suite 100, Birmingham, AL 35244, USA
e-mail: lcianfrini@gmail.com; dmdpri@aol.com

C. Block, M.S.
Department of Psychology, University of Alabama at Birmingham,
1300 University Boulevard, Campbell Hall Ste 415, Birmingham,
AL 35294, USA
e-mail: cblock@uab.edu

T.R. Deer et al. (eds.), *Treatment of Chronic Pain by Integrative Approaches: the AMERICAN ACADEMY of PAIN MEDICINE Textbook on Patient Management*, DOI 10.1007/978-1-4939-1821-8_7,
© American Academy of Pain Medicine 2015

pain. We will examine not just the specialized techniques used within the purview of trained pain/health psychologists but will also introduce brief therapeutic strategies that can be implemented within any medical practice.

Background and History

> The mind is its own place and in itself, can make a Heav'n of Hell, a Hell of Heav'n.
>   – John Milton, *Paradise Lost*

Like in the old Hallmark card commercial, we now accept readily that, "It's the thought that counts." A person can make what they will of any given situation. We have all seen friends, loved ones, coworkers, and patients exacerbate stress through worry, rumination, passivity, or aggression. Conversely, we have witnessed inspiring resilience in the face of personal traumas, environmental disasters, and debilitating chronic illnesses. Although laypersons, the medical pain management community, and third-party payors have increasingly recognized the impact of psychosocial factors and behavioral medicine interventions on the pain experience over the past 30 years, this was actually a battle long fought.

Historically, the biomedical, dualistic disease model of pain, dating back to the ancient Greeks and promulgated by Descartes in the seventeenth century, was the dominant conceptualization. Depending on philosophical and career orientation, pain was typically viewed in one of two ways: (a) as an organic phenomenon solely within the sensory domain of the body, to be treated by physicians and surgeons, or (b) as uniquely "of the mind" and thus beyond the scope of physical treatment. Philosophers, religious leaders, and physicians of each era provoked a pendulum swing from one extreme perspective to the other. Integrative models of pain have followed several key paradigm shifts throughout the last several decades, away from the unidimensional physiological model to the gate control theory conceived of by Melzack and Wall [1] to the more broadly encompassing biopsychosocial perspective of illness [2], to the current zeitgeist regarding the dynamic and elegant concept of neuroplasticity.

Scientific Foundation

> When we wish to perfect our senses, neuroplasticity is a blessing; when it works in the service of pain, plasticity can be a curse.
>   – Norman Doidge

To understand the role of psychology in the treatment of pain, we must rewind and first clarify the difference between nociception and pain. Nociception begins with the activation of peripheral nociceptors via the process of transduction. Impulses are transmitted to the dorsal horn of the spinal cord where they can and often do undergo modulation. Depending upon the particular set of circumstances, these impulses may be up- or downregulated. The gate control theory introduced by Melzack and Wall [1], and later refined by Melzack and Casey [3], provided a heuristic foundation for understanding some of the sources of nociceptive modulation, including "top-down" cognitive processes such as anxiety, attention, or distraction that may influence the gate. The resulting nociceptive activity is propagated to higher centers via ascending tracts. Somatotopic organization is carried out in thalamic structures with subsequent activation of multiple higher cortical centers including the somatosensory, cingulate, and prefrontal cortices. The dynamic interplay among the various cortical structures involved as well as stimulation of the descending modulatory system influences an individual's overall experience of pain, which is subject to change *despite* stable peripheral stimulation. Put simply, the scientific evidence suggests that pain isn't pain until the brain *says* it's pain. Indeed, one can experience "pain" without the activation of peripheral nociceptors. While we understand nociception to be the electrochemical journey of impulses working toward the brain, the noted neurologist V.S. Ramachandran clarified that "Pain…is created by the brain and projected onto the body" ([4], p. 190).

As early as 1959, Beecher advanced the realization that pain is influenced by more than pure nociceptive input. In the context of his study with wounded World War II soldiers, secondary gain and cognitive appraisals (e.g., the wound pain is tolerable because it represents a reprieve from the battlefield) emerged as strong correlates of self-reported pain intensity and requests for opioid analgesia [5]. Almost 40 years later, Rainville and colleagues [6] demonstrated through a unique hypnosis study design that an emotional or affective component of pain could be independently manipulated from the sensory or intensity component.

These early studies, taken together with our increased understanding of anatomical brain structure and function assisted by advances in technology [e.g., functional magnetic resonance imaging (fMRI)], the mapping of interconnecting neural pain pathways, and our ever-expanding awareness of the plasticity of neuronal connections, help to account for some of the vast intra- and interindividual differences in the perception of and reaction to pain. When we pause to critically analyze the reciprocal connections between limbic, thalamic, and sensorimotor areas of the brain (see Fig. 7.1), it becomes obvious that what we experience as *pain* is larger than the sum of its sensory-discriminative, affective-motivational, and cognitive-evaluative components. The pain "maps" in the brain are in constant flux secondary to both afferent and efferent processes, including peripheral injury, continued nociceptive input, central and peripheral sensitization, and input fed from the limbic system and higher cortical connections.

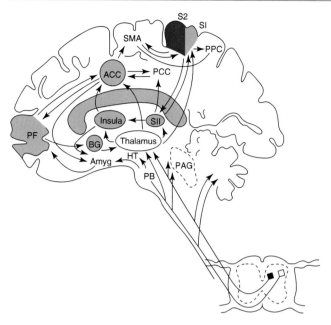

Fig. 7.1 The pain matrix (Reprinted with permission from Bushnell and Apkarian [7]). *ACC* anterior cingulate cortex, *Amyg* amygdala, *BG* basal ganglia, *HT* hypothalamus, *PAG* periaqueductal gray matter, *PB* parabrachial nucleus, *PCC* posterior cingulate cortex, *PF* prefrontal cortex, *PPC* posterior parietal cortex, *S1* primary somatosensory cortex, *S2* secondary somatosensory cortex, *SMA* supplementary motor area

Given the significant degree of reciprocal overlap between the limbic/emotional and pain-processing areas of the cortex evident in Fig. 7.1, intuitively, any treatment which influences one is likely to affect the other. Pharmacological therapies are well known to influence neurotransmitter activity. But, what about the psychological/behavioral therapies? Over a decade ago, psychiatrist and Nobel Laureate Eric Kandel ([8], p. 460) proposed the following:

> Insofar as psychotherapy or counseling is effective and produces long-term changes in behavior, it presumably does so through learning, by producing changes in gene expression that alters the strength of synaptic connections and structural changes that alter the anatomical pattern of interconnections between nerve cells of the brain. As the resolution of brain imaging increases, it should eventually permit quantitative evaluation of the outcome of psychotherapy.

This assertion was certainly prescient, given what we now know about the influence of psychological techniques on brain neuroplasticity. For example, using PET scan technology, Goldapple and colleagues [9] compared the effects of antidepressant treatment with paroxetine to that of cognitive behavioral therapy (CBT). CBT was found to have a modality-specific effect, producing unique blood flow changes in the frontal cortex, anterior cingulate cortex, and hippocampus. Thus, the effect of CBT was largely to normalize the metabolic activity of the prefrontal lobes. Other

studies have also documented similar cortical changes facilitated by psychotherapeutic intervention for disorders including posttraumatic stress disorder, specific phobia, depression, and anxiety [10–14]. Such studies led to Dr. Kandel's revised view, several years later, that "There is no longer any doubt that psychotherapy can result in detectable changes in the brain" [15].

Despite the appeal of the biopsychosocial model, medical pain specialists often unwittingly promote the "pain-as-functional-or-structural-abnormality" concept. The hope of surgeons and patients alike is that once the physical cause of the pain is identified and treated appropriately, the pain will be eliminated. The focused quest for a "pain generator" as well as the predominance of purely medical/physical modalities suggested as first-line options in published treatment guidelines from medical societies can lead some patients down an unsatisfying and incomplete path. This occurs especially if the somatic treatment recommended and attempted is ineffective, partially effective, or when a direct physiological cause cannot be immediately localized. Patients are often left to "just deal with" the residual, incurable symptoms on their own.

Psychological processes of learning and memory, mood and affect, social withdrawal and isolation, past traumatic events, pain beliefs, anticipation of pain exacerbation, and coping style can all play a role in an individual's adjustment to chronic pain. All of these factors have the potential to influence the pain experience at several phases: at the onset of pain, during the seeking and receiving of healthcare and support, and in the development of chronic pain-related disability and work loss [16]. Recognizing the contribution of psychosocial factors to an individuals' pain opens the door for the implementation of psychologically oriented cognitive and behavioral self-management strategies to address the remaining pain complaints and provide a more comprehensive, holistic approach to improving quality of life despite persistent pain.

Of note, acknowledging that psychological factors are involved with the pain experience does not mean that the pain is "in the patient's head," that is to imply, psychogenic or factitious in origin. As expressed by Andrew Miller in his novel *Ingenious Pain*, "All pain is real enough to those who have it; all stand equally in need of compassion" [17]. International studies show that nearly half of people with chronic pain still experience negative cognitive, emotional, and physical effects despite conventional medical therapies, as well as poor social and occupational functioning and overall lower quality of life [18, 19]. For example, the most potent drugs only decrease pain levels by 30–40 % in fewer than half of patients [20]. Surgical techniques such as artificial disk implantation or implantable drug delivery systems also provide modest pain reduction [20]. In addition to pain relief of limited clinical significance in inadequately screened patients, implantable devices also run the risk of adverse side effects [20, 21]. However, patients who participate in various forms of psychological interventions as a complement or adjunct to medical treatment have been found to significantly improve. Improvements in pain intensity, mood, coping, daily activity, and social functioning have all been reported [22, 23] without the risk of adverse physical consequences.

The inefficiency of even our best medical interventions may be due, in part, to the fact that many of the reasons for the inadequate responses to medical treatments are indeed psychological. Relevant psychological factors may include underreporting or exaggeration of pain intensity, inadequate communication skills between physician and patient, unrealistic or inappropriate expectations for outcomes, fears of addiction, fear of stigma, noncompliance to physical therapy exercise regimens, or other health behaviors. Addressing these psychological barriers can improve medical treatment outcomes and assist the patient in coping with any residual pain in the long term. Put simply, the goal of the psychological therapies is to help patients develop a satisfactory quality of life, whatever they define that to be within their own values and abilities, *despite* the persistent pain.

Clinical Examples and Usefulness in Clinical Practice

There are several evidence-based psychological therapies effectively implemented in clinical pain populations. These include but are not limited to (a) behavioral therapies modeled on operant and classical conditioning paradigms, such as exposure and desensitization to avoided activities; (b) cognitive behavioral therapy and acceptance-based therapies; (c) biofeedback and relaxation training; (d) group therapies; and (e) motivational enhancement therapy. Another technique that falls under the "psychological therapy" umbrella is hypnosis, which is covered elsewhere in this book. Insight-oriented and psychodynamic approaches, which are predicated on the belief that pain may be a manifestation of emotional distress and which emphasize the influence of early childhood experi-

ences on the experience of pain in adulthood, will not be reviewed here in the interest of space and paucity of well-designed outcomes studies in pain populations. Some newer therapies such as narrative therapy [24] show promise in the management of chronic mental and medical illnesses, but as of yet there is very little literature on the efficacy of this modality among individuals with chronic physical pain. We will begin with some of the classic behavioral psychology conceptualizations and associated therapies.

Classical and Operant Conditioning Techniques

The most useful piece of learning for the uses of life is to unlearn what is untrue.

– Antisthenes

Most everyone with an undergraduate Psych 101 class under their belt is familiar with the concept of Pavlovian conditioning, also known as "classical" conditioning. In the landmark experiment, dogs were trained to salivate (conditioned response) at the sound of a ringing bell (conditioned stimulus) after numerous repeated pairings of the bell with meat powder (unconditioned stimulus). Thus, the dogs were eventually conditioned to anticipate food and salivate at the mere sound of the bell. Pavlov's studies supported Aristotle's observations of the "law of association by contiguity," essentially paraphrased as "If a person experiences two environmental events (stimuli) at the same time or one right after the other (contiguously), those events will become associated in the person's mind, such that the thought of one will, in the future, tend to elicit the thought of the other."

This type of associative learning occurs in patients with chronic pain as well. Take, for example, a patient who has an unpleasant reaction like a spinal headache following a lumbar epidural block. This patient may develop a conditioned fear response to further epidurals, and the fear may even generalize to other contextual cues (e.g., needles) or other stimuli (e.g., other suggested interventional procedures). See Table 7.1 for an overview of classical conditioning terminology.

Table 7.1 Classical conditioning basic terminology and examples

Term	Definition	Example
Unconditioned stimulus (US)	A stimulus that naturally triggers a response	A dental procedure that involves drilling
Unconditioned response (UR)	A response that occurs naturally in response to the unconditioned stimulus	The increased heart rate and muscle tension that arises during the painful dental procedure
Conditioned stimulus (CS)	A neutral stimulus, that when paired with an unconditioned stimulus, begins/triggers a conditioned response	The smell and sounds of the dentist's office experienced during the procedure
Conditioned response (CR)	A learned response to a previously neutral (conditioned) stimulus	Increased heart rate and muscle tension while sitting in the dentist's waiting room at the next visit, exposed only to the smell and sounds of the office

Therapeutic interventions based upon the premise of classical conditioning aim to replace the conditioned response through techniques that involve gradual exposure to the feared stimulus paired instead with a neutral or calming stimulus. In other words, individuals are taught to "unlearn" the anxiety symptoms. Techniques such as systematic desensitization are often and effectively used to treat panic disorder, specific phobias, and posttraumatic stress disorder [25]. Together with the provider, the patient who fears a needle would develop a hierarchy of increasingly anxiety-provoking scenarios (e.g., seeing a needle in the room, watching others receive a needle stick, feeling the prick on their own skin, and so on) and would be guided through the steps combined with deep breathing, other relaxation techniques, or pleasant thoughts. These steps are initially performed covertly using imagined scenarios until the patient's subjective ratings of distress are tolerable; the patient then progresses to in vivo exposure to real-life situations.

Another promising desensitization therapy, called eye movement desensitization and reprocessing (EMDR), is also described by its developer [26] as both an information processing and an "integrative" form of psychotherapy. It was developed initially for work with specific traumas, involves multiple phases of therapy, and can lead to rapid resolution of negative emotions. The goal is to associate/pair calmer emotions with the traumatic memories and images; the individual recalls the event, but it is less upsetting. Techniques such as bilateral stimulation (alternating taps or auditory tones) or rapid lateral eye movements and substitution of neutral beliefs regarding the trauma are used. Most of the applied research and randomized controlled trials have been conducted with trauma samples like adult survivors of sexual abuse or assault, as well as natural disaster- and combat-related posttraumatic stress disorder [27–29]. However, there is some compelling early evidence that EMDR may be successful in the reduction

and elimination of phantom limb pain and associated psychological consequences of amputation [30–33]. While intriguing, most of the studies using EMDR to treat pain have been case series with small sample sizes, and large-scale randomized controlled studies are, to date, lacking.

> The consequences of an act affect the probability of it's occurring again.
>
> – B.F. Skinner

If you have ever disciplined a child, either through time-outs, spanking, taking away TV or video game time, or raising your voice, or if you've given in to a demand for a toy in a store checkout line to avoid a tantrum and stares of passersby, you have felt the influence of another type of conditioning known as operant conditioning. Operant conditioning involves the use of reinforcement-based techniques—giving praise, taking away aversive conditions—to either increase the likelihood of a future positive behavior (e.g., doing homework) through reward or to decrease the potential for a negative behavior (e.g., checkout line tantrums) through aversive consequences. There is evidence indicating that, compared to healthy controls, patients with chronic pain have increased sensitivity to operant conditioning factors such as reinforcement and punishment [34]. Indeed, the word "pain" has etymological roots with the words *punishment* and *penalty* [35]. Table 7.2 provides an overview of operant conditioning principles.

One of the most common applications of operant conditioning in chronic pain patients is in the behavioral modification of overt pain behaviors. William Fordyce [36] was the first to recognize the effects of environmental factors in shaping the pain experience and to apply these principles to the treatment of chronic pain. Without standardized diagnostic procedures to quantify an individual's unique experience of pain, clinicians are compelled to ask for self-reports,

Table 7.2 Operant conditioning basic terminology and examples

Term	Definition	Example	Potential result
Positive reinforcement	An increase in the probability of a behavior being repeated due to the addition of a positive consequence	After Mr. Smith *displayed several verbal and nonverbal pain behaviors* (B), his wife pays him *increased attention* (C)	Increased likelihood that Mr. Smith will display pain behaviors in order to solicit support and attention
Negative reinforcement	Increase in the probability of a behavior being repeated due of the stopping or avoiding of a negative consequence	Mr. Smith *takes a few extra oxycodone* (B) which *reduces his pain* (C)	Increased likelihood that Mr. Smith will continue to self-adjust his medications in order to avoid anticipated pain
Extinction	Decreases the probability of a behavior being repeated due to absence of expected consequence	Rather than responding to Mr. Smith's pain behaviors, his wife instead *ignores them* (B)	Decreased likelihood that Mr. Smith will display pain behaviors around his wife
Punishment	Decreases the probability of the behavior being repeated due to application of negative consequence	Mr. Smith's physician, upon seeing another *failed urine drug screen* (B), *declines to prescribe* (C) Mr. Smith opioid medications any longer	Decreased likelihood that Mr. Smith will violate his pain treatment contract in the future

B behavior, *C* consequence

monitor overt signals (e.g., in-office postures, facial expressions, and affect), and make inferences about the patient's pain from their verbal comments and observable behaviors.

Pain behaviors include (a) *verbal responses* such as moaning or gasping; (b) *nonverbal responses* including limping, grimacing, guarding painful limbs, and wincing; (c) *generally reduced activity level* including sitting and lying down; and (d) *increased or prolonged use of therapies* such as medications or a TENS unit to control pain [37]. These behaviors, either with conscious intent or more often unwittingly, elicit responses from observers. Family members may then acknowledge the patient's pain through overly solicitous attentive responses, for example, taking over chores or rubbing the patient's back. Physicians may respond with ordering unnecessary procedures or increasing medication doses. As a result of receiving these desirable consequences (i.e., positive reinforcement), the patient learns that their message has been received and the likelihood is increased that the patient will continue to exhibit the behaviors to obtain desired responses in the future. In addition, more adaptive well behaviors (e.g., working, doing laundry) may be overlooked and may extinguish with time.

Therapy based on operant conditioning principles has multiple goals: (a) making patients aware of their overt behaviors, (b) helping them realize more assertive ways of communicating about their pain, (c) educating spouses and families on how to respond with positive attention to desirable well behaviors or ignore/withdraw attention from unhealthy behaviors, and (d) reducing maladaptive or ineffective overt pain behaviors. Efficacy has been observed for this therapy across several chronic pain disorders, including low back pain [38] and fibromyalgia [39], although a more recent review indicates that it is not superior to cognitive or cognitive behavioral treatments for low back pain [40].

Interestingly, solicitous responses from spouses to nonverbal pain behaviors have been shown to be significant predictors of greater pain and physical disability in patients [41]. For example, women with chronic pain who have highly solicitous husbands show lower pain tolerance, greater pain-related interference, poorer performance on functional activity tasks, and greater use of opioid medications [42]. These results underscore the need to include the spouse/partner in clinical interviews and observe the interpersonal interactions. Intervention using couples therapy is warranted for patients with aggressive or overly solicitous spouses; couples can be educated on the operant conditioning model, and spouses can be trained to respond in more appropriate ways to improve the function of the patient.

Over time, you may notice that some patients start to restrict an expanding number of situations and activities (e.g., leave work, stop engaging in hobbies). Not only is an activity like work or exercise *associated* with an exacerbation of pain, the active person is, in effect, *punished* by the increase in pain intensity and discomfort. The individual learns to anticipate and fear the consequence and may choose to avoid the pain-provoking activity. Obviously, this process may reduce compliance to exercise and physical therapy and prevent engagement in adaptive household chores and social activities. The restricted movement may then become reinforcing because the aversive stimulus is avoided, increasing the likelihood of further activity avoidance.

A team of neuroscientists recently presented evidence that fear memories in adult rats are protected from erasure by compounds in the extracellular matrix of the amygdala [43]. In adult animals, fear conditioning induces a permanent memory that is resilient to erasure. In contrast, during early postnatal development, extinction of conditioned fear leads to memory erasure. This suggests that fear memories are actively protected in adults. Compounds called chondroitin sulfate proteoglycans (CSPGs) organize into perineuronal nets in the amygdala, and this coincides with the developmental switch in fear memory resilience. So, not only can avoidance of pain lead to worse functional outcomes, but the avoidance behavior can also strengthen the fear of pain, and our adult brains may take over to actively protect and preserve these fear memories.

Intuitively, avoidance may subsequently lead to muscle deconditioning, increased muscle tension, and amplification of pain. This concept has been promoted in the literature under a variety of constructs: anticipatory avoidance, fear-avoidance, and kinesiophobia, among others. The fear-avoidance model has been used to explain why a minority of acute low back pain sufferers develop a chronic pain problem [44]. It is also the force behind the use of quota-based exercise programs that proliferated in the early multidisciplinary behavioral pain programs [45], in which there is a gradual buildup of exposure to exercises and repetitions. However, more recent studies have called into question the hypothesized consequences of fear-avoidance for daily functioning [46], and sophisticated longitudinal design and statistical analysis suggest that fear-avoidance beliefs do not limit activity and cause pain/disability in a global manner [47].

Traditionally, operant conditioning therapies took place within inpatient pain rehabilitation environments to promote consistency, but there are no limitations to the settings where operant and classical conditioning can be effectively applied. Mental health providers may work with patients individually or with couples in outpatient or residential therapy settings. Physical therapists can apply reinforcement techniques and graded exposure during exercise sessions. Nurses and medical assistants often talk a patient through blood draws in a calming manner to reduce fear associations.

There are several ways for physicians to implement these behavioral techniques during office visits, on rounds, or even during quick consultations:

- Avoid basing treatment plans solely on patient pain behaviors (e.g., "She's not writhing on the floor, so she must not be a 9/10") and conversely attempt to attend to and praise well behaviors. It has been shown that pain severity and other physical symptoms were significantly underestimated in patients with major depressive episode or panic disorder symptoms [48], who may appear excessive in their behavioral presentations. We do not want to reward or punish the patient with dramatic presentation nor undertreat the stoic patient.
- Suggest time-contingent medication dosing rather than pain-contingent dosing and clearly explain the rationale and recommended time schedule (e.g., write q8h rather than t.i.d.).
- Encourage activity pacing (remember the motto "Take a break *before* you need a break and then get back to it") to break up the overactivity-pain-rest cycle and reassociate activity with positive outcomes.
- Consider playing comforting music in post-procedure recovery rooms to associate a calming stimulus with a possibly uncomfortable and disorienting experience.

Classical and operant conditioning and their associated therapies are primarily subsumed under the umbrella of behavioral theories. You may be using them already more than you realize. While these therapies can be quite useful in addressing specific activity avoidance, overt pain behaviors, and overly solicitous spousal reactions, they fail to address an important factor in the development of maladaptive adjustment to chronic pain: cognition. This "second wave" of psychological therapies incorporates mental processes and responses and is known as cognitive behavioral therapy.

Cognitive Behavioral Therapy for Pain

If you don't like something, change it; if you can't change it, change the way you think about it.

– Mary Engelbreit

Imagine that you're sitting in a chair in the corner of a dimly lit room, ruminating on life's burdens, financial and social stressors, and uncomfortable physical symptoms. It's not difficult to imagine that your mood would change, posture might slump, facial expression draw into a frown, and muscles become tense. Why, then, is it such a surprise that the opposite is true—that one's mood could lift while in a sunny space, surrounded by supportive friends, distracted by enjoyed activities, or with kind words of self-encouragement? However, individuals with chronic pain often get stuck in a habitual cycle of negative thoughts about themselves, the world around them, and the future.

The cognitive part of cognitive behavioral therapy (CBT) for chronic pain management involves modifying such negative and maladaptive thoughts related to pain. Familiar negative statements include "This pain is killing me," "I'm

worthless because of the pain," "No one understands my pain," and "I can't do *anything* because of this pain."

CBT also focuses on increasing a person's productive functioning in rewarding activities—the behavioral part, if you will. Cognitive behavioral treatment emphasizes active patient participation. Both didactic methods and Socratic dialogue are employed between therapist and patient. The four essential components of all CBT interventions are reviewed in further detail below and include (a) education, (b) skills acquisition, (c) cognitive and behavioral rehearsal, and (d) generalization and maintenance.

The best prescription is knowledge.

– C. Everett Koop

The *education* phase presents a credible rationale for the CBT intervention for chronic pain, encourages patients to believe they can actively manage their pain and mood, and integrates the CBT model with general health issues. Educational topics might cover pain mechanisms, activity pacing, sleep hygiene, proper use of pain medications, the pain-mood-behavior interaction, barriers to compliance, stress management, weight management, assertiveness and other communication skills, smoking cessation, and other health-related topics. In addition, before CBT techniques are implemented, the patient must learn and accept the cognitive behavioral model and be trained to identify thoughts, moods/emotions, environmental triggers, behavioral response patterns, and habitual belief systems.

During the next therapeutic phase called *skills acquisition*, maladaptive thoughts, feelings, and behaviors are slowly replaced with healthier and more effective alternatives. Behavioral skills include active relaxation training and controlled diaphragmatic breathing exercises to target reductions in autonomic arousal (discussed later in this chapter), attentional diversion from pain, training in assertiveness and problem-solving skills, pleasant activity scheduling, pacing activities to break the overactivity-pain-rest cycle, and other active health behavior strategies (e.g., implementing an exercise program, smoking cessation).

The negative thoughts of pain patients commonly fall into one or more of several categories. Some of the most common forms of distorted thinking or erroneous beliefs are seen in Table 7.3. One type of distorted negative thinking warrants special mention. You have seen a patient who is engaging in pain *catastrophizing* if you've heard the phrases, "My pain is killing me," "I can't cope with this," and/or "My pain is always a 10 out of 10 and will never get better." Defined both as a maladaptive appraisal or coping style and a stable dispositional trait, pain catastrophizing is most readily defined by its three components [49]: (a) magnification (exaggerated symptom perception), (b) rumination (inability to direct attention away from painful sensations), and (c) helplessness (feeling unable to cope with the pain given one's present resources).

Table 7.3 Common types of pain-related cognitive distortions

Cognitive distortion	Examples
Dichotomous/all-or-none thinking	"Unless my pain is cured, my life will never be good"
	"If I can't dig in my garden, I won't get outside at all"
Fortune telling/prediction	"I can't go to church because I will end up experiencing more pain and be miserable the entire time"
Mind reading	"Everyone at the store thought I was lazy because I was using the scooter"
Imperative thinking/shoulds and musts	"I shouldn't have to ask for help"
	"I should be able to mow my lawn in an hour like I used to"

Pain catastrophizing is a particularly influential construct that has been shown to be a potent predictor of pain-related disability [50], quality of life [51], suicidal ideation [52], observable pain behavior and spousal response [53, 54], as well as postsurgical pain ratings and narcotic usage [55], often exceeding the contribution of depression itself to these outcomes. Pain catastrophizing has also been implicated as a predictor for poor response to minimally invasive procedures such as radiofrequency lesioning and injection treatments [56], as well as a predictor or persistent pain at two years following total knee arthroscopy [57]. With regard to mechanism of action, there is recent evidence that catastrophizing affects supraspinal endogenous pain-inhibitory and pain-facilitatory processes [58], is associated with dysfunctional cortisol responses [59], and may be linked to altered neuro-immunologic responses to pain [for an excellent critical review of the pain catastrophizing literature [60]].

Thus, during the cognitive skills acquisition phase, the patient is taught to monitor their thoughts, identify any irrational beliefs or thought distortions, and restructure the thought pattern toward more adaptive and realistic appraisals of the situation. For example, to "decatastrophize," a patient would be guided to evaluate the realistic probability of her worst case imagined scenario and identify resources to cope with it. A therapist might ask, "What's the worst thing that could happen with your pain?" "How sure are you that this will occur?" and "If so, then what? Could you cope with that?" With a teamwork approach and techniques such as modeling, role-playing exercises, and a careful questioning dialogue, a therapist will assist the patient with challenging their negative thoughts and encourage them to create alternatives. It is important to note that CBT is not about "putting on rose-colored glasses" and adopting a "Pollyanna personality," which is just as distorted as one who habitually thinks through a negative filter. Rather, it is about adopting a realistic and neutral view of the pain and other situations.

> Act the way you'd like to be and soon you'll be the way you act.
> – George W. Crane

The *cognitive and behavioral rehearsal* phase is a practice component to help the patient consolidate and master the newly learned skills in their natural environment. Homework assignments are often used with graded tasks to enhance the patient's sense of self-efficacy or confidence in one's abilities to use the new skills effectively and to reinforce their efforts.

The ultimate goal is *generalization and maintenance*, in which skills used for specific situations, such as coping with pain, generalize to everyday stressors across multiple environmental and social settings.

For example, we recall one particular patient who insisted that she felt angry and depressed following any type of exercise session. When asked what she was thinking about during her time on the treadmill, she responded that she aimed a rhythmic mantra toward the machine, "I hate this thing. I hate this thing. I hate this thing." One may then see how this became a self-fulfilling prophecy in which the patient essentially talked herself into "hating" the exercise session and her mood shortly followed suit. Once she identified the negative thought, she was guided to create an alternative to use during her exercise sessions, for example, "This is good for me, I'm proud of myself for exercising." She was asked to experiment with the alternative mental tapes during her session and track her thoughts, physical sensations, and mood before and after the exercise sessions in a diary format. When presented with the evidence that she felt better both physically and emotionally when she substituted the positive mantra, her efforts were reinforced and she began to look forward to the exercise sessions.

Evidence for Cognitive Behavioral Efficacy

The application of CBT for patients with chronic pain began nearly simultaneously with its advent in the early 1970s, although CBT and its close theoretical companion, rational emotive behavior therapy (REBT), were originally created with the intent to address more traditional psychological problems [61–63]. According to a review by Turk and colleagues [20], CBT—as a stand-alone treatment or when embedded within the framework of an interdisciplinary pain rehabilitation program—has shown strong empirical evidence of success in the treatment of chronic pain.

Several meta-analyses have indicated medium to large effect sizes for CBT-based interventions in both adult and child chronic pain populations [23, 64]. In addition to statistical significance by means of effect sizes, these studies also demonstrate clinical significance for pain reduction. For example, in one study a reduction of up to 68 % in headache frequency was observed from pre- to post-CBT treatment, as compared to 56 % for biofeedback and 20 % for a wait-list control condition [65].

CBT has been noted to produce significant changes in cognitive coping and appraisals, health-related quality of life, depression, social support, reported pain intensity, pain-related interference, return to work, and reductions in the behavioral expression of pain [22, 23, 65]. Improvements in physiological measures like heart rate, both at rest and in response to stress, have also been observed [65]. In general, CBT has strong empirical support as an effective treatment for chronic pain patients across a variety of conditions, including cancer pain [66], sickle-cell pain [67], low back pain [68–70], knee pain [71], rheumatoid arthritis [72, 73], vulvodynia [74], and temporomandibular joint pain [75], among others. Studies have compared treatment groups to waiting list controls, placebo medication conditions, and other treatment conditions such as physical therapy alone, education alone, and medical interventions alone. Improved outcomes have been shown to last at least 1 year or more, even among patients reporting long-term, preintervention disability [22, 23, 65, 76, 77]. There is also evidence from cross-lagged panel design studies that positive changes in cognitive process variables—including pain catastrophizing, helplessness, and pain anxiety—*precede* changes in pain-related outcomes in the context of multidisciplinary pain management programs [78].

CBT is also a cost-effective adjunct to medical interventions, associated with shorter hospital stays [79], and particularly when offered in group format. Brach and colleagues [80] performed an economic evaluation of 174 patients with rheumatoid arthritis randomly and blindly assigned to either a CBT group or client-centered supportive-experiential group (SET). Each group was performed as an adjunct module to a standard 2-week inpatient rehabilitation program. At 12-month follow-up, patients in the CBT group had fewer internist visits, fewer inpatient days, fewer day-care treatments, utilized fewer assistive devices, had lower medication costs, had fewer sick days, and required less caregiving from friends/relatives as compared to the SET group. All in all, the cost of adding either the CBT or SET group to the rehabilitation program was €47 per patient or about €282 per group [80].

Evidence for the efficacy of CBT has also come in the form of neuroimaging. Techniques such as magnetic resonance imaging (MRI), functional magnetic resonance imaging (fMRI), and positron-emission tomography (PET) have documented neuroplastic changes produced by components of CBT. deLange and colleagues [81] examined volumetric changes after CBT in 22 patients with chronic fatigue syndrome (CFS) and 22 healthy controls. At baseline, CFS patients had significantly lower gray matter volume than controls. After CBT, these patients experienced an increase in gray matter volume, specifically in the lateral prefrontal cortex. Neuroplasticity

secondary to cognitive behavioral treatment has been observed for a variety of disorders including specific phobia [13, 14] as well as depression, anxiety, posttraumatic stress disorder, and obsessive-compulsive disorder [10, 12, 82]. More specific to chronic pain, observed neuroplastic changes have been shown to especially involve neural regions implicated in the descending pain-inhibitory system: the anterior cingulate cortex (ACC), medial and lateral prefrontal cortex (particularly the dorsal lateral PFC), insula, periaqueductal gray, and ventromedial hypothalamus.

For example, enhanced perceived self-control over pain has been associated with increased activation of the prefrontal cortex in addition to attenuated activation in the ACC, insula, and secondary somatosensory centers, associated with reduced subjective pain perception [83]. Similarly, Salomons and colleagues [84] observed that individuals with greater perceived controllability of pain showed activation of the ventral lateral prefrontal cortex and reported less pain. Research indicates that endogenous opioid systems may be involved in cognitive pain coping—the opioid antagonist naloxone has been shown to block the beneficial analgesic effects of cognitive pain coping [85].

> Pain is inevitable; suffering is optional
>
> – Unknown
>
> …You have already borne the pain. What you have not done is feel all you are beyond the pain.
>
> – Saint Bartholomew [c. 1st century]

Acceptance-Based Therapy

As noted above, the traditional focus in CBT has been on teaching coping methods that emphasize control or change in the content of psychological experiences. The connotation of cognitive and behavioral coping skills training is that pain is an entity against which we must fight, control, or win. The constant struggle against pain is understandably exhausting and often frustrating. Acceptance and Commitment Therapy (ACT) is a recently evolved treatment model, one of the "third wave" or "third generation" behavioral and cognitive therapies that encompasses and extends CBT processes to instead engender a goal of "psychological flexibility" rather than control [86]. There are six important processes utilized in ACT, three of which have been studied in the context of chronic pain, including (1) *acceptance* [87, 88], (2) *mindfulness-based methods* that support awareness without judgment and "contact with the present moment" [89], and (3) *values-related processes* in relation to patient functioning [90] (for a full description of the six specific processes used in ACT, see [91]). In each of these studies, the ACT processes are significantly associated with improved emotional, physical, and social functioning [92].

In summary, CBT can target maladaptive thoughts and dysfunctional behaviors in a time-limited manner, either individually in outpatient therapy sessions or in a group setting. However, there are several brief interventions available to physicians in clinical practice:

- Listen to the content *and* context of patient's words. Suggest that they replace "shoulds and musts" with phrases that begin with "I'd like to." Model for them to replace "I can't..." with "I could if...."
- If they are being particularly harsh on themselves or indecisive, ask them to identify how they might talk to a friend with a similar problem.
- Ask them to rank their most cherished values (e.g., family, church, creative pursuits) and encourage them to focus their efforts on those goals despite pain.
- Consider giving a brief screening instrument for depression, anxiety, or catastrophizing in your office.
- Most importantly, be aware of the power of *your own* descriptors and prognostic statements.

During a recent intake interview, one of our patients commented, "My doctor told me he didn't think the SI joint injection would work, but he'd do it anyway. He was right... it didn't work." That patient was unwittingly set up ahead of time for a treatment failure simply from the force of the physician's comment. Similarly, phrases such as "You have the back of an 85-year-old," or "Your back is crumbling to dust" can create powerful and persistent imagery, and said to a patient already prone to catastrophizing, might influence patient mood, behaviors, and future treatment outcomes.

Biofeedback and Relaxation Therapies

We have writing and teaching, science and power;
we have tamed the beasts and schooled the lightning... but we have still to tame ourselves.
– Wells, H.G.

Head and feet keep warm, the rest will take no harm.
– Thomas Fuller

Stare into a mirror and smile. Adjust your facial muscles until you create the most comfortable looking smile. Congratulations, you've just performed biofeedback. Biofeedback and the various forms of self-management relaxation therapies are generally classified as psychophysiological interventions. These therapies involve a systematic approach to increasing awareness of one's cognitive and physiological responses to achieve a state of full body and mental relaxation and peace. Biofeedback is a procedure in which the therapist monitors an individual's physiological responses through a feedback device (e.g., a computer, temperature gauge, heart rate monitor). Processes such as heart rate variability, electrodermal responses, skin temperature, brain waves through electroencephalography (EEG), and respiratory rate can all be tracked. The feedback is provided

in real time as the patient uses various cognitive and behavioral techniques to learn how to control the bodily response. Forms of relaxation therapy include autogenic training, diaphragmatic breathing, guided imagery, and progressive muscle relaxation.

Biofeedback has been shown to be especially effective in the treatment of migraine, tension-type, and vascular headaches [93, 94]. A recent meta-analysis [95] revealed medium to large effect sizes, as well as reductions in frequency of headache attacks. Biofeedback promotes higher perceived self-efficacy and reductions in anxiety, depression, muscle tension, and analgesic use [64, 96]. Intention-to-treat and publication-bias analyses have also shown that these treatment effects remain stable for at least 14 months posttreatment, even when patients who withdrew were treated as nonresponders [64, 96]. Research in this area has demonstrated that biofeedback is more effective than headache monitoring, placebo, and other relaxation therapies, and its effects are enhanced when home training is combined with clinic-based therapies [97]. Biofeedback is effective for a variety of other conditions, including temporomandibular disorders, arthritis, fibromyalgia, and traumatic brain injury [98, 99].

Biofeedback involving electromyographical (EMG) responses has been used as an adjunct therapy to standard exercise in patients experiencing low back pain [100, 101], with resulting improvement in the strength and tone of lumbar paraspinal muscles. However, some evidence is suggestive that EMG biofeedback is not superior to other relaxation treatments or even treatment as usual [102, 103]. Neurofeedback, which involves control over neuroelectrophysiological processes, has primarily been used to treat attention deficit/hyperactivity disorder (ADHD), learning disabilities, seizures, depression, head injury, substance abuse, and anxiety; however, it has also been recently applied to chronic pain. For example, Siniatchkin and colleagues [104] utilized neurofeedback in ten children suffering from migraine without aura. During these sessions, participants attempted to self-regulate slow cortical potentials. Results indicated reductions in cortical excitation and in number of days with migraines. Two recent studies using neurofeedback with fibromyalgia patients were equivocal. In one study [105], neurofeedback was shown to produce improvements in pain intensity, fatigue, depression, and anxiety ratings and scores on the Fibromyalgia Impact Questionnaire compared with patients taking escitalopram (Lexapro). However, in a study using a sham control group versus treatment with an EEG biofeedback system [106], no significant differences were observed at 3- and 6-month follow-up. For additional information on neurofeedback, see Evans and Abarbanel [107] and Demos [108].

In a novel application of real-time fMRI, deCharms and colleagues [109] first utilized thermal heat stimulus to show eight healthy participants activation in the rostral anterior cingulate cortex. During intermittent pain stimuli, participants were asked to change their brain activity while watching a visual representation of their rACC activation, using suggestions such as changing focus of attention or altering the pain's emotional value. Eight participants with chronic pain were also run through the training, using their own spontaneous pain rather than externally induced pain. By the end of the experiment, pain participants (vs. control) experienced a 64 % decrease in pain ratings on the McGill pain questionnaire as well as 44 % decrease in pain ratings on a visual analogue scale. Healthy participants (vs. control) experienced a 23 % enhancement in control over pain intensity as well as a 38 % enhancement in control over pain unpleasantness. Although the research is compelling that individuals can gain such control over brain activation and pain control [109–112], widespread clinical use of this method is not realistic or cost-effective at this time.

Additional reviews have evidenced efficacy for other relaxation therapies that do not use the equipment of biofeedback. One study of postoperative outcomes for 44 adults undergoing head and neck procedures found that listening to a 28-min guided imagery CD prior to the procedure resulted in reduced postoperative anxiety, pain intensity, and shorter length of stay in the postoperative anesthesia care unit [113]. Another study examined 15 women with interstitial cystitis (IC) who listened to a 25-min guided imagery CD twice a day for 8 weeks versus a group of women with IC instructed to rest; results indicated reductions in mean pain scores as well as reductions in reported IC-related symptoms [114]. Other studies have shown guided imagery to be effective for increasing self-efficacy for managing pain and fibromyalgia symptoms although no effect was noted for reduction in pain intensity [115].

Another form of relaxation therapy is *progressive muscle relaxation* (PMR), or the systematic tensing and relaxing of sets of muscle groups to decrease overall muscular tension. While some research has not shown any beneficial effects for PMR [116], other studies have demonstrated efficacy, for example, in reducing pain intensity for hip/knee osteoarthritis after 2 months of weekly 30-min PMR sessions [117]. Emery and colleagues [118] examined the effects of PMR on descending modulation of nociception, as measured by the nociceptive flexion reflex, in 55 healthy young adults. Compared with controls, participants in the PMR group experienced a significant increase in their reflex threshold and reported reduced stress, although pain ratings themselves did not change. Patients with certain types of chronic musculoskeletal pain should be cautioned against vigorously engaging in this form of relaxation since overtensing muscles in terms of both duration and intensity may exacerbate their pain.

Autogenic training (AT) combines elements of deep breathing, progressive relaxation, and guided imagery, whereby the patient attends to various muscle groups and visualizes sensations of warmth, tension reduction, or calm to induce feelings of relaxation—for example, noting internally "my legs feel heavy and warm" and/or "my heartbeat is gradually slowing down." This type of relaxation therapy may be more amenable to patients with chronic pain who cannot engage in PMR. However, research is equivocal to date. One study found no difference between AT groups and usual care groups for the treatment of reflex sympathetic dystrophy [119], while another study revealed significantly decreased mean headache frequency and intensity in women who suffered from migraine without aura [120].

Neuroimaging research utilizing MRI indicated that expert mindfulness meditation practitioners showed enhanced thickness in regions of the prefrontal cortex [121]. Similar research has also associated meditation with increased gray matter density in the brainstem [122], as well as increased gray matter concentration in the right anterior insula, left inferior temporal gyrus, and right hippocampus [123]. Using fMRI, transcendental meditation practitioners showed 50 % less activation of pain-processing brain regions during painful heat stimulation than controls, even when not in a meditative state. Even more interesting was the finding that controls could achieve the same results with just 5 months of training [124]. Xiong and Doraiswamy [125] suggest several potential mechanisms for these beneficial effects, including reduced stress-induced cortisol secretion, neuroprotection via increased levels of brain-derived neurotrophic factor, reduced oxidative stress, improved lipid profiles, and/or strengthened neuronal connections with increased cognitive reserve capacity.

Johnston and Vogele [126] examined 38 preparation-for-surgery outcomes studies grouped by type of intervention (e.g., procedural, sensory, behavioral, cognitive, relaxation) and found that an array of therapies such as relaxation, guided imagery, hypnosis, and education had an average effect size of 0.85 for pain reduction and 0.61 for improvements in recovery time. However, as helpful as these therapies may be for general stress reduction and pain coping, we still need to further our understanding in terms of their mechanisms of action and potential role in pain modulation.

There are a number of ways physicians can provide relaxation resources to complement existing medical therapies:
- Monitor blood pressure in-office while having the patient perform deep breathing.
- Purchase inexpensive finger temperature monitors and have patients attempt to raise their own hand temperature by a few degrees in the waiting area.
- Recommend portable biofeedback devices such as the *RESPeRATE* breathing trainer or the *emWave* personal stress reliever for use at home. These are moderately expensive options but may help with practice in between in-office biofeedback sessions.
- Research and locate a certified biofeedback therapist in your area through organizations such as the Biofeedback Certification International Alliance (BCIA, www.bcia.org).
- Educate patients on the physical and psychological benefits of relaxation. This can be done easily by providing

educational literature in the form of flyers and handouts in your clinic waiting room that include brief "how to" guidelines for practice at home and contact information for local resources (e.g., yoga or Tai Chi classes, massage).

Pain Groups

'Tis not enough to help the feeble up, but to support them after.
– William Shakespeare

Individual commitment to a group effort--that is what makes a team work, a company work, a society work, a civilization work.
– Vince Lombardi

As mentioned above, CBT and education can also be conducted in a cost-effective manner within group settings. This may be particularly important for chronic pain populations, as individuals with pain often gravitate to patient-led support groups. There are some advantages to using group therapy or support forums compared to individual counseling. Pain is often an isolating and alienating experience, and groups provide a sense that patients are not alone in this endeavor. The realization that one shares common problems (e.g., recurrent depression, physiological dependency on pain medications, unsupportive family members) can reduce the experience of helplessness and provide a sense of belonging. Patients may accept suggestions from others they perceive as sharing and appreciating their daily suffering, although they may resist similar feedback from therapists who they perceive as healthy.

Additionally, groups can serve as a place for sharing information about helpful procedures, treatments, specific skills for management of pain, tangible support, and to disconfirm chronic pain biases and myths. Research shows that social support has a beneficial impact on reducing morbidity and mortality from chronic health conditions [127–130]. For example, Holt-Lundstad and colleagues [127] performed a meta-analysis involving 148 studies and 308,849 total participants, followed for an average of 7.5 years. Results indicated a 50 % greater likelihood of survival (OR = 1.5; 95 % CI = 1.42–1.59) in individuals with increased social relationships as compared to those with poor/insufficient relationships. The authors noted that the magnitude of the observed effect was not only comparable to quitting smoking but exceeded many other renowned risk factors for mortality such as obesity and sedentary lifestyle.

Although reimbursement for group therapy and educational sessions varies widely, pain groups provide the opportunity for enhanced cost-effectiveness by allowing the therapist to treat a greater number of patients than would be feasible with more individualized treatment approaches [131]. Studies have shown pain groups to be effective across a variety of pain populations, including mixed chronic pain conditions [132], low back pain [133], rheumatoid arthritis [72], sickle-cell disease [134], fibromyalgia [135], and for subgroups of individuals with migraine headaches [136]. The group modality was found to be efficacious for adolescents [134], for the elderly [132, 137], and even for couples [138]. Pain groups have been shown to reduce reported pain intensity and disability scores [139]. Although formal group therapy is often conducted within the context of residential pain program or grant funded projects, physicians can do the following to promote the benefits of supportive group settings:

- Let patients know they are not alone in coping with this chronic condition. Assist in normalizing some of the associated emotions and thoughts.
- Use your local resources, such as newspapers, city guides, recreational centers, or local chapters of national organizations to find the patient-led chronic pain support groups in your area.
- Contact the American Chronic Pain Association (ACPA; www.acpa.org) to find local group leaders—this organization will provide training and excellent materials for interested patient group leaders. Post flyers or brochures advertising the local groups in your waiting room.

Motivational Interviewing

Motivation is like food for the brain. You cannot get enough in one sitting.
It needs continual and regular top ups.
– Peter Davies

Motivation is the art of getting people to do what you want them to do because they want to do it.
– Dwight D. Eisenhower

For many chronic pain patients, making the required substantial lifestyle changes such as starting an exercise program, learning to pace daily activities, taking medications on a time-contingent regimen, and practicing relaxation techniques constitutes an overwhelming hurdle. As health providers, we hope and expect that patients who sought our expertise and advice will automatically be compliant with the agreed-upon treatment plan. However, in clinical practice, we also realize that absolute adherence is the ideal and not reality. Medication compliance, even for short-term antibiotic regimens, is notoriously low [140]. Simple strategies (e.g., varying type of exercise, providing incentives) for improving adherence to physical therapy have been largely unsuccessful, especially for home-based exercise programs [141]. We also understand the limitations in being able to predict and identify aberrant opioid-related behaviors, despite the availability of reasonable risk screening measures [142]. Treatment dropout is also a common problem in psychotherapy, due to low motivation, external social difficulties, dissatisfaction with the therapist, or feelings of improvement [143]. Some individuals just need an extra "push" to engage in necessary self-management approaches.

Motivational interviewing (MI) is an evidence-based clinical treatment approach initially developed for the treatment of alcoholic patients [144, 145] that has been adapted to help pain patients explore and resolve ambivalence about behavior change and boost their intrinsic motivation to adopt a self-management approach to their pain concerns [146]. Motivation is loosely defined by Miller and Rolnick [144] as "the probability that a person will enter into, continue, and adhere to a specific strategy" and is emphasized by the patient's actions rather than verbal assurances. One of the key assumptions of MI is that people already know *how* to engage in adaptive behaviors—they simply vary in the degree to which they are *prepared* to engage in those behaviors [147]. In the case of chronic pain, for example, one may assume that nearly all patients know how to walk for exercise, and thus, a lack of knowledge does not sufficiently explain the lack of exercise behavior. Motivational interviewing, then, can work synergistically with CBT to address lack of motivation or behavioral readiness by providing an environment conducive to increased readiness for change [148].

Prochaska and DiClemente [149] developed a *Stages of Change* model for identifying the specific stages people go through as they change from maladaptive to adaptive behaviors. According to this transtheoretical model, each stage poses a set of different challenges that must be addressed before progressing to the next stage (Fig. 7.2) [150]. Although there is a conflicting evidence regarding the exact number, nature, and clinical relevance of subscales using the primary measure called the Pain Stages of Change Questionnaire (PSOCQ) [151], five subscales generally emerge that are consistent with the original stages of change model as applied to chronic pain populations [152, 153]. The beginning stage,

precontemplation, describes patients who do not see the need for change and may even be resistant to change. For example, a pain patient who smokes 2 packs of cigarettes per day may irritably resist the surgeon's recommendation to quit smoking prior to a lumbar fusion. *Contemplators*, on the other hand, see the need for change but have not yet committed to action. In our current example, perhaps the patient understands and accepts that their tobacco use is why the surgery has been delayed. In the *preparation* phase, there exists both the intent to change and initial steps to do so, although the full range of self-care behaviors is absent. Here, the smoker may verbalize their intent to quit and set a target quit date. In the final stage, *action*, patients take on modification of their behavior and/or environment with the intent of creating change. The smoker throws away the final pack of cigarettes, buys some chewing gum, and stops smoking. This stage may either be maintained (*maintenance* stage) or individuals are susceptible to *relapse*, where they may exit the cycle and reenter at any point. Although the clinical utility of the stage classification has been questioned in use with chronic pain patients [154], identification with the various stages, as measured by scores on the PSOCQ, has been associated with pain intensity reports, disability, and depression [151, 155].

Treatment is longitudinal in nature given that a patient's stage of change is dynamic across time. MI is problem-focused, clinician-directed but patient-centered, interpersonal in nature, and can be tailored to the individual's stage of readiness with increasingly specific recommendations as the stages progress. At early stages, a supportive environment is key; the therapist must exhibit empathy and reflect patients' emotions. MI techniques help patients clearly recognize their problems, perform personal cost-benefit analyses of their behaviors (i.e., "decisional balance analysis"), develop consistency between their therapeutic goals and motivation, and increase patient's sense of self-efficacy and personal responsibility.

Meta-analytic review has indicated that MI is effective in improving both physiological (72 %) and psychological symptoms (73 %) [156], as well as health behaviors such as diet and exercise [157]. Changes in readiness to self-manage pain have been seen post-multidisciplinary pain treatment programs, with increases in action and maintenance behaviors over the course of the program, concurrent with changes in pain coping strategies and function [154].

In summary, MI is a useful complementary set of techniques to enhance patient motivation, promote adherence to treatment recommendations, and increase readiness to adopt self-driven health and pain management behaviors. Mental health professionals often weave in MI techniques during a course of cognitive behavioral therapy, teach the skills during educational sessions, or focus on them during a multidisciplinary pain program. However, physicians can be a powerful source of encouragement and motivation in their office visits or pre-procedure consultations:

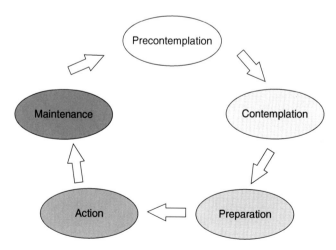

Fig. 7.2 Stages of change model (Adapted from Jensen [147], Miller and Rollnick [144], and Prochaska and DiClemente [149])

- By simply asking the patient what their goals are (in person or even on a medical visit paper-and-pencil form), you are heightening their awareness of what is important to them.
- Ask them about both their healthy and not-so-healthy coping behaviors (*we must admit that even smoking, over-eating, and social withdrawal are still attempts to cope, albeit maladaptive*) and listen without judgment.
- Patients expect their physician to educate them about the negative consequences of their unhealthy behaviors (e.g., nicotine has a damaging effect on discs, bone, and wound healing) but consider turning the advice on its head. That is, focus on the "pros" of adopting the healthier behavior (e.g., "If you quit smoking, you are more likely to have faster postsurgical healing and bone fusion"). This subtle twist on the necessary health advice can help frame the desired behavior in a more positive light.
- Allow room within the traditionally paternalistic physician-patient relationship for the patient to take more personal responsibility for their behaviors and hold them accountable for their actions.

Conclusions

It is our duty to remember at all times and anew that medicine is not only a science, but also the art of letting our own individuality interact with the individuality of the patient.
– Albert Schweitzer

It would be a great thing to understand pain in all its meanings.
– Peter Mere Latham

This chapter has highlighted the need to consider pain as a personal experience influenced not only by physical pathology but also synergistically by prior learning history, cognitive belief systems, social influences, and behavioral motivators. These factors help to explain the wide variability of patient's responses to pain that we see in clinical practice. Given the strength of the emotional and psychosocial components involved in pain perception and modulation, it is critical to give the evidence-based psychological therapies a place in the whole-person management of pain.

One interesting recent suggestion is to match our knowledge of the primary cortical areas involved in the processing and modulation of pain with the goals of psychological pain therapies to provide a thoughtful scientific-based treatment plan for each individual patient. Jensen [158] called this a "neuropsychological model of pain," and some examples are summarized in Table 7.4.

We all have that "Oh no, so-and-so's on the schedule today" gut-drop feeling from time to time. Of course, psychological referrals for patients with suicidal ideation and disruptive personality disorders are certainly warranted, but the scope of psychological therapy for pain is much broader. Collaborate not only with the mental health providers in your area but also with the patient. Several studies have demonstrated that patients who are involved in making medical decisions fare better and are more satisfied than patients who do not [159–161]. Explain to your patient that your recommendation for a psychological referral does not mean you think the pain is "all in their head." Help them set realistic expectations for their treatment and frame the psychological therapies as additional neuroplastic modifiers.

Whether you collaborate with psychologists in the community through a referral process, or if you have one on staff, the integration of therapeutic modalities within the biopsychosocial perceptive is the goal. The incremental benefit of combined treatments can address the limitations that we have seen with pain monotherapies. Instead of the traditional step approach of progressing to more invasive treatments in a sequential manner after each successive treatment failure, consider using psychological treatments as an adjunct all the way through the process, from initial assessment to opioid monitoring to improving compliance with physical therapy recommendations to preinterventional screening, and so on.

Table 7.4 Using the neuropsychological model of pain in treatment planning

Behavioral/psychological symptom	Associated brain area	Appropriate psychological intervention
Maladaptive pain-related cognitions or treatment goals	Prefrontal cortex	Cognitive restructuring
		Operant conditioning
		Motivational interviewing
		Acceptance-based therapy
Elevated affective pain component ("suffering")	Anterior cingulate cortex (ACC)	Operant conditioning
		Motivational interviewing
		Acceptance-based therapy
Perceptions of physical pathology that needs to be fixed; feelings that the sensory experience is inconsistent with physical safety	Insula	Self-hypnosis
		Relaxation training
Reports of very high pain intensity	Sensory cortex	Self-hypnosis
		Relaxation training

Summarized from Jensen [158]

As you have also noticed in this chapter, you are likely already using some of these techniques in a modified way on a daily basis in your practice. As Dennis Turk stated simply in reference to the integration of medical and psychological therapies for pain, "Perhaps 1+1 does = 3" [162].

References

1. Melzack R, Wall PD. Pain mechanisms: a new theory. Science. 1965;150:971–9.
2. Engel GL. The clinical application of the biopsychosocial model. Am J Psychiatry. 1980;137:535–44.
3. Melzack R, Casey KL. Sensory, motivational, and central control determinants of pain. In: Kensalo DR, editor. The skin sense. Springfield: Thomas; 1968. p. 423–39.
4. Doidge N. The brain that changes itself: stories of personal triumph from the frontiers of brain science. New York: Penguin; 2007.
5. Beecher HK. Measurement of subjects responses. New York: Oxford University Press; 1959.
6. Rainville P, Duncan GH, Price DD, Carrier B, Bushnell MC. Pain affect encoded in human anterior cingulate but not somatosensory cortex. Science. 1997;277:968–71.
7. Bushnell MC, Apkarian AV. Representation of pain in the brain. In: McMahon SB, Koltzenburg M, editors. Wall and Melzack's textbook of pain. 5th ed. Philadelphia: Churchill Livingstone (Elsevier); 2005. p. 107–24.
8. Kandel E. A new intellectual framework for psychiatry? Am J Psychiatry. 1998;155:457–69.
9. Goldapple K, Segal Z, Garson C, et al. Modulation of cortical-limbic pathways in major depression. Arch Gen Psychiatry. 2004;61:34–41.
10. Frewen PA, Dozois DJ, Lamius RA. Neuroimaging studies of psychological interventions for mood and anxiety disorders: empirical and methodological review. Clin Psychol Rev. 2008;28:228–46.
11. Letizia B. Neuroanatomical changes after Eye Movement Desensitization and Reprocessing (EMDR) treatment in posttraumatic stress disorder. J Neuropsychiatry Clin Neurosci. 2007;19:475–6.
12. Linden DEJ. How psychotherapy changes the brain – the contribution of functional neuroimaging. Mol Psychiatry. 2006;11:528–38.
13. Paquette V, Levesque J, Mensour B, et al. Change the mind and you change the brain: effects of cognitive-behavioral therapy on the neural correlates of spider phobia. Neuroimage. 2003;18:401–9.
14. Straube T, Glauer M, Dilger S, Hans-Joachim M, Miltnera WHR. Effects of cognitive-behavioral therapy on brain activation in specific phobia. Neuroimage. 2006;29:125–35.
15. Etkin A, Pittenger C, Polan HJ, Kandel ER. Toward a neurobiology of psychotherapy: basic science and clinical applications. J Neuropsychiatry Clin Neurosci. 2005;17(2):145–58.
16. Barker S. Pain and psychosocial factors. In: Van Griensven HV, editor. Pain in practice: theory and treatment strategies for manual therapists. New York: Elsevier; 2005. p. 107–30.
17. Miller A. Ingenious pain. London: Sceptre; 1997.
18. Breivik H, Collett B, Ventafridda V, Cohen R, Gallacher D. Survey of chronic pain in Europe: prevalence, impact on daily life, and treatment. Eur J Pain. 2006;10:287–333.
19. Moulin DE, Clark AJ, Speechley M, Morley-Forster PK. Chronic pain in Canada – prevalence, treatment, impact, and the role of opioid analgesia. Pain Res Manag. 2002;4:179–84.
20. Turk DC, Swanson KS, Tunks ER. Psychological approaches in the treatment of chronic pain patients – when pills, scalpels, and needles are not enough. Can J Psychiatry. 2008;53:213–23.
21. Ives TJ, Chelminsky PR, Hammett-Stabler CA, et al. Predictors of opioid misuse in patients with chronic pain: a prospective cohort study. BMC Health Serv Res. 2006;4:46.
22. Hoffman BM, Papas RK, Chatkoff DK, Kerns RD. Meta-analysis of psychological interventions for chronic low back pain. Health Psychol. 2007;26:1–9.
23. Morley S, Eccleston C, Williams A. Systematic review and meta-analysis of randomized controlled trials of cognitive behaviour therapy and behaviour therapy for chronic pain in adults, excluding headache. Pain. 1999;80:1–13.
24. Roe D, Hasson-Ohayon I, Kravetz S, Yanos PT, Lysaker PH. Call it a monster for lack of anything else: narrative insight in psychosis. J Nerv Ment Dis. 2008;196:859–65.
25. Olatunji BO, Cisler JM, Deacon BJ. Efficacy of cognitive behavioral therapy for anxiety disorders: a review of meta-analytic findings. Psychiatr Clin North Am. 2010;33(3):557–77.
26. Shapiro F. Eye movement desensitization and reprocessing: basic principles, protocols, and procedures. 2nd ed. New York: Guilford Press; 2001.
27. Taylor S, Thordarson DS, Maxfield L, Fedoroff IC, Lovell K, Ogrodniczuk J. Comparative efficacy, speed, and adverse effects of three PTSD treatments: exposure therapy, EMDR, and relaxation training. J Consult Clin Psychol. 2003;71:330–8.
28. Bradley R, Greene J, Russ E, Dutra L, Westen D. A multidimensional meta-analysis of psychotherapy for PTSD. Am J Psychiatry. 2007;162(2):214–27.
29. Bisson J, Andrew M. Psychological treatment of post-traumatic stress disorder (PTSD). Cochrane Database Syst Rev. 2007;(3):CD003388. doi:10.1002/14651858.CD003388.pub3.
30. Ray AL, Zbik A. Cognitive behavioral therapies and beyond. In: Tollison CD, Satterthwaite JR, Tollison JW, editors. Practical pain management. 3rd ed. Philadelphia: Lippincott; 2001. p. 189–208.
31. Russell M. Treating traumatic amputation-related phantom limb pain: a case study utilizing eye movement desensitization and reprocessing (EMDR) within the armed services. Clin Case Stud. 2008;7:136–53.
32. Schneider J, Hofmann A, Rost C, Shapiro F. EMDR in the treatment of chronic phantom limb pain. Pain Med. 2008;9:76–82.
33. Wilensky M. Eye movement desensitization and reprocessing (EMDR) as a treatment for phantom limb pain. J Brief Ther. 2006;5:31–44.
34. Flor H, Knost B, Birbaumer N. The role of operant conditioning in chronic pain: an experimental investigation. Pain. 2002;95:111–8.
35. Bingham B, Ajit SK, Blake DR, Samad TA. The molecular basis of pain and its clinical implications in rheumatology. Nat Clin Pract Rheumatol. 2009;5:28–37.
36. Fordyce WE. Behavioral methods for chronic pain and illness. Saint Louis: The C.V. Mosby Company; 1976.
37. Stiles TC, Wright D. Cognitive-behavioural treatment of chronic pain conditions. Nord J Psychiatry. 2008;62:30–6.
38. Vlaeyen JW, Haazen IW, Schuerman JA, Kole-Snijders AM, van Eeek H. Behavioural rehabilitation of chronic low back pain: comparison of an operant treatment, an operant-cognitive treatment and an operant-respondent treatment. Br J Clin Psychol. 1995;34:95–118.
39. Thieme K, Gromnica-Ihle E, Flor H. Operant behavioral treatment of fibromyalgia: a controlled study. Arthritis Rheum. 2003;49:(3)314–20.
40. Henschke N, Ostelo RW, van Tulder, MW, et al. Behavioural treatment for chronic low-back pain. Cochrane Database Syst Rev. 2010;(7):CD002014.

41. Romano JM, Turner JA, Jensen MP, et al. Chronic pain patient-spouse behavioral interactions predict patient disability. Pain. 1995;63:353–60.

42. Fillingim RB, Doleys DM, Edwards RR, Lowery DD. Spousal responses are differentially associated with clinical variables in women and men with chronic pain. Clin J Pain. 2003;19:217–24.

43. Gogolla N, Caroni P, Lüthi A, Herry C. Perineuronal nets protect fear memories from erasure. Science. 2009;325:1258–61.

44. Vlaeyen JW, Linton SJ. Fear-avoidance and its consequences in chronic musculoskeletal pain: a state of the art. Pain. 2000;85:317–32.

45. Doleys DM, Crocker MF, Patton D. Responses of patients with chronic pain to exercises quotas. Phys Ther. 1982;62:1111–4.

46. Hasenbring MI, Verbunt JA. Fear-avoidance and endurance-related responses to pain: new models of behavior and their consequences for clinical practice. Clin J Pain. 2010;26(9):747–53.

47. Leonhardt C, Lehr D, Chenot JF. Are fear-avoidance beliefs in low back pain patients a risk factor for low physical activity or vice versa? A cross-lagged panel analysis. Psychosoc Med. 2009;29:1–12.

48. Zastrow A, Faude V, Seyboth F, Niehoff D, Herzog W, Lowe B. Risk factors of symptom underestimation by physicians. J Psychosom Res. 2008;64(5):543–51.

49. Sullivan MJ, Bishop SR, Pivik J. The Pain Catastrophizing Scale: development and validation. Psychol Assess. 1995;7:524–32.

50. Severeijns R, Vlaeyen JW, van den Hout MA, Weber WE. Pain catastrophizing predict pain intensity, disability, and psychological distress independent of the level of physical impairment. Clin J Pain. 2001;17(2):165–72.

51. Lame IE, Peters ML, Vlaeyen JW, Kleef M, Patijn J. Quality of life in chronic pain is more associated with beliefs about pain, than with pain intensity. Eur J Pain. 2005;9:15–24.

52. Edwards RR, Smith MT, Kudel I, Haythornthwaite J. Pain-related catastrophizing as a risk factor for suicidal ideation in chronic pain. Pain. 2006;126:272–9.

53. Sullivan MJ, Adams H, Sullivan ME. Communicative dimensions of pain catastrophizing: social cueing effects on pain behavior and coping. Pain. 2004;107(3):220–6.

54. Keefe FJ, Lefebvre JC, Egert JR, Affleck G, Sullivan MJ, Caldwell DS. The relationship of gender to pain, pain behavior, and disability in osteoarthritis patients: the role of catastrophizing. Pain. 2000;87(3):325–34.

55. Roth ML, Tripp DA, Harrison MH, et al. Demographic and psychosocial predictors of acute perioperative pain for total knee arthroplasty. Pain Res Manag. 2007;12(3):184–94.

56. Van Wijk RM, Geurts JW, Lousberg R, et al. Psychological predictors of substantial pain reduction after minimally invasive radiofrequency and injection treatments for chronic low back pain. Pain Med. 2008;9(2):212–21.

57. Forsythe ME, Dunbar MJ, Hennigar AW, Sullivan MJ, Gross M. Prospective relation between catastrophizing and residual pain following knee arthroplasty: Two-year follow-up. Pain Res Manag. 2008;13(4):335–41.

58. Weissman-Fogel I, Sprecher E, Pud D. Effects of catastrophizing on pain perception and pain modulation. Exp Brain Res. 2008;186(1):79–85.

59. Johansson AC, Gunnarsson LG, Linton SJ, et al. Pain, disability and coping reflected in the diurnal cortisol variability in patients scheduled for lumbar disc surgery. Eur J Pain. 2008;12(5):633–64.

60. Quartana PJ, Campbell CM, Edwards RR. Pain catastrophizing: a critical review. Expert Rev Neurother. 2009;9(5):745–58.

61. Beck AT. Cognitive therapy and the emotional disorders. New York: Penguin; 1979.

62. Beck AT, Rush AJ, Shaw BF, et al. Cognitive therapy of depression. New York: Guilford; 1979.

63. Ellis A, Grieger RM. Handbook of rational-emotive therapy. New York: Springer; 1977.

64. Trautmann E, Lackschewitz H, Kröner-Herwig B. Psychological treatment of recurrent headache in children and adolescents – a meta-analysis. Cephalalgia. 2006;26:1411–26.

65. Martin PR, Forsyth MR, Reece J. Cognitive-behavioral therapy versus temporal pulse amplitude biofeedback training for recurrent headache. Behav Ther. 2007;38:350–63.

66. Syrjala KL, Donaldson GW, Davis MW, Kippes ME, Carr JE. Relaxation and imagery and cognitive-behavioral training reduce pain during cancer treatment: a controlled clinical trial. Pain. 1995;63:189–98.

67. Chen E, Cole SW, Kato PM. A review of empirically supported psychosocial interventions for pain and adherence outcomes in sickle cell disease. J Pediatr Psychol. 2004;29:197–209.

68. Bland P. Group CBT is a cost-effective option for persistent back pain. Practitioner. 2010;254:7.

69. Lamb SE, Hansen Z, Lall R, et al. Group cognitive-behavioral treatment improves chronic low back pain in a cost-effective manner. Lancet. 2010;375:916–23.

70. Turner JA, Clancy S. Comparison of operant behavioral and cognitive-behavioral group treatment for chronic low back pain. J Consult Clin Psychol. 1988;56:261–6.

71. Keefe FJ, Caldwell DS, Williams DA, et al. Pain coping skills training in the management of osteoarthritis knee pain: a comparative study. Behav Ther. 1990;21:49–62.

72. Bradley LA, Young LD, Anderson KO, et al. Effects of psychological therapy on pain behavior of rheumatoid arthritis patients: treatment outcome and six-month follow-up. Arthritis Rheum. 1987;30:1105–14.

73. Sharpe L, Sensky T, Timberlake N, Ryan B, Brewin CR, Allard S. A blind, randomized, controlled trial of cognitive-behavioural intervention for patients with recent onset rheumatoid arthritis: preventing psychological and physical morbidity. Pain. 2001;89:275–83.

74. Masheb RM, Kerns RD, Lozano C, Minkin MJ, Richman S. A randomized clinical trial for women with vulvodynia: cognitive-behavioral therapy vs. Supportive psychotherapy. Pain. 2009;141:31–40.

75. Turner JA, Mancl L, Aaron LA. Short-and long-term efficacy of brief cognitive-behavioral therapy for patients with chronic temporomandibular disorder pain: a randomized, controlled trial. Pain. 2006;12:181–94.

76. Nicholas MK. On adherence to self-management strategies. Eur J Pain. 2009;13:113–4.

77. Williams AC, Nicholas MK, Richardson PH, Pither CE, Fernandes J. Generalizing from a controlled trial: the effects of patient preference versus randomization on the outcome of inpatient versus outpatient chronic pain management. Pain. 1999;83:57–65.

78. Burns JW, Glenn B, Bruehl S, et al. Cognitive factors influence outcome following multidisciplinary chronic pain treatment: a replication and extension of a cross-lagged panel analysis. Behav Res Ther. 2003;41(10):1163–82.

79. Thomas VJ, Wilson-Barnett J, Goodhart F. The role of cognitive-behavioural therapy in the management of pain in patients with sickle cell disease. J Adv Nurs. 1998;27:1002–9.

80. Brach M, Sabariego C, Herschbach P, Berg P, Engst-Hastreiter U, Stucki G. Cost-effectiveness of cognitive-behavioral group therapy for dysfunctional fear of progression in chronic arthritis patients. J Public Health. 2010;32(4):547–54. Epub 2010 Apr 8.

81. deLange FP, Koers A, Kalkman JS. Increase in prefrontal cortical volume following cognitive behavioural therapy in patients with chronic fatigue syndrome. Brain. 2008;131:2172–80.

82. Roffman JL, Marci CD, Glick DM, Dougherty DD, Rauch SL. Neuroimaging and the functional neuroanatomy of psychotherapy. Psychol Med. 2005;35:1385–98.

83. Wiech K, Kalisch R, Weiskopf N, Pleger B, Stephan KE, Dolan RJ. Anterolateral prefrontal cortex mediates the analgesic effects

of expected and perceived control over pain. J Neurosci. 2006;26:11501–9.

84. Salomons TV, Johnstone T, Backonia MM, Shackman AJ, Davidson RJ. Individual differences in the effects of perceived controllability on pain perception: critical role of the prefrontal cortex. J Cogn Neurosci. 2007;19:993–1003.

85. Bandura A, O'Leary A, Taylor CB, Gauthier J, Gossard D. Perceived self-efficacy and pain control: opioid and nonopioid mechanisms. J Pers Soc Psychol. 1987;53:563–71.

86. Hayes SC. Acceptance and commitment therapy, relational frame theory, and the third wave of behavior therapy. Behav Ther. 2004;35:639–65.

87. McCracken LM, Eccelston C. A prospective study of acceptance of pain and patient functioning with chronic pain. Pain. 2005;118:164–9.

88. McCracken LM, Vowles KE. Acceptance of chronic pain. Curr Pain Headache Rep. 2006;10:90–4.

89. McCracken LM, Gauntlett-Gilbert J, Vowles KE. The role of mindfulness in a contextual cognitive-behavioral analysis of chronic pain-related suffering and disability. Pain. 2007;131:63–9.

90. McCracken LM, Yan SY. The role of values in a contextual cognitive-behavioral approach to chronic pain. Pain. 2006;123:137–45.

91. Hayes SC, Luoma J, Bond F, Masuda A, Lillis J. Acceptance and commitment therapy: model, processes, and outcomes. Behav Res Ther. 2006;44:1–25.

92. Vowles KE, Wetherell JL, Sorrell JT. Targeting acceptance, mindfulness, and values-based action in chronic pain: findings of two preliminary trials of an outpatient group-based intervention. Cogn Behav Pract. 2009;16:49–58.

93. Andrasik F. Biofeedback in headache: an overview of approaches and evidence. Cleve Clin J Med. 2010;77:S72–6.

94. Cott A, Parkinson W, Fabich M, Bédard M, Marlin R. Long-term efficacy of combined relaxation: biofeedback treatments for chronic headache. Pain. 1992;51:49–56.

95. Nestoriuc Y, Martin A, Rief W, Andrasik F. Biofeedback treatment for headache disorders: a comprehensive efficacy review. Appl Psychophysiol Biofeedback. 2008;33:125–40.

96. Nestoriuc Y, Rief W, Martin A. Meta-analysis of biofeedback for tension-type headache: efficacy, specificity, and treatment moderators. J Consult Clin Psychol. 2008;76:379–96.

97. Nestoriuc Y, Martin A. Efficacy of biofeedback for migraine: a meta-analysis. Pain. 2007;128:111–27.

98. Yucha C, Montgomery D. Evidence-based practice in biofeedback and neurofeedback. Wheat Ridge: Association for Applied Psychophysiology and Biofeedback; 2008.

99. Pulliam CB, Gatchel RJ. Biofeedback 2003: its role in pain management. Crit Rev Phys Rehab Med. 2003;15:65–82.

100. Asfour SS, Khalil TM, Waly SM, Goldberg ML, Rosomoff RS, Rosomoff HL. Biofeedback in back muscle strengthening. Spine. 1976;15:510–3.

101. Nouwen A, Bush C. The relationship between paraspinal EMG and chronic low back pain. Pain. 1984;20:109–23.

102. Bush C, Ditto B, Feuerstein M. A controlled evaluation of paraspinal EMG biofeedback in the treatment of chronic low back pain. Health Psychol. 1985;4:307–21.

103. Stuckey SJ, Jacobs A, Goldfarb J. EMG biofeedback training, relaxation training, and placebo for the relief of chronic back pain. Percept Mot Skills. 1986;63:1023–36.

104. Siniatchkin M, Hierundar A, Kropp P, Kuhnert R, Gerber WD. Self-regulation of slow cortical potentials in children with migraine: an exploratory study. Appl Psychophysiol Biofeedback. 2000;25:13–32.

105. Kayiran S, Dursun E, Dursun N, Ermutlu N, Karamürsel S. Neurofeedback intervention in fibromyalgia syndrome: a randomized, controlled, rater blind clinical trial. Appl Psychophysiol Biofeedback. 2010;35(4):293–302.

106. Nelson DV, Bennett RM, Barkhuizen A, et al. Neurotherapy of fibromyalgia? Pain Med. 2010;11:912–9.

107. Evans JR, Abarbanel A. Introduction to quantitative EEG and neurofeedback. San Diego: Academic; 1999.

108. Demos JN. Getting started with neurofeedback. New York: WW Norton; 2005.

109. deCharms RC, Maeda F, Flover GH. Control over brain activation and pain learned by using real-time functional MRI. Proc Natl Acad Sci USA. 2005;102:18626–31.

110. Caria A, Veit R, Sitram R, et al. Regulation of anterior insular cortex activity using real-time fMRI. Neuroimage. 2007;35: 1238–46.

111. deCharms RC, Christoff K, Glover GH, Pauly JM, Whitfueld S, Gabrieli JD. Learned regulation of spatially localized brain activation using real-time fMRI. Neuroimage. 2004;21:436–43.

112. Weiskopf N, Sitaram R, Josephs O, et al. Real-time functional magnetic resonance imaging: methods and applications. Magn Reson Imaging. 2007;25:989–1003.

113. Gonzalez EA, Ledesma RJ, McAllister DJ, Perry SM, Dyer CA, Maye JP. Effects of guided imagery on postoperative outcomes in patients undergoing same-day surgical procedures: a randomized, single-blind study. AANA J. 2010;78:181–8.

114. Carrico DJ, Peters KM, Diokno AC. Guided imagery for women with interstitial cystitis: results of a prospective, randomized controlled pilot study. J Altern Complement Med. 2008;14: 53–60.

115. Menzies V, Taylor AG, Bourguignon C. Effects of guided imagery on outcomes of pain, functional status, and self-efficacy in persons diagnosed with fibromyalgia. J Altern Complement Med. 2006;12:23–30.

116. Hasson D, Arnetz B, Jelveus L, Edelstam B. A randomized clinical trial of the treatment effects of massage compared to relaxation tape recordings on diffuse long-term pain. Psychother Psychosom. 2004;73:17–24.

117. Gay MC, Philippot P, Luminet O. Differential effectiveness of psychobiological interventions for reducing osteoarthritis pain: a comparison of Erickson hypnosis and Jacobsen relaxation. Eur J Pain. 2002;6:1–16.

118. Emery CF, France CR, Harris J, Norma G, Vanarsdalen C. Effects of progressive muscle relaxation on nociceptive flexion reflex threshold in healthy young adults: a randomized trial. Pain. 2008;138:375–9.

119. Fialka V, Korpan M, Saradeth T, et al. Autogenic training for reflex sympathetic dystrophy: a pilot study. Complement Ther Med. 1996;4:103–5.

120. Juhasz G, Zsombok T, Gonda X, Nagyne N, Modosne E, Bagdy G. Effects of autogenic training on nitroglycerin-induced headaches. Headache. 2007;47:371–83.

121. Lazar SW, Kerr CE, Wasserman RH, et al. Meditation experience is associated with increased cortical thickness. Neuroreport. 2005;16:1893–7.

122. Vestergaard-Poulsen P, van Beek M, Skewes J, et al. Long-term meditation is associated with increased gray matter density in the brainstem. Neuroreport. 2009;20:170–4.

123. Hölzel BK, Ott U, Gard T, et al. Investigation of mindfulness meditation practitioners with voxel-based morphometry. Soc Cogn Affect Neurosci. 2008;3:55–61.

124. Orme-Johnson DW, Schneider RH, Son YD. Neuroimaging of meditation's effect of brain reactivity to pain. Neuroreport. 2006;17:1359–63.

125. Xiong GL, Doraiswamy PM. Does meditation enhance cognition and brain plasticity? Ann N Y Acad Sci. 2009;1172:63–9.

126. Johnston M, Vogele C. Benefits of psychological preparation for surgery: a meta-analysis. Ann Behav Med. 1993;15:245–56.

127. Holt-Lundstad J, Smith TB, Layton B. Social relationships and mortality risk: a meta-analytic review. PLoS Med. 2010; 7:1–20.

128. House JS, Landis KR, Umberson D. Social relationships and health. Science. 1988;241:540–5.

129. Mookadam F, Arthur HM. Social support and its relationship to morbidity and mortality after acute myocardial infarction. Arch Intern Med. 2004;164:1514–8.

130. Pinquart M, Duberstein PR. Associations of social networks with cancer mortality: a meta-analysis. Crit Rev Oncol Hematol. 2010;75:122–37.

131. Thorn BE, Kuhajda MC. Group cognitive therapy for chronic pain. J Clin Psychol. 2006;62:1355–66.

132. Ersek M, Turner JA, McCurry SM, Gibbons L, Kraybill BM. Efficacy of a self-management group intervention for elderly persons with chronic pain. Clin J Pain. 2003;19:156–67.

133. Cole JD. Psychotherapy with the chronic pain patient using coping skills development: outcome study. J Occup Health Psychol. 1998;3:217–26.

134. Thomas VJ, Dixon AL, Milligan P. Cognitive-behaviour therapy for the management of sickle cell disease pain: an evaluation of a community-based intervention. Br J Health Psychol. 1999;4:209–29.

135. Keel PJ, Bodoky C, Gerhard U, Müller W. Comparison of integrated group therapy and group relaxation training for fibromyalgia. Clin J Pain. 1998;14:232–8.

136. Thorn BE, Pence LB, Ward LC, et al. A randomized clinical trial of targeted cognitive behavioral treatment to reduce catastrophizing in chronic headache sufferers. J Pain. 2007;8:938–49.

137. Ersek M, Turner JA, Cain KC, Kemp CA. Results of a randomized controlled trial to examine the efficacy of a chronic pain self-management group for older adults. Pain. 2008;138: 29–40.

138. Langelier RP, Gallagher RM. Outpatient treatment of chronic pain groups for couples. Clin J Pain. 1989;5:227–31.

139. Bezalel T, Carmeli E, Katz-Leurer M. The effect of a group education programme on pain and function through knowledge acquisition and home-based exercise among patients with knee osteoarthritis: a parallel randomised single-blind clinical trial. Physiotherapy. 2010;96:137–43.

140. Greenberg RN. Overview of patient compliance with medication dosing: a literature review. Clin Ther. 1984;6(5):592–9.

141. McLean SM, Burton M, Bradley L, Littlewood C. Interventions for enhancing adherence with physiotherapy: a systematic review. Man Ther. 2010;15(6):514–21. Epub 2010 Jul 14.

142. Chou R, Fanciullo GJ, Fine PG, Miaskowski C, Passik SD, Portenoy RK. Opioids for chronic noncancer pain: prediction and identification of aberrant drug-related behaviors: a review of the evidence for an American Pain Society and American Academy of Pain Medicine clinical practice guidelines. J Pain. 2009;10(2):131–46.

143. Bados A, Balaguer G, Saldana C. The efficacy of cognitive-behavioral therapy and the problem of drop-out. J Clin Psychol. 2007;63(6):585–92.

144. Miller WR, Rollnick S. Motivational interviewing: preparing people to change addictive behavior. 2nd ed. New York: Guilford Press; 2002. p. 33–42.

145. Miller WR, Zweben A, DiClemente CC, Rychartik RG. Motivational enhancement therapy manual: a clinical research guide for therapists treating individuals with alcohol abuse and dependence (DHHS publication no. ADM 92–1894). Washington, D.C.: U.S. Government Printing Office; 1992.

146. Kerns RD, Rosenberg R. Predicting responses to self-management treatments for chronic pain: application of the pain stages of change model. Pain. 2000;84:49–55.

147. Jensen MP. Enhancing motivation to change in pain treatment. In: Gatchel RJ, Turk DC, editors. Psychological approaches to pain management: a practitioner's handbook. New York: Guilford Press; 1996. p. 78–111.

148. Hettema J, Steele J, Miller WR. Motivational interviewing. Annu Rev Clin Psychol. 2005;1:91–111.

149. Prochaska JO, DiClemente CC. Stages of change in the modification of problem behaviors. In: Hersen M, Eisler RN, Miller PN, editors. Progress in behavior modification. Sycamore: Sycamore Press; 1982. p. 184–214.

150. Prochaska JO, DiClemente CC, Norcross JC. In search of how people change: applications to addictive behaviors. Am Psychol. 1992;47:1102–14.

151. Kerns RD, Rosenberg R, Jamison RN, Caudill MA, Haythornthwaite J. Readiness to adopt a self-management approach to chronic pain: the Pain Stages of Change Questionnaire (PSOCQ). Pain. 1997;72(1–2):227–34.

152. Keefe FJ, Lefebvre JC, Kerns RD, Rosenberg R, Beaupre P, Prochaska J, et al. Understanding the adoption of arthritis self-management: stages of changes profiles among arthritis patients. Pain. 2000;87:303–13.

153. Dijkstra A, Vlaeyen JWS, Rijnen H, Nielson W. Readiness to adopt the self-management approach to cope with chronic pain in fibromyalgic patients. Pain. 2001;90:37–45.

154. Jensen MP, Nielson WR, Turner JA, Romano JM, Hill ML. Changes in readiness to self-manage pain are associated with improvement in multidisciplinary pain treatment and pain coping. Pain. 2004;111:84–95.

155. Strand EB, Kerns RD, Haavik-Nilsen K, et al. Higher levels of pain readiness to change and more positive affect reduce pain reports – a weekly assessment study on arthritis patients. Pain. 2007;127(3):204–13.

156. Rubak S, Sandbæk A, Lauritzen T, Christensen B. Motivational interviewing: a systematic review and meta-analysis. Br J Gen Pract. 2005;55:305–12.

157. Burke B, Arkowitz H, Mechola M. The efficacy of motivational interviewing: a meta-analysis of controlled clinical trials. J Consult Clin Psychol. 2003;71:843–61.

158. Jensen MP. A neuropsychological model of pain: research and clinical implications. J Pain. 2010;11(1):2–12.

159. Singh JA, Sloan JA, Atherton PJ, Smith T, Hack TF, Huschka MM, et al. Preferred roles in treatment decision making among patients with cancer: a pooled analysis of studies using the Control Preferences Scale. Am J Manag Care. 2010;16(9):688–96.

160. Petrella RJ, Petrella M. A prospective, randomized, double-blind, placebo controlled study to evaluate the efficacy of intraarticular hyaluronic acid for osteoarthritis of the knee. J Rheumatol. 2006;33(5):951–6.

161. Greenfield S, Kaplan S, Ware Jr JE. Expanding patient involvement in care: effects on patient outcomes. Ann Intern Med. 1985;102(4):520–8.

162. Turk DC. Combining somatic and psychosocial treatment for chronic pain patients: perhaps 1+1 does = 3. Clin J Pain. 2001;17:281–3.

Billing Psychological Services for Patients with Chronic Pain

8

Geralyn Datz and Daniel Bruns

Key Points

- It is important for mental health professionals to be knowledgeable about current regulations and rationale for psychological billing in the context of pain management.
- Understanding of correct billing procedures allows psychologists to accurately code their services, as well as receive reimbursement.
- Health and behavior codes provide an opportunity for psychologists delivering primarily medically related services, including psychological pain treatment, to accurately code and receive reimbursement.
- Psychological testing is an essential component in assessing surgical readiness, psychiatric comorbidity, and/or risk evaluation for chronic opioid use. It is vital for psychologists to be informed of appropriate coding and recording procedures of this service.
- Correct documentation is a valuable tool for obtaining timely reimbursement, as well as successfully capturing the patient encounter. Incorrect docmentation can result in denial of services.

Money is better than poverty,
if only for financial reasons.

– Woody Allen

*Billing codes and requirements are subject to change and modification. The authors would recommend conversations with your local carrier for billing updates and clarification.

G. Datz, Ph.D. (✉)
Southern Behavioral Medicine Associates,
1 Commerce Drive, Suite 106, Hattiesburg, MS 39402, USA
e-mail: southernbmed@gmail.com

D. Bruns, PsyD
Health Psychology Associates,
1610 29th Avenue Place, Suite 200, Greeley, CO 80634, USA
e-mail: daniel.bruns@healthpsych.com

Introduction

Billing and coding is the means through which a clinical service gains economic value. Within the practice of pain medicine, knowledge of psychological billing methods is a matter of particular importance to anyone wishing to employ a psychologist or provide psychological services within a pain medicine practice, medical center, outpatient health services, or surgery center. Unfortunately, billing for psychological services is poorly understood Understanding of correct billing procedures allows psychologists to accurately code their services, as well as receive reimbursement. Health and behavior codes provide an opportunity for psychologists delivering primarily medically related services, including psychological pain treatment, to accurately code and receive reimbursement. Psychological testing is also an essential component for developing treatment plans, and appropriate coding and recording procedures of this service are also reviewed. Psychologists, medical providers, billing agencies, and the insurance companies that reimburse psychological services all may be confused or differ with regard to billing for psychological procedures. At minimum, this leads to delays in patient care, inconvenience to patients and providers, and lost revenue. At worst, a lack of billing knowledge leads to psychological services not being reimbursed and as a result not being provided. Without the availability of psychological evaluation services to address psychological screening requirements for various medical treatments, these treatments might not be funded either. Beyond that, without these psychological services, there is an increased risk of improper selection of patients for procedures or therapies, patient nonadherence to medical instructions, decline of patient health or recovery due to undetected or untreated psychiatric comorbidity, or worsening of chronic pain due to influences of biopsychosocial factors.

Psychological Assessment of Patients with Chronic Pain

Surprisingly, despite the essential nature of billing knowledge, most psychologists and medical professionals graduate with no training at all about billing for psychology services in a medical setting. Psychological services are products whose nature is defined by the Current Procedural Terminology (CPT) [1]. The CPT, somewhat ironically, is a work in which psychologists have extremely limited input. As a result, the rules and procedures of billing for psychological services are sometimes counterintuitive. As such, understanding the methods of billing and the perspective of business is essential to enable psychologists and their colleagues to define a suite of services that not only meet the needs of patients but also conform to established requirements of billing procedures. Only then can psychological services become the foundation of an economically viable practice.

The rationale for this chapter is to educate providers about the role and practice of psychological billing in the pain medicine environment. A caveat here is that the information below may change over time and may vary by region, payor, and policy. While the information below is believed to be accurate at the time of this writing, a cornerstone of business practice is that a clinician should verify the terms of a particular policy before service delivery and, as is often necessary, preauthorize the services requested.

Business Considerations

It has been noted that at the present time, most of health care remains divided between general medicine and mental health. This distinction permeates our culture to a remarkable degree, manifesting itself in the form of professional organizations (American Medical Association vs. American Psychological Association), treatment guidelines (medical treatment guidelines vs. mental health treatment guidelines), and law (medical laws vs. mental health laws). Unfortunately, the science is clear that this premise is not true for chronic medical conditions generally [2, 3] and for chronic pain in particular [4]: Medical health and mental health are not separate and distinct, but are inseparably intertwined.

Traditionally, psychologists have provided psychotherapy as a separate service from medical care. When physicians referred medical patients to psychologists, or psychiatrists, it was after no organic cause had been found. In those cases, it was assumed that lacking an obvious medical cause, the report of symptoms must be due to psychopathology, drug seeking, attention-seeking, or malingering. This belief arose from seeing the body and mind as separate, a direct result of the biomedical model of training that many physicians receive [5]. The biomedical model also influences reim-

bursement, as most private insurance policies employ a two-payor system, which separates or "carves out" mental health services from medical services and creates separate funding sources for each of these types of services. This can create challenges for the psychologist who is treating patients with pain, as the psychologist is using psychological methods to treat a medical condition. These techniques, which are often referred to as "behavioral medicine," include psychological methods that identify, diagnose, treat, and rehabilitate illness and disease. Several of the psychological specializations that use behavioral medicine techniques are health psychologists, pain psychologists, medical psychologists, behavioral health consultants, and behavioral medicine specialists.

Beyond psychologists, physicians, nurse practitioners, and other professionals may also use some or all of psychological procedure codes to supplement the practice of pain medicine. The purpose of this chapter is to educate healthcare professionals working in the pain medicine environment about two of the most useful but often misunderstood areas of psychological services to pain medicine: health and behavior (H&B) code services and psychological testing services. H&B services are reimbursed for several non-physician specialists. In contrast, psychological testing codes may be used by psychologists, physicians, and sometimes other professions as well. In pain medicine specifically, physicians will benefit from becoming familiar with psychological evaluation and treatment practices and billing methods. Together, these will make it possible to develop an economically sustainable means of detecting significant adjustment issues [6] or comorbid psychopathology [7–9] and to develop strategies for risk mitigation in patients with chronic pain [10]. In the text that follows, the background and logistics of code usage will be explained, and clinical vignettes will illustrate their proper use.

Health and Behavior Codes

The belief that psychological and physical health is entirely separate leads to the mistaken assumption that psychological services would have no impact on "real" medical conditions. Nothing could be further from the truth. A recent study determined that the leading causes of death in this country are modifiable behaviors, such as smoking, improper diet, lack of physical activity, and substance abuse, which in turn cause heart disease, stroke, pulmonary disease, diabetes, and many forms of cancer [11]. Because of this, for 7 of the top 10 leading causes of death, the primary means of prevention and/or treatment involves behavior change [12]. Since psychologists specialize in assessing and modifying behaviors, they can play a valuable role in the treatment of medical disorders. The application of psychological services to the treatment of medical disorders is called "behavioral medicine."

Table 8.1 Health and behavior code descriptions and reimbursement estimates

Service	CPT code	Description	Approximate Medicare 2012 payment
Assessment – initial	96150	An assessment service that includes a clinical interview, behavioral and psychophysiological assessment, and the administration of health-oriented questionnaires	15 min (1 unit): $20.42 1 h (4 units): $81.68
Reassessment	96151	A reassessment to evaluate the patient's condition and determine the need for further treatment	15 min (1 unit): $19.74 1 h (4 units): $78.96[a]
Intervention – individual	96152	Intervention services provided to an individual to modify the psychological, behavioral, cognitive, and social factors affecting the patient's physical health and well-being	15 min (1 unit): $18.72 1 h (4 units): $74.88
Intervention – group (per person)	96153	An intervention service provided to a group Group must be two or more people	15 min (1 unit): $4.42 60 min (4 units): $17.68 10 members (4 units): $176.80
Intervention – family with patient present	96154	An intervention service provided to family to improve patients health and well-being, with education and skills training of family members	15 min (1 unit): $18.38 1 h (4 units): $73.52
Intervention – family without patient present	96155	An intervention service provided to family members of a patient, designed to improve patient health, adaptation to illness, and enhance familial coping	15 min (1 unit): $0[a] 1 h (4 units): $0

[a]Note: Medicare and some private payors do not currently reimburse this service

In January 2002, the Centers for Medicaid and Medicare services adopted six new codes reflecting health and behavior intervention services, and these were added to the Current Procedural Terminology (CPT®) code book (Table 8.1) [1, 13]. These "health and behavior" (H&B) codes are designed to address the behavioral, social, and psychophysiological procedures to prevent, treat, or manage physical health problems and are intended for use by non-physician healthcare clinicians operating within their scope of practice. This includes psychologists (PhDs), nurses (RN, NPs), and other non-physician specialists.

The H&B assessment procedures are offered to patients with an established illness or medical symptoms. The codes make it possible for psychologists and others to provide services to patients with chronic pain without having to diagnose the patient with some type of psychological disorder. In contrast to traditional psychological services, which must be paired with psychiatric diagnosis for billing, the H&B codes are psychological services that are paired with a medical diagnosis for billing. Consequently, it has been noted that, "Clinically, for the first time, practitioners working inside of medicine now have a tool to conceptualize psychology as medical service and have a mechanism to pay for it" [14].

It is noteworthy that, prior to CPT 2002, there was no way for psychologists to adequately capture these types of services. This sometimes led to ethical and professional quandaries for psychologists who worked in medical settings [15]. Medicare and other insurance companies have disallowed psychologists from using evaluation and management (E/M codes, CPT 99201–99205; 99211–99215; all CPT codes ©2012 American Medical Association. All rights reserved) on the basis of their training and the fact that these codes require medical management. Neuropsychological test codes

(CPT 96100–96117) are not appropriate because they reflect testing of cognitive function and response of the central nervous system, which does not necessarily pertain to physical illness. Psychotherapy codes (CPT 90801–90809) are designed for use by psychologists and psychiatrists, but require a mental health diagnosis, which may not be present in medical patients. "The difficulties associated with acute or chronic medical illness, prevention of physical illness and disability, and maintenance of health, in many instances, do not meet criteria for a psychiatric diagnosis" [15]. Nonetheless, traditional psychotherapy codes were often used in this context, which could create a clinical dilemma. In the past, some providers used psychotherapy codes to bill for behavioral medicine services, as it was "administratively mandated," while observing that it was also "not an accurate reflection of the patient encounter" [14]. Counseling and risk factor reduction codes (CPT 99401–99429) are not useful in this context as they require the *absence* of a physical health diagnosis, illness, or symptoms, which is clearly contraindicated for health and behavior interventions. In any case, these procedure codes are generally not reimbursable for psychologists. Similarly, psychological assessment codes (CPT 90801 for the interview and 96101–96103 for testing and report) were also developed in the context of a mental illness/psychiatric diagnosis. While appropriate for some clinical assessments of medical patients, they may be problematic if the primary assessment is related only to the medical condition and its impact on functioning (e.g., herniated lumbar disc, cancer-related pain), as opposed to identifying psychiatric disorders (e.g., depression, anxiety, addiction, or PTSD) or psychiatric complications (e.g., malingering or symptom magnification). It should be noted here though that the ICD-9-CM, the ICD-10-CM, and the DSM-IV-TR all include a diagnosis for "pain disorder," which includes those patients whose pain reports are judged to be affected by psychosocial factors. Thus, for those patients exhibiting chronic pain with symptoms that exceed what would be expected given the objective medical findings, a diagnosis of pain disorder coupled with psychological assessment CPT codes may be applicable. These are discussed in greater detail below.

The principle advantage of health and behavior coding is that they allow psychologists to provide behavioral medicine services without utilizing psychiatric diagnoses. These codes were intended to be funded through medical, not mental, health carve outs, and this offers several advantages over traditional psychological service codes (CPT 90801–90806 and 96101–96103). Most importantly, health and behavior codes are not subject to Medicare's "Outpatient Mental Health Treatment Limitation," whereby Medicare reduces its copayment for mental health services from 80 to 50 %. This reduction only applies to services provided to outpatients with a "mental, psychoneurotic, or personality disorder identified by an ICD-9-CM diagnosis code between 290 and 319" [16]. As such, reimbursement for H&B codes occurs at a rate of 80 %, as it is considered a covered service under the medical portion of insurance. By 2014, though, it is expected that mental health services will be paid at the same 80 % level as physical health services [17]. Secondly, outside of Medicare, the use of psychological codes by psychologists will generally involve billing the mental health insurer, not the medical insurer, and the involvement of a second insurance company can add an additional complication administratively. Third, as above, the use of psychological codes requires a psychiatric diagnosis, and while psychiatric disorders are common in patients with chronic pain, they are not always present.

Logistics of Code Use

There are six H&B codes: two for assessment (initial and reassessment) and four for intervention (individual, group, family with and without patient present). All health and behavior codes only account for face-to-face time spent between a provider and patient. H&B codes are billed in 15-min increments, with no "rounding up." Therefore, if less than 15 min of services is provided the lesser increment must be used (e.g., 28 min of intervention = 1 unit = 15 min). Under Medicare rules, psychiatric treatment codes (CPT 90801–90809 and 96101–96103) and H&B treatment codes cannot be billed on the same day. If both services are needed on the same day, only the predominant service should be billed. With respect to identifying physical health diagnosis, only existing medical diagnoses as reported by the patient's physician should be reported. These codes rely on coding a

physical health diagnosis from the International Classification of Diseases, 9th Edition [18]. Obtaining the physical diagnosis requires a review of medical records or communication with the patients' referring physician. While multiple ICD-9-CM diagnoses may also be present (e.g., 722.81 post laminectomy syndrome, lumbar, 723.1 cervicalgia), the physical diagnosis that is primary focus of treatment that day should be reported. While a direct referral from a physician is not necessary to utilize these codes, non-physician practitioners should not attempt to diagnose a patient's medical condition without medical collaboration as that is outside the scope of practice. Table 8.2 provides a description of Axis I diagnoses codes that are typically used with these codes.

With respect to goals of these codes, "The elements of a health and behavior assessment and intervention are designed to improve a patient's health, ameliorate specific disease processes, and improve overall well-being" [15]. Performance of an H&B *assessment* may include a health-focused clinical interview, behavioral observations, psychophysiological monitoring, use of health-oriented questionnaires, and assessment data interpretation. Elements of a H&B *intervention* may include cognitive, behavioral, social, and psychophysiological procedures that are designed to improve the patient's health, ameliorate specific disease-related problems, and improve overall well-being. A detailed description of these services is provided below in clinical vignettes. The patients with chronic pain who may benefit from use of these codes include those with needs for monitoring adherence to medical treatment and medication regimens, overall adjustment issues secondary to pain diagnosis, and those suffering from the physical and emotional discomfort of chronic pain. In addition, patients suffering from chronic pain with a need for training in adaptive coping behaviors (i.e., relaxation, biofeedback, pacing, problem solving), and/or reduction in potentially harmful or risk taking behaviors (including over-medicating, excessive sedentary behavior, and social isolation), would also be excellent candidates for treatment with these codes. Established illnesses that may benefit from use of these codes include cancer, low back pain, neck pain, shoulder pain, postsurgical pain, post laminectomy syndrome, fibromyalgia, phantom limb pain, and myofascial pain, to name a few.

Since 2006 almost all medicare-assisted contractors reimburse H&B codes. In addition, although many private carriers also reimburse these codes, there are exceptions, so it is always recommended to check with the specific carriers in the state of practice. It is notable that Medicare, and most private carriers, does not reimburse for services provided without the patient present (CPT 96155), despite the fact that a fee has been established for this code. As a guideline, nationwide Medicare reimbursement rates, without geographic adjustments, are listed in Table 8.1.

Table 8.2 Commonly used diagnoses for patients with pain

ICD-9-CM/ICD-10-CM diagnosis[a]	DSM-IV-TR diagnosis[b]	ICD-9-CM/ICD-10-CM diagnostic code
Pain disorder related to psych. factors/pain disorder with related psych. factors	Pain disorder with associated [psychological factors] and [medical condition] (code physical diagnosis on Axis III)	307.89/F45.42
Psychogenic pain/pain disorder exclusively related to psychological factors	Pain disorder associated with psychological factors	307.80/F45.41
Somatization disorder [Briquet's disorder]	Somatization disorder	300.81/F45.0
Undifferentiated somatoform disorder	Undifferentiated somatoform disorder	300.82/F45.1
Other specified psychophysiological malfunction/somatoform autonomic dysfunction		306.8/F45.8
Unspecified adjustment reaction	Adjustment disorder unspecified	309.9/F43.20
Psychic factors associated with diseases classified elsewhere/psychosomatic disorder, NOS	[specified psychological factor] Affecting [indicate medical condition]	316.00F45.9
Other unknown and unspecified causes of morbidity and mortality	Diagnosis deferred	799.90
Noncompliance with medical treatment	Personal history of noncompliance with treatment, presenting hazards to health	V15.81
	DSM 5c: Proposed Complex Somatic Symptom Disorder will incorporate previous diagnoses of somatization disorder, undifferentiated somatoform disorder, hypochondriasis, pain disorder associated with both psychological factors and a general medical condition, pain disorder associated with psychological factors, and factitious disorder, and has no equivalent in the ICD-9 or ICD-10	

DSM-IV-TR © 2000 American Psychiatric Association. All rights reserved
DSM 5 © 2010 American Psychiatric Association. All rights reserved
[a]Note: ICD-10-CM scheduled to become effective October 1, 2013 [44]
[b]Note: All DSM-IV-TR Dx use the equivalent ICD-9-CM Dx codes
[c]Note: DSM-IV-TR is current APA manual for psychiatric disorders. DSM 5 is currently in revision and expected to become effective in 2013

Troubleshooting Issues

Psychiatric Comorbidity. Use of the H&B codes is not precluded in a patient with an existing mental health diagnosis. However, H&B treatment in a patient with comorbid psychopathology must focus on the physical illness/disease that is present and the patients' biopsychosocial adjustment to their disease/illness, *not* their needed mental health treatment. A general rule of thumb is that if you spend greater than 50 % of time discussing concerns and offering treatment for physical illness, bill the H&B code. Conversely, if greater than 50 % of time is spent in counseling and providing support and techniques for treatment of mental illness, then the psychotherapy codes should be used, and the documentation should reflect this.

Assessment. When using the H&B assessment or reassessment codes (96150, 96151), a variety of health-oriented questionnaires can be included along with a clinical interview. These can include traditional standardized psychological measures, along with a variety of nonstandardized checklists and physical and coping strategy measures. A few examples of nonstandardized measures specific to pain assessment are included in Table 8.3, and standardized measures are listed in Table 8.4. Note that this code does not

Table 8.3 Commonly used non- and partly standardized assessment tools

Assessment tool	Abbreviation
Beck Anxiety Inventory	BAI
Beck Depression Inventory – II	BDI-II
Brief Pain Inventory	BPI
Coping Strategies Questionnaire	CSQ
Current Opioid Misuse Measure	COMM
Chronic Pain Acceptance Questionnaire	CPAQ
McGill Pain Questionnaire	MPQ
Multidimensional Pain Inventory	MPI
Numerical Rating Scales	NRS
Opioid Risk Tool	ORT
Oswestry (Low Back Pain) Disability Questionnaire	ODQ
Pain Anxiety Symptoms Scale	PASS
Pain Catastrophizing Scale	PCS
Patient Health Questionnaires	PHQ
Screener and Opioid Assessment for Patients in Pain – Revised	SOAPP-R
Visual Analog Scales, Verbal Rating Scales	VAS, VRS

include indirect, or non-face-to-face time, and as a result, measures used in this assessment are generally brief and focused and may include nonstandardized clinical checklists.

Table 8.4 Resources for psychologists

APA Practice Directorate: Phone number: 202-336-5889. For advocacy and support with claims denials of H&B codes by managed care companies

APA Practice Central: www.apapractice.org includes section on H&B coding, psychological testing, and practice tips. Look under the "Reimbursement" and "Billing and Coding" subsections

Health Psychology and Rehabilitation: www.healthpsych.com go to the "Practitioner's Toolbox" for valuable strategies about "Resolving Issues with Medical Payors"

2006 Psychological Testing Codes Toolkit from the APA Practice Organization, available at http://www.apapractice.org/apo/toolkit.html#

When more extensive testing (personality, psychopathology) is warranted, the psychological testing codes (96101–96103) should be employed.

Group Therapy. H&B groups provide psychoeducation and social support as relating to physical health, health behaviors, and medical illness (e.g., distinguishing acute from chronic pain, explaining the pathophysiology of pain signal, teaching how to increase activity level despite pain), not mental health (e.g., management of depression, anxiety, trauma). H&B group therapy is reasonable in medical or psychological settings that already use group-based treatments, including intensive outpatient pain management settings, multidisciplinary pain programs, medical or mental health-based office-based settings, and hospital settings. H&B groups often have a cognitive behavioral component, instructing patients how to practice psychological coping skills for modulating chronic pain, improving quality of life despite pain, or for coping with functional limitations. This treatment is different than mental health groups (CPT 90853) that focus on mental illness and may use non-evidence-based methods (e.g., process, support, or psychodynamic approaches).

Payor Issues. While H&B services are sorely needed in the field of pain medicine, in practice, reimbursement problems can occur. In most insurance policies, mental health reimbursement has been "carved out" of the medical insurance contract and provided for under a separate contract. This sometimes creates a problem when attempting to get H&B services authorized, as H&B services can violate contractual boundaries. The mental health insurer will say "We can't reimburse you for this because [contractually] we can't pay for medical diagnoses or medical CPT codes. You should call the medical insurer." Similarly, the medical insurer will say "We can't reimburse you for this because [contractually] we can't reimburse psychologists. Call the mental health insurer." If these problems occur, several resources are available to support and advocate for practitioners and are listed in Table 8.4 and are also available online [19]. In practice, handling this issue sometimes entails educating the payors about these codes and their purpose and pointing out any discrepancy in their policy. In particular, it is ironic that while many payors now require psychological evaluations prior to spinal surgery, spinal cord stimulator implants, or inrathecal pump implants, these same payors

may not have made arrangements to reimburse these evaluations. When this type of difficulty is encountered, it is often useful to begin by speaking with the payor's provider relations representative and to inquire about gaining in-network status for providing health and behavior services or making other arrangements for reimbursement. In the case of some private payors, reimbursement of H&B services for psychologists must go through the mental health payor. Paradoxically, this will require the assignment of a DSM-IV-TR psychiatric diagnosis for a medical patient who may have no known psychiatric condition. A method of addressing this matter suggested by some payors is to assign a DSM-IV-TR diagnosis as follows: On Axis III, list the medical diagnosis and ICD-9-CM code. On Axis I and II, list "DSM-IV 799.90 Diagnosis Deferred," as the purpose of H&B services are neither to assess nor treat psychiatric disorders. Having this DSM-IV code on the forms, however, may facilitate the mental health payor's ability to process the claim.

Clinical Vignettes

96150 Initial Evaluation

A 42-year-old male, military veteran, undergoing treatment for irritable bowel syndrome and fibromyalgia pain is referred for biopsychosocial assessment of pain and psychological distress that developed after fibromyalgia diagnosis. Reduced quality of life due to pain and inability to return to work are also noted.

A 56-year-old male who fell 200 ft off of an oil rig, sustained injuries to both cervical and lumbar spine regions, and is status post two cervical spine surgeries and a lumbar discectomy. He is referred for persisting distress and refractory pain that has not optimally responded surgical and pharmacological interventions. The patient feels worthless and useless as he has never been unemployed before and strongly identifies with his work.

A 16-year-old female is referred for chronic pelvic pain secondary to endometriosis and has dropped out of school due to constant pain and embarrassment over her condition. She has trouble tolerating short-acting opioid analgesics, and her family also has cultural discomfort with the use of pain medicines.

Procedure Description

Patients are assessed with either standardized tests or less formal clinical questionnaires, and a structured clinical interview, which includes both the patient and family members. The clinician assesses the impact of pain condition on activities of daily living, sleep, mood, and quality of life in the following ways. During the interview, medical, psychiatric, and substance abuse histories are assessed, and behavioral observations are made. Medical records are also reviewed, and the overall impressions are formulated into a case conceptualization and treatment plan that is made explicit in the documentation. When appropriate, patients are recommended for individual and/or group cognitive behavioral therapy services emphasizing non-pharmacological coping skills, psychological adjustment to chronic pain and disability, and relaxation training or biofeedback for chronic pain.

96152 Individual Intervention

A 35-year-old female, diagnosed with ankle pain after a fall at work, is referred for assessment and follow-up treatment including coping strategies for chronic pain and assistance in return to work. Initial assessment included clinical interview, psychosocial assessment, and review of medical records. It was determined that the patient had significant concerns about returning to work due to the possibility of re-injury, as well as conflicts with her employer over requested accommodations, and a concern about lax safety policies that led to her injury in the first place.

A 68-year-old male who is status post 5 lumbar surgeries, most recently a fusion of L5 to S1, is seen for 8 months of cognitive behavioral therapy focusing on his distress at his inability to perform daily activity including yard work and manual tasks related to the maintenance of his 75-acre farm. Initial assessment via clinical interview, test results, and corroboration from medical providers revealed him as resistant to taking any form of pain medication and to have continual problems in pacing and accepting his pain diagnosis.

Procedure Description

Patients are provided weekly or bimonthly cognitive behavioral therapy, relaxation response training, and cognitive restructuring focused on teaching abilities to self-manage pain. Patients are taught how to adjust activity level, take medications correctly, and address psychological maladjustment (anger, denial) regarding injuries. Patients are given knowledge about their disease process and educated about which factors assist and limit their recovery. Weekly assessments demonstrate progress in treatment and individualized therapy goals.

96153 Group Intervention

A psychologist runs an 8-week outpatient H&B pain management group that meets twice a week for 90 min. The psychologist uses a treatment manual [20] to design a cognitive behavioral intervention for 8–10 chronic patients with chronic pain who are referred by their physicians for learning problem solving and self-management strategies for adapting to their chronic pain conditions. The psychologist treats a variety of pain syndromes in the group including low back, neck, and leg pain.

A psychologist runs a 12-week outpatient H&B treatment group for 60 min once weekly for patients with chronic pain secondary to fibromyalgia. The group consists of four to eight female patients referred by a rheumatologist who observed that many of her female patients were suffering with a variety of behavioral and psychological issues including sleep disturbance, depression secondary to pain and disability, poor pacing, and chronic tension which appeared to worsen the patients underlying pathology. Topics include activity scheduling, cognitive restructuring, relaxation training, and cognitive behavioral therapy for insomnia.

A psychologist runs a six-session medication compliance group for patients with chronic pain being maintained on chronic opioid therapy. A board-certified pain physician who offers long-term medication management for patients with chronic pain and requires the group as part of his opioid treatment agreement. The group meets once weekly for 6 weeks for 60 min. Topics include explaining risks and side effects of medications, medical adherence principles, motivational enhancement strategies, and discussing the concepts of addiction, tolerance, withdrawal, and physical dependence. Strategies for safeguarding medications and how to report and manage side effects are also discussed.

A psychologist runs a biweekly 12-session smoking cessation group for patients with chronic pain who are being considered for chronic opioid therapy. Internal medicine and pain medicine specialists in a hospital-based setting provide referrals. Based on evidence that nicotine use in this population is correlated with greater presence of aberrant opioid behaviors, the physician group requires abstinence from nicotine prior to initiating pharmacotherapy. The group occurs once weekly for 8 weeks, 60 min per session, and topic includes identifying smoking triggers, how to develop a quitting plan, and preventing relapse. Referring physicians also collaborate in prescribing nicotine replacement therapies and/or pharmacotherapies for smoking cessation.

Procedure Description

For each group, the rationale for the group is fully explained in the documentation. Each group includes psychoeducation, cognitive behavioral components, and social support elements. Patients are given outcome assessments prior to, during, and at the termination of the group, and these are recorded in the patients' therapy notes. Behavioral observations are made of the patients, their responses to the treatments, and their completion of assignments and behavioral tasks. Topics covered at each session and the progress of each patient are recorded and individualized.

96151 Reassessment

A 52-year-old male, a former commercial builder who fell off a roof, received 8 months of cognitive behavioral (96152) therapy and made significant gains in treatment. He recently reinjured his low back while vacationing with his son. His pain increased, and he began to regress, exhibiting unsanctioned dose escalations of his Lortab. He admits he became very anxious when realizing his physical limitations outside of work and states, "I wasn't going to just give into the pain." He is referred for reevaluation of psychosocial adjustment and coping skills training.

A 25-year-old female nurse who sustained a crush injury to her right upper extremity as a result of a mounted television falling on her while at work is being treated as an individual in an outpatient mental health setting. She is reassessed after 6 months of treatment, as she is not progressing as expected. Additionally, FCE results indicate she has significant upper extremity impairment and may not be able to return work in her former capacity. She has significant catastrophizing and is developing psychosocial distress at the prospect of not returning to work, as she is a single mother.

Procedure Description

Initial assessment measures are reviewed on both patients. Additional tests are administered based on the patients' reactions to new stressors. Patient's psychological status, medical compliance, use of cognitive behavioral strategies, relaxation and meditation practices are assessed. Current functioning is compared to initial evaluation and last outcome measurement. The need for further treatment is evaluated and supported.

96154 Family with Patient Present

A 21-year-old male who was run over by a commercial forklift. He sustained significant and debilitating injuries to right lower extremity and is status post nine leg surgeries. Although his limb was preserved, the patient was having significant difficulty adjusting to his injury. His mother encourages his passivity, bringing him everything he needs, and even bathing and clothing him, activities his physical therapist states he can do on his own with adaptations which were ordered for the home (rails and supports). The mother reported feel-

ing extreme sympathy for son. The father and older sister have become resentful of patient and mother, stating that they feel "ignored" and "unimportant." At the same time, the mother feels unsupported by family members and appears to increase her focus on son in response to reactions from husband and daughter. The sister and the patient frequently fight, with the sister calling him a "baby," and the patient feeling shamed by his sisters' judgments and experiencing self-pity stating, "No one will ever marry me."

Procedure Description

A family systems approach is sometimes utilized to treat the multiple interactions of the patient's pain problem with the family of origin. For example, a mother could be taught which activities require the most assistance and how to emotionally support her son without catering to his every whim. At the same time, her son could be encouraged to develop physical as well as emotional independence from his mother, which is something that he wants, but does not know how to implement. The son's recreational activity is also increased including church attendance and community involvement. During treatment, the sister and father's feelings of resentment and frustration are openly aired and cognitive restructuring and behavioral assignments are used to assist family members in developing new relationships with each other. Communication skills and assertiveness techniques are also emphasized which reduce conflicts at home.

96155 Family Without Patient Present

A 49-year-old female diagnosed with metastatic breast cancer is being aggressively treated with both pharmacotherapy and radiation therapy status post right-sided mastectomy. The patient is referred for treatment by her oncologist for pain management via behavioral methods including biofeedback and imagery, as well as impact of disease on her quality of life, physical image, and family of two teenage sons and husband.

Procedure Description

The patient's husband and sons are enrolled in treatment as the patient has trouble attending psychologist appointments due to the distance that she lives from the treatment facility and the severity of her pain. The husband works approximately 1 mile from treatment facility and is able to come for therapy in the mornings prior to his workday, while the sons attend as they are able. In treatment, the family members are taught relaxation, communication strategies, emotional support, and cognitive restructuring techniques to assist the patient in managing her pain at home. This allows family members to become active agents in the treatment of their mother's problem, as previously they felt marginalized and helpless as they watched their mother suffer.

Psychological Assessment

In pain medicine, the purposes of psychological assessment include (1) assessing the patient for presence of psychopathology, (2) as a supplement to determining surgical readiness (which may also be required by the insurance carrier), and (3) for assessing potential substance abuse, including any aberrant behaviors or personality variables associated with increased risk of medication misuse.

The prevalence of psychopathology in patients with chronic pain is well recognized [7, 8, 21]. In one study, 77 % of patients with chronic pain met lifetime diagnostic criteria for at least one Axis I diagnosis, and 59 % demonstrated current symptoms [22]. The most common diagnoses preceding chronic low back pain were major depression (54 %), substance abuse (94 %), and anxiety disorders (95 %). Beyond affective disturbances, at least one personality disorder was present in 51 % of the patients [22]. Other studies show that anxiety decreases pain thresholds and tolerances [23], depression is linked to poor treatment outcome with traditional medical approaches [24], and anxiety and depression are associated with magnification of medical symptoms [25]. In general, psychopathology increases pain intensity and disability, contributing to a negative cycle, where functional limitations are perpetuated [26]. As a result, it is not surprising that unrecognized and untreated psychopathology can interfere with successful rehabilitation [27].

The concept of psychological testing for use in assisting medical decision-making is not new. Psychological selection has been used in several arenas for assessing surgical appropriateness and readiness, including for spinal cord stimulation [9], bariatric surgery [28, 29], spine surgery [9, 30], heart surgery [31, 32], and intrathecal pump placement [33]. Overall, results suggest that attitudinal (e.g., expectations) and mood factors (e.g., depression, anxiety) are strongly predictive of surgical outcome, including need for anesthesia, length of hospital stay, functional recovery, and patient ratings of recovery [34]. Recently, Wasan and colleagues utilized psychological assessment to identify outcome for medial branch nerve blocks [35]. They found that the presence of psychiatric comorbidity, in particular high levels of depression and anxiety, predicted diminished pain relief from steroid injection at 1-month follow-up.

In addition, the use of psychological assessment is part of an emerging application of patient selection methodology that is helpful in identifying patients most appropriate for opioid use. Several guidelines have recognized that a comprehensive opioid screening requires assessment of substance abuse, addiction potential, psychopathology, and medical compliance [35–38]. In practice, this is achieved via a multifaceted approach that includes psychological testing, as part of a "universal precautions" approach to risk assessment [39, 40]. In summary, there is a strong rationale for the use of psychological testing to pain medicine, and physicians are encouraged to use experienced assessment practitioners to supplement their chronic pain treatments in this way.

Although either a clinical psychologist or a physician can bill psychological testing codes and perform supervision for these types of tests, psychologists generally have the greatest expertise in the area. Clinical psychologists must indicate who ordered the testing on the bill for services, however. Some other non-physician practitioners are also allowed to conduct these tests, including nurse practitioners, clinical nurse specialists, and physician assistants, but doing so must be consistent with their training and experiences and within their scope of practice as defined in their state. For example, nurse practitioners and specialists offering this service typically must do so in collaboration with a physician.

The CPT codes for psychological assessment include 90801 (diagnostic interview) and three codes for psychological testing (see Table 8.5). CPT 96101 was revised in 2008 to distinguish the actual services of the psychologist or the physician (interview, report writing, integration) from those performed by technicians (96102) or computers (96103 for unassisted computer administration and scoring). In theory, all of these codes can be used in various combinations for an evaluation. In practice, however, some private payors and policies have idiosyncratic rules, including ones that may redefine CPT codes and how they are used. For example, the policy of some payors dictates that while they will preauthorize multiple hours of testing during an evaluation, their system does not allow reimbursement of more than one psychological service on any given day. This policy requires the clinician to bill all hours under a single CPT code, such as 96101. Another area of variance is that the definition of "technician" varies under differing states and coverage policies and should be investigated prior to billing these codes. Types of psychological tests that pertain to psychological evaluations for pain medicine that commonly meet the standards of utilization review are listed in Table 8.6. When submitting psychological testing claims for payment, physicians, psychologists, and non-physician practitioners

Table 8.5 Psychological testing codes and use

96101	Psychological testing, per hour, and interpretation and reporting, per hour, by a qualified professional (clinical or independent psychologist, physician, nurse, clinical nurse specialist, or physician assistant)
96102	Psychological testing per hour by a technician, with per hour interpretation and reporting by a qualified professional (psychologist of physician)
96103	Psychological testing per unit by a computer, with interpretation and reporting by a psychologist or physician. Can only be billed once no matter how many instruments are administered

Table 8.6 Commonly used standardized psychological tests used for pain assessment

Assessment tool	Abbreviation
Battery Health Improvement-2	BHI2™
Brief Battery for Health Improvement	BBHI2™
Millon Behavioral Medicine Diagnostic	MBMD™
Minnesota Multiphasic Personality Inventory-2	MMPI-2™
Minnesota Multiphasic Personality Inventory-2 Revised Form	MMPI-2-RF™
Millon Multiaxial Clinical Inventory-III	MCMI-III™
Pain Patient Profile	P3®

must use both the CPT codes utilized reporting the health-care practitioner service(s) and the DSM-IV-TR/ICD-9-CM diagnosis codes for documenting the suspected or diagnosed mental illness condition. In addition, the medical necessity of these tests must be established (see Documentation section for meeting these criteria). The ICD-9-CM diagnosis code ranges that can be used to support psychological testing codes and medical necessity include 290.0–299.80 (dementias through pervasive developmental disorders), 300.00–319 (anxiety, dissociative, and somatoform disorders through unspecified mental retardation), and 347.00–347.01 (narcolepsy and aphasia through aphonia).

The CPT codes of 96101 and 96102 are based on 1-h units of service. In practice, though, the actual amount of time spent providing the service will vary and will need to be rounded off. The accepted means of rounding the time for these codes for some payors is as follows: If the actual time spent providing the service is 31–90 min, 1 h is charged. Similarly, if the actual time spent providing the service is 91–150 min, 2 h are charged. Since under these rules, the reimbursement for 31 min of time is the same as for 90 min, clinicians need to be mindful of the financial impact of rounding rules. Sometimes, though, a brief psychological assessment may take less than 31 min. Is this case, the modifier "-52" can be appended to the code (e.g., 96101–52). This modifier indicates a reduced service and thus allows for billing for the use of brief measures when less than 31 min is spent. This practice can make it possible to get reimbursed for the use of brief psychological tests, and this is especially useful in medical offices where patients are seen at a fast pace.

Case Vignettes

A patient is referred to a psychologist for a presurgical spinal cord stimulator evaluation. The patient cannot tolerate oral medication and severe neuropathic pain in left lower extremity. The psychologist spends 60 min in face-to-face contact with the patient, taking a psychological and medical history, a substance use history, and assessing motivation and understanding of procedure. In addition, 135 min is spent reviewing medical records, report writing, and integration. The MMPI-2-RF and the BHI 2 tests are administered via computer and scored on the computer. Billing: 90801 is billed for the interview, 1 unit of 96103–59 computer administration is billed for the testing [note that Medicare and others may require the modifier "-59" to be appended to this procedure code when it is used on the same day as 96101 to indicate that it is a separate service], and 2 units of 96101 are billed of psychologist time to write the report that integrates the test results with the interview and the medical records.

A physician is considering a patient for an intrathecal pump placement. The patient has exhausted all conservative treatments. The patient is administered a MMPI-2-RF via paper and pencil, unattended, for 2 h. The results are scored via computer, entered by a nurse. The report is given to the physician, who interprets profile, discusses the results with the patient, and determines that the patient is appropriate for the procedure, given test results and the patients history, which is well known to the provider. Under this scenario, no units could be billed. As no report is generated and no integration of results occurs, 96101 cannot be billed. As the computer is only used for scoring and not for administration, 96103 cannot be billed either. Consideration of additional data, however, and additional time spent with the patient may allow the MD to bill for a more extensive E/M service.

A patient is being considered for chronic opioid therapy. She evidences aberrant behavior in the form of recent unsanctioned dose escalations. The patient is referred to a psychologist for assessment of risk for medication misuse. The MBMD, PAI, and SOAPP-R are administered via paper, for 3 h, while a technician observes patient and is available to assist the patient as needed. The technician scores the measures and presents to psychologist. The psychologist interviews patient for 90 min and spends 2 h in report writing, integration, and consultation with the referring provider about patient behavior. Billing: 90801 is billed for a 75 min interview, 96101 is billed for 2 h of testing of psychologist time (2 units), and 96102 is billed for 3 h of technician time (3 units).

A patient being treated for fibromyalgia has not responded as expected to treatment and cries frequently during the interview. The physician suspects depression and uses a computer-administered BBHI 2 to assess the patient. Since the patient is a delayed recoverer (which could suggest a DSM-IV pain disorder) and also exhibits signs of depression, there are two separate justifications for ordering a psychological test. The physician bills for 96103 computerized test administration in addition to the E&M code.

Table 8.7 Health and behavior documentation guidelines

Session start and end time	Behavioral factors affecting physiological function
Estimated # of sessions	Emotional factors affecting physiological function
Presence of physical illness	Cognitive factors affecting physiological function
Psychological factor/status	Social factors affecting physiological function
Measurement of goals	Treatment, prevention, and management of physical health problem or disability

Table 8.8 Psychological testing guidelines

Where testing and interview (if applicable) occurred	Patient has symptoms consistent with mental illness
Test administrator	Interpretation of test(s): if by computer, add summary of test administrator
Face-to-face time spent administering, interpreting, and reporting test results	Summarize results including:
Time spent incorporating test results, clinical interpretation, and writing report	1. Treatment, including how test results affect the prescribed treatment
Appropriate test(s) selected and how tests scored	2. Follow-up/administration of test to measure efficacy of procedure
Medical necessity of test(s) described (supported through documented diagnosis)	3. Outcomes/measurement 4. Any recommendation for further testing
Documentation of physical condition(s)	

Documentation

The importance of proper documentation cannot be overemphasized. Documentation substantiates the services being billed, quantifies the payment being billed, and may be requested by the carrier in many cases. In the case of H&B codes, documentation should include stating the medical necessity of services, outlining a plan of care and its specific elements, monitoring progress in treatment, and documenting the outcome of services provided. For psychological testing, the need for testing should be provided (e.g., suspicion of depression, anxiety, addictive behavior), test results should be summarized, and recommendation for treatment should be made. For all codes used, it is important that the general structure of each clinical contact should include a discussion of the rationale for service, the primary diagnosis being treated, the intervention provided, the overall plan of care, and either the start and end times or duration of visit (Tables 8.7 and 8.8).

Medical Necessity

In many cases, establishing medical necessity is required. CMS defines medical necessity as "always based on the patient's condition. When documenting medical necessity, identify the skilled service and the reason this skilled service is necessary for the beneficiary in objective terms." Services are medically necessary if they are (a) proper and needed for diagnosis and treatment of a medical condition; (b) furnished for the purpose of diagnosis, direct care, and treatment of a medical condition; (c) meet good clinical practice standards; and (d) are not primarily for the convenience of the patient [41].

If medical necessity is not established, claims for services will be denied. Further, if Medicare or another payor determines that services were medically unnecessary after payment has already been made, it will be treated as an overpayment and the payer will insist that the money be refunded, typically with interest. Additionally, if a provider routinely demonstrates a pattern of delivering services that are not medically necessary, the provider may face monetary penalties, exclusion from insurance programs, and even criminal prosecution.

Notes Versus Records

When documenting health and behavior interventions, practitioners must decide whether they wish to keep additional psychotherapy notes. Under the Privacy Rule of the Health Insurance Portability and Accountability Act (HIPAA), behavioral therapy and psychotherapy notes have special status, while psychotherapy records do not. *Psychotherapy notes* means "notes recorded (in any medium) by a health care provider who is a mental health professional documenting or analyzing the contents of conversation during a private counseling session or a group, joint, or family counseling session" and that are separated from the rest of the individual's medical record. "Such notes are to be used only by the therapist who wrote them, maintained separately from the medical record, and not involved in the documentation necessary for health care treatment, payment, or operations" [42].

Psychotherapy notes "exclude medication prescription and monitoring, counseling session start and stop times, the modalities and frequencies of treatment furnished, results of clinical tests, and any summary of the following items: diagnosis, functional status, the treatment plan, symptoms, prognosis, and progress" to date. These elements are referred to as psychotherapy records (see Table 8.7) [43]. HIPAA singles out behavioral therapy notes for special handling and leaves all other types of psychotherapy records to be handled the same as all other protected health information (PHI). If a provider chooses to also keep psychotherapy notes, these must be kept separate from the rest of patients' medical records, which can make patients feel more secure about their privacy. Note that even though H&B treatment may not be psychotherapy from the clinical perspective, notes generated from H&B services can still be classified as psychotherapy notes as defined by HIPAA.

Conclusion

This chapter reviews the use of two groups of psychological treatment codes, H&B and psychological testing, as they pertain to pain medicine. Assessments and interventions that these codes support are reviewed, and case discussions are provided. Psychologists can offer a valuable service to medical providers. Although it is doubtful that anyone goes into the field of medicine with hopes of mastering the CPT, doing so is a practical necessity, without which services cannot be reimbursed. When the complexities of billing and coding for psychological services are mastered, the rendering of mental health care is able to become an economically sustainable and integral aspect of pain treatment.

References

1. Beebe M, Dalton JA, Espronceda M. CPT 2009 professional edition (current procedural terminology, professional ed.). Washington, D.C: American Medical Association; 2008.
2. Havelka M, Lucanin JD, Lucanin D. Biopsychosocial model – the integrated approach to health and disease. Coll Antropol. 2009;33(1):303–10.
3. Adler RH. Engel's biopsychosocial model is still relevant today. J Psychosom Res. 2009;67(6):607–11.
4. Gatchel RJ, Peng YB, Peters ML, Fuchs PN, Turk DC. The biopsychosocial approach to chronic pain: scientific advances and future directions. Psychol Bull. 2007;133(4):581–624.
5. American College of Occupational and Environmental Medicine. Occupational medicine practice guidelines. 2nd ed. Beverly Farms: OEM Press; 2004.
6. Turner JA, Jensen MP, Romano JM. Do beliefs, coping, and catastrophizing independently predict functioning in patients with chronic pain? Pain. 2000;85(1–2):115–25.
7. Dersh J, Polatin PB, Gatchel RJ. Chronic pain and psychopathology: research findings and theoretical considerations. Psychosom Med. 2002;64(5):773–86.
8. McWilliams LA, Cox BJ, Enns MW. Mood and anxiety disorders associated with chronic pain: an examination in a nationally representative sample. Pain. 2003;106(1–2):127–33.
9. Bruns D, Disorbio JM. Assessment of biopsychosocial risk factors for medical treatment: a collaborative approach. J Clin Psychol Med Settings. 2009;16(2):127–47.
10. Ives TJ, Chelminski PR, Hammett-Stabler CA, et al. Predictors of opioid misuse in patients with chronic pain: a prospective cohort study. BMC Health Serv Res. 2006;6:46.
11. Mokdad AH, Marks JS, Stroup DF, Gerberding JL. Actual causes of death in the United States, 2000. JAMA. 2004;291(10):1238–45.
12. Wiggins JG. Would you want your child to be a psychologist? Am Psychol. 1994;49(6):485–92.
13. APA Government Relations Staff. Health and behavior assessment and intervention CPT codes. 2010. http://www.apapracticecentral.org/reimbursement/billing/health-behavior.aspx. Accessed 21 Oct 2010.
14. Kessler R. Integration of care is about money Too: the health and behavior codes as an element of a new financial paradigm. Fam Syst Health. 2008;26(2):207–16.
15. American Medical Association. Health and behavior assessment/intervention. CPT assistant, vol. 15. Washington, DC: AMA Press; 2005. p. 1–15.
16. Department of Health and Human Services: Centers for Medicare and Medicaid Services. CMS manual system. Transmittal 1843. Outpatient mental health treatment limitation. Washington, D.C.: Department of Health and Human Services; 2009.
17. Department of Health and Human Services: Centers for Medicare & Medicaid Services (CMS). CMS manual system: Transmittal #1843. Outpatient mental health treatment limitation. 2009. https://www.cms.gov/transmittals/downloads/R1843CP.pdf. Accessed 1 Nov 2010.
18. American Medical Association. ICD-9-CM, 1996: international classification of diseases, 9th revision, clinical modification : volumes 1 and 2, color-coded, illustrated ICD-9 CM codes. Dover: American Medical Association; 1995.
19. Bruns D. A step-by-step guide to obtaining reimbursement for services provided under the health and behavior codes. 2009; http://www.healthpsych.com/tools/resolving_h_and_b_problems.pdf. Accessed 5 Nov 2010.
20. Thorn BE. Cognitive therapy for chronic pain : a step-by-step guide. New York: Guilford Press; 2004.
21. Dersh J, Gatchel RJ, Polatin P, Mayer T. Prevalence of psychiatric disorders in patients with chronic work-related musculoskeletal pain disability. J Occup Environ Med. 2002;44(5):459–68.
22. Polatin PB, Kinney RK, Gatche RJ, Lillo E, Mayer TG. Psychiatric illness and chronic low-back pain. The mind and the spine – which goes first? Spine. 1993;18(1):66–71.
23. Cornwall A, Donderi DC. The effect of experimentally induced anxiety on the experience of pressure pain. Pain. 1988;35(1):105–13.
24. Burns JW, Johnson BJ, Mahoney N, Devine J, Pawl R. Cognitive and physical capacity process variables predict long-term outcome after treatment of chronic pain. J Consult Clin Psychol. 1998;66(2):434–9.
25. Katon W, Ciechanowski P. Impact of major depression on chronic medical illness. J Psychosom Res. 2002;53(4):859–63.
26. Holzberg AD, Robinson ME, Geisser ME, Gremillion HA. The effects of depression and chronic pain on psychosocial and physical functioning. Clin J Pain. 1996;12(2):118–25.
27. Gatchel R. Psychological disorders and chronic pain: cause and effect relationships. In: Gatchel RJ, Turk DC, editors. Psychological approaches to pain management: a practitioner's handbook. New York: Guilford; 1996. p. 33–54.
28. Sarwer DB, Thompson JK, Mitchell JE, Rubin JP. Psychological considerations of the bariatric surgery patient undergoing body contouring surgery. Plast Reconstr Surg. 2008;121(6):423e–34.
29. Mechanick JI, Kushner RF, Sugerman HJ, et al. Executive summary of the recommendations of the American Association of Clinical Endocrinologists, the Obesity Society, and American Society for Metabolic & Bariatric Surgery medical guidelines for clinical practice for the perioperative nutritional, metabolic, and nonsurgical support of the bariatric surgery patient. Endocr Pract. 2008;14(3):318–36.
30. den Boer JJ, Oostendorp RA, Beems T, Munneke M, Oerlemans M, Evers AW. A systematic review of bio-psychosocial risk factors for an unfavourable outcome after lumbar disc surgery. Eur Spine J. 2006;15(5):527–36.
31. Burg MM, Benedetto MC, Soufer R. Depressive symptoms and mortality two years after coronary artery bypass graft surgery (CABG) in men. Psychosom Med. 2003;65(4):508–10.
32. Burg MM, Benedetto MC, Rosenberg R, Soufer R. Presurgical depression predicts medical morbidity 6 months after coronary artery bypass graft surgery. Psychosom Med. 2003;65(1):111–8.
33. Van Dorsten B. Psychological considerations in preparing patients for implantation procedures. Pain Med. 2006;7(s1):S47–57.

34. Rosenberger PH, Jokl P, Ickovics J. Psychosocial factors and surgical outcomes: an evidence-based literature review. J Am Acad Orthop Surg. 2006;14(7):397–405.

35. Wasan AD, Jamison RN, Pham L, Tipirneni N, Nedeljkovic SS, Katz JN. Psychopathology predicts the outcome of medial branch blocks with corticosteroid for chronic axial low back or cervical pain: a prospective cohort study. BMC Musculoskelet Disord. 2009;10:22.

36. Trescot AM, Helm S, Hansen H. Opioids in the management of chronic non-cancer pain: an update of American Society of the Interventional Pain Physicians' (ASIPP) guidelines. Pain Physician. 2008;11(2S):S5–62.

37. Federation of State Medical Boards. Model policy for the use of controlled substances for the treatment of pain. J Pain Palliat Care Pharmacother. 2004;19:73–8.

38. Chou R, Fanciullo GJ, Fine PG, et al. Clinical guidelines for the use of chronic opioid therapy in chronic noncancer pain. J Pain. 2009;10(2):113–30.

39. Gourlay DL, Heit HA, Almahrezi A. Universal precautions in pain medicine: a rational approach to the treatment of chronic pain. Pain Med. 2005;6(2):107–12.

40. Passik SD, Kirsh KL. The interface between pain and drug abuse and the evolution of strategies to optimize pain management while minimizing drug abuse. Exp Clin Psychopharmacol. 2008;16(5):400–4.

41. Department of Health and Human Services: Centers for Medicare & Medicaid Services (CMS). Medicare glossary: definition of medically necessary. 2010. http://www.medicare.gov/Glossary/ShowTerm.asp?Language=English&term=medically+necessary. Accessed 1 Nov 2010.

42. Department of Health and Human Services. Federal Register. 1999;64(212):59938. http://frwebgate2.access.gpo.gov/cgi-bin/PDFgate.cgi?WAISdocID=zT6q9W/1/2/0&WAISaction=retrieve. Accessed 1 Nov 2010.

43. Department of Health and Human Services. Federal Register. 2000;65(250):82497. http://frwebgate2.access.gpo.gov/cgi-bin/PDFgate.cgi?WAISdocID=zT6q9W/1/2/0&WAISaction=retrieve. Accessed 1 Nov 2010.

44. World Health Organisation. ICD-10 Classifications of Mental and Behavioural Disorder: Clinical Descriptions and Diagnostic Guidelines. 1992. Geneva. World Health Organisation.

Hypnosis and Pain Control

9

David Spiegel

Key Points

- Hypnosis is a state of highly focused attention, coupled with dissociation of peripheral awareness and heightened response to suggestion.
- Hypnotizability is a stable trait – most children and about two-thirds of the adult population are hypnotizable. Hypnosis can help people establish control over both acute and chronic pain.
- Hypnosis reduces pain perception in parts of the brain that affect both sensation and suffering.
- Hypnotic analgesia involves sensory transformation via change in perception of the nature of the pain (temperature, etc.) sensory accommodation, inducing physical relaxation rather than fighting the pain.
- Patients can be taught self-hypnosis and learn to manage pain on their own.

Introduction

Hypnosis, begun as a therapeutic discipline in the eighteenth century, was the first Western conception of psychotherapy [1]. It is a powerful analgesic, and there is compelling clinical documentation of its effectiveness as far back as the mid-nineteenth century. The British surgeon James Esdaile reported that 80 % of subjects obtained anesthesia with hypnosis during major surgical procedures such as amputations [2]. Hypnosis has been proven effective in treating pain and anxiety in the medical setting using randomized prospective trial methodology among both adults [3] and children [4]. Hypnosis is a state of highly focused attention coupled with

a suspension of peripheral awareness [5, 6]. This ability to attend intensely while reducing awareness of context allows one to alter the associational network linking perception and cognition. The hypnotic narrowing of the focus of attention [7] is analogous to looking through a telephoto lens rather than a wide-angle lens – one is aware of content more than context. This can also facilitate reduced awareness of unwanted stimuli, such as pain, or of problematic cognitions, such as depressive hopelessness, that can amplify pain [5, 8]. Such a mental state enhances openness to input from others – often called suggestibility – and can increase receptivity to therapeutic instruction. Yet despite much clinical and neurobiological evidence, hypnosis is rarely used as an analgesic for adults or children.

Background or History That Makes This Chapter Significant

Pain can be either exacerbated or diminished by the emotional, cognitive, and social environment that surrounds it. As Fig. 9.1 illustrates, pain signals can be modulated from the top down as well as the bottom up. When Melzack and Wall [9, 10] promulgated their "gate control" theory of pain, antedating the discovery of endogenous opiate receptors in the spinal cord and periaqueductal gray, they emphasized bottom-up modulation of pain signals. Yet they had noticed that in Pavlov's original experiments, dogs seemed to habituate to constant pain, implying a top-down pain modulation system as well. Cortical signals can amplify or inhibit pain input. Indeed, pain usually occurs within the context of subjective distress that is associated with a major medical illness or physical trauma. Thus, the "pain experience" represents a combination of both tissue damage and the emotional reaction to it. In fact, the intensity of pain is directly associated with its meaning, as Beecher showed when comparing opiate levels required to control post-injury pain on the Anzio Beachhead (very low levels) and among less seri-

D. Spiegel, M.D. (✉)
Department of Psychiatry and Behavioral Sciences,
Stanford School of Medicine, 40th Quarry Road,
Stanford, CA 94305, USA
e-mail: aspiegel@stanford.edu

T.R. Deer et al. (eds.), *Treatment of Chronic Pain by Integrative Approaches: the AMERICAN ACADEMY
of PAIN MEDICINE Textbook on Patient Management*, DOI 10.1007/978-1-4939-1821-8_9,
© American Academy of Pain Medicine 2015

Fig. 9.1 Pain processing

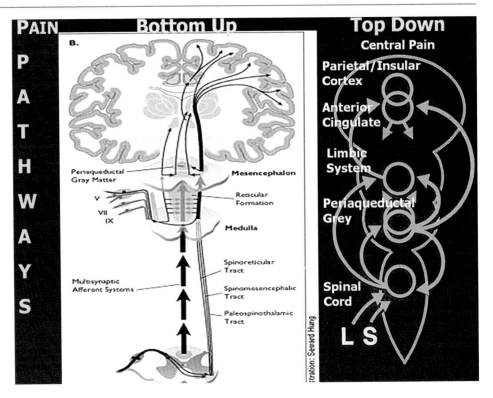

ously injured civilian trauma casualties (high levels) [11]. Those cancer patients who believe the pain represents a worsening of their disease experience more pain [12]. Indeed, the meaning of the pain and associated anxiety and depression accounts for more variance in pain than site of metastasis. Pain is often intensified by the helplessness that accompanies it. Many chronic pain patients acknowledge that they could live with their discomfort if they could just keep it within certain boundaries. The combination of pain and its perceived uncontrollability serves to amplify it. The desire for control is a critical component of pain management. Hypnosis provides an excellent opportunity for many to modulate or even eliminate pain.

While there is a common misperception that hypnosis primarily involves relinquishing control and constitutes mindless submission to suggestion, hypnosis is actually a normally occurring state of highly focused attention, with a relative diminution in peripheral awareness [4–6]. Being hypnotized is akin to being so caught up in a good movie, play, or novel that one loses awareness of surroundings and enters the imagined world, a state termed "absorption" [7]. Indeed, people who have such states spontaneously are more likely to be highly hypnotizable on formal testing, indicating that native hypnotic ability is mobilized spontaneously in the service of intense engagement in a variety of activities [8]. Although the suspension of disbelief involved in such absorption may make hypnotized people appear more suggestible, that is, responsive to the instructions of the person inducing hypnosis, in fact all hypnosis is self-hypnosis, a

means of focusing attention, whether self-induced or suggested by someone else. Thus, the very state that would appear to engender loss of control can be utilized quite effectively to enhance control, especially over unwanted sensations such as pain, which can be placed at the periphery of awareness, altered, or even eliminated.

Pain is the ultimate psychosomatic phenomenon. It is composed of both a somatic signal that something is wrong with the body and interpretation of the meaning of that signal involving attentional, cognitive, affective, and social factors. Many athletes and soldiers sustain serious injuries in the heat of sport or combat and are unaware of the injury until someone points out bleeding or swelling. On the other hand, others with comparatively minor physical damage report being totally overcome with pain. A single parent with a sarcoma complained of severe unremitting pain as well as concern about her failure to discuss her terminal prognosis with her adolescent son. When an appropriate meeting was arranged to plan for his future and discuss her prognosis with him, the pain resolved [11].

Indeed, anxiety and depression are often associated with pain [13–15]. Depression is the most frequently reported psychiatric diagnosis among chronic pain patients. Reports of depression among chronic pain populations range from 10 to 87 % [16]. Patients with two or more pain conditions have been found to be at elevated risk for major depression, whereas those patients with only one pain condition did not show such an elevated rate of mood disorder in a large sample of health maintenance organization (HMO) patients. The relative severity of the depression observed in chronic pain patients was illustrated by Katon and Sullivan [17] who showed that 32 % of a sample of 37 pain patients met criteria for major depression and 43 % had a past episode of major depression.

Anxiety is especially common among those with acute pain. Like depression, it may be an appropriate response to serious trauma through injury or illness. Pain may serve a signal function or be part of an anxious preoccupation, as in the case of the woman with the sarcoma cited above. Similarly, anxiety and pain may reinforce one another, producing a snowball effect of escalating and mutually reinforcing central and peripheral symptoms.

Scientific Foundation of This Topic to Pain Care

There is considerable evidence that hypnosis affects clinically important aspects of somatic functioning. The oldest and best established effect is on pain, dating back to the pioneering work of Esdaile [2]. This finding has been replicated in numerous studies [3, 12–15, 18–23]. We conducted a randomized controlled clinical trial among 241 patients undergoing invasive radiological procedures and demonstrated that, compared to either routine care or structured attention, hypnosis produced significant reductions in pain, anxiety, complications, and procedure time while requiring only half of the total analgesic medication (Fig. 9.2a, b) [3].

Hypnosis in combination with group therapeutic support has been proven highly effective in reducing chronic pain as well. In two randomized clinical trials involving women with metastatic breast cancer, this treatment resulted in a significant reduction in pain over a 1-year period while patients were on the same and low amounts of analgesic medication (Fig. 9.3) [16, 24].

Neuroimaging and Hypnosis

Hypnotic analgesia results in reduced amplitude of the somatosensory event-related potential, including early (p100) as well as later (p200 and p300) components [17]. There is evidence from other laboratories that hypnotic analgesia involves both sensory and affective aspects of pain and that changes in the wording of hypnotic instructions alter parts of the brain involved in hypnotic analgesia, from reduced perception (somatosensory cortex) to reduced concern with the pain (anterior cingulate cortex) [25–27]. Many studies have demonstrated that hypnotic alteration of perception changes perceptual processing in the brain. Changing the wording of a pain-directed hypnotic instruction from "you will feel cool, tingling numbness more than pain" to "the pain will not bother you" shifts activation from the

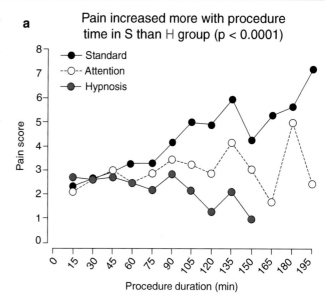

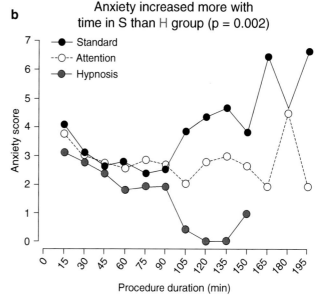

Fig. 9.2 (**a**) Pain increased more with procedure time in S than H group, and (**b**) anxiety increased more with time in S than H group (Adapted from Lang et al. [3])

somatosensory cortex to the dACC [25, 27]. Similarly, in a PET study, hypnotic suggestion to add or subtract color was shown to alter blood flow in color processing regions of the brain in comparable directions [28]. Hypnotized subjects were asked to see a grayscale pattern in color; under hypnosis, color areas in the ventral visual processing stream were activated, whether they were shown colors or the grayscale stimulus. Believing was seeing. Raij et al. found that DLPFC, dACC, and frontoinsular activation correlated with the degree of pain experienced under hypnotic suggestion [29]. Using PET, Faymonville implicated many regions including the dACC and DLPFC in hypnosis and hypnotic reduction in pain perception [30].

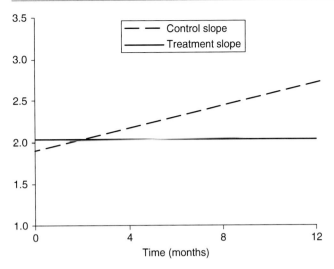

Fig. 9.3 Slopes and mean scores for pain and suffering over the first 12 months and analyzed separately for education only (control) and group therapy plus education (treatment) conditions

Several studies have tested the idea that endogenous opiates account for hypnotic analgesia. But, with one partial exception [31], studies with both volunteers [32] and patients in chronic pain [33] have shown that hypnotic analgesia is not blocked and reversed by a substantial dose of naloxone, an opiate receptor blocker, given in double-blind, crossover fashion. Therefore, the cortical attention deployment mechanism is at the moment the most plausible explanation for hypnotic reduction of pain.

Clinical Examples and Usefulness in Clinical Practice

Utilizing Hypnosis

It is wise to commence pain treatment utilizing hypnosis with two types of measurement: of pain and of hypnotizability. Patients can reliably report their pain experience on a 0–10 analog scale, and this provides a benchmark for assessing the subsequent effectiveness of various hypnotic techniques.

The term "hypnotizability" refers to the individual's degree of responsiveness to suggestion during hypnosis [34]. Hypnotizability is a highly stable and measurable trait [5]. In one study, hypnotizability was found to have a 0.7 test-retest correlation over a 25-year interval, making it a more stable trait than IQ over such a long period of time [34]. The trait of hypnotizability is a crucial moderating variable in pain treatment response, both that involving hypnosis directly [35] and in augmenting placebo response [36]. Although not all patients are sufficiently hypnotizable to benefit from these techniques, two out of three adults are at least somewhat hypnotizable [4], and it has been estimated that hypnotic

capacity is correlated at a 0.5 level with effectiveness in medical pain reduction [37]. Furthermore, clinically effective hypnotic analgesia is not confined to those with high hypnotizability [25].

One especially useful way of introducing hypnosis into the therapy is through the use of a clinical hypnotizability scale, such as the Hypnotic Induction Profile [5] or the Stanford Hypnotic Clinical Scale [38]. This form of initial hypnotic induction has several advantages:

1. It provides useful information about the patient's degree of hypnotizability. About one in four adults are not hypnotizable, and one in ten is extremely responsive [5]. Patients' performance on a hypnotizability test provides either a tangible demonstration of their hypnotic ability, which is a good starting point for therapy and is often surprising to patients, or it demonstrates that hypnosis is unlikely to be useful, in which case other techniques can be employed. Thus, the hypnotic induction can be turned into a rational deduction about the patient's resources for change [37].

2. The atmosphere of testing enhances the treatment alliance and defuses anxieties about loss of control. The therapist's responsibility is to provide a clinically appropriate setting and give instructions for the systematic exploration of the patient's hypnotic capacity. This is not a power struggle in which the therapist tries to "get the patient into a trance" and the patient succumbs or resists. The therapist is interested in finding out the results of the test, not in proving how successful he or she is at hypnotizing a patient. Thus, the atmosphere becomes something of a Socratic dialogue, in which both discover what the patient already "knows" (hypnotic capacity) but about which there may be little conscious awareness or prior experience. The hypnotic test can be used as a means of providing a sense of physical comfort and safety that is dissociated from the pain experience itself, demonstrating to the patient in a neutral way their ability to alter perception and motor function. It is also useful to teach patients from the beginning to enter the state of hypnosis as a state of self-hypnosis so that they feel in control of the transition to this altered mental state. The instructions can be simple: "All hypnosis is really self-hypnosis." Now that we have demonstrated that you have a good capacity to use hypnosis, let me show you how to use it to work on a problem. While there are many ways to enter a state of self-hypnosis, one simple means is to count from one to three. On "one," do one thing: look up. On "two," do two things: slowly close your eyes, and take a deep breath. On "three," do three things: let the breath out, let your eyes relax but keep them closed, and let your body float. Then, let one hand or the other float up in the air like a balloon, and that will be your signal to yourself and to me that you are ready to concentrate [5]. Once in a state of self-hypnosis, patients can be taught to produce a physical

sensation of floating, lightness, or buoyancy. Their sense of physical comfort can be reinforced by having them initially imagine that they are somewhere safe and comfortable, such as floating in a bath, a lake, a hot tub, or space. This enhances their sense of control over their body.

Hypnotic Analgesia

Hypnosis and similar techniques work through three primary mechanisms: muscle relaxation, perceptual alteration, and cognitive distraction. Pain is often accompanied by reactive muscle tension. Patients frequently splint the part of their body that hurts. Yet, because muscle tension can by itself cause pain in normal tissue and because traction on a painful part of the body can exacerbate pain, techniques that induce greater physical relaxation reduce pain. Therefore, having patients enter a state of hypnosis and concentrate on an image that connotes physical relaxation such as floating or lightness often produces physical relaxation and reduces pain.

The second major component of hypnotic analgesia is perceptual alteration. Patients can be taught to imagine that the affected body part is tingling or numb. Temperature metaphors are often especially useful, which is not surprising since pain and temperature sensations are part of the same neurosensory system, conducted through small poorly myelinated C fibers to the lateral spinothalamic tract in the spinal cord. Thus, imagining that an affected body part is cooler or warmer using an image of dipping it in ice water or warming it in the sun can often help patients transform pain signals. This is especially useful for extremely hypnotizable individuals who can, for example, relive an experience of dental anesthesia and reproduce the drug-induced sensations of numbness in their cheek, which they can then transfer to the painful part of their body. Rather than "fighting" the pain, they can transform it, concentrating on competing sensations. The third approach involves cognitive alteration, changing the context in which pain is experienced or understood. They can also simply "switch off" perception of the pain with surprising effectiveness [27, 28]. Some patients prefer to imagine that the pain is a substance with dimensions that can be moved or can flow out of the body as if it were a viscous liquid. Others like to dissociate, imagining that they can step outside their body to, for example, visit another room in the house. Less hypnotizable individuals often do better with distraction techniques that help them focus on competing sensations in another part of the body.

The effectiveness of the specific technique employed depends upon the degree of hypnotic ability of the subject. For example, while most patients can be taught to develop a comfortable floating sensation on the affected body part, highly hypnotizable individuals may simply imagine a shot of Novocain (procaine hydrochloride) in the affected area,

producing a sense of tingling numbness similar to that experienced in dental work. Other patients may prefer to move the pain to another part of their body or to dissociate the affected part from the rest of the body. As an extreme form of hypnotically induced, controlled dissociation, some highly hypnotizable patients may imagine themselves floating above their own body, creating distance between themselves and the painful sensation or experience. To some more moderately hypnotizable patients, it may be easier to focus on a change in temperature, either warmth or coolness. Low hypnotizable subjects often do better with simple distraction, focusing on sensations in another part of their body, such as the delicate sensations in their fingertips.

It is useful to take stock both during and after the hypnotic session regarding pain ratings: "Now with your eyes closed, and remaining in this state of concentration, please describe how your body is feeling." Then ask, "On a scale of 0–10, please rate your level of discomfort right now."

The images or metaphors used for pain control employ certain general principles [1]. Sensory transformation. The first is that the hypnotically controlled image may serve to "filter the hurt out of the pain." They learn to transform the pain experience. They acknowledge that the pain exists, but there is a distinction between the signal itself and the discomfort the signal causes. The hypnotic experience, which they create and control, helps them transform the signal into one that is less uncomfortable. So patients expand their perceptual options by having them change from an experience in which either the pain is there or it is not to an experience in which they see a third option, in which the pain is there but transformed by the presence of such competing sensations as tingling, numbness, warmth, or coolness [2]. Sensory accommodation. Patients are taught not to fight the pain. Fighting pain only enhances it by focusing attention on the pain, enhancing related anxiety and depression, and increasing physical tension that can literally put traction on painful parts of the body and increase the pain signals generated peripherally.

For patients undergoing painful procedures, such as bone marrow aspirations, the main focus is on the hypnotic imagery per se rather than relaxation. This works especially well with children since they are so highly hypnotizable and easily absorbed in images [29, 30]. Patients may be guided through the experience while the procedure is performed, or a given scenario can be suggested, and later the patient can undergo the experience hypnotically while the procedure is under way. This enables them to restructure their experience of what is going on and dissociate themselves psychologically from pain and fear intrinsic to their immediate situation. A large-scale randomized trial compared hypnosis with nonspecific emotional support and routine care during invasive radiological procedures. All patients had access to patient-controlled intravenous analgesic medication consisting of midazolam and fentanyl. The hypnosis condition provided significantly greater analgesia and relief of anxiety, despite patient use of one-half the medication. Furthermore, with hypnosis, there were fewer procedural complications such as hemodynamic instability; the procedures took on average 18 min less time, and the overall cost was reduced by $348 per procedure [38].

Self-Hypnosis

Hypnotic techniques can easily be taught to patients for self-administration [5, 6]. Pain patients can be taught to enter a state of self-hypnosis in a matter of seconds with some simple induction strategies, such as looking up while slowly closing their eyes, taking a deep breath and then letting the breath out, their eyes relax, and imagining that there is body floating and that one hand is so light it can float up in the air like a balloon. They are then instructed in the pain control exercise, such as coolness or warmth, tingling, or numbness, and taught to bring themselves out by reversing the induction procedure, again looking up, letting the eyes open, and letting the raised hand float back down. Patients can use this exercise every 1–2 h initially and any time they experience an attack of pain [5, 13]. It is useful to provide them with a written summary of the hypnotic induction, analgesic technique employed, and means of exiting the hypnotic state. As with any pain treatment technique, hypnosis is more effective when employed early in the pain cycle, before the pain has become so overwhelming that it impairs concentration. Patients should be encouraged to use this technique early and often because it is simple and effective [34] and has no side effects [35].

Hypnotic Analgesia in Children

Hypnotic techniques are likely to be even more effective among children with pain than adults, since children are more hypnotizable than adults and are thus easily absorbed in images [39, 40]. In using hypnosis with children, some find it helpful to play in an imaginary baseball game and to picture themselves going to another room in the house or watching a favorite TV show. This enables children to restructure their experience of what is occurring and dissociate themselves psychologically from pain and fear of the procedure. This approach utilizes the intense focus in hypnosis to help children dissociate their attention and imagination from their immediate physical surroundings and experiences. It is also helpful to have parents assist and rehearse the procedure so that the children do not encounter anything unfamiliar.

There is evidence that hypnosis can provide anxiety and pain relief to children with medical conditions [41–43], including with cancer [31, 32, 44, 45], cystic fibrosis [33], pain problems [46, 47], pulmonary symptoms

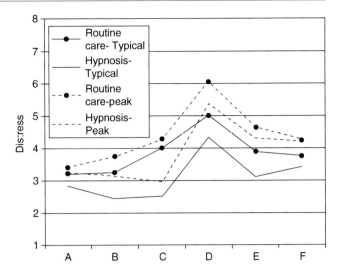

Fig. 9.4 Observer ratings of typical and peak distress levels over phases of the procedure by condition. *A* getting to the table, *B* initial x-ray, *C* catheterization, *D* cleaning and catheterization, *E* bladder infusion and x-rays, *F* voiding and catheter removal

[48], abdominal pain [49–56], and postoperative course [57]. Additionally, hypnosis is a noninvasive intervention with minimal risk, which returns control of the experience to the child [58, 59].

We have considerable experience utilizing hypnosis as an analgesic with children experiencing acute pain. In one randomized clinical trial of the use of hypnosis for children undergoing voiding cystourethrograms, those randomized to the hypnosis condition were given a 1-h training session in self-hypnotic visual imagery by a trained therapist. Parents and children were instructed to practice using the imaginative self-hypnosis procedure several times a day in preparation for the upcoming procedure (Fig. 9.4). The therapist was also present during the procedure to conduct similar exercises with the child. Results indicate significant benefits for the hypnosis group, compared to the routine care group in the following four areas: (1) Parents of children in the hypnosis group, compared to those in the routine care group, reported that the procedure was significantly less traumatic for their children compared to their previous VCUG procedure. (2) Observational ratings of typical distress levels during the procedure were significantly lower for children in the hypnosis condition compared to those in the routine care condition. (3) Medical staff reported a significant difference between groups in the overall difficulty of conducting the procedure, with less difficulty reported for the hypnosis group. (4) Total procedural time was significantly shorter – by almost 14 min – for the hypnosis group compared to the routine care group (Fig. 9.5a, b). Moderate to large effect sizes were obtained on each of these four outcomes [4].

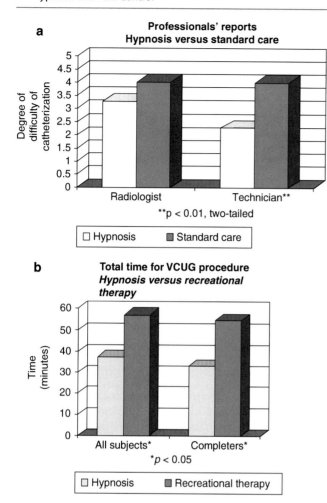

Fig. 9.5 (**a**) Professional's reports: hypnosis versus standard care. (**b**) Total time for VCUG procedure: hypnosis versus recreational therapy

Future Directions for This Topic

Hypnosis is one of the oldest, safest, and most effective analgesic techniques, and there is growing evidence supporting its use [60, 61]. One interesting new direction is coupling hypnosis with technology that enhances sensory immersion, such as computer-based virtual reality systems [35, 62]. These can enhance analgesic effects and make the most of a given individual's hypnotizability.

Secondly, more can be learned about the neural basis of hypnotic trance and hypnotic analgesia. Knowing specific regions of the brain that are coactivated in hypnosis may help us to better design hypnotic techniques.

Third, application of hypnosis to novel settings can expand and improve its use. Recently, hypnosis has been effectively utilized during breast biopsy [61, 63], and even during lumpectomy for breast cancer [63, 64]. Such techniques have great promise in making medical treatment more effective and humane [6, 65].

Summary

Hypnosis is a safe, effective, and comforting adjunct to the management of both acute and chronic pain. Most individuals are sufficiently hypnotizable to obtain at least some benefit from it, and some will experience substantial relief. It is a means of teaching control over discomfort and can be coupled with other analgesic treatment approaches. Those clinicians utilizing hypnosis for analgesia should have training in this technique along with primary training and licensure in their clinical discipline, be it medicine, dentistry, psychology, or other health-care profession. Referral to a good clinician can be obtained from such professional organizations as the Society for Clinical and Experimental Hypnosis (www.SCEH.US) or the American Society of Clinical Hypnosis (www.ASCH.net). While many types of pain intervention are being developed, it is worth remembering that the strain in pain lies mainly in the brain.

References

1. Ellenberger HF. Discovery of the unconscious: the history and evolution of dynamic psychiatry. New York: Basic Books; 1970.
2. Esdaile J. Hypnosis in medicine and surgery (ed Reprinted 1957). New York: Julian Press; 1846.
3. Lang E, Benotsch E, Fink L, et al. Adjunctive non-pharmacological analgesia for invasive medical procedures: a randomised trial. Lancet. 2000;355:1486–90.
4. Butler LD, Symons BK, Henderson SL, et al. Hypnosis reduces distress and duration of an invasive medical procedure for children. Pediatrics. 2005;115:e77–85.
5. Spiegel H, Spiegel D. Trance and treatment: clinical uses of hypnosis. Washington, D.C.: American Psychiatric Press; 2004.
6. Spiegel D. The mind prepared: hypnosis in surgery. J Natl Cancer Inst. 2007;99:1280–1.
7. Spiegel D. Hypnosis and implicit memory: automatic processing of explicit content. Am J Clin Hypn. 1998;40:231–40.
8. Yapko M. Hypnotic intervention for ambiguity as a depressive risk factor. Am J Clin Hypn. 2001;44:109–17.
9. Melzack R. From the gate to the neuromatrix. Pain Suppl. 1999;6:S121–6.
10. Melzack R, Wall PD. Pain mechanisms: a new theory. Science. 1965;150:971–9.
11. Beecher HK. Relationship of significance of wound to pain experienced. J Am Med Assoc. 1956;161:1609–13.
12. Jensen M, Patterson DR. Hypnotic treatment of chronic pain. J Behav Med. 2006;29:95–124.
13. Patterson DR, Jensen MP. Hypnosis and clinical pain. Psychol Bull. 2003;129:495–521.
14. Frenay MC, Faymonville ME, Devlieger S, et al. Psychological approaches during dressing changes of burned patients: a prospective randomised study comparing hypnosis against stress reducing strategy. Burns. 2001;27:793–9.
15. NIH Technology AP. Integration of behavioral and relaxation approaches into the treatment of chronic pain and insomnia. NIH technology assessment panel on integration of behavioral and relaxation approaches into the treatment of chronic pain and insomnia. JAMA. 1996;276:313–8.

16. Butler LD, Koopman C, Neri E, et al. Effects of supportive-expressive group therapy on pain in women with metastatic breast cancer. Health Psychol. 2009;28:579–87.

17. Spiegel D, Bierre P, Rootenberg J. Hypnotic alteration of somatosensory perception. Am J Psychiatry. 1989;146:749–54.

18. Cardenas DD, Jensen MP. Treatments for chronic pain in persons with spinal cord injury: a survey study. J Spinal Cord Med. 2006;29:109–17.

19. Jensen MP, Barber J, Hanley MA, et al. Long-term outcome of hypnotic-analgesia treatment for chronic pain in persons with disabilities. Int J Clin Exp Hypn. 2008;56:156–69.

20. Jensen MP. The neurophysiology of pain perception and hypnotic analgesia: implications for clinical practice. Am J Clin Hypn. 2008;51:123–48.

21. Molton IR, Graham C, Stoelb BL, et al. Current psychological approaches to the management of chronic pain. Curr Opin Anaesthesiol. 2007;20:485–9.

22. Oneal BJ, Patterson DR, Soltani M, et al. Virtual reality hypnosis in the treatment of chronic neuropathic pain: a case report. Int J Clin Exp Hypn. 2008;56:451–62.

23. Spiegel D. Hypnosis with medical and surgical patients. Gen Hosp Psychiatry. 1983;5:265–77.

24. Spiegel D, Bloom JR. Group therapy and hypnosis reduce metastatic breast carcinoma pain. Psychosom Med. 1983;45:333–9.

25. Rainville P, Duncan GH, Price DD, et al. Pain affect encoded in human anterior cingulate but not somatosensory cortex. Science. 1997;277:968–71.

26. Rainville P, Hofbauer RK, Paus T, et al. Cerebral mechanisms of hypnotic induction and suggestion. J Cogn Neurosci. 1999;11:110–25.

27. Rainville P, Carrier B, Hofbauer RK, et al. Dissociation of sensory and affective dimensions of pain using hypnotic modulation. Pain. 1999;82:159–71.

28. Kosslyn SM, Thompson WL, Costantini-Ferrando MF, et al. Hypnotic visual illusion alters color processing in the brain. Am J Psychiatry. 2000;157:1279–84.

29. Raij TT, Numminen J, Narvanen S, et al. Strength of prefrontal activation predicts intensity of suggestion-induced pain. Hum Brain Mapp. 2009;30:2890–7.

30. Faymonville ME, Laureys S, et al. Neural mechanisms of antinociceptive effects of hypnosis. Anesthesiology. 2000;92:1257–67.

31. Zeltzer L, LeBaron S. Hypnosis and nonhypnotic techniques for reduction of pain and anxiety during painful procedures in children and adolescents with cancer. J Pediatr. 1982;101:1032–5.

32. Zeltzer LK, Dolgin MJ, LeBaron S, et al. A randomized, controlled study of behavioral intervention for chemotherapy distress in children with cancer. Pediatrics. 1991;88:34–42.

33. Belsky J, Khanna P. The effects of self-hypnosis for children with cystic fibrosis: a pilot study. Am J Clin Hypn. 1994;36:282–92.

34. Green JP, Barabasz AF, Barrett D, et al. Forging ahead: the 2003 APA Division 30 definition of hypnosis. Int J Clin Exp Hypn. 2005;53:259–64.

35. Patterson DR, Wiechman SA, Jensen M, et al. Hypnosis delivered through immersive virtual reality for burn pain: a clinical case series. Int J Clin Exp Hypn. 2006;54:130–42.

36. McGlashan TH, Evans FJ, Orne MT. The nature of hypnotic analgesia and placebo response to experimental pain. Psychosom Med. 1969;31:227–46.

37. Spiegel H, Spiegel D. Induction techniques. In: Burrows GD, Dennerstein L, editors. Handbook of hypnosis and psychosomatic medicine. Amsterdam: North-Holland/Biomedical Press; 1980.

38. Hilgard ER, Hilgard JR. Hypnosis in the relief of pain. Los Altos: William Kauffman; 1975.

39. Morgan AH, Hilgard ER. Age differences in susceptibility to hypnosis. Int J Clin Exp Hypn. 1972;21:78–85.

40. Hilgard JR. Personality and hypnosis: a study of imaginative involvement. Chicago: University of Chicago Press; 1970.

41. Kuttner L. Management of young children's acute pain and anxiety during invasive medical procedures. Pediatrician. 1989;16:39–44.

42. Kuttner L, Bowman M, Teasdale M. Psychological treatment of distress, pain, and anxiety for young children with cancer. J Dev Behav Pediatr. 1988;9:374–81.

43. Kuttner L. Managing pain in children. Changing treatment of headaches. Can Fam Physician. 1993;39:563–8.

44. Hilgard ER. Hypnotic susceptibility and implications for measurement. Int J Clin Exp Hypn. 1982;30:394–403.

45. Liossi C, Hatira P. Clinical hypnosis versus cognitive behavioral training for pain management with pediatric cancer patients undergoing bone marrow aspirations. Int J Clin Exp Hypn. 1999;47:104–16.

46. Zeltzer L, Tsao JC, Stelling C, et al. A phase I study on the feasibility and acceptability of an acupuncture/hypnosis intervention for chronic pediatric pain. J Pain Symptom Manage. 2002;24:437–46.

47. Dinges DF, Whitehouse WG, Orne EC, et al. Self-hypnosis training as an adjunctive treatment in the management of pain associated with sickle cell disease. Int J Clin Exp Hypn. 1997;45:417–32.

48. Anbar RD. Hypnosis in pediatrics: applications at a pediatric pulmonary center. BMC Pediatr. 2002;2:11.

49. Vlieger AM, Menko-Frankenhuis C, Wolfkamp SC, et al. Hypnotherapy for children with functional abdominal pain or irritable bowel syndrome: a randomized controlled trial. Gastroenterology. 2007;133:1430–6.

50. Tsao JC, Zeltzer LK. Complementary and alternative medicine approaches for pediatric pain: a review of the state-of-the-science. Evid Based Complement Alternat Med. 2005;2:149–59.

51. Simons LE, Logan DE, Chastain L, et al. Engagement in multidisciplinary interventions for pediatric chronic pain: parental expectations, barriers, and child outcomes. Clin J Pain. 2010;26:291–9.

52. Kroner-Herwig B. Chronic pain syndromes and their treatment by psychological interventions. Curr Opin Psychiatry. 2009;22:200–4.

53. Kohen DP, Olness KN, Colwell SO, et al. The use of relaxation-mental imagery (self-hypnosis) in the management of 505 pediatric behavioral encounters. J Dev Behav Pediatr. 1984;5:21–5.

54. Jay SM, Elliott C, Varni JW. Acute and chronic pain in adults and children with cancer. J Consult Clin Psychol. 1986;54:601–7.

55. Galili O, Shaoul R, Mogilner J. Treatment of chronic recurrent abdominal pain: laparoscopy or hypnosis? J Laparoendosc Adv Surg Tech A. 2009;19:93–6.

56. Banez GA. Chronic abdominal pain in children: what to do following the medical evaluation. Curr Opin Pediatr. 2008;20:571–5.

57. Lambert SA. The effects of hypnosis/guided imagery on the postoperative course of children. J Dev Behav Pediatr. 1996;17:307–10.

58. Hockenberry MJ, Cotanch PH. Hypnosis as adjuvant antiemetic therapy in childhood cancer. Nurs Clin North Am. 1985;20:105–7.

59. Olness K, Kohen D. Hypnosis and hypnotherapy with children. 3rd ed. New York: Guilford; 1996.

60. Stoelb BL, Molton IR, Jensen MP, et al. The efficacy of hypnotic analgesia in adults: a review of the literature. Contemp Hypn. 2009;26:24–39.

61. Lang EV, Berbaum KS, Faintuch S, et al. Adjunctive self-hypnotic relaxation for outpatient medical procedures: a prospective randomized trial with women undergoing large core breast biopsy. Pain. 2006;126:155–64.

62. Askay SW, Patterson DR, Sharar SR. Virtual reality hypnosis. Contemp Hypn. 2009;26:40–7.

63. Montgomery GH, Bovbjerg DH, Schnur JB, et al. A randomized clinical trial of a brief hypnosis intervention to control side effects in breast surgery patients. J Natl Cancer Inst. 2007;99:1304–12.

64. Schnur JB, Bovbjerg DH, David D, et al. Hypnosis decreases presurgical distress in excisional breast biopsy. Anesth Analg. 2008;106(2):440–4, table of contents.

65. Spiegel D. Wedding hypnosis to the radiology suite. Pain. 2006;126:3–4.

Acupuncture

Ji-Sheng Han

Key Points

- The essence of acupuncture analgesia is to make use of endogenous neurotransmitters and neuropeptides, such as endorphins, to suppress pain and interrupt the vicious cycle of pain mechanisms with little aversive side effects.
- Aside from its placebo effect, acupuncture does have a strong physiological effect in the treatment of acute and chronic pain.
- Acupuncture significantly reduces, but not abolishes, surgically induced pain. Acupuncture can also significantly reduce postoperative pain and vomiting.
- The selection of an optimal frequency is a major issue for the effectiveness of electroacupuncture in the treatment of various kinds of chronic pain.
- Acupuncture-induced endogenously mobilized pain-killing mechanisms combined with exogenously induced pharmacological mechanisms can result in synergistic therapeutic effect for the best of pain patients.
- A design of a proper control group is important in the clinical study of acupuncture analgesia.

Introduction

Acupuncture is an ancient Chinese medical technique with a history of over 2,000 years. The term "acupuncture" is derived from the word *acus*, meaning a sharp point, and *punctura*, meaning to pierce. It can be defined as a technique of inserting and manipulating fine filiform needle into specific points on the body to relieve pain and for various therapeutic purposes.

J.-S. Han, M.D. (✉)
Department of Neurobiology, Neuroscience Research Institute, Peking University, 38 Xue Yuan Road, Beijing 100083, China
e-mail: hanjisheng@bjmu.edu.cn

According to the original acupuncture technique, after the insertion of the needle into the skin, it should be manipulated in an up-and-down and rotating movement, termed as "manual needling," in an attempt to reopen the hypothetical channel or meridian so that the obstructed Qi can resume its path. Since the hypothetical "meridian" has not been materialized so far, people tried to find other media for its execution, such as nerves, blood vessels, lymphatic, and connective tissues. In modern times, new methods of stimulating the acupuncture points (acupoints) have been introduced, including (a) applications of electric current to the needles inserted into the acupoints (electroacupuncture, EA), or via skin electrodes placed over the acupoints (transcutaneous electrical acupoint stimulation, TEAS); (b) injection of chemicals into the acupoints; or (c) finger-pressure massage on selected acupoints(acupressure). Concerning the site of stimulation, in addition to the original 362 acupoints, many new acupoints have been described on specific body parts, leading to, for instance, scalp acupuncture, hand acupuncture, and ear acupuncture.

Revival of acupuncture started in the late 1950s when a group of surgeons in China thought, if acupuncture can ameliorate the existing pain, why not use acupuncture preemptively to prevent the inevitable pain as a result of surgical procedures? The clinical trial of using acupuncture to replace anesthetics during surgical operations was termed "acupuncture anesthesia," now widely accepted as "acupuncture analgesia." Research in this field was encouraged by the Chinese medical authorities in the 1960s and being conducted in major hospitals and in most medical schools. A journalist, Mr. James Reston, reported in the *New York Times* on his own experience of having acupuncture to reduce the postoperative pain in Beijing in 1971. This was followed by the visit of the US President, Richard Nixon, to China in 1972, which then surged the popularity of acupuncture in the USA and around the world. The National Institute of Health (NIH)-sponsored Consensus Conference on Acupuncture held in Bethesda, Maryland, in 1997 marked another

T.R. Deer et al. (eds.), *Treatment of Chronic Pain by Integrative Approaches: the AMERICAN ACADEMY of PAIN MEDICINE Textbook on Patient Management*, DOI 10.1007/978-1-4939-1821-8_10,
© American Academy of Pain Medicine 2015

milestone of acupuncture: treatment of pain, nausea, and vomiting was endorsed to acupuncture as clinically effective and scientifically valid [1].

Half a century has passed since the first practice of acupuncture anesthesia in a surgical theater in 1958. In this chapter, the established findings – both scientifically and in practice – will be summarized, starting from introduction of the scientific foundation of acupuncture effects, followed by some clinical applications. The key of this chapter is to capture the basic phenomena and the principal mechanisms of acupuncture analgesia and to help clinicians to decide whether they would like to try acupuncture and related techniques in their own practice. Several review articles are listed for the better understanding of the background and the general picture of acupuncture analgesia [2–6].

Scientific Foundation

Basic Phenomenon

To ascertain whether acupuncture stimulation would indeed lower pain sensitivity, acupuncture was administered to human volunteers [7]. To measure the nociceptive threshold of the skin, the potassium iontophoresis method was used, whereby the minimal intensity of an anode (5 mm diameter) current needed to produce a clear pain sensation was recorded, usually by 1 mA. A total of eight body sites, distributed over the head, neck, chest, abdomen, legs, and back, was selected to test pain sensitivity. An acupuncture needle was inserted into the Hegu (large intestine 4, LI4) point, located at the thenar muscle of the hand, considered to be the most powerful for its analgesic effect. Following the continuous manipulation of the needle, a gradual increase of the pain threshold was observed. It took 30 min for the pain threshold to increase from 1 to around 2 mA, and leveled off thereafter. When the needle was poured off, the pain threshold started to decrease exponentially, with a half-life of around 16 min. The time course of slow onset and slow decay, as well as an entire body elevation of the pain threshold, suggested a mechanism of chemical mediation (Fig. 10.1).

In above mentioned study, it was also noted that acupuncture did not work for every subject. While the majority (approximately 85 %) were responders, a small percentage were low or nonresponders, with no significant increase of the pain threshold during the period of stimulation. Interestingly, this type of distribution is reproducible, at least in a period of 1 week. Similar phenomena were observed in the rodent when they were administered with acupuncture at the Zusanli point (ST36) near the knee joint, and the nociceptive threshold was assessed by the tail-flick latency. The experiment was repeated within 1 week, and the results were highly reproducible. The closer the two tests, the higher the reproducibility. This suggests that the magnitude of the analgesic response toward acupuncture stimulation depends on constitutional factors on one hand, and some temporary acting factors on the other.

Preliminary Analysis of the Possible Mechanisms

While the nature of the "meridian" or the "channel" was still in question, one may ask whether the nervous system or chemical mediators were involved. The results obtained in the human study were so straightforward that the analgesic effect could be totally prevented when the local anesthetic procaine was infiltrated into the deeper structures under the point, but not by its subcutaneous injection. The results suggest that it is the nervous tissue in the muscle and tendon that senses the stimulation. It was later made clear that the small-

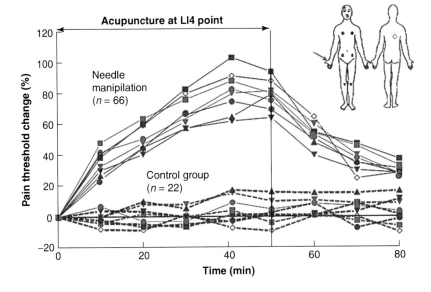

Fig. 10.1 Pain threshold changes in response to acupuncture at LI4 point located at the thenar eminence. Eight representative skin points were identified for the measurement of pain threshold by potassium iontophoresis method. The needle was manipulated continuously for 50 min. The slow rising during the stimulation period and the slow decay after the removal of the needle suggest the involvement of neurochemical mechanisms (Modified from Research Group of Acupuncture Analgesia, Beijing Medical College [7])

Fig. 10.2 Cross infusion of cerebroventricular fluid between two rabbits. The donor rabbit was subject to acupressure stimulation at the kunlun point near the Achilles tendon. The perfusate of the donor was injected into the lateral ventricle of the recipient rabbit. Latency of the radiant heat-induced head jerk was taken as the nociceptive threshold (Modified from Research Group of Acupuncture Anesthesia, Beijing Medical College [9])

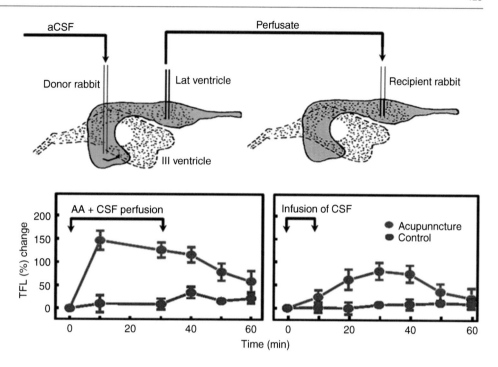

myelinated nerve fibers (Aβ fibers and a small part of the Aδ fibers) are responsible for the transmission of afferent impulses to the spinal cord [8].

Another important step made in the study of the mechanisms of acupuncture analgesia was the cerebrospinal fluid (CSF) cross-perfusion study [9]. In order to test the hypothesis of whether there are chemical mediators produced in the brain that may be responsible for the analgesic effect, stainless steel cannulae were implanted into the lateral ventricle of the rabbit so that the brain ventricle can be perfused with artificial CSF, and the perfusate was then infused immediately to the cerebroventricle of the recipient rabbit. When acupuncture was administered to the donor rabbit, the pain threshold increased dramatically. During this period, the CSF was drawn from the donor rabbit and injected into the brain of the recipient. A significant increase of the pain threshold was observed in the recipient rabbit (Fig. 10.2), although no acupuncture was given to this animal. These results suggested that during the acupuncture, some chemical substance(s) with analgesic potency might have been produced, which can be removed from the donor rabbit to the recipient. This finding triggered the interest to explore the neurochemical mechanisms of acupuncture effects.

Classical Neurotransmitters

A literature search revealed serotonin, or 5-hydroxytryptamine (5-HT), to be a candidate for the mediators of the analgesic effect. Studies performed in rats and rabbits showed that increase of the availability of 5-HT in brain or spinal cord potentiated acupuncture analgesia, whereas blockade of 5-HT synthesis or receptor activation resulted in a significant decrease of the analgesic effect. All of the results pointed to the conclusion that 5-HT in the central nervous system plays an important role in the mediation of acupuncture analgesia [10].

In contrast to the unique effect of 5-HT in the entire central nervous system, the role played by norepinephrine (NE) was much more complicated. Most of the information suggested that NE in the spinal cord played a facilitatory role for acupuncture analgesia, in contrast to the antagonistic role in the brain [11].

Opioid Peptides and the Frequency Specific Release (Fig. 10.3)

The discovery of enkephalins in the pig brain in 1975 triggered a huge storm in the biomedical field. Every researcher in this field tried to find some relation with endogenous opioid peptides, and there was no exception for researchers of acupuncture analgesia. David Mayor [12] was the first to step into this field. He used the opioid receptor antagonist naloxone as the research tool and found that the analgesic effect of acupuncture for dental pain can be prevented by the subcutaneous injection of naloxone, suggesting the involvement of endogenous opioid substances. Since opioid receptors can be divided into three types, μ, δ, and κ, and naloxone is a nonspecific antagonist for all three kinds of opioid receptors, this pharmacological tool can hardly be used to make a further receptor-type differentiation. Using a specific antagonist for the three types of opioid receptor, Han and colleagues were able to find

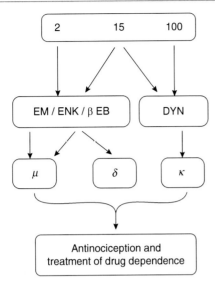

Fig. 10.3 Frequency-dependent release of opioid peptides in the central nervous system. Shown are four kinds of opioid peptides (*EM* endorphins, *ENK* enkephalins, *βEP* β-endorphin, *DYN* dynorphins), three kinds of opioid receptors (*μ*, *δ*, *κ*), and three representative frequency of electroacupuncture (2, 15, and 100 Hz)

that the analgesic effect of 2-Hz stimulation is mediated by *μ* and *δ* receptor, whereas at 100 Hz, the effect is mediated by *κ* receptors [13]. Further studies using radioimmunoassay revealed that 2 Hz increased the release of enkephalins and endorphins in the CNS to interact with *μ* and *δ* receptors, whereas 100 Hz increased the release of dynorphin in the spinal cord to interact with *κ* receptors (Fig. 10.3) [13].

An interesting question was that if low- or high-frequency stimulation can only accelerate the release of a fraction of the opioid peptide family, can we design a pattern of frequency which can accelerate the release of all four kinds of opioid peptides. This may have a practical impact since there are reports showing that simultaneous activation of two types of opioid receptors may cause a synergistic effect [14, 15]. After a series of exhausting experiments performed in the rat, it was revealed that a frequency automatically alternating between 2 and 100 Hz, each lasting for 3 s, produced a significantly more potent analgesic effect than pure low or pure high frequency alone [13]. This is reasonable since a fraction of the enkephalins released during the low-frequency period may survive to the next period of high-frequency stimulation when dynorphin is released. The coexisting enkephalin and dynorphin may interact at the receptor sites to produce a synergistic effect.

Anti-opioid Peptides and Acupuncture Tolerance

In performing animal experiments of acupuncture analgesia, two basic phenomena called our attention. One is the marked individual variation or the unpredictability of the acupunc-

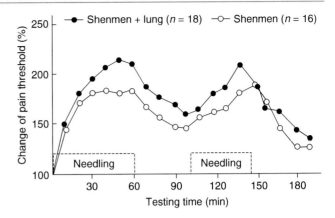

Fig. 10.4 Influence of manual needling at ear acupoint Shenmen (*n* = 16) or Shenmen plus lung (*n* = 18) on pain threshold of the skin over the chest and abdomen in humans. The pain threshold increased during the period of needle manipulation and started to decrease when the needle is staying in situ (Modified from Research Group of Ear Acupuncture, Jiangsu College of New Medicine [77])

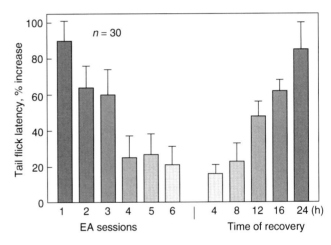

Fig. 10.5 Repeated electroacupuncture to the rat produced a decrease of the analgesic effect, referred to as acupuncture tolerance. It took 24 h for a full recovery of the acupuncture analgesia (Modified from Han et al. [16])

ture effect, and the other is the gradual fading of the analgesic effect with time if acupuncture is administered too often in a short period of time. As a general rule, acupuncture analgesia needs time (about 30 min) to build up to its full potential, and the effect would decay when the acupuncture needle is poured off (Fig. 10.1) or left unattended (Fig. 10.4). If EA is given 30 min/h, for 4–5 h, the analgesic effect would decrease gradually (Fig. 10.5) [16]. This is not due to the local tissue damage caused by repeated needle insertion and manipulation, since the situation would remain even if the needle is inserted into a new point of the body without any tissue damage.

In searching for the possible mechanisms, a hypothesis was raised that, according to the concept of Yin and Yang balance in the Chinese philosophy, the existence of a natural pain-killing substance (endorphin) might be accompanied by the existence of another substance with an antagonistic effect (anti-opioid substance). After a careful survey, this putative anti-opioid substance was identified as cholecystokinin octapeptide (CCK-8) [17]. In fact, repeated EA produced an increase of the production and release of opioid peptides, and in the same time, there is a gradual increase of the CCK-8 in the central nervous system which plays an antagonistic role against opioids, thereby reduces the effect of EA. This phenomenon is termed "acupuncture tolerance," to mimic the situation of "morphine tolerance" produced by repeated injection of morphine. It was interesting to find that for rats with CCK predominates over opioid peptides in the central nervous system, they can be a nonresponder toward acupuncture, or a weak responder but quickly developing into acupuncture tolerance. The situation can be reversed if (a) CCK antagonist is injected intracerebroventricularly or intrathecally to the rat, or (b) the gene expression of CCK is blocked by the antisense probe against preproCCK administered centrally. In that case, the nonresponder of acupuncture analgesia can be changed into responder and the diminished analgesic effect can be revived [17, 18]. The lesson learned from this mechanism is that acupuncture should not be given too often, or last too long in one session.

Neural Pathways

From neurophysiological point of view, acupuncture analgesia can be taken as a reflex action. The afferent comes from the nerve fibers (mostly $A\beta$ fibers) innervating the acupoint, and the efferent is the descending pathway modulating the sensitivity of the dorsal horn neurons not only in the same segment but also in heterogenous segments. Studies in the rat revealed that 100-Hz stimulation of the acupoint would trigger the release of dynorphin in the spinal cord. After the destruction of the parabrachial nucleus of the brain stem, high-frequency EA would no longer produce an analgesic effect [19]. Conversely, 2-Hz EA induces the release of β-endorphin in the brain and enkephalin in the whole central nervous system. After the destruction of the arcuate nucleus of the hypothalamus (where β-endorphin neurons aggregated), 2-Hz EA would no longer elicit analgesic effect. Taken together, a diagram could be constructed to show the hypothetical neural pathway for acupuncture analgesia (Fig. 10.6). Neither low- nor high-frequency EA would work if a lesion is placed at the periaqueductal gray (PAG) of the midbrain [19].

Other neural pathways have also been proposed. For example, 100-Hz stimulation can evoke supraspinal long-term depression not only in normal rats [20] but also in sham operated rats subject to neuropathic pain [21], contributing to the mechanisms of high-frequency EA-induced analgesic effect.

A hypothetical diagram was proposed by Han, which gives a general picture of the neural network underlying acupuncture analgesia, at least for the control of the acute pain [6].

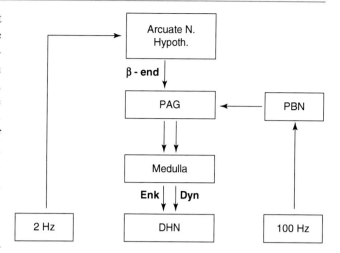

Fig. 10.6 The neural pathway for the analgesic effect induced by electroacupuncture of different frequencies. *Arcuate N. Hypoth.* arcuate nucleus of hypothalamus, *PAG* periaqueductal gray of the midbrain, *DHN* dorsal horn neuron of the spinal cord, *PBN* parabrachial nucleus, *β-end* β-endorphin, *ENK* Enkephalin, *DYN* dynorphin

Functional magnetic resonance imaging (fMRI) was used to characterize the possible brain areas being involved in mediating the acupuncture effect. Since stimulation of any of the body sites would cause extensive changes in the brain MRI picture, it is hard to characterize the brain sites responsible for acupuncture-induced analgesic effect. Zhang et al. [22] tried to correlate the magnitude of acupuncture-induced BOLD signal change observed in identified brain area with the magnitude of the analgesic effect induced by 2- or 100-Hz EA stimulation,respectively. The results showed that the analgesic effect induced by low and high frequencies seems to be mediated by different, though partially overlapping brain networks. In either frequency, the averaged fMRI activation levels of bilateral secondary somatosensory area and insula, contralateral anterior cingulate cortex, and thalamus were positively correlated with the EA-induced analgesic effect. In the 2-Hz EA group, positive correlation was observed only in contralateral primary and supplementary motor areas, while negative correlation was observed in bilateral hippocampi. In 100-Hz EA group, positive correlations were observed in contralateral inferior parietal lobule and ipsilateral anterior cingulate cortex, while negative correlation was found in contralateral amygdale. These results suggest that functional activation of certain brain areas might be correlated with the effect of EA analgesia in a frequency-dependent manner. More work is needed in order to figure out the complicated neural network controlling acupuncture-induced analgesic effect.

Mode of Stimulation (MA, EA, TEAS)

In clinical practice, various kinds of methods have been used to secure the optimal stimulation of the acupoint. Manual needling (MA) is the classical technique, with the characteristics of preciseness, capable of directing the needle in various angles to find the maximal deqi sensation and freely adjusting the needle movement to obtain a specific effect termed "warm," "cold," etc.

Studies show that various kinds of manual needling produce different pattern of afferent impulses in the sensory nerves and activation of the dorsal horn neurons. Out of 12 different kinds of needle manipulation, Wang et al. [23] studied three most popularly used modes, that is, twist, drag-plug, and gradual mode, respectively. Single-unit recordings of the dorsal horn neuron of the rat showed clearly different patterns in the inter-spike intervals (ISI). Based on the reconstructed phase space, they analyzed the spatiotemporal behavior of the time series. The largest Lyapunov exponent, which is an important parameter for describing the nonlinear system behavior, varies significantly in different modes of acupuncture. However, various types of manual needling technique (e.g., "burning mountain" for hot, "frozen sky" for cold) need years to learn and to master.

Compared to manual needling, electroacupuncture (EA) is a modern approach based on the basic finding that the effect of acupuncture is relied on the integrity of the nervous system [7] and that delivering specific forms of electric impulses is the easiest way to activate the afferent nerves in a predictable manner, with the added advantage of time saving and very high reproducibility. Aside from the great time saving and the reproducibility of the treatment, a significant advantage of using EA is that you can try, in certain degree, to change the internal environment of the central nervous system according to the ever changing need of the body system, for example, the use of low frequency (2–4 Hz) for the production and release of enkephalins in the central nervous system and high frequency (80–120 Hz) for dynorphins in the spinal cord [13]. The clinical effects produced by EA of different frequencies can be very different. Study shows that for treatment of rat model of neuropathic pain produced by lumbar nerve ligation, 2 Hz is much effective than 100 Hz, with the involvement of mu opioid receptors [24]. In contrast, for the treatment of patients with spinal cord injury-induced muscle spasm, it is only 100 Hz, but not 2 Hz, which works [25], with the involvement of kappa opioid receptors [26]. In these extreme cases, one frequency may serve as the control of the other. Here, the credibility of the design for "control" is nearly perfect, since no one knows which frequency is better, even for the care provider. This frequency-specific design can be served as an example to show the specificity of the EA treatment, rather than a design of using a nonspecific skin touch for psychological "believing." However, the frequency specificity does not apply for every disease. For example, for the treatment of rat model of complete adjuvant-induced arthritis, both high- and low-frequency EA work at a similar efficacy [27].

Unlike electroacupuncture (EA) which uses percutaneous (invasive) approach, the transcutaneous electric acupoint stimulation (TEAS) is a noninvasive way of stimulating the acupoint by the use of skin pads placed on the skin surface overlying the acupoint in lieu of the needle. This is also called "acupuncture without a needle." Since the skin electrode is usually 4×4 cm in size, it would never miss the "acupoint." Since all the parameters are shown on the LED screen precisely, it can also be used by the patient or family under the instruction of the acupuncturist or the physician, thereby reduces the number of visit to the doctor.

The efficacy of EA in pain control has repeatedly been shown to be no less than manual needling. Wang et al. [28] had done a careful study in the rat experiment, comparing the analgesic effect produced by EA or TEAS, with the conclusion that TEAS is at least as effective, if not more effective, than EA. The analgesic effect produced by either method can be blocked by naloxone at the same degree, suggesting a similar underlying mechanism of action. Given that these forms of acupoint stimulation may have similar therapeutic effect and underlying mechanisms, we will make clear statement separately for MA, EA, and TEAS in the following text when clinical applications are to be mentioned.

In the recent literature, there is another term called "percutaneous electrical nerve stimulation (PENS)" in contrast to "transcutaneous electrical nerve stimulation (TENS)" [29]. In a commentary put forwarded by Cummings [30], the author mentioned that "PENS is neither different in principle nor in practice from EA. While the term accurately reflects the nature of the treatment, there is no substantial justification for referring to PENS as a novel therapy."

Clinical Examples and the Usefulness in Clinical Practice

Acupuncture Anesthesia During the Surgical Procedure

In the late 1950s up to 1970s, there was a large-scale clinical practice in China of using acupuncture in lieu of anesthetics for surgical procedures, named "acupuncture anesthesia." In fact, in most hospitals, acupuncture was used in combination with anesthetics to form a "complex acupuncture anesthesia," or "acupuncture-assisted anesthesia (AAA)." To take a few examples, in the Tiantan hospital of Beijing specialized for brain surgery, Wang et al. [31] reported that in a series of cranial operations, they can reduce the dosage of enflurane by 45–48 % while fulfilling all the requirements of a successful anesthesia. This may be especially interested by the new trend of "anesthesia for awake neurosurgery" [32]. Qu et al. [33] performed kidney transplantation under combined acupuncture/

epidural anesthesia in the Shanghai First People's Hospital. They reported a reduction of procaine usage for 48 % with robust satisfaction. Almost all the reports concerning the complex acupuncture anesthesia stressed the benefits of earlier recovery, less postoperative pain and other complications, and shortened hospitalization. Sim et al. [34] reported 90 patients randomly assigned to one of three groups: group I – placebo EA, group II – preoperative EA for 45 min, and group III – 45 min of postoperative EA. The results showed that preoperative EA leads to a reduced intraoperative alfentanil consumption and has a morphine-sparing effect during the early postoperative period. However, this was not universally confirmed by report from other group [35].

Postoperative Pain

In contrast to some controversy whether acupuncture can reduce the anesthetic use during the surgical procedure, there is a unanimous agreement that acupuncture could significantly reduce the postoperative pain. Paul White's group published the first paper of a series of studies in 1997 [36], using the electronic device (HANS) for transcutaneous electrical acupoint stimulation (TEAS) to assess if it can reduce the postoperative PCA requirement for hydromorphone (HM). In a single-blind controlled study, they found that compared to the blank control of "PCA only" group, the HM used in the sham TEAS group showed a 22 % reduction. For the real TEAS group, they used two levels of intensity, the threshold level (4–5 mA) and the double threshold level (9–12 mA), resulting in a 34 % ($P < 0.05$) and 65 % ($P < 0.001$) reduction, respectively. The postoperative side effects (nausea, dizziness, pruritis, and sedation) were also significantly reduced. Similar results were reported for reduction of postoperative pain [37–40], nausea, and vomiting [40–42].

Since acupuncture or its several variants are shown by evidence-based medicine to be so cost effective for controlling postoperative pain, nausea, vomiting, and lack of clinical toxicity, Dr. White called on more clinicians to incorporate these acustimulation techniques into their perioperative therapeutic armamentarium [43]. In an accompanying editorial, the editor in chief suggested that, "once the mechanism of action is understood, claims of clinical efficacy for acustimulation will no longer be extraordinary" [44].

Low Back Pain

Low back pain (LBP) is one of the most common causes for primary care clinic visits, only second to common cold, and it is the second most common cause of absence from work in adults who are over 55 years of age. According to the National Center of Complementary and Alternative Medicine (NCCAM), NIH, people use acupuncture for various types of pain, and back pain is the most commonly reported, followed by joint pain, neck pain, and headache [2].

In a study reported by Ghoname et al. [45], 60 patients of LBP were divided into four groups to compare the effectiveness of PENS (equivalent to EA) with sham-PENS, TENS, and exercise. PENS is significantly more effective in decreasing the VAS pain scores after each treatment than the other three groups. The average daily oral intake of non-opioid analgesics (2.6 ± 1.4 pills/day) was decreased to 1.3 ± 1.0 pills/day with PENS ($P < 0.008$) compared with 2.5 ± 1.1, 2.2 ± 1.0, and 2.6 ± 1.2 pills/day with sham-PENS, TENS, and exercise, respectively. Compared with the other three modalities, 91 % of the patients reported that PENS was the most effective in decreasing their LBP. The PENS therapy was also significantly more effective in improving physical activity, quality of sleep, and sense of well-being ($P < 0.05$ for each).

The SF-36 survey confirmed that PENS improved post-treatment function more than sham-PENS, TENS, and exercise [45]. In another study, 68 LBP patients secondary to degenerative lumbar disc diseases were treated with EA of different frequencies: 4 Hz, alternating 15 and 30 Hz, 100 Hz, and 0 Hz serving as control. Each treatment was administered for a period of 30 min, three times per week for 2 weeks. In contrast to the control group which produced little improvement, all other groups produced significant decreases in the severity of pain and improvement in the quality of life. Of the three frequencies, 15/30 Hz was the most effective in decreasing pain. Therefore, the alternative low and high frequency was more effective than with low or high frequency alone [46]. This replicates what we found in the rat experiment where 2/100 Hz was significantly better than only 2 or 100 Hz alone in the antinociceptive effect [47].

Further studies revealed that as far as analgesic effect is concerned, needle insertion plus electrical stimulation (EA) is much better than needle staying without stimulation [46, 48], acupuncture-like TENS is better than ordinary TENS [49], and dermatomal stimulation (lumbar region for back pain, neck region for neck pain) is better than stimulation at the distal sites [50].

In summary, while most of the studies showed that acupuncture or EA are effective for low back pain, there are negative reposts [51]. Concerning the life span of the therapeutic effect, it may be short lasting [52] or longer lasting for at least 3 months [48], depending on the design of the protocol, especially the number of treatment being used.

Osteoarthritis of the Knee

Acupuncture seems to be effective for osteoarthritis, especially in the area of the knee. However, controversy exists on the clinical effectiveness. Moreover, difference in the design, sample size, and protocol of the studies made it hard to draw any definitive conclusions. Here, we make comparison of two articles using acupuncture for the treatment of osteoarthritis of the knee joint, both published in the Annals of Internal Medicine, one got negative result [52] and another positive result [53]. We hope to find out some meaningful differences in experimental design, data collection, and interpretation.

From the comparisons made above, we can see that in order to depict a difference between the true and placebo acupuncture groups, one should consider the following: (a) to strengthen the effect of true acupuncture by more treatment sessions. Compared to Berman et al. who used 23 sessions, Scharf et al. used only 10. (b) Berman et al. [53], but not Scharf et al. [54], used EA to supplement manual needling (1 vs. 0) and (c) to weaken the effect of placebo or sham acupuncture by reducing the number of needle insertion (2 vs. 10). Aside from that, there are several related issues need to be considered in the future studies (Table 10.1).

Concerning the possible mechanisms of action, a recent publication [55] seemed to give some clue. Patients with chronic osteoarthritis were given EA of 20–25 min per session, once a day for 10 days, and the control group was given sham needle insertion at nonpoints without electrical stimulation. The EA group showed a significant improvement in pain, stiffness, and disability as shown by the WOMAX index and VAS value. In the meantime, there was a significant increase in plasma β-endorphin ($P = 0.001$) and a significant fall in plasma stress hormone cortisol ($P = 0.016$).

In February 2008, the OARSI recommendation for the management of hip and knee osteoarthritis, Part II: OARSI evidence-based, expert consensus guidelines, was released [56]. The purpose was to develop concise, patient-focused, up-to-date, evidence-based, expert consensus recommendations for the management of hip and knee osteoarthritis (OA). As a result, 20 out of 51 treatment modalities were universally recommended. The non-pharmacological modalities (totaling 12, including TENS and acupuncture) and the pharmacological (totaling eight) modalities were considered equally effective. Therefore, a combination of non-pharmacological and pharmacological treatments was recommended. Out of that, they also identified five surgical modalities. However, the National Institute of Health and Clinical Excellence (NICE) published a new guideline on the

Table 10.1 Comparison of the conditions applied and results obtained by Berman et al. [53] and Scharf et al. [54], using acupuncture for the treatment of osteoarthritis of the knee joint

	Berman et al. [53]	Scharf et al. [54]
Treatment centers (number of physicians)	Three clinics in one University (7 acupuncturists)	Multicenters (320 physicians)
Trial size	570	1,039
% drops	31.4 % drop by 26 weeks	57.5 % drop by 26 weeks
Concealment of allocation	Letter from central statistical core	Centralized telephone randomization
Pain scale	WOMAC (0–10)	WOMAC (0–10)
Treatment duration (sessions)	26 weeks (23)	6 weeks (10)
Manual acupuncture group (depth of needle insertion)	4 distal points (1 in); 5 local points (1.5 in). Two points in abdominal area for non-insertion intervention	6 local obligatory points 2 of 16 defined acupoints could be chosen A maximum of 4 Ah shi points were allowed
EA	One point for EA (8 Hz, 20 min)	No EA
"No acupuncture" group	Six 2-h sessions of education	10 physician visits
Placebo acupuncture group	Mock needles on each of the 9 leg points, mock EA unit with light and sound 2 needle insertion in abdominal nonpoints	10 non-acupoints at lower and upper limb, superficial needling up to 5 mm without Qi, no manual needle movement
Standard care	Continue to receive analgesics from their primary care physicians	Oral NSAID, up to 6 physiotherapy
Summary for "true" group	Inserted needles with 2 manual stimulations, plus EA at one local point	Inserted needles with 2 manual stimulations, without EA
Summary for "placebo" group	9 placebo needles (no insertion) Only 2 true needles inserted in abdomen	10 needles inserted in upper and lower limbs
Evaluation	8th and 26th week	13th and 26th week
Primary outcomes	WOMAC and functional scores	WOMAC and functional scores
Secondary outcomes	Functional improvement: patient global assessment, 6 min walk, SF-36	Functional improvement: global patient assessment, SF-12 physical subscale, SF-12 mental subscale
Results	True acup > Placebo acup > No acup Pain improved in 14 week versus placebo. Improvement of functional score since 8th week, but not PGA score	Taking 36 % improvement in WOMAC as success: True acup (53.1) = Placebo acup (51.0) >No acup (29.1)

care and management of osteoarthritis, which stated that there is insufficient evidence to recommend acupuncture for the treatment of OA [57]. This raised controversy [58, 59] which needs time to reconcile with.

Diabetic Neuropathic Pain

Diabetic patient can develop neuropathic changes that affect peripheral nerve function, leading to symmetrical lower extremity pain. The pain could be very severe to affect a normal life, and no satisfactory treatment is currently available. Abuaisha et al. [60] conducted a relatively long-term study to explore the effectiveness of acupuncture for its treatment. Forty-six diabetic patients with chronic painful peripheral neuropathy were treated with classical acupuncture, 20 min per session, six sessions in 10 weeks. Seventy-seven percent showed significant improvement in their primary and/or secondary symptoms ($P < 0.01$). After 18–52 weeks of follow-up, 67 % were able to stop or significantly reduce their medication and only 24 % required further acupuncture treatment. These data suggest that acupuncture is a safe and effective therapy for painful diabetic neuropathy, although the mechanism of action remains speculative. Hamza et al. [61] used EA (PENS) at 15–30-Hz frequency for the treatment of 50 type 2 diabetic patients with peripheral neuropathic pain over 6-month duration, with sham EA (needle insertion without movement or electrical stimulation) as control. EA was given at 10 acupoints at the lower extremities, 30 min per session, three times a week, for 3 weeks. After a 1-week washout period, all patients were switched to the other modality. VAS was used to assess pain, physical activity, and quality of sleep before each session. A significant reduction of the pain score ($P < 0.001$) and improvement of physical activity, sense of well-being, and quality of sleep while reducing the need for oral non-opioid analgesic medication were observed in the EA group, whereas the control group was of no significant change. While the design of this study is more convincing than the previous one and the results are encouraging, more study is needed to uncover its long-term therapeutic effect.

Neuropathic pain is usually resulted from a nerve injury leading to the hypersensitivity or sensitization of the central nociceptive mechanisms. Acupuncture or electroacupuncture of low frequency (2 Hz) may produce a long-term depression at the spinal cord dorsal horn level [21], thereby reduces the sensitization, an effect mediated by opioid receptors and NMDA receptors.

Migraine

Migraine is a frequent and disabling episodic headache with autonomic disturbance. Pharmacological interventions are used to treat the acute attack and to prevent its relapse with limited success. Acupuncture has been reported to be effective in prophylactic and therapeutic purposes. Endres et al. [62] reviewed the existing data and came to the conclusion that a 6-week course (10 sessions) of acupuncture is not inferior to a 6-month prophylactic drug treatment, although the Chinese point selection and the depth of needle insertion is not as important as had been thought to be. They therefore suggested that acupuncture should be integrated into the existing migraine treatment protocol. For the treatment of acute attack of migraine, Li et al. [63] took 175 migraine patients and divided them into three groups. The verum group received acupuncture in 10 points with continuous manipulation for 30 min to induce deqi sensation, whereas the two control groups receive needle insertion in various nonpoints and staying there without movement, hence no deqi sensation. The degree of pain was assessed by the VAS (0–10) 0.5, 1, 2, and 4 h after the removal of the needles. A decrease of VAS by 1.0, 0.5, and 0.1 cm was observed after 4 h in the verum acupuncture group and the sham 1 and sham 2 acupuncture groups, respectively. Most patients in the acupuncture group experienced complete pain relief (40.7 %) and did not experience recurrence or intensification of pain (79.6 %). The results indicated that the true acupuncture group with deqi sensation is significantly better than the nonpoint groups. It is obvious that while the result of one treatment is moderate, the therapeutic effect may show a cumulative trend in the consecutive treatments.

Facco et al. [64] checked the effectiveness of a true acupuncture treatment in migraine without aura, comparing it to a standard mock acupuncture protocol, an accurate mock acupuncture-healing ritual and untreated controls. All groups were provided with standard rizatriptan treatment. The results showed that the true acupuncture group was significantly better than the control groups 6 months after the starting of the trial ($P < .0001$). Jena et al. [65] investigated the effectiveness of acupuncture in addition to routine care in patients with primary headache with more than 12-months history of two or more episodes per month. They found that acupuncture plus routine care was associated with marked clinical improvements compared with routine care alone ($P < .001$).

After reviewing all the reports, Diener [66] stated that application of the procedure in daily life would be impractical. The idea of patients leaving the workplace with a mild headache to see a person performing acupuncture is difficult to conceive. In fact, Diener's concern has been solved by technical improvement. It is time to try if transcutaneous electrical acupoint stimulation (TEAS) would induce similar therapeutic and prophylactic effect. If so, then it can be performed by the patient under the direction of the physician, saving a considerable amount of time, especially for the prophylactic purpose.

Muscle Spastic Pain

Spinal trauma is a condition often occurred in car accidents and falls. In the United States, the annual incidence of spinal cord injury (SCI) is around 12,000, with a prevalence of over 259,000 persons [67]. Severe spinal cord injury often induces flaccid muscle paralysis, which may turn into muscle spasm accompanied by cramping pain, and is hard to treat. Wang et al. [68] used transcutaneous electrical acupoint stimulation (TEAS) for the treatment of the spastic pain. The electrical stimulation was delivered to the skin over the two acupoints at the hand (LI4 on the dorsum of the hand and the other at the center of the palm) to form a circuit and two acupoints at the opposite leg (ST36 near the knee joint and BL57 at the calf muscle) to form a circuit. Wang et al. tried the low and high frequencies and found that only 100 Hz, but not 2-Hz stimulation, suppressed the muscle spasticity. The effect recorded at the end of one session (30 min) lasted for only 20–25 min. However, after a prolonged stimulation protocol (once a day, five times a week for 4 weeks), a cumulative therapeutic effect appeared in the second week, shown as a gradual decrease of the ankle clonus score and the Ashworth score accompanied by a reduction of pain score and an improvement of well-being. The therapeutic effect reached a plateau at the third and fourth week. The effect was sensitive to naloxone, suggesting that opioid peptides were involved. Animal studies revealed that implantation of a wax ball into the cervical spinal cord of the rat produced an increase of the muscle tonicity assessed by H reflex, accompanied by a decrease of the dynorphin content of the spinal cord [26]. Electroacupuncture at 100 Hz applied on the acupoint ST36 near the knee joint and SP6 near the ankle joint produced an increase of the dynorphin content and a decrease of the muscle tonicity. Intrathecal injection of the kappa opioid agonist U-50488 produced a similar spasmolytic effect [26]. Summarizing from the clinical observation and the rat experiment, we reached a hypothesis that spinal trauma produced a decrease of dynorphin in the spinal cord and an increase of muscle tonicity and the development of muscle spasm. This pathological status can be partially reversed by 100-Hz peripheral stimulation as a result of increased production and release of dynorphin which can be mimicked by the intrathecal injection of the kappa agonist U-50488. This preliminary study is certainly worth further clinical exploration.

Fibromyalgia

Fibromyalgia affect 2 % of population, with a man to women ratio of 1:7, and no cure is known. Acupuncture has been tried with uncertain effect. Four systemic reviews published in 2007–2009 showed pessimistic results, ranging from "no" to "mixed" or "moderate" effect. However, there are several papers showing optimistic results. One is from the Mayo Clinic [69]. They recruited 50 patients with fibromyalgia and evenly divided to two groups. One group used real acupuncture at 18–20 points, with 2- or 10-Hz stimulation for 20 min. The control group received mock needle without skin penetration. The patients received six sessions of treatment in a period of 2–3 weeks. The symptoms were measured by the Fibromyalgia Impact Questionnaire (FIQ) immediately, 1 and 7 months after the treatment. Acupuncture group showed a significant pain relief and a reduction of fatigue and anxiety. The effect was most marked in 1 month ($P = 0.007$) and gradually faded in seventh month. Harris et al. [70] at the University of Michigan observed the severity of the symptom of FM and the availability of mu opioid receptors in the brain, assessed by the positron emission tomography (PET) using ^{11}C-labeled carfentanyl as the tracer. A negative correlation was revealed in the severity of the syndrome and the availability of mu receptors, especially in the brain region known to play a role in pain modulation, such as nucleus accumbens, the amygdale, and the dorsal cingulate gyrus. This result may explain why morphine is not very effective in reducing the pain of FM patients. In the second study [71], they observed the effect of acupuncture for the treatment of FM. In the meantime, they used PET scan to assess the ^{11}C carfentanyl-binding potential of the brain regions relevant to pain control (nucleus accumbens, cingulate, caudate, amygdale). Single session of manual acupuncture applied at nine acupoints located at the head and all four extremities produced a mild increase of the receptor-binding potential (short-term effect). After 1 month of acupuncture treatment (eight sessions), the brain binding potential of ^{11}C carfentanyl increased dramatically (long-term effect), which was associated with a decrease of the FM symptoms. These effects were not found in patients receiving sham acupuncture (skin pricking without needle penetration). The results indicate that the therapeutic effect of acupuncture for FM is related with the increase of the binding potential of the morphine receptors in the brain. The work of Harris and associates not only confirmed the therapeutic effect of acupuncture on FM but also demonstrated that the effect of acupuncture is related with its ability of increasing the binding potential of the brain to mu agonists.

Future Directions

Design of Appropriate Control Group

To make an overview on research in acupuncture analgesia, one can see that the main issues of controversy focused on the question whether the effect of acupuncture is superior over the control group. Unlike the pharmacological experiment where a pill or an injection which looks identical yet contains inert substance can be used to replace the real one, acupuncture is a sophisticated procedure which is extremely difficult to imitate. In designing a clinical trial, at least two factors should be considered. One is the selection of the site of stimulation (the right acupoint), and the other is the technique of needle manipulation. For the selection of the site of stimulation, one can use (a) the real acupoint, as documented in the ancient book marked with points along the hypothetical line on the skin, named "meridian"; (b) irrelevant point, which has been used for other purpose not related with the disease under study; and (c) non-acupoint, which can be located several millimeters away from the real acupoint, or midway between two meridians, or where no meridians are known, for example, in the area along the armpits where no meridians passing by. Acupuncture at (b) and (c) can be regarded as sham acupuncture. For the control of the stimulation, one can use (a) minimal stimulation, such as inserting the needle to a small depth, using a weak twisting, or even leaving the needle unattended so that no "deqi" sensation is produced; (b) a blunt needle or a tooth stick to prick the skin without penetration (placebo); and (c) a pseudo-intervention such as a beam of laser light which is switched off immediately. The procedure of placebo acupuncture can be done covert to the patient, or being done in an overt manner. In the later case, a special device is needed so that the patient sees the needle being taped into the skin but actually is withdrawn into a hollow space [72]. All these designs are considered inert to the subject, only to produce a psychological effect to imitate the acupuncture procedure. However, none of these are technically perfect. Lund et al. [73] pointed out that even light touch of the skin can stimulate the mechanoreceptors coupled to slow-conducting unmyelinated (C) afferent fibers, resulting in the activation of the insular region of the brain, but not in the somatosensory cortex. Activity in these C tactile fibers has been suggested to induce emotional and hormonal reactions commonly seen after caressing and a sense of well-being. In one word, they are not "inert." The authors listed results from published papers that for the treatment of migraine which has an important affective component, minimal acupuncture stimulation can produce the same therapeutic effect as real acupuncture. However, for the treatment of osteoarthritis of the knee with a more pronounced sensory component, minimal acupuncture is usually ineffective.

With the advance of technology, acupuncture has been developed into more sophisticated forms, such as EA and transcutaneous electric acupoint stimulation (TEAS). In these cases, the design of the control group has more flexibility. For example, in order to provide minimal electrical stimulation, one can use the threshold stimulation, that is, the intensity is adjusted to a level barely sensible to the patient. To further weaken the stimulation, one can adjust the current output to 1 min on and 2 min off, thereby to cut the time of stimulation to one third of the original level, yet the subject still feels the sensation come-and-go. In a study to test the feasibility of TEAS for reducing the urge to smoking, Han's group revealed that when they reduce the intensity from 10 to 5 mA, the effect remained. However, when the intermittent 5 mA is used, it could no longer reduce the urge to smoking [74].

Comparison of the neural correlates of acupuncture and placebo effect would show that while acupuncture pathway is from bottom up (afferent comes from spinal cord to brain), placebo effect is from up down (from brain to the cord). But they use similar descending pathways including opioid and monoaminergic mechanisms. Brain imaging study showed that amygdale, insula, and hypothalamus may demonstrate some acupuncture specificity, whereas dorsolateral prefrontal cortex (DLPFC) and rostral anterior cingulate cortex (rACC) may support nonspecific brain expectancy related with placebo effect [75].

To summarize, placebo effect is common in biomedical practice and acupuncture is of no exception. Therefore, great care should be taken for the interpretation of the experimental results. When one finds the effect of placebo acupuncture to be similar with verum acupuncture, it should not be simply interpreted to mean that acupuncture is of no effect. Indeed, placebo analgesia and acupuncture analgesia may use the same opioid mechanism [76]. Conversely, when the mechanisms of placebo and nocebo are made clear, one may like to strengthen the placebo effect and to reduce the nocebo effect, in order to intensify the therapeutic capacity for the good of the patients [76].

Primary Outcome, Secondary Outcome, and Long-Term Effect

Primary outcome of pain alleviation is usually assessed by the visual analog scale. While the immediate analgesic effect is important, the follow-up long-term effect is even more desirable. Compared to oral pills, acupuncture treatment usually takes more time to achieve a visible therapeutic effect. So if the effect of acupuncture is short lasting, the superiority for this treatment modality would be greatly diminished. Likewise, research on the mechanisms of acupuncture effect should also put more emphasis on its long-term effect A good example was made by Harris et al. who used a PET scan to show that one session of acupuncture produced an immediate increase of morphine-binding potential in the brain. This elevation was even stronger when eight sessions of acupuncture were delivered to FM patient in 1 month of time [71]. Long-lasting analgesic effect would naturally induce simultaneous changes in sleep quality, physical activity, quality of life, and sense of well-being. These secondary outcomes are supplementary evidence to support the primary outcome.

Summary and Conclusions

Acupuncture is getting more and more popular in the medical field. This technology can be used for the treatment of distinctive diseases, or an array of conditions such as acute and chronic pain. One of the mechanisms is that it can increase the production and release of opioid peptides [13] and also increase the opioid receptor availability [71] in the discrete regions of the central nervous system. Conversely, acupuncture may just strengthen the homeostasis or activate the self-healing process via modulation of endocrine/immune systems, thereby improving the health status.

While the authentic form of acupuncture is manual needling, the demarcation between manual needling, electroacupuncture (EA), and transcutaneous electric acupoint stimulation (TEAS) is gradually fading. From neurobiological point of view, acupuncture can be regarded as a special form of peripheral stimulation for neuromodulatory effect. For example, during the pharmacological anesthesia for surgical operation, why not make use of the endogenous opioid system to reduce the postoperative pain and nausea/vomiting, simply by putting the skin electrodes on the acupoints prior to chemical anesthesia and leaving the TEAS device kept on for the whole period of surgery. During the treatment of migraine, for example, why not combine the drug intervention with the TEAS, simply by training the patient with the use of the portable TEAS device together with the self-sticky skin electrodes. This way, we can contribute to the global effort of increasing the therapeutic efficiency and, in the meanwhile, lowering the medical cost.

Looking at the future, when the clinical efficacy of acupuncture is made clear and the mechanisms of its action are better elucidated, one would expect that patients, physicians, and insurance providers would show more interest for the use of acupuncture in the clinical practice.

References

1. NIH Consensus Development Conference on Acupuncture. 3–5 Nov 2007. NIH continuing Medical Education. See: Ramsay DJ, Bowman MA, Greenman PE, et al. NIH Consensus Development Panel Acupuncture. JAMA. 1998;280:1518–24.
2. NCCAM, NIH. Get the facts. Acupuncture for pain. Web site: nccam.nih.gov.
3. Nahin RL, Barness PM, Straussman BJ, et al. Costs of complementary and alternative medicine (CAM) and frequency of visits to CAM practitioners: United States, 2007. Natl Health Stat Rep. 2009;18:1–16.
4. Wang SM, Kain ZN, White P. Acupuncture analgesia: I. The Scientific Basis. Pain Med. 2008;106:602–21.
5. Zhao ZQ. Neural mechanisms underlying acupuncture analgesia. Prog Neurobiol. 2008;85(4):355–75.
6. Butler MJ, Sidall PJ. Neurochemical and neurophysiologic effect of needle insertion: clinical implications. In: Cousins J, Carr DB,
7. Horlocker TT, Bridenbaugh PO, editors. Cousins and Bridenbaugh's "neural blockade in clinical anesthesia and pain medicine". 4th ed. Philadelphia: Lippincott, Williams & Wilkins; 2009. p. 763–76.
7. Research Group of Acupuncture Analgesia, Beijing Medical College. The effect of acupuncture on pain threshold of the skin on human volunteers. Chin Med J. 1973;3:151–7.
8. Lu GW, Liang RZ, Xie JQ, et al. Role of peripheral afferent by needling point Zusanli. Sci Sin. 1979;22:680–92.
9. Research Group of Acupuncture Anesthesia. Beijing Medical College: the role of some neurotransmitters of brain in acupuncture analgesia. Sci Sin. 1974;17:112–30.
10. Han JS, Chou PH, Lu CH, et al. The role of central 5-HT in acupuncture analgesia. Sci Sin. 1979;22:91–104.
11. Xie CW, Tang J, Han JS. Central norepinephrine in acupuncture analgesia. Differential effects in brain and spinal cord. In: Takagi H, Simon EJ, editors. Advances in endogenous and exogenous opioids. Tokyo: Kodansha; 1981. p. 288–90.
12. Mayer DJ, Price DD, Raffi A. Antagonism of acupuncture analgesia in man by narcotic antagonist naloxone. Brain Res. 1977;121: 368–72.
13. Han JS. Acupuncture: neuropeptide release produced by electrical stimulation of different frequencies. Trends Neurosci. 2003;26: 17–22.
14. Huang L, Ren MF, Lu JH, et al. Mutual potentiation of the analgesic effects of met-enkephalin, dynorphin A(1–13) and morphine in the spinal cord of the rat. Acta Physiol Sinica. 1987;39:454–46.
15. Sutters KA, Miaskowski C, Taiwo YO, et al. Analgesic synergy and improved motor function produced by combinations of μ-δ- and μ-κ-opioids. Brain Res. 1990;530:290–4.
16. Han JS, Li SJ, Tang J. Tolerance to electroacupuncture and its cross tolerance to morphine. Neuropharmacology. 1981;20:593–6.
17. Tang NM, Dong HW, Wang XM, et al. Cholecystokinin antisense RNA increases the analgesic effect induced by electroacupuncture or low dose morphine: conversion of low responder rats into high responders. Pain. 1997;71(71):81.
18. Han JS. Opioid and anti-opioid peptides: a model of Yin-Yang balance in acupuncture mechanisms of pain modulation. In: Stux G, Hammerschlag R, editors. Clinical acupuncture, scientific basis. Berlin/Heidelberg: Springer; 2001. p. 51–68.
19. Han JS, Wang Q. Mobilization of specific neuropeptides by peripheral stimulation of identified frequencies. News Physiol Sci. 1992;7:176–80.
20. You HJ, Tjolsen A, Arent-Nielson L. High frequency conditioning stimulation evokes supraspinal independent long-term depression but not long term potentiation of the spinal withdrawal reflex in rats. Brain Res. 2006;1090:116–22.
21. Xing GG, Liu FY, Qu XX, et al. Long term synaptic plasticity in the dorsal horn neuron and its modulation by electroacupuncture in rats with neuropathic pain. Exp Neurol. 2007;208:323–32.
22. Zhang WT, Jin Z, Cui GH, et al. Relations between brain network activation and analgesic effect induced by low versus high frequency electrical acupoint stimulation in different subjects: a functional magnetic resonance imaging study. Brain Res. 2003;982: 168–78.
23. Wang L, Fei XY, Zhu B. Chaos analysis of the electrical signal time series evoked by acupuncture. Chaos Solition Fractals. 2007;33: 901–7.
24. Sun RQ, Wang HC, Wan Y, et al. Suppression of neuropathic pain by peripheral electrical stimulation in rats: mu opioid receptor and NMDA receptor implicated. Exp Neurol. 2004;187:23–9.
25. Wang JZ, Zhou HJ, Liu GL, et al. Han's acupoint nerve stimulator for the treatment of spinal cord injury induced muscle spasticity. Chin J Pain Med. 6:217–24.
26. Dong HW, Wang LH, Zhang M, et al. Decreased dynorphin A (1–17) in the spinal cord of spastic rats after the compressive injury. Brain Res Bull. 2005;67:189–95.

27. Liu HX, Tian JB, Luo F, et al. Repeated 100 Hz TENS for the treatment of chronic inflammatory hyperalgesia and suppression of spinal release of substance P in monoarthritic rats. Evid based Complement Alternat Med. 2006;3:101–16.

28. Wang Q, Mao LM, Han JS. Comparison of the antinociceptive effects induced by electroacupuncture and transcutaneous electrical nerve stimulation in the rat. Int J Neurosci. 1992;65:117–29.

29. Ahmed HE, Craig WF, White PF, et al. Percutaneous electrical nerve stimulation: an alternative to antiviral drugs for acute herpes zoster. Anesth Analg. 1998;87:911–4.

30. Cumming M. Percutaneous electrical nerve stimulation – electroacupuncture by another name? A comparative review. Acupunct Med. 2001;19:32–5.

31. Wang BG, Wang EZ, Chen XZ, et al. Acupuncture anesthesia combined with enflurane for cranial operations. Integr Chin West Med China. 1994;14:10–3 (In Chinese).

32. Billota F, Rosa G. "Anesthesia" for awake neurosurgery. Curr Opin Anaesthesiol. 2009;22:560–5.

33. Qu GL, Zhuang XL, Xu GH, et al. Clinical study on kidney transplantation under complex acupuncture and drug anesthesia. Acupunct Res. 1997;4:275–9.

34. Sim CK, Xu PC, Pua HL, et al. Effects of electroacupuncture on intraoperative and postoperative analgesic requirement. Acupunct Med. 2002;20:56–65.

35. Morioka N, Akca O, Doufas AG, et al. Electroacupuncture at the Zusali, Yanlinquan and Kunlun points does not reduce anesthetic requirement. Anesth Analg. 2002;95:98–102.

36. Wang BG, Tang J, White PF, et al. Effect of the intensity of transcutaneous acupoint electrical stimulation on the postoperative analgesic requirement. Anesth Analg. 1997;85:406–13.

37. Chen L, Tang J, White PF, et al. The effect of location of transcutaneous electrical nerve stimulation: acupoint versus nonacupoint stimulation. Anesth Analg. 1998;87:1129–34.

38. Lin ZG, Lo MW, Hsieh CL, et al. The effect of high and low frequency electroacupuncture in pain after lower abdominal surgery. Pain. 2002;99:509–14.

39. White PF, Hamza MA, Recart A, et al. Optimal timing of acustimulation for antiemetic prophylaxis as an adjunct to ondansetron in patients undergoing plastic surgery. Anesth Analg. 2005;100:367–72.

40. Grube T, Uhlemann C, Weiss T, et al. Influence of acupuncture on postoperative pain, nausea and vomiting after cisceral surgery: a prospective, randomized comparative study of metamizole and standard treatment. Schmerz. 2009;23(4):370–6.

41. Korinenko Y, Vincent A, Cutshall SM, et al. Efficacy of acupuncture in prevention of postoperative nausea in cardiac surgery patients. Ann Thorac Surg. 2009;88:637–42.

42. Zarate E, Mingus M, White PF, et al. The use of transcutaneous Acupoint electrical stimulation for preventing nausea and vomiting after laparoscopic surgery. Anesth Analg. 2001;92:629–35.

43. White PF. Use of alternative medical therapies in the perioperative period: is it time to get on board? Anesth Analg. 2007;104:251–4.

44. Shafer SL. Did our brains fall out? Anesth Analg. 2007;104:247–8.

45. Ghoname EA, et al. Percutaneous electrical nerve stimulation for low back pain: a randomized crossover study. J Am Med Assoc. 1999;281:818–23.

46. Ghoname EA, Craig WF, White PF, et al. The effect of stimulus frequency on the analgesic response to percutaneous electrical nerve stimulation in patients with chronic low back pain. Anesth Analg. 1999;88:841–6.

47. Chen XH, Guo SF, Chang CG, Han JS. Optimal conditions for eliciting maximal electroacupuncture analgesia with dense-and-disperse mode stimulation. Am J Acupunct. 1994;22:47–53.

48. Sator-Katzenschager SM, Scharbert G, Kozek-Langenecker SA, et al. The short and long-term benefit in chronic low back pain through adjuvant electrical versus manual auricular acupuncture. Pain Med. 2004;98:1359–64.

49. Gadsby JG, Flowerdew MW. Transcutaneous electrical stimulation and acupuncture-like transcutaneous electrical nerve stimulation for chronic low back pain. Cochrane Database Syst Rev. 2006;(1): CD000210.

50. White PF, Craig WF, Vakharia AS, et al. Percutaneous neuromodulation therapy: does the location of electrical stimulation effect the acute analgesic response? Anesth Analg. 2000;91:949–54.

51. Ernst E, White A. Acupuncture for back pain: a meta-analysis of randomized controlled trials. Arch Intern Med. 1998;158: 2235–41.

52. Yokoyama M, Sun XH, Oku S, et al. Comparison of percutaneous electrical nerve stimulation with transcutaneous electrical nerve stimulation for long-term pain relief in patients with chronic low back pain. Anesth Analg. 2004;98:1552–6.

53. Berman BM, Lao LX, Langenberg P, et al. Effectiveness of acupuncture as adjunctive therapy in osteoarthritis of the knee. Ann Intern Med. 2004;141:901–10.

54. Scharf HP, Mansmann U, Stretberger K, et al. Acupuncture and knee osteoarthritis. A tree-armed randomized trial. Ann Intern Med. 2006;145:12–20.

55. Ahsin S, Saleem S, Bhatti AM. Clinical and endocrinological changes after electroacupuncture treatment in patients with osteoarthritis of the knee. Pain. 2009;147(1-3):60–6.

56. Zhang W, Moslowitz RW, Nuki G, et al. OARSI recommendations for the management of hip and knee osteoarthritis, Part II: OARSI evidence-based, expert consensus guidelines. Osteoarthritis Cartilage. 2008;16(2):137–62.

57. Conaghan PG, Dickson J, Grant RL. Guideline Development Group. Care and management of osteoarthritis in adults: summary of NICE guidance. BMJ. 2008;336(7642):502–3.

58. White A. NICE guideline on osteoarthritis: is it fair to acupuncture? No. Acupunct Med. 2009;27:70–2.

59. Latimer N. NICE guideline on osteoarthritis: is it fair to acupuncture? Yes. Acupunct Med. 2009;27:72–5.

60. Abuaisha BB, Costanzi JB, Boulton AJM. Acupuncture for the treatment of chronic painful peripheral diabetic neuropathy: a long term study. Diabetic Res Clin Pract. 1998;39:115–21.

61. Hamza MA, Proctor TJ, White PF, et al. Percutaneous electrical nerve stimulation: a novel analgesic therapy for diabetic neuropathic pain. Diabetes Care. 2000;23:365–70.

62. Endres HG, Diener HC, Molsberger A. Role of acupuncture in the treatment of migraine. Expert Rev Neurother. 2007;7:1121–34.

63. Li Y, Liang F, Yang X, et al. Acupuncture for treating acute attacks of migraine: a randomized controlled trial. Headache. 2009;49: 805–16.

64. Facco E, Liguori A, Petti F, et al. Traditional acupuncture in migraine: a controlled randomized study. Headache. 2008. doi:10.1111/j.1526-4610.2007.00916.x.

65. Jena S, Will CM, Brinkhaus B, et al. Acupuncture in patients with headache. Cephalalgia. 2008;28:969–79.

66. Diener HC. Migraine: is acupuncture clinically viable for treating acute migraine? Nat Rev Neurol. 2009;5:469–70.

67. Spinal Cord Injury Information Network. Updated 2009.

68. Wang JZ, Zhou HJ, Liu GL, et al. Post-traumatic spinal spasticity treated with Han's Acupoint Nerve Stimulator (NASS). Chin J Pain Med. 2000;6:217–24.

69. Martin DP, Sletten CD, Williams BA, et al. Improvement in fibromyalgia symptom with acupuncture: results of a randomized controlled trial. Mayo Clin Proc. 2006;81:749–57.

70. Harris RE, Clauw DJ, Scott DJ, et al. Decreased central mu-opioid availability in fibromyalgia. J Neurosci. 2007;27:10000–6.

71. Harris RE, Zubieta JK, Scott DJ, et al. Traditional Chinese acupuncture ad placebo (sham) acupuncture are differentiated by their effect on mu-opioid receptors (MORs). Neuroimage. 2009;47:1077–85.

72. Streitberger K, Kleinhenz J. Introducing a placebo needle into acupuncture research. Lancet. 1998;352:364–5.

73. Lund I, Naslund J, Lundeberg T. Minimal acupuncture is not a valid placebo control in randomized controlled trials of acupuncture: a physiologist's perspective. Chin Med. 2009;4:1–9.

74. Lambert C, Berlin I, Lee TL, et al. A Standardized transcutaneous electric acupoint stimulation for relieving tobacco urges in dependent smokers. eCAM. 2008;1093:1–9.

75. Dhond R, Kettner N, Napadow V. Do the neural correlates of acupuncture and placebo effects differ? Pain. 2007;128:8–12.

76. Enck P, Benedetti F, Schedlowski M. New insights into the placebo and nocebo response. Neuron. 2008;59:195–206.

77. Research Group of Ear Acupuncture, Jiangsu College of New Medicine. The effect of ear acupuncture on the pain threshold of the skin at thoracic and abdominal region. In: Theoretical study on acupuncture anesthesia. Shanghai: Shanghai People's Press; 1973. p. 27–32.

Manual Therapies

11

John F. Barnes, Albert L. Ray, and Rhonwyn Ullmann

Key Points

- Manual therapies are an essential part of functional restoration and pain treatment in people with persistent pain.
- Several therapeutic techniques can help with neuroplastic positive changes in brain function (retraining the brain).
- The most critical element in improving function is to find a technique that "fits" the patient best since they all have common elements for brain change.
- The common feature of successful long-term improvement via manual therapies seems to be simultaneous multiple inputs to the brain; some of which incorporate mindful focused attention coupled with sensory and/or motor activities.
- The therapeutic improvements from the manual therapies discussed in this chapter demonstrate long-term effectiveness, unless the person is re-traumatized in body, mind, or both.

J.F. Barnes, PT, LMT, NCTMP (✉)
Myofascial Release Treatment Centers and Seminar,
222 West Lancaster Avenue, Suite 100, Paoli, PA 19301, USA
e-mail: paoli@myofascialrelease.com

A.L. Ray, M.D.
Medical Director, The LITE Center, 5901 SW 74 St, Suite 201,
South Miami, FL 33143, USA

Clinical Associate Professor, University of Miami Miller School
of Medicine, Miami, FL, USA
e-mail: aray@thelitecenter.org

R. Ullmann, BS, M.S.
The LITE Center,
5901 SW 74 St, Suite 201, South Miami, FL 33143, USA
e-mail: bearrab@aol.com

Introduction

Manual therapy is an essential and critical part of interdisciplinary functional restoration and pain treatment. There are multiple types of manual therapies. This chapter will present a select few, all of which have clinically shown themselves to be effective for such treatment. Some of these techniques have been in existence for centuries, while others are more recent. However, all of them have evolved over time and experience of the main therapists behind their names and styles, based on what has been the most effective for those suffering from chronic pain. They all have experience and time-testing behind them. Some of the literature is scant in terms of modern "evidence-based" studies for various reasons: some were started and developed long before double-blind randomized controlled trials were considered necessary; some have evolved by therapists who have reported techniques that they find work and were meant to be shared with other practitioners as practical and useful ways to improve function without intending to "prove" their worthiness to a scientific community; some have simply evolved because patients respond to them; and, especially in today's economic climate, research funding to create and implement double-blind randomized trials of these techniques is rare, if available at all. There is, however, crucial and critical thinking behind all of the techniques that will be presented in this chapter. The purpose of this chapter is to present an overview of various manual therapy techniques in order to raise awareness on the part of our readers as to what is available, and we submit that there is much more specific information, as well as courses, available to all who desire a more involved learning of these topics or wish to be able to practice these various techniques.

There is no one particular manual therapy technique that is, by development, superior to others. Different patients respond differently, and whichever technique a person is able to utilize to help themselves is the important discriminator. However, in these authors' experience, those techniques which include more than one "brain input" at a time seem to be the techniques that offer the most effective opportunities to alter neuroplastic patterns in the brain, and that is why this list of therapies have been chosen for discussion. This mind-body connection "release" via multiple simultaneous brain "inputs" also seems to be one characteristic which makes these techniques more effective than single-modality "traditional" physical therapy for those suffering from persistent pain.

We will now turn to specific manual therapies and begin with the John Barnes technique. Within this section is a more detailed discussion related to the fascia and the mind-body connection within this "connective" tissue system. The principles related to fascial characteristics, however, are applicable to the other therapeutic techniques that follow as well.

John F. Barnes Myofascial Release

Myofascial release is a whole body, hands-on approach for the evaluation and treatment of the human structure. Its focus is the fascial system. Pain associated with physical trauma, an inflammatory or infection process, surgical procedures, or structural imbalance from dental malocclusion, osseous restriction, leg-length discrepancy, and pelvic rotation may all create inappropriate fascial strain.

Trauma and inflammatory responses create myofascial restrictions that can produce tensile pressures of approximately 2,000 lb/in.^{2} on pain-sensitive structures that do not show up in any of the standard tests (x-rays, myelograms, CT scans, electromyography, etc.).

This enormous pressure acts like a "straightjacket" on muscles, nerves, blood vessels, and osseous structures producing the symptoms of pain, headaches, and restriction of motion. Myofascial release allows the chronic inflammatory response to resolve and eradicate the enormous pressure of myofascial restrictions exerted on pain-sensitive structures to alleviate symptoms and to allow the body's natural healing capacity to function properly.

Fascia, an embryologic tissue, reorganizes along the lines of tension (called tensegrity) imposed on the body, adding support to misalignment and contracting to protect the individual from further trauma (real or imagined). This has the potential to alter organ and tissue physiology significantly. Fascial strains can slowly tighten, causing the body to lose its physiologic adaptive capacity. Flexibility and spontaneity of movement are lost, setting the body up for more trauma, pain, and limitation of movement. These powerful fascial restrictions begin to pull the body out of its three-dimensional alignment.

Janet Travell's [1] detailed description of the myofascial element indicates that there is a smooth fascial sheath which surrounds every muscle of the body, so that every muscular fascicle is surrounded by fascia, every fibril is surrounded by fascia, and every microfibril down to the cellular level is surrounded by fascia. Therefore, it is the fascia that ultimately determines the length and function of its muscular component, and muscle becomes an inseparable component of fascia. Because fascia covers the muscle, bones, nerves, organs, and vessels down to the cellular level, malfunction of the system due to trauma, surgery, poor posture, or inflammation can bind down the fascia, resulting in abnormal pressure on any or all of these body components.

As Travell [1] has explained, restrictions of the fascia can create pain or malfunction throughout the body, sometimes with bizarre side effects and seemingly unrelated symptoms that do not always follow dermatome zones. An extremely high percentage of people suffering with pain, loss of motion, or both may have fascial restriction problems.

John F. Barnes Myofascial Release (JFBMFR), along with therapeutic exercise and movement therapy, improves the vertical alignment and lengthens the body, providing more space and less pressure for the proper functioning of osseous structures, neuromatrix system, blood vessels, and organs.

Thus, for example, with an injury to the lumbosacral area, patients have been known to experience distant symptoms such as occipital headaches, upper cervical pain and dysfunction, feelings of tightness around the thoracic area, lumbosacral pain, and tightness and lack of flexibility in the posterior aspect of the lower extremity. During trauma, or with development of a structural imbalance, a proprioceptive memory pattern of pain is established in the central nervous system. Beyond the localized pain from injured nerves, these reflex patterns remain to perpetuate the pain during and beyond healing of the injured tissue, similar to the experience of phantom limb pain.

Once fascia has tightened and is creating symptoms distant from the injury, appropriate traditional localized treatments may produce temporary results; however, they do not treat the "straightjacket" of pressure that is causing the symptoms. Myofascial release (JFBMFR) techniques are performed in conjunction with specific systematic treatment. The gentle tractioning forces applied to the fascial restrictions will elicit heat from a vasomotor response which increases blood flow to the affected area, enhancing lymphatic drainage of toxic metabolic wastes, realignment of fascial planes, and, most importantly, reset the soft tissue proprioceptive sensory mechanism. The activity seems to reprogram the central nervous system, enabling the patient to perform a normal, functional range of motion without eliciting the previous pain patterns [2].

The goal of this form of myofascial release is to remove fascial restrictions and restore the body's equilibrium. When the structure has been returned to a balanced state, it is realigned with gravity. When these aims have been accomplished, the body's inherent ability to self-correct returns, thus restoring optimum function and performance with the least amount of energy expenditure [3]. A more ideal

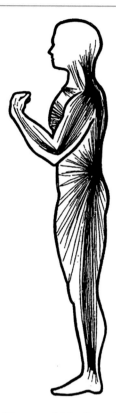

Fig. 11.1 Fascia man (Courtesy of John Barnes)

environment to enhance the effectiveness of concomitant systematic work therapy is also created (Fig. 11.1).

The trained JFBMFR therapist finds the cause of symptoms by evaluating the fascial system. The technique requires continuous reevaluation during treatment, including observation of vasomotor responses and their location as they occur after a particular restriction has been released.

When the location of the fascial restriction is determined, gentle pressure is applied in its direction. It is hypothesized that this has the effect of pulling the elastocollagenous fibers straight. When hand or palm pressure is first applied to the elastocollagenous complex, the elastic component is engaged, resulting in a "springy" feel. The elastic component is slowly stretched until hands stop at what feels like a firm barrier. This is the collagenous component. This barrier cannot be forced; it is too strong. Instead, the therapist continues to apply gentle sustained pressure, and soon, the firm barrier will yield to the previous melting or springy feel as it stretches further. This yielding phenomenon is related to viscous flow; that is, a low load (gentle pressure) applied slowly will allow a viscous medium to flow to a greater extent than a high load (quickly applied) pressure [4, 5]. The viscosity of the ground substance has an effect on the ground collagen since it is believed that the viscous medium that makes up the ground substance controls the ease with which collagen fibers rearrange themselves (Jenkins DHR). As this rearranging occurs, the collagenous barrier releases, producing a change in tissue length [4].

JFBMFR techniques and myofascial unwinding seem to allow for the complete communication of mind with body and body with mind, which is necessary for healing. The body remembers everything that ever happened to it, and Hameroff's research [6] indicates that the theory of "quantum coherence" points toward the storing of meaningful memory in the microtubules, cylindrical protein polymers that we find in the fascia of cells. Mind-body awareness and healing are often linked to the concept of "state-dependent" memory, learning, and behavior [7, 8]. For example, a certain smell or the sound of a particular piece of music may create a flashback phenomenon, a visual, sensorimotor replay of a past event or an important episode in our lives with such vividness that it is as if it were happening at that moment. Work based on the writings of and expanded upon by Barnes, Hameroff, and colleagues [6] includes position-dependent memory, learning, and behavior, with the structural position being the missing component in Selye's state-dependent theory as it is currently described [7, 8].

During periods of trauma, people form subconscious indelible imprints of the experience that have high levels of emotional content and which could not be processed at the time of occurrence. The body can hold information below the conscious level, as a protective mechanism, so that memories tend to become dissociated, or amnesiac, called memory dissociation, or reversible amnesia. Subconscious holding patterns eventually form for specific muscular tone or tension patterns, and the fascial component then tightens into these habitual positions of strain as a compensation to support misalignment that results (tensegrity effect). Therefore, the repeated postural insults of a lifetime, combined with the tensions of emotional and psychological origin, seem to result in tense, contracted, bunched, and fatigued fibrous tissue. A combination of mental and physical stresses may alter the neuromyofascial and skeletal structure, creating a visible, identifiable physical change which, itself, generates further stress, such as pain, joint restrictions, general discomfort, and fatigue. A chronic stress pattern produces long-term muscular contraction which, if prolonged, can cause energy loss, mechanical inefficiency, pain, cardiovascular pathology, and hypertension [9]. Memories are state (or position) dependent and can therefore be retrieved when the person later repeats that particular state (or position). This information is not available in the normal conscious state, and the body's protective mechanisms keep us away from the positions that our mind-body awareness construes as painful or traumatic.

It has been demonstrated consistently that when a myofascial release technique takes the tissue to a significant position, or when myofascial unwinding allows a body part to assume a significant position three-dimensionally in space, the tissue not only changes and improves, but memories, associated emotional states, and belief systems rise to the conscious level. This awareness, through the positional reproduction of a past event or trauma, allows the individual to grasp the previously hidden information that may be creating or maintaining symptoms or behavior that deter improvement. With the repressed and stored information now at the conscious level, the individual is in a position to learn which holding or bracing patterns have been impeding progress and why. The release of the tissue with its stored emotions and hidden information creates an environment for change. As such, no longer do patients habitually find themselves holding or stiffening to protect themselves from future pain or trauma. Release of fear and emotion takes place simultaneously with physical fascial release and physiologic release of the associated stress hormones.

Fascia and New Explanatory Paradigms

Clinical evidence has demonstrated that restrictions in the fascial system are of considerable importance in relieving pain and restoring function [10]. Myofascial release becomes vitally important when we realize that these restrictions can exert tremendous tensile forces on the neuromuscular-skeletal systems and other pain-sensitive structures, creating the very symptoms that we have been trying to eliminate [11].

An important component of the theory behind the mind-body connection is the ability for people to transmit natural bioelectrical currents along the endogenous electromagnetic fields of the three-dimensional network of the fascial system of another person [4]. Medical applications of exogenous bioelectromagnetics (like x-ray) are very common. Endogenous bioelectromagnetic field, natural within all living beings, has only more recently been studied [4, 12].

Increasingly, medical researchers and experienced health professionals are beginning to view the body as a self-correcting mechanism with bioelectric healing systems. According to Cowley [13], some scientists are starting to explore the body's sensitivity to electromagnetic energy. Electromagnetic fields "trigger the release of stress hormones... [and] can affect such processes as bone growth, communication among brain cells, and even the activity of white cells" [13].

Copper wire is a well-known conductor of electricity. If copper wire becomes twisted or crushed, it loses its ability to conduct energy properly. It is thought that fascia may act like copper wire when it becomes restricted through trauma, inflammatory processes, or poor posture over time. Then, its ability to conduct the body's bioelectricity seems to be diminished, setting up structural compensations and, ultimately, symptoms or restrictions of motion [4]. Just like untwisting a copper wire, myofascial release techniques seem to restore the fascia's ability to conduct bioelectricity, thus creating the environment for enhanced healing. Release techniques can also structurally eliminate the enormous pressures that fascial restrictions exert on nerves, blood vessels, and muscles [4].

Fascial "Memory"

It appears that not only the myofascial element but also every cell of the body has a consciousness that stores memories and emotions [4, 14]. Research findings suggest that the mind and body act on each other in often remarkable ways. With the help of sophisticated new laboratory tools, investigators are demonstrating that emotional states can translate into altered responses in the immune system, the complex array of organs, glands, and cells that comprises the body's principal mechanism for repelling invaders. The implications of this loop are unsettling. To experts in the field of psycho-neuroimmunology, the immune system seems to behave almost as if it had a brain of its own. This is creating a revolution in medicine in the way we view physiology. More than that, it is raising profound and tantalizing questions about the nature of behavior, about the essence of what we are [15].

Fascia is not accessed by traditional mechanical methods such as point mobilization modalities or traditional stretching methods. Fascia, instead, responds to the combination of the intentional application of endogenous bioelectromagnetic energy fields and the sustained mechanical pressure at the myofascial barrier from within the therapist. Through the palms and fingers of the therapist's hands, this gentle, sustained mechanical pressure seems to open memories and experiences in restricted fascia, for upon the release of restrictions, patients commonly become transported back to an injurious experience and with similar emotion, relating the experience in three-dimensional detail [4]. Once the trauma is completely experienced and fascial restrictions have given way, healing can commence. We have yet to learn the cellular mechanism of the healing process, it is believed that as restrictions are removed from fascia, body energy, blood, lymph, neurotransmitters, neuropeptides, and steroids are free to flow, restoring balance, homeostasis, and overall health to the system [4].

Myofascial release is not offered to replace traditional physical therapy techniques, but rather to supplement and enhance them as a complementary approach in evaluating and treating patients with pain, restriction of motion, and structural symptoms.

Yoga

Yoga historically evolved from a Hindu spiritual and ascetic discipline which utilizes specific body postures (asana) along with breath control (prana) and simple meditation to achieve unity of body and mind. Asana is the Sanskrit term for the physical postures of yoga. (Interestingly, many "traditional" Western physical therapy stretches and exercises are based in yoga tradition, but they do not incorporate the mindful focus in addition.) However, asana is only one of eight "limbs" of yoga, the majority of which are more concerned with mental and spiritual well-being rather than the physical. This technique is about creating balance in the body through development of strength and flexibility, including stretching. One style, vinyasa, utilizes the poses quickly in succession to create body heat through movement, while other styles go more slowly to focus on increasing stamina and perfect alignment of the pose.

Yoga has been found to be effective in the treatment of low back pain. In looking at randomized trials of yoga in low back pain with pain level as a mandated outcome measure, five RCTs suggested yoga significantly reduced low back pain compared to usual care, education, or conventional therapeutic exercises [16]. An 8-week yoga program demonstrated reduced pain, reduced catastrophizing, increased acceptance and mindfulness, and increased cortisol levels in women with fibromyalgia [17]. Positive results are shown in primary dysmenorrhea in reducing the pain intensity and duration [18]. In children with functional abdominal pain and irritable bowel syndrome, yoga has reduced pain and frequency, especially in children between 8 and 11 years old [19]. In a yogic prana (breathing) energization technique (YPET) study of fresh simple fractures of extra-articular long and short bones, patients within the yoga treatment showed significant improvement over controls in pain reduction, tenderness reduction, swelling, and increased fracture time density and number of cortices united [20].

Feldenkrais Method or Awareness Through Movement®

Feldenkrais Method is a form of somatic education developed by Dr. Moshe Feldenkrais, a physicist, judo expert, mechanical engineer, and educator who utilized this knowledge base to design a method of gentle movement and directed attention to improve movement and enhance human functioning. Another name for this treatment method is Awareness Through Movement®. It is based on the principles of physics, biomechanics, and an empirical understanding of learning. It has been successfully utilized in all age groups in both physically challenged and physically fit groups, including professional athletes. It is claimed to be useful for helping those with chronic pain, those wishing to improve their self-awareness and self-image, and in central nervous conditions such as multiple sclerosis, cerebral palsy, and stroke.

Literature is scarce for treatment of chronic pain with Feldenkrais Method, but one study of 14 women with nonspecific neck and shoulder pain in a self-report study model demonstrated significant improvement and found the technique "wholesome, but difficult." Additionally, they reported positive changes in posture, balance, a feeling of release, and increased self-confidence, and these positive effects remained after 4–6-month follow-up [21]. In a study comparing Body Awareness Therapy (BAT), Feldenkrais Method (FM), and conventional physiotherapy in patients with nonspecific musculoskeletal disorders, both the BAT and FM groups improved over conventional therapy in pain and quality of life, and they remained stable over time, while the conventional therapy group deteriorated at 1-year follow-up [22].

Pilates

Pilates exercises were developed by Joseph Pilates in the 1920s. There are six principles to Pilates exercises which emphasize precision of movement over quantity of exercise, and these include centering, control, flow, breath, precision, and concentration. Core muscle strength is the foundation of this technique, and these include the deep muscles of the abdomen and back. Pilates exercises are done either on a mat or on specialized equipment that utilizes pulleys and the patient's own body weight for resistance.

Literature review for Pilates-based treatment of chronic pain produced mixed results. One 4-week study for treatment of nonspecific chronic low back pain looked at pain reduction and functional disability, and demonstrated a significant decrease in pain and disability which continued at 12-month follow-up, compared to a control group receiving usual care [23]. Another study compared Pilates training in people with fibromyalgia with a home exercise program of stretching/relaxation found significant improvement in both pain and FIQ (Fibromyalgia Impact Questionnaire) at 12 weeks, but only in FIQ at 24 weeks in the Pilates group [24]. Multiple studies did literature reviews of RCTs including nonspecific low back pain with varied results. In a systematic review and meta-analysis, Lim concluded that Pilates-based exercises are superior to minimal intervention for pain relief, but not superior to other forms of exercise to reduce pain and disability [25]. The La Touche [24] review also found positive effects for reducing pain in nonspecific chronic low back pain but cautions that no studies have identified which specific parameters are to be applied when prescribing Pilates exercises [26]. However, Posadzki's literature review found "some evidence" supporting effectiveness of Pilates in management of low back pain, they point out that no definite conclusions could be drawn, and further research is needed due to the sample sizes, heterogeneity of inclusion/exclusion criteria, etc. [27]. On the contrary, one literature review found no improvement in pain or functionality in low back pain patients when compared to control and lumbar stabilization exercise groups. However, the Pilates group was no worse either [28].

Alexander Technique

The Alexander technique is focused on movement and release of tension in the body. It is designed to improve the ease and freedom of movement, balance, support, and coordination. This technique improves the efficiency with which we move and decreases the energy and effort required. It is more a reeducation of the mind and body, rather than an exercise program, but it is a useful manual therapy. Like Feldenkrais Method, Alexander technique is based on tension patterns in our movement that develop from about age 3–4 years on, and both techniques are designed to reinstate better movement, more "childlike" to make improvement. Both utilize awareness as a major part of change, and both are based on learning philosophies. The Alexander technique is utilized in painful conditions based on the body tensions, usually out of our awareness, involved in painful conditions.

The medical literature regarding treatment of pain with Alexander technique provides supportive evidence for this treatment. One study found Alexander technique alone superior to either massage or massage combined with Alexander technique for chronic back pain [29]. In fact, those patients reported being able to manage their back pain better utilizing Alexander teachings without the excuses made for difficulty in standard exercising, because it "made sense" and they could perform it while carrying out everyday activities or relaxing [30]. Two studies found Alexander lessons effective for chronic pain at 1-year follow-up [31, 32]. A literature review by Ernst found two good studies that demonstrated Alexander technique to be useful in reducing disability in patients suffering from Parkinson's disease and improving pain behavior and disability in patients with back pain. They recommend further study of this technique, as the evidence was not "convincing" [33].

Aquatic Therapy

Water is an excellent medium for recovery from minor to major injuries and chronic pain. It addresses muscle imbalances and postural problems and is also less threatening to patients who are afraid of exercise, pain, and/or reinjury. By creating a safe environment, one in which the patient can feel more in control and one that may not increase pain, can be a stepping-stone to changing the patients perception of pain and of movement.

The properties of water make it ideal for achieving therapeutic goals in a safe and effective environment [34, 35]:

- Buoyancy. Buoyancy is the upward pressure exerted by the fluid in which the body is immersed. Buoyancy opposes the force of gravity, allowing the body to move more freely and easily than on land.
- Decreased compressive forces. This is due to the effects of buoyancy. The deeper one is in water, the greater the decrease in the compressive or weight-bearing forces on all joints, as well as the discs of the spine.
- Even hydrostatic pressure on submerged body parts. There is equal pressure from the water on the body that increases with depth. This is helpful for swelling around the joints or circulatory problems because the static fluid around the joints is forced upward toward the heart by hydrostatic pressure.
- Temperature. Aquatic therapy can be affected in any comfortable water temperature, but heated water (89–91 °F) has been found to be demonstrably more effective, especially for persons with arthritic conditions.

Many patients who are unable or not emotionally or psychologically ready to exercise in a conventional clinic setting can successfully participate in water exercise programs. In addition to the physical benefits (below), the safe environment builds confidence and trust in their ability to move and to exercise:

- Safety. One of the attractions to water as a therapeutic modality is the safety. Water is supportive through its buoyancy, resistive in nature, and equal in hydrostatic pressure on the submerged body part.
- Flexibility/range of motion. Due to the decrease of gravitational forces in water, the body moves freely, and overall weight is diminished so that a body part can be lifted and stretched without as much pain.
- Strengthening. The body in water is working against resistance, yet the patient feels supported and safe in this environment. As strength and endurance improve, resistive devices are available that enable the person to "turn up" the intensity of the exercise, further increasing cardiovascular strength and endurance aspects of reconditioning.
- Muscle reeducation. When movement patterns have been altered due to injury and/or pain, reeducating the whole body as well as the brain can be accomplished effectively in water.
- Balance. The environment in water is ever-changing, and the patient is constantly challenged.

Functional Movement/Restoration

What is "functional movement" and how does it differ from "traditional" physical therapy?

Functional movement is a "functional approach" to exercise and restoration, meaning that it is designed to address "real-world" movements and mimics the broad range of daily movements one might normally do. It teaches the body how to actually move, use, and increase available strength utilizing everyday movement patterns [36, 37]. Basically, it is directed toward the way a patient works, plays, and lives.

Its goal is to get the patient back to work, play, and normalized life.

Once an injury and/or pain begins (particularly if it began quite a while ago), the way a patient moves changes due to compensation and fear of pain. This puts stress on more than just the injured area. Changes and pain begin to be noticed in other areas of their body as well. Treating just the injured area, as is often done, does not treat the patient. As patients begin to feel pain in other areas, it frequently affects not just their body, but their mind and their spirit. Treating only the injured area is often not the answer. Integration of mind, body, and spirit simultaneously restores functionality and retrains the brain by creating new and/or restoring normal movement patterns that can help return patients back to life.

Summary

In this chapter, we have reviewed some of the most important manual therapy techniques that are utilized for reducing pain and restoring functionally improved mechanical abilities and mindful peacefulness. The utilization of touch should be apparent in all of these techniques, some of which allow for direct touching as a way to transfer information and energy between the pain sufferer and the therapist helping them, while others do it with indirect touching and "self-touching" of energy (as in yoga). The most important common denominator that we have found among all of these manual techniques is the useful application of mindful focus coupled with simultaneous sensory and/or motor involvement. This double stimulation of the brain seems to us to be the link that alters the brain in a positive way in either depotentiating the long-term potentiation that occurred by sensitization of the pain pathways or those that "clogged" the information transfer ability of the body's connective tissue system, especially the fascia. Once these problems are reversed, our mind-body connections are able to optimize their functions, and we see improvement that not only helps the person feel and function better but is permanent unless new problems develop. This is the important part of the manual therapies presented here, and why they become significantly important adjuncts to more traditional type physical therapies, which do not seem to make the same permanent improvements in persons with persistent pain. Traditional physical therapies are much more effective in treating the type of eudynia where pain is still a symptom of an underlying mechanical problem such as an acute injury, postsurgical problems, or flare-ups of arthritic conditions. Once maldynia develops, the manual therapies reviewed in this chapter become much more useful, because they are effective in changing the neuroplastic dysfunctional brain states that have developed and in "clearing out" longstanding dysfunctional conditions within the soft tissue, especially, as mentioned, the fascia.

References

1. Travell J. Myofascial pain and dysfunction. Baltimore: Williams & Wilkins; 1983.
2. Barnes J. Myofascial release: the search for excellence. In: Davis C, editor. Complementary therapies in rehabilitation. Thorofare: Slack Inc; 2004. p. 60.
3. Barnes JF, Smith G. The body is a self-correcting mechanism. Phys Ther Forum. July 1987;27.
4. Oschman JL. Energy medicine: the science basis. New York: Churchill Livingstone; 2000.
5. Jenkins DHR. Ligament injuries and their treatment. Rockville: Aspen Publications; 1985.
6. Hameroff SR. Quantum coherence in microtubules: a neural basis for emergent consciousness. J Conscious Stud. 1994;1(1):91–118.
7. Selye H. History and present status of the stress concept. In: Goldberger L, Breznitz S, editors. Handbook of stress. New York: Macmillan; 1982. p. 7–20.
8. Selye H. The stress of life. New York: McGraw-Hill; 1976.
9. Chaitow L. Neuro-muscular technique – a practitioner's guide to soft tissue mobilization. New York: Thorsons; 1985. p. 13–5.
10. Barnes JF. The significance of touch. Phys Ther Forum. 1988;7:10.
11. Popper KR, Eccles JC. The self and its brain. Berlin: Springer; 1977.
12. National Institutes of Health (U.S.). Alternative medicine: expanding medical horizons. Report to the NIH on alternative medical systems of practices in the United States. Pittsburgh: US Government Printing Office, Superintendent of Documents; 1992. p. 48–50.
13. Cowley G. An electromagnetic storm. Newsweek. 1989;114(2): p. 77.
14. Pert CB. Molecules of emotion: the science behind mind-body medicine. New York: Touchstone; 1997.
15. Kurtz R. Body centered psychotherapy: the Hakomi therapy. Ashland: The Hakomi Institute; 1988.
16. Posadski P, Ernst E. Yoga for low back pain: a systematic review of randomized clinical trials. Clin Rheumatol. 2011;30(9):1257–62.
17. Curtis K, Osadchuk A, Katz J. An eight-week yoga intervention is associated with improvements in pain, psychological functioning and mindfulness, and changes in cortisol levels in women with fibromyalgia. J Pain Res. 2011;4:189–201.
18. Rakhshaee Z. Effect of three yoga poses (cobra, cat and fish poses) in women with primary dysmenorrheal: a randomized clinical trial. J Pediatr Adolesc Gynecol. 2011;24(4):192–6.
19. Brands MM, Purperhart H, Deckers-Kocken JM. A pilot study of yoga treatment in children with functional abdominal pain and irritable bowel syndrome. Complement Ther Med. 2011;19(3):109–14.
20. Oswal P, et al. The effect of add-on yoga prana energization technique (YPET) on healing of fresh fractures: a randomized control study. J Altern Complement Med. 2011;17(3):253–8.
21. Ohman A, Aström L, Malmgren-Olsson EB. Feldenkrais® therapy as group treatment for chronic pain – a qualitative evaluation. J Bodyw Mov Ther. 2011;15(2):153–61.
22. Malmgren-Olsson EB, Bränholm IB. A comparison between three physiotherapy approaches with regard to health-related factors in patients with non-specific musculoskeletal disorders. Disabil Rehabil. 2002;24(6):308–17.
23. Rydeard R, Leger A, Smith D. Pilates-based therapeutic exercise: effect on subjects with nonspecific chronic low back pain and functional disability: a randomized controlled trial. J Orthop Sports Phys Ther. 2006;36(7):472–84.
24. Altan L, et al. Effect of pilates training on people with fibromyalgia syndrome: a pilot study. Arch Phys Med Rehabil. 2009;90(12):1983–8.
25. Lim EC, et al. Effects of Pilates-based exercises on pain and disability in individuals with persistent nonspecific low back pain: a

systematic review with meta-analysis. J Orthop Sports Phys Ther. 2011;41(2):70–80.

26. La Touche R, Escalante K, Linares MT. Treating non-specific chronic low back pain through the Pilates Method. J Bodyw Mov Ther. 2008;12(4):364–70.

27. Posadski P, Lizis P, Hagner-Derengowska M. Pilates for low back pain: a systematic review. Complement Ther Clin Pract. 2011; 17(2):85–9.

28. Pereira LM, et al. Comparing the Pilates method with no exercise or lumbar stabilization for pain and functionality in patients with chronic low back pain: systematic review and meta-analysis. Clin Rehabil. 2012;26(1):10–20. Epub 2011 Aug 19.

29. Beattie A. Participating in and delivering the ATEAM (Alexander technique lessons, exercise, and massage) interventions for chronic back pain: a qualitative study of professional perspectives. Complement Ther Med. 2010;18(3–4):119–27.

30. Yardley L, et al. Patients' views of receiving lessons in the Alexander technique and an exercise prescription for managing back pain in the ATEAM trial. Fam Pract. 2010;27(2):198–204.

31. Ehrlich GE. Alexander technique lessons were effective for chronic or recurrent back pain at 1 year. Evid Based Med. 2009;14(1):13.

32. Little P, et al. Randomised controlled trial of Alexander technique lessons, exercise, and massage (ATEAM) for chronic and recurrent back pain. Br J Sports Med. 2008;42(12):965–8.

33. Ernst E, Canter PH. The Alexander technique: a systematic review of controlled clinical trials. Forsch Komplementarmed Klass Naturheilkd. 2003;10(6):325–9.

34. Suomi R, Collier D. Effects of arthritis exercise programs on functional fitness and perceived ADL measures in older adults with arthritis. Arch Phys Med Rehabil. 2003;84(11):1589–94.

35. Hinman R, Haywood S, Day A. Aquatic PT for hip and knee OA: results of a single blind randomized control trial. J Am Phys Ther Assoc. 2007;87:32–42.

36. Chek P. Functional exercises from the inside out in "Live with Paul Chek" series. New York: C.H.E.K. Institute; 2003.

37. Santana JC. Functional training: an old concept with a new name. Boca Raton: The Institute of Human Performance (IHP); 2009.

Treatment of Chronic Painful Musculoskeletal Injuries and Diseases with Regenerative Injection Therapy (RIT): Regenerative Injection Therapy Principles and Practice

12

Felix S. Linetsky, Hakan Alfredson, David Crane, and Christopher J. Centeno

Key Points

- Focuses on treatment of pain related to pathology of the connective tissue
- Provides detail explanation of mechanism of action
- Emphasizes neurolytic properties of chemical injectates
- Describes biologic injectates in details
- Compares and explains the significant resemblance of pain maps derived from the interspinous ligaments with those from the spinal and pelvic synovial joints
- Provides a step by step approach to differential diagnosis and treatment
- Describes future directions for regenerative injection therapy

F.S. Linetsky, M.D. (✉)
Department of Osteopathic Principles and Practice,
Nova Southeastern University of Osteopathic Medicine,
Clearwater, FL, USA
e-mail: linetskyom@gmail.com

H. Alfredson, M.D., Ph.D.
Sports Medicine Unit, University of Umea,
Gosta Skoglunds Vag 3, Umea 90738, Sweden
e-mail: hakan.alfredson@idrott.umu.se

D. Crane, M.D.
Regenerative Medicine, Crane Clinic Sports Medicine,
219 Chesterfield Towne Center, Chesterfield, MO 63005, USA
e-mail: dcranemd@earthlink.net

C.J. Centeno, M.D.
Physical Medicine and Rehabilitation and Pain Medicine,
Regenerative Medicine, Centeno-Schultz Clinic,
403 Summit Blvd, Broomfield, CO 80021, USA
e-mail: centenooffice@centenoclinic.com

Introduction

Regenerative injection therapy (RIT), also known as prolotherapy or sclerotherapy, is a treatment for chronic musculoskeletal pain caused by connective tissue diathesis utilizing chemical or biologic substances [1]. Steroidal and nonsteroidal anti-inflammatory medications are useful in degenerative disease processes with concomitant inflammatory changes or fibrosis which tethers adjacent structures such as nerves or tendons. In such instances, hydrodissection with injectates containing corticosteroid may also prove useful. RIT is a viable, type-specific treatment for chronic conditions that involve collagen destruction or degeneration. Multiple controlled and uncontrolled studies indicated effectiveness of RIT in treating painful degenerative musculoskeletal conditions. Advances in imaging technology such as MRI and diagnostic ultrasound made it possible to visualize soft tissue pathology in the muscles, ligaments, and tendons. Tendinosis is frequently present in the appendicular and axial tendons. The diagnosis of tendinosis requires therapeutic interventions different from corticosteroids. There is literally an army of capable doctors who need biologically active substances to repair or regenerate degenerative pathologic changes. Old and newer injectates used for RIT such as polidocanol, platelet-rich plasma, and stem cells meet these requirements and are rendering impressive results.

The published pain patterns from ligaments, muscles, intervertebral discs, and synovial joints in the cervical thoracic and lumbar regions overlap significantly (Figs. 12.1, 12.2, 12.3, 12.4, 12.5, and 12.6) [2–4, 10–16]. Nonetheless, ligaments and tendons of these regions are rarely included in differential diagnosis. This chapter is addressing the diagnostic and therapeutic approaches to chronic musculoskeletal pain related to the pathology of fibrous collagenous connective tissue that could benefit from RIT.

T.R. Deer et al. (eds.), *Treatment of Chronic Pain by Integrative Approaches: the AMERICAN ACADEMY of PAIN MEDICINE Textbook on Patient Management*, DOI 10.1007/978-1-4939-1821-8_12,
© American Academy of Pain Medicine 2015

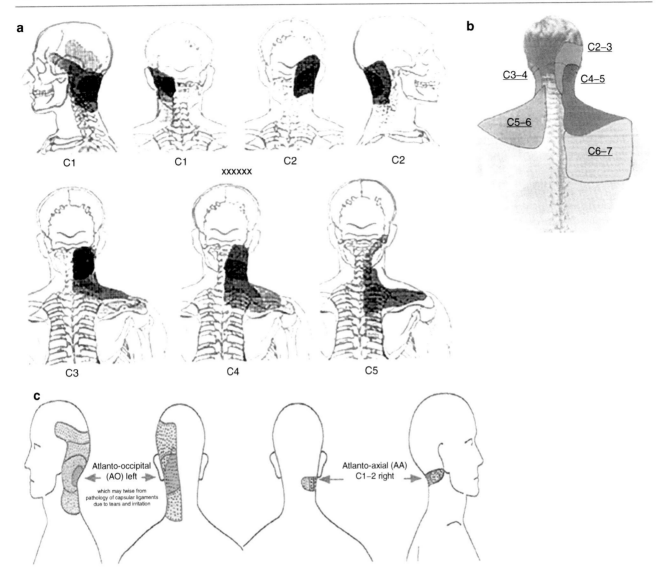

Fig. 12.1 Modified comparative composition of pain distribution in the cervical region provoked by injections of hypertonic saline in to the interspinous ligaments (**a**) Feinstein et al. [2]. Synovial joints: (**b**) (**c**) Significant overlap of these pain maps is due to the fact that injected structures are innervated by the cervical dorsal rami specifically the medial branches (MBDR). Similar relations exist in the thoracic, lumbar, and sacral regions (With permission from Dwyer et al. [3]; and Dreyfuss et al. [4])

Evolution of Terminology

Prior to 1930s, this treatment was called "injection treatment" with addition of a pathologic descriptor such as of injection treatment of varicose veins or injection treatment of hydroceles [17]. Biegeleisen coined the term "sclerotherapy" in 1936 [18].

Concluding that sclerotherapy implied scar formation, Hackett coined the term prolotherapy as "the rehabilitation of an incompetent structure by the generation of new cellular tissue." Hackett's supposition that "… prolotherapy is a treatment to permanently strengthen the 'weld' of disabled ligaments and tendons to bone" led to treatment with injections at the fibro-osseous junctions [11]. More recent work found significant amount of degenerative changes in the midsubstance of the ligaments and tendons as well as ruptures at the fibro-muscular interfaces, and intersubstance changes.

Further, current understanding of the basic science is such that regeneration and repair extend beyond the proliferative stage which is only a short phase of the healing process. More so, proliferation is an integral part of a malignant unsuppressed growth as well as degenerative changes which are present in the bones, synovium, intervertebral discs, ligaments, tendons, and fascial connective tissues. Regenerative injection therapy was coined by Dr. Linetsky because it is a more appropriate nomenclature for the treatment modality which promotes natural healing [1, 19–22].

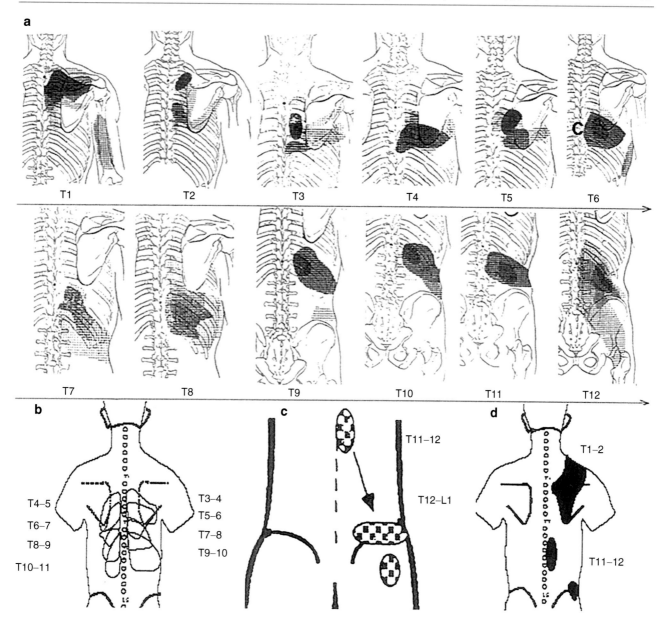

Fig. 12.2 A modified, comparative composition of pain distribution in the thoracic region provoked by injections of hypertonic saline into the interspinous ligaments by Feinstein et al. [2] (Upper two rows – **a**) and thoracic Z-joints (**b**) by Dreyfuss et al. [4], (**c**) by Dussault and Kaplan [5], and (**d**) by Fukui et al. [6]. Significant resemblance of the pain patterns and their overlaps is due to the fact that injected structures receive the same segmental innervated by the thoracic dorsal rami specifically the medial branches (MBDR)

Local Anesthetics in the Diagnosis of Musculoskeletal Pain

Differential diagnosis of musculoskeletal pain based on infiltration of procaine at the fibro-osseous junctions was pioneered in the 1930s by Leriche [16, 19, 22]. Steindler and Luck described that posterior primary rami provide sensory supply to muscles, tendons, thoracolumbar fascia, ligaments, and aponeuroses and their origins and insertions; therefore, no definite diagnosis could be made based on clinical presentation alone. They established the following criteria to prove a causal relationship between the structure and pain symptoms: reproduc-

tion of local and referral pain by needle contact, suppression of local tenderness, and referral/radiating pain by procaine infiltration [23]. Haldeman and Soto-Hall [24] infiltrated procaine in to posterior sacroiliac and interspinous ligaments, zygapophyseal joint capsules producing a field block with a marked relaxation of spastic musculature facilitating a routine use of sacroiliac and facet joint manipulations. They have introduced manipulation of axial joints under local anesthesia [24].

The same basic principles have been employed over all of the anatomic areas since the inception of RIT. Local anesthetic diagnostic blocks are still the best available objective confirmation of the precise source of pain in clinical diagnosis [3, 4, 11–17, 22–25].

Fig. 12.3 Modified comparative composition of pain distribution in the lumbar region provoked by injections of hypertonic saline into the (**a**) lumbar interspinous ligaments dots in the midline from Kellgren et al. [7], from lumbar Z-joints, Mooney and Robertson [8] (**b**), and from asymptomatic subjects (**c**) of symptomatic patients (*paravertebral dots*); significant resemblance of the pain patterns and their overlaps is due to the fact that injected structures receive the same segmental innervated by the lumbar dorsal rami specifically the medial branches (MBDR)

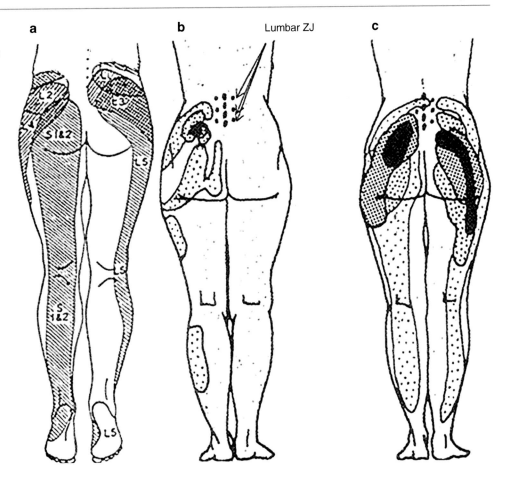

Anatomic Biomechanical and Pathologic Considerations

Ligaments are dull white, dense connective tissue structures that connect adjacent bones. They may be intra-articular, extra-articular, or capsular. Collagen fibers in ligaments may be parallel, oblique, or spiral, each of these orientations contains specific cross-linking formations. Such orientations represent adaptation to specific directions in restriction of joint displacements. Under a light microscope, ligaments have a crimped, wavelike appearance which unfolds during initial loading of collagen [22, 26–28]. When elongated up to 4 % of original length, ligaments and tendons return to their original crimped wave appearance. Beyond 4 % of elongation, they lose elasticity and become permanently laxed, causing joint hypermobility. In degenerated ligaments, subfailure was reported at earlier stages of elongation. At its best, natural healing may restore connective tissue to their pre-injury length, but only 50–75 % of its pre-injury tensile strength [22, 27–30].

There are three types of nerve terminals in posterior spinal ligaments: free nerve endings and the Pacini and the Ruffini corpuscles. A sharp increase in the quantity of free nerve endings at the tips of lumbar spinous processes was documented (Fig. 12.7) [29].

Collagenous tissues are deleteriously affected by nonsteroidal anti-inflammatory drugs (NSAIDs), steroid administrations, inactivity, and denervation. A single corticosteroid injection into a ligament or tendon has been reported to have debilitating effects on the strength of collagen contained therein [27].

In the presence of repetitive microtrauma with insufficient time for recovery, use of NSAIDs and steroids, tissue hypoxia, metabolic abnormalities, and other less defined causes, connective tissues lose their homeostasis and cycle toward an accelerated degenerative pathway [17, 22, 27, 30, 32–34]. Therefore, a cautious use of anti-inflammatory therapy continues to be a useful, but an adjunctive, therapy [32]. It should be noted that unless homeostasis is reestablished in a joint which the ligament protects, further progressive degenerative changes occur with time when continued laxity is present. A well-known example of this is the development of osteoarthrosis in the knee joint following ACL injury with associated laxity of the joint capsule.

As opposed to ligaments, tendons are glistening whitish collagenous bands interposed between muscle and bone that transmit tensile forces during muscle contraction.

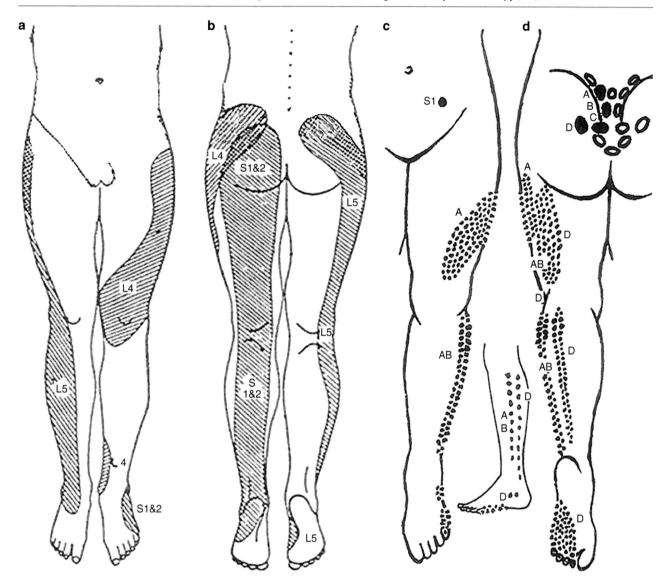

Fig. 12.4 Modified comparative composition of pain distribution from lumbosacral region provoked by injections of hypertonic saline into the (**a**, **b**) interspinous ligaments from L4–5 to S1–2 from Kellgren et al. [7]. (**c**, **d**) Referred pain maps from posterior sacroiliac ligament enthesopathies and sacroiliac joint instability (*AB* from the upper fibers, *CD* lower fibers ileum and sacrum) (Reproduced from Hackett [9]). Hackett published these maps after abolishing pain with local anesthetic infiltration in more than 7,000 injections over 17 years. Significant resemblance of the pain patterns and their overlaps is due to the fact that injected structures receive the same segmental innervated by the lumbar dorsal rami (Prepared for publication by Felix Linetsky M.D.)

There are considerable variations in shape and structure of fibro-osseous attachments and myotendinous junctions. A normal tendon with a cross section of 10 mm in diameter can support a load of 600–1,000 kg [22, 26, 33].

Collagenous tissue response to trauma is inflammatory/regenerative/reparative in nature and varies with the degree of injury. In the presence of cellular damage, regenerative pathway takes place; in the case of extracellular matrix damage, a combined regenerative/reparative pathway takes place. Both are controlled by hormones, chemical, and growth factors [17, 22, 27, 30, 32–34]. Central denervation, such as in quadriplegia, paraplegia, or hemiplegia, leads to a statistically high, accelerated tendon degeneration [33]. Radiofrequency procedures may not be an exception. Corticosteroids do not arrest or slow the course of degenerative process. Neoneurogenesis and neovasculogenesis are also integral components of degeneration.

The presence of vascular and neural ingrowth into degenerated intervertebral discs, posterior spinal ligaments, the hard niduses of fibromyalgia, and tennis elbow tendinopathies have been known for some time. Presence of neuropeptides in the facet joint capsules and articular and periarticular tissue of the sacroiliac joints with the absence of inflammatory markers are also well established, rendering

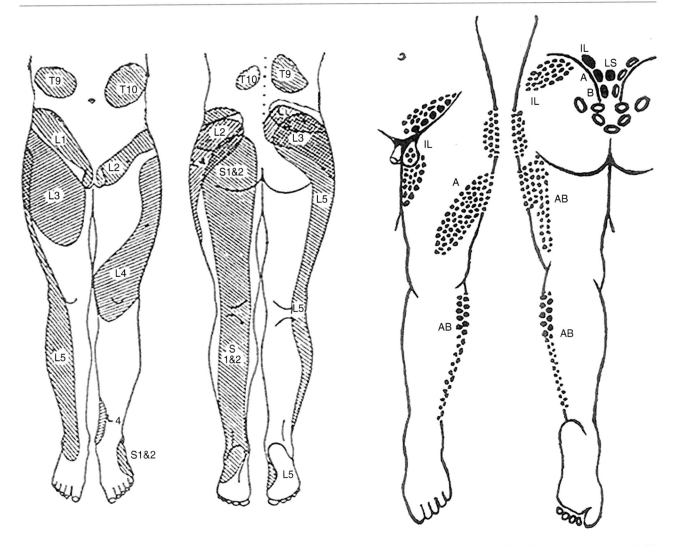

Fig. 12.5 Modified comparative composition of pain distribution from lumbosacral region provoked by injections of hypertonic saline into the (**a, b**) interspinous ligaments from L1–2 to S1–2 from Kellgren et al. [7]. (**c, d**) Trigger areas and referred pain from iliolumbar (*IL*) and posterior sacroiliac (upper *AB*) ligaments (lumbosacral (*LS*) and sacroiliac joint instability). Hackett published these maps after abolishing pain with local anesthetic infiltration in more than 7,000 injections over 17 years. Significant resemblance of the pain patterns and their overlaps is due to the fact that injected structures are innervated by the same segmental lumbar dorsal rami (From Hackett [9]. Prepared for publication by Felix Linetsky M.D.)

the aforementioned structures nociceptive; nonetheless, corticosteroid injections are still the advocated therapeutic interventions [35–39].

More recently, research dedicated to sports medicine shed light on degenerative changes in tendinosis and tendinopathy as a distinct pathologic and clinical entity [40]. The neurovascular ingrowth was studied extensively in Achilles, patellar, and supraspinatus tendinosis. Intratendinous microdialysis of these tendons found normal prostaglandin E_2 (PGE$_2$) levels in chronic painful tendinosis. Analyses of biopsies showed no upregulation of pro-inflammatory cytokines. The neurotransmitter glutamate, a potent modulator of pain in the central nervous system, was found in tendinosis. Microdialysis demonstrated significantly higher glutamate

levels in chronic painful tendinosis in comparison with pain-free control tendons [41–44]. Significantly, higher lactate levels were found in chronic painful tendinosis in comparison with pain-free normal tendons, implicating either hypoxia or a higher metabolic rate in pathophysiology of tendinosis [45].

Biopsies from the areas with tendinosis and neovascularization followed by immunohistochemical analyses of specimens showed substance P (SP) in the nerves juxtapositioned to the vessels and in the nervi vasorum together with calcitonin gene-related peptide (CGRP) juxtapositioned to the vascular walls [46, 47]. The neurokinin-1 receptor (NK-1R), that is known to have a high affinity for SPP, has been found in the vascular wall [48]. The findings of neuropeptides indicate

Fig. 12.6 Trigger areas and needle positions for diagnosis and treatment of cervical enthesopathies with small fiber neuropathies and neuralgias with their respective referral pain maps from ligaments and tendons. (*A–C*) Between superior and inferior nuchal lines. *ART* ZJ articular ligaments and periarticular tendons, *IS* Interspinous ligaments (From Hackett [9])

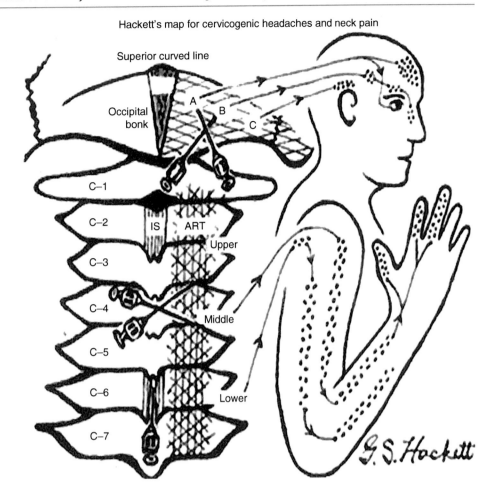

the presence of a so-called neurogenic inflammation mediated by (SP) – like neuropeptides. The use of diagnostic ultrasound is very helpful in evaluation of tendinosis and other musculoskeletal pathology and will be described under radiologic evaluation.

Rationale

The rationale for RIT in chronic painful pathology of ligaments and tendons evolved from clinical, experimental, and histological research performed for injection treatment of hydroceles and hernia. In hydroceles, hypertrophied subserous connective tissue layer reinforced capillary walls and prevented further exudate formation. The same principle is employed in the treatment of chronic bursitis. Conversely in hernias, proliferation and subsequent regenerative/reparative response lead to a fibrotic closure of the defect [17–22].

A similar ability to induce a proliferative regenerative repetitive response in ligaments and tendons was demonstrated in experimental and clinical studies, with a 65 % increased diameter of collagen fibers [18, 49–51]. Multiple recent studies demonstrated that injecting polidocanol in to

the neovascularity proximal to Achilles, patellar, and supraspinatus tendinosis under color Doppler (CD) ultrasound guidance produced an ultrasound-documented resolution of tendinosis and neovascularity, allowing patients return to a full painless activities. Thus, the sclerosing agent acting directly on neovessels is capable of restoring connective tissue homeostasis by modulation of local hemodynamic [52–55].

Clinical Anatomy in Relation to RIT

The shape of a human body is irregularly tubular. This shape, cross-sectionally and longitudinally, is maintained by continuous compartmentalized fascial stacking that incorporates, interconnects, and supports various ligaments, tendons, muscles, neurovascular, and osseous structures. Collagenous connective tissues, despite slightly different biochemical content, blend at their boundaries and at the osseous structures, functioning as a single unit. This arrangement provides bracing and a hydraulic amplification effect to the muscles, increasing contraction strength up to 30 % (Fig. 12.7) [22, 26, 56–62].

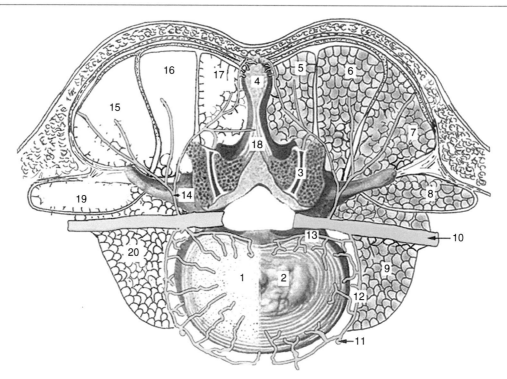

Fig. 12.7 Cross-sectional semi-schematic drawing of lumbar area illustrates *1* vertebral body, *2* intervertebral disc, *3* zygapophyseal joint (*ZJ*), *4* spinous process, *5* multifidus, *6* longissimus thoracis, *7* iliocostalis lumborum, *8* quadratus lumborum, *9* psoas major, *10* ventral ramus, *11* sympathetic trunk, *12* gray ramus communicant, *13* sinuvertebral nerve, *14* dorsal ramus, *15* lateral branch of the dorsal ramus (*LBDR*) in longissimus thoracis compartment, *16* intermediate branch of the dorsal ramus (*IBDR*) in iliocostalis lumborum compartment, *17* medial brunch of the dorsal ramus (*MBDR*) in multifidus compartment, *18* interspinous ligament, *19* quadratus lumborum compartment, and *20* psoas major compartment. MBDR innervates ZJ, multifidi, and interspinous ligaments and forms a several fold increase of the free unmyelinated nerve fibers at the tips of the spinous processes (Modified from Sinelnikov [31]. Modified and prepared for publication by Tracey James. All rights reserved. No part of this picture may be reproduced or transmitted in any form or by any means without written permission from Felix Linetsky M.D.)

Movements of the extremities, spine, and cranium are achieved through various well-innervated articulations, which are syndesmotic, synovial, and symphysial. For the ease of radiologic evaluation, spinal joints were allocated to the anterior, middle, and posterior columns. Syndesmotic joints are anterior and posterior longitudinal ligaments, anterior and posterior atlantooccipital membranes (ALL and PLL), supraspinous and interspinous ligaments (SSL and ISL), and ligamentum flavum (LF).

Symphysial joints are the intervertebral discs (IVD), which are absent at the cranio-cervical and sacral segments, but present from the sacrococcygeal segments caudally.

Spinal synovial joints are the atlantoaxial (AA), atlanto-occipital (AO), zygapophyseal (ZJ), costotransverse (CTJ), and costovertebral (CVJ); sacroiliac (SI) joint is a combined synovial–syndesmotic joint [22, 26, 56, 57].

Differential diagnosis is based on understanding of the regional and segmental anatomy, pathology, as well as segmental, multisegmental, and intersegmental innervation of the compartments and their contents around the spine; this is provided by ventral rami (VR), dorsal rami (DR), gray rami communicants (GRC), sinuvertebral nerves (SVN), and the sympathetic chain (SC) (Fig. 12.7) [22, 26, 56, 57].

Lumbar interspinous ligaments receive innervation from the medial branches of the dorsal rami (MBDR). Three types of nerve terminals in posterior spinal ligaments have been confirmed microscopically. They are the free nerve endings and the Pacini and Ruffini corpuscles. These nerve endings arise from lumbar MB [29]. A sharp increase in the quantity of free nerve endings at the lumbar spinous processes attachments (enthesis) was documented, rendering them putatively nociceptive (Fig. 12.7) [29]. Experimental and empiric observations suggest that a similar arrangement exists at the cervical and thoracic spinous processes, especially at the C2, C7, and T1, rendering them putatively nociceptive (Fig. 12.8) [2, 10, 28, 56]. Willard demonstrated that cervical, thoracic, and lumbar MBs on their distal course are located very close to the bone descending to the very apex of the spinous process, innervating the multifidus and cervical interspinales muscles [28, 56]. A formal recent anatomic study by Zhang et al. reconfirmed these observations in the cervical region [62]. Proximal to the origin, cervical MB is located in the gutter formed by the neighboring ZJ capsules under the semispinalis capitis (SSCa) tendon and supplies twigs to ZJ capsules. Thereafter, MB continues dorsomedially supplying on its course the semispinalis cervices (SSCe) and SSCa.

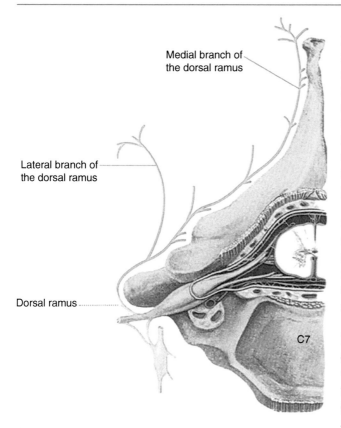

Medial branch of
the dorsal ramus

Lateral branch of
the dorsal ramus

Dorsal ramus

C7

Fig. 12.8 The course of the dorsal ramus proper and its lateral (LBDR) and medial branches (MBDR) represented semi-schematically at the level of C7 (Modified from Sinelnikov [31]. Modified and prepared for publication by Tracey James. All rights reserved. No part of this picture may be reproduced or transmitted in any form or by any means without written permission from Felix Linetsky M.D.)

At the mid-lamina level, MB innervates the multifidi and continues adjacent to every spinous process bilaterally below C2 to become a

Thus, MBs do not exclusively supply innervation to the cervical, thoracic, and lumbar ZJ but also to the structures that have enthesis at the spinous processes. This explains the similarity of clinical presentations and the significant overlap of the known pain patterns (Figs. 12.1, 12.2, 12.3, 12.4, 12.5, 12.6, 12.7, and 12.8) [2–4, 10–13, 28, 56, 62].

Current prevailing trends in diagnostic efforts address discogenic, facetogenic, and neurocompressive components of spinal pain. The therapy is directed toward neuromodulation or neuroablation with radiofrequency generators or corticosteroid injections [25]. Example, cervical ZJ is responsible for 54 % of chronic neck pain after whiplash injury; the prevalence may be as high as 65 % [58]. In patients with headaches after whiplash, more than 50 % of the headaches stem from the C2 to C3 z-joint [25, 58]. Intraarticular corticosteroid injections are ineffective in relieving chronic cervical z-joint pain [59]. These statistical data strongly suggest the presence of nociceptors other than ZJ and IVD [22, 25, 58, 59].

Spondyloarthropathies with enthesopathies and muscular, ligamentous, and tendinous pain are rarely, if ever, included in the differential diagnosis or therapeutic plan. The unspoken reasons for this are economical. Major insurance carriers identify the MBDR block as a ZJ block. Any other injections are considered trigger point or ligament injections, and only two ligament or tendon injections or a maximum of three trigger point injections with corticosteroids are reimbursed during the same office visit at a very low rate. The fact that there may be several nociceptors in the same area in the same patient at the same time is disregarded.

The other reason can be explained by the spinal uncertainty principle. In a simple example of two motion segments, the disc, facets, and musculotendinous compartments are each considered as one putative nociceptive unit, the total number of clinically indistinguishable combinations rises to 63 possibilities. It is practically impossible to address such a magnitude of possibilities under fluoroscopic guidance.

In the majority of cases, RIT can be done without radiologic guidance, taking innervation into account. Therefore, it can afford evaluation of many putative nociceptors from the variety of pain presentations and offers a practical advantage that can be accomplished during the same procedure (Fig. 12.9). The syndromes and conditions treated with RIT are listed in Table 12.1 [11, 17–22, 39, 52–55, 57, 60–84].

Clinical Presentation and Evaluation

The list of syndromes and conditions gives the reader the idea that there is a wide variety of presenting complaints including headaches, neck pain, low back pain, pain between the shoulders, mid-scapular pain, pain mimicking pleurisy or various radiculopathies, thoracolumbar area pain, occipital and suboccipital pain, low back and hip pain, neck and shoulder pain, sharp pain with difficulty breathing, tail bone pain with difficulty seating, and any combination of these symptoms. The intensity, duration, and quality of pain are variable, and the onset may be sudden or gradual. The evaluation may reveal postural abnormalities, functional asymmetries, and combinations of kyphoscoliosis, flattening of cervical and lumbar lordosis, and arm or leg length discrepancies. A wide range of increased or restricted passive and active range of motions as well as frank deformities of axial or peripheral joints may be present.

Contractions against resistance usually denote a tendon-related pain, whereas passive attempts to bring a joint to the anatomic range indicate a ligament-related pain. The most reliable, objective clinical finding is tenderness which may be present at the fibro-osseous junction (enthesis) or at the mid-substance of a muscle, ligament, or tendon. Such areas of tenderness are identified and marked and become the subject of ultrasound investigation and eventually needle probing "needling" and local anesthetic block. The needle placement

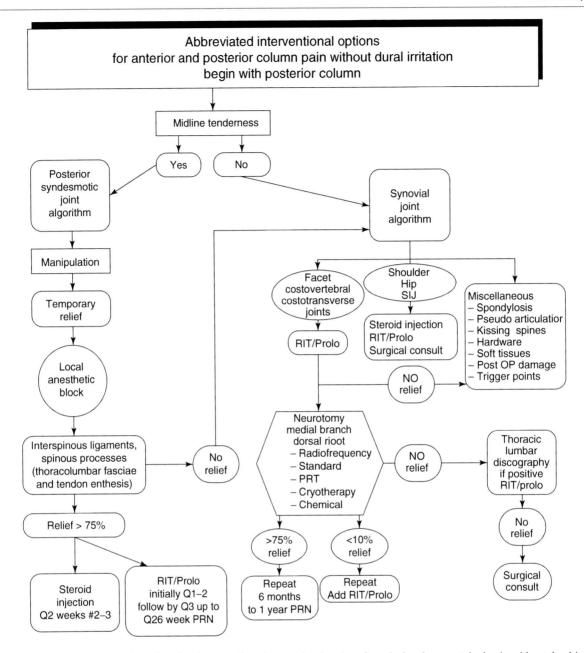

Fig. 12.9 Self-explanatory, modified, abbreviated excerpt from interventional options for spinal and paravertebral pain without dural irritation including large synovial joints (From Linetsky et al. [57])

at the areas of maximum tenderness usually reproduces the pain that becomes temporarily worse during infiltration of local anesthetic and usually subsides within 10–15 s after infiltration. Such diagnostic blocks may be performed with or without fluoroscopic or ultrasound guidance. Abolishment or persistence of tenderness and or local or referred pain concludes the clinical examination and becomes the basis for clinical diagnosis (Figs. 12.9 and 12.10) [11, 22, 57, 63–65].

Radiologic Evaluation Relevant to RIT

Plain Radiographs

Plain radiographs are of limited diagnostic value in painful pathology of the connective tissue, but may indirectly suggest the presence of such pathology by detecting structural or

Table 12.1 The syndromes and conditions treated with RIT

Barre–Lieou syndrome	Acromioclavicular sprain/arthrosis
Cervicocranial syndrome (cervicogenic headaches)	Scapulothoracic crepitus
Temporomandibular pain and dysfunction syndrome	Rotator cuff syndrome: supraspinatus, infraspinatus, subscapularis tendinosis, or impingement
Whiplash injury syndrome, spasmodic torticollis	Proximal and distal biceps tendinosis
Cervical and cervicothoracic spinal pain of "unknown" origin	Tennis and golfer's elbow
Cervicobrachial syndrome (shoulder/neck pain)	Baastrup's disease – kissing spine
Snapping scapulae syndrome or scapulothoracic crepitus	Recurrent shoulder dislocations
Hyperextension/hyperflexion injury whiplash syndromes	Myofascial pain syndrome
Cervical, thoracic, and lumbar facet syndromes	Ehlers–Danlos syndrome
Cervical, thoracic, and lumbar sprain/strain	Marie–Strumpell disease
Cervical, thoracic, and lumbar disc syndrome	Internal disc derangement
Slipping rib syndrome	Failed back surgery syndrome
Costotransverse and costovertebral joint arthrosis pain and subluxations	Low back pain syndrome
Sternoclavicular arthrosis and repetitive sprain and subluxations	Iliac crest syndrome
Acromioclavicular arthrosis and instability	Friction rib syndrome
Repetitive thoracic segmental dysfunction	Sacroiliac joint sprain/strain and instability
Costosternal arthrosis/arthritis	Groin pull/sprain/strain
Tietze's syndrome/costochondritis/chondrosis	Coccydynia syndrome
Interchondral arthrosis	Groin sprains
Xiphoidalgia syndrome	Snapping hip syndrome
	Gluteus minimus and medius tendinosis
	Trochanteric tendinosis
	Patellar tendinosis
	Osgood Schlatter disease
	Achilles tendinosis

positional osseous abnormalities, like anterior or posterior listhesis on flexion/extension lateral views and degenerative changes in general with deformities of the osseous and articular components such as osteophyte formations in various parts of the skeleton, ectopic calcifications, and improperly healed fractures [66].

Magnetic Resonance Imaging (MRI)

MRI may detect the pathology of intervertebral disc, ligamentous injury, interspinous bursitis, enthesopathy, ZJ disease, SIJ pathology, neural foramina pathology, bone contusion, infection, fracture, or neoplasia. Magnetic resonance imaging may exclude or confirm spinal cord disease and pathology related to extramedullary, intradural, and epidural spaces. MRI detects cartilage abnormality, degenerative tendon and ligament pathology, tendinosis, joint effusions, bursitis, soft tissue edema, hematoma, ligament tendon and muscle rupture, and vascular abnormalities [66, 67].

Computed Tomography Scans (CT)

CT scan may detect small avulsion fractures of facets, laminar fracture, fracture of vertebral bodies and pedicles,

and neoplastic or degenerative changes in the axial or appendicular skeleton [66].

Bone Scan

Bone scans are useful in assessing entire skeleton to evaluate for metabolically active disease processes [66].

Diagnostic Ultrasound

Gray scale (GS) ultrasound can detect in real time joint effusions, bursitis, cystic formations, synovial hypertrophy, cartilage abnormality, muscle atrophy, attenuation or partial disruptions of ligaments, tendons or muscles, ectopic calcifications, tendon enlargement, inhomogeneity in tendinosis, and nerve hypertrophy like in carpal tunnel syndrome. Nerve and tendon subluxations or impingements are evaluated with dynamic ultrasound. GS ultrasound provides real-time needle guidance during various diagnostic or therapeutic injections including aspirations, nerve blocks, and percutaneous needle tenotomy. Ultrasound is becoming a more useful tool in the assessment of myofascial and osseous pain sources because it allows a dynamic pattern recognition as well as direct evaluation and patterning in superficial collagenous

Fig. 12.10 Schematic drawing demonstrating sites of tendon origins and insertions (enthesis) of the paravertebral musculature in the cervical, thoracic, lumbar, and pelvic regions with parts of the upper and lower extremities. Clinically significant enthesopathies with small fiber neuropathies and neuralgias are common at the locations identified by *dots*. *Dots* also represent most common locations of needle insertion and RIT injections (Note: Not all of the locations are treated in each patient) (Modified from Sinelnikov [31]. Modified and prepared for publication by Tracey James. All rights reserved. No part of this picture may be reproduced or transmitted in any form or by any means without written permission from Felix Linetsky M.D.)

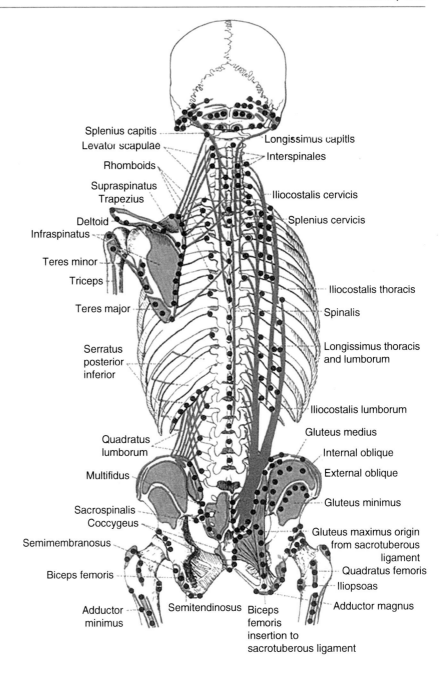

Splenius capitis
Levator scapulae
Rhomboids
Supraspinatus
Trapezius
Deltoid
Infraspinatus
Teres minor
Triceps
Teres major
Serratus posterior inferior
Quadratus lumborum
Multifidus
Sacrospinalis
Coccygeus
Semimembranosus
Biceps femoris
Adductor minimus
Semitendinosus
Biceps femoris insertion to sacrotuberous ligament

Longissimus capitis
Interspinales
Iliocostalis cervicis
Splenius cervicis
Iliocostalis thoracis
Spinalis
Longissimus thoracis and lumborum
Iliocostalis lumborum
Gluteus medius
Internal oblique
External oblique
Gluteus minimus
Gluteus maximus origin from sacrotuberous ligament
Quadratus femoris
Iliopsoas
Adductor magnus

structures. Ultrasound is now a preferred method to evaluate rotator cuff pathology in the office setting and is gaining popularity in knee joint evaluation prior to arthroscopy.

The color Doppler (CD) ultrasound can detect neovascularities to be injected, when present, in tendinosis or synovitis and delineate positions of large vessels and nerves to be avoided during injections [52–55, 68, 69]. Unless the practitioner is very experienced in MSK, ultrasound correlations with plain radiographs, MRI, CT scans, and palpation are highly advisable. There are a multitude of weekend courses in musculoskeletal ultrasound; the industry is promoting the methodology, but the high quality hands on supervised

training is not yet available at the academic institutions for the practicing physicians. Gaining a supervised high-quality experience takes time.

Solutions for Injections

Local anesthetics are an important component of the solutions used for RIT and were described under the heading of *Local Anesthetics in the Diagnosis of Musculoskeletal Pain*. When contemporary local anesthetics are combined with hyperosmolar injectates, they provide long-lasting diagnostic/therapeutic blocks, and the reasons for this scientifically proven effect will be described below.

Five types of injectates are used for RIT, and they are:
1. Osmotic shock agents such as hypertonic dextrose, glycerin, or distilled water
2. Chemical irritants such as phenol
3. Chemotactic sclerosing agents such as sodium morrhuate, Sotradecol, or polidocanol
4. Particulates such as pumice suspension
5. Biologic agents such as whole blood, platelet-rich plasma (PRP), autologous conditioned serum (ACS), platelet-poor plasma (PPP), adipose-derived and bone marrow aspirate concentrates with their mesenchymal and hematopoietic biocellular components, and isolated and cultured mesenchymal stem cells

The injectates in groups 1–4 have been used as a single agent in various concentrations or in various combinations with other chemical agents, and their concentrations are mixed with local anesthetics, by the virtue of being injected into connective tissue, all of them become irritants [57, 60, 61, 63–65, 71–74]. Injectates in group 5 are also used as a single injectate agent in various concentrations or in various combinations of the agents and their concentrations.

Experimental studies demonstrated that any solution with osmolality greater than a 1,000 mOsm/l is *neurolytic*, causing separation of the myelin lamellae in myelinated nerve fibers and total destruction in unmyelinated fibers, after soaking for 1 h in solutions with osmolality greater than 1,000 mOsm/l or a distilled water. Hypoosmolar solutions produce a reversible conduction block of rabbit vagus nerve and potentiate the local anesthetics. C fibers showed evidence of axonal damage characterized by accumulation of macrophages and proliferation of Schwann cells. Osmotic fragility of axons is similar to that of erythrocytes after exposure to 0.4 and 0.5 dilutions of normal saline. When administered intrathecally, local anesthetics are more effective in hypobaric solution than in hyperbaric solution [85–88]. In humans, intrathecal hypertonic saline produced good results in chronic intractable pain and is currently used in epidurolysis of adhesions [17, 89–91]. Hypertonic/hyperosmolar dextrose has been successfully used for treatment of enthesopathies with small fiber neuropathies, spondyloarthropathies, and internal disc derangements [1, 11, 17, 19–22, 57, 73, 74].

Pharmacologic *properties of phenol, glycerin, and hypertonic dextrose are both neurolytic and inflammatory*. Various concentrations of water- and glycerin-based phenol solutions have been used to treat pain. The literature suggests that perineural phenol glycerin combinations produce a better regenerative/reparative response; these experimental findings support the use of phenol glycerin or phenol glycerin dextrose solutions in treatment of axial and peripheral enthesopathies with small fiber neuropathies and neuralgias [92–102].

Neurolytic intra-articular injections of a 10 % aqueous phenol, diluted to 5 % with omnipaque or omniscan contrast and local anesthetic, are used in the Pain Management Department of Mayo Clinic to facilitate nursing care in severely debilitated patients [103].

Diluted 5 % phenol in 50 % glycerin solution is used for the treatment of spinal enthesopathies and injections at donor harvest sites of the iliac crest for neurolytic and regenerative/reparative responses. Prior to injection, 1 ml of this solution is mixed with 4 ml of local anesthetic 1,086 mOsm/l [63, 64]. The most common solutions contain lidocaine/dextrose mixtures in various concentrations. Lidocaine is available in 0.5–2 %; dextrose is available in a 50 % concentration.

To achieve a 10 % dextrose concentration, dilution is made with lidocaine in 4:1 proportions (i.e., 4 ml of 1 % lidocaine is mixed with 1 ml of 50 % dextrose) and will produce a 0.8 % lidocaine with osmolality of 555 mOsm/l (*hyperosmolar block*).

To achieve a 12.5 % dextrose concentration, dilution is made with lidocaine in 3:1 proportions (i.e., 3 ml of 1 % lidocaine mixed with 1 ml of 50 % dextrose) and will produce a 0.75 % lidocaine with osmolality of 694 mOsm/l (*hyperosmolar block*).

To achieve a 20 % dextrose concentration, dilution is made with lidocaine in 3:2 proportion (i.e., 3 ml of 1 % lidocaine mixed with 2 ml of 50 % dextrose) and will produce a 0.6 % lidocaine with osmolality of 1,110 mOsm/l (*hyperosmolar neurolytic block*). In two studies, this solution produced a 50 % reduction in low back pain lasting for 2 years.

A 1:1 dilution makes a 25 % dextrose concentration with 0.5 lidocaine solution with osmolality of 1,388 mOsm/l (*hyperosmolar neurolytic block*). In two studies, this solution was used for intradiscal injections.

Dextrose/phenol/glycerin (DPG) solution is referred to as DPG or P2G and contains dextrose and glycerin in equal 25 % amounts, 2.5 % phenol and water. Prior to injection, DPG is diluted in concentrations of 1:2 = 1,368 mOsm/l, 1:1 = 2,052 mOsm/l, or 2:3 = 1,641 mOsm/l with a local anesthetic.

When dextrose-containing solutions are not controlling pain and dysfunction, progression to stronger solutions such as sodium morrhuate, Sotradecol, or polidocanol has been used in various dilutions up to a full strength.

Five percent sodium morrhuate is a mixture of sodium salts of saturated and unsaturated fatty acids of cod liver oil and 2 % benzyl alcohol (chemically very similar to phenol), which acts as both a local anesthetic and a preservative. This is very well tolerated in selective patients with rheumatoid arthritis or ankylosing spondyloarthropathies, personal observation of the senior author.

Sotradecol® (sodium tetradecyl sulfate injection) is a sterile nonpyrogenic solution for intravenous use as a sclerosing agent. Three percent (30 mg/ml) with 2 % benzyl alcohol: Each mL contains sodium tetradecyl sulfate 30 mg and benzyl alcohol 20 mg. It can be used interchangeably with sodium morrhuate; clinical results are similar, but there is a lesser possibility of allergic reactions.

Polidocanol is a nonionic detergent, containing a polar hydrophilic (dodecyl alcohol) and an apolar hydrophobic (polyethylene oxide) chain as active ingredients. On March 31, 2010, the US Food and Drug Administration (FDA) approved polidocanol injection for the treatment of small varicose veins. Polidocanol is a local anesthetic and antipruritic component of ointments and bath additives. The substance is also used as a sclerosant, an irritant injected to treat varicose veins. Professor Alfredson has extensively used 1 % polidocanol in 1–2 ml increments for the treatment of tendinosis [52–55].

Pumice suspension: Pumice is a substance of volcanic origin consisting chiefly of complex silicates of aluminum, potassium, and sodium. Pumice is insoluble in water and is not attacked by acids or alkali solutions. It is used in this preparation as a material irritant to stimulate the fibrosing process. Extra fine grade is defined as one that passes a 325 mesh sieve at 84 % or more, and only a trace is retained by a 200 mesh sieve:

- Pumice (extra fine grade) – 1.0 g.
- Glycerin – 5.0 ml.
- Polysorbate 80–0.09 ml (2 standard drops).
- Preservatives q.s.
- Lidocaine 1–2 % q.s. ad 100 cc.
- Place in a multidose bottle, sterilize, and shake well before use.

Two to three milliliter of this suspension is drawn in a 10-ml syringe mixed with dextrose formula of a choice or alone. Drawing in to the syringe should be done through the same gage needle that will be used for injection. Suspension was developed by Dr. Gedney for injections of sacroiliac ligaments to stabilize SI and lumbosacral joints [19–22].

Biocellular autografts include whole blood, platelet-rich plasma (PRP), autologous conditioned serum (ACS), platelet-poor plasma (PPP), and adipose- and bone marrow-derived aspirate concentrates with mesenchymal and hematopoietic components [104–109]. Widely popularized and accepted in recent years, these autografts are composed of three ingredients used separately or together:

1. PRP or ACS provides platelet concentrates with cytokines and growth factors.
2. Autologous fat cells provide a living collagen bioscaffold with its intrinsic stromal vascular tissue transferred in the form of a graft or a lyophilized collagen in the form of an injectate which may be utilized as a cellular bioscaffold matrix.
3. Lipoaspirates or adipose tissue plus/minus bone marrow aspirate concentrate provides stromal vascular fraction with supporting mesenchymal stem cells.

PRP is a platelet concentrate of four- to eight-fold above baseline levels that contain signal proteins, platelet-derived growth factors, chemokines, and cytokines that control inflammatory cascade. Autologous conditioned serum (ACS or ACP) contains platelet concentrations of two to three-fold baseline levels, and whole blood contains platelet levels at baseline. It remains a point of debate in the literature which autograft provides a superior collagen growth. It may depend on the structure to be regenerated which level of chemokine and cytokine concentration or MSC concentration or pure scaffold regeneration proves most helpful.

PRP is a reach source of important signal proteins (cytokines) and a variety of growth factors (GF) critical to initiation and maintenance of the entire inflammatory cascade in vivo. Many studies have shown the effectiveness of these GFs in healing.

Bone marrows concentrate with or without supporting matrix releases chemokines and cytokines. Growth factors are known to be a major player in vascular remodeling. The platelets in a bone marrow concentrate upon activation secrete stromal-derived factor (SDF-1). This supports primary adhesion and migration of progenitor cells to the site of injury. Bone marrow stroma contains plastic adherent cells (colony-forming unit fibroblast, CFU-F) that can give rise to a broad spectrum of fully differentiated connective tissues [105–107].

Adipose-derived mesenchymal stem cells (AD-MSCs) also contribute to the growth factor load through direct secretion of growth factors (autocrine amplification system), such as vascular endothelial growth factor (VEGF), insulin-like growth factor 1 (IGF-1), IGF-2, and hepatocyte growth factor. Additional benefits of adipose tissue comparing to bone marrow are greater concentration of mesenchymal stem cells, ready availability, ease and rapidity of harvesting, lower morbidity, and diminished cost. In addition, adipose tissues possess properties which serve as an ideal living bioscaffold or matrix [106, 107].

PRP concentrates are obtained by venous blood draw of 20–120 cc. Centrifugation produces the buffy coat fraction. Various manufacturers utilize proprietary techniques to remove the neutrophils with the intent of maintaining the monocyte fraction along with the platelet fraction of spun cells. The amount of cytotoxicity of neutrophils in vivo is currently a point of contention in the literature. It is therefore up to the practitioner to decide if they wish to manufacture platelet concentrates via a two spin centrifugation technique or utilize a proprietary solution on the market [108, 109].

Bone marrow aspirates are obtained via 12-ga. multiport aspiration needle with a stylet placed within the iliac crest or other appropriate marrow cavity, and 60–120 cc of marrow is aspirated in small aliquots obtained from multiple positions within the marrow cavity. This gives variable numbers of CD34+ cells in a matrix of total nucleated cells. The total number of cells is based on the aspiration and centrifugation technique. Manufacturer and independent tests are available to measure cell counts [105].

Lipoaspirates, or autologous fat grafting (AFG), are used extensively in aesthetic and reconstructive surgery over the past 20 years. A closed syringe system (Tulip Medical) and cell-friendly microcannulas allow a safe and effective harvest of volumes ranging from 10 to 20 cc. Combined with thrombin-activated PRP, this injectate is accurately placed by guided ultrasonography into damaged muscular, tenoligamentous, and cartilaginous tissue [107].

Practical note: The physician should examine the state and federal laws of their respective practice location to determine what level of cellular processing is permissible under current law.

Isolated and Expanded Stem Cells

Mesenchymal stem cells (MSCs), also known as marrow stromal cells, derive from mesodermal tissues and are pluripotent adult stem cells with therapeutic potential in regenerative medicine [110–116]. It has been shown recently that MSCs are a heterogeneous population of similar cells rather than one distinct cell type [117]. As a result, outside of the ability to select cells via adhesion culture and a handful of hallmark surface markers, there is still no uniformly accepted definition of an MSC [118].

As stated above, MSCs can be easily isolated from many different tissues, including a whole bone marrow aspirate, marrow mobilized whole blood, muscle biopsy, adipose liposuction aspirate, and other tissues [110]. As a rule, the closer the graft source to the treated tissue, the more efficient are the MSCs to differentiate into to the treated tissue type. For example, Vidal compared equine MSCs derived from the bone marrow to ones derived from adipose tissue for their chondrogenic potential and found that bone marrow MSCs produced a more hyaline-like matrix and had improved glycosaminoglycan production [119]. Animal studies demonstrated that bone marrow MSC produced better repair of a tibial osteochondral defect when compared to adipose MSCs [120]. Yoshimura determined that MSCs derived from the synovial tissue of the knee (closest to the target tissue of cartilage defect) produced a better chondrogenesis than bone marrow MSCs [121].

MSC Culture Expansion

A limited amount of cells can be obtained from any tissue. In many instances, the number that can be harvested from the source tissue is less than the quantity of cells needed for tissue repair. One method to obtain larger numbers of cells is to culture them. A delicate balance exists between length of time in culture (which produces more cells) and adverse consequences to the cells (such as genetic transformation).

MSCs are usually expanded in a culture via monolayer. MSCs are placed into a specialized flask and allowed to attach to a plastic surface and fed with a nutrient broth. Because MSCs are contact inhibited, they will grow on this surface until they become confluent at which point they abruptly stop growing. To keep MSCs proliferating in culture, when the colonies are near confluence, the nonadherent cells in the media are discarded and an enzyme is used to detach the MSCs from the plastic surface. The MSCs are then replated in a similar flask, and fresh media is added. Most MSCs are grown in culture for 11–17 days, because some studies have shown decreased differentiation if MSCs are grown for prolonged periods in culture with a higher chance of genetic mutation [122–125].

How Do the MSCs Affect Tissue Repair?

Animal studies have demonstrated the multipotency of MSCs and their ability to differentiate into muscle, bone, cartilage, tendon, and various cells of internal organs. However, these cells also act via paracrine mechanisms to assist in tissue repair. In this context, paracrine is defined as the production of certain growth factors and cytokines by the MSCs which can assist in tissue repair [126].

Donor Versus Autologous MSC Sources

Obviously, autologous stem cells do not have the risk of communicable disease transmission as donor allogeneic cells. However, there are reasons why donor cells are attractive. For example, some studies have shown a decreased differentiation potential for MSCs obtained from older patients [127]. In addition, somatic genetic variants (i.e., trisomy V and VII) have been demonstrated in the MSCs and osteoprogenitors of some patients with osteoarthritis [128].

Use of MSC in Musculoskeltal Diathesis

MSCs have been used in animal and early clinical studies to repair meniscal tissue, cartilage, and intervertebral discs. Izuta et al. demonstrated meniscus repair after MSCs transplant on a fibrin matrix [129]. Horie reported that synovial-derived MSCs after injection into massive rat meniscus tears were able to differentiate and repair meniscal tissue [130]. Yamasaki et al. repopulated devitalized meniscus with MSCs and demonstrated biomechanical properties approximating the normal meniscus [131].

The earliest models of cartilage repair used autologous, cultured chondrocytes [132]; others used MSCs because MSCs have shown innate cartilage repair properties through both differentiation and paracrine signaling [133]. In these studies, an osteochondral defect (OCD) was created, and the MSCs were implanted into the lesion, often in a hydrogel or other carrier or at times through local adherence [134–137]. Partial to robust healing of the OCD takes place over weeks to months [110]. The cartilage produced by these cells was very much like native hyaline cartilage, but subtle differences have been observed [138].

Traditional spinal surgery on degenerated intervertebral discs (IVDs) continues to show disappointing results [139–141]. Conversely, animal studies have shown robust repair of acutely injured IVDs [142–148]. For example, Sakai et al. have published animal models whereby MSCs are combined with atelocollagen and achieved disc repair with improvements in hydration, height, and disc morphology demonstrated on MRI [149]. Richardson et al. and Risbud et al. investigating the coculturing of MSCs with cells from the nucleus pulposus (NP) demonstrated that this technique can produce partially differentiated cells that are capable of repopulating the NP in an animal model [150, 151]. Finally, Miyamoto et al. recently demonstrated that intra-discal transplantation of synovial-derived MSCs prevented disc degeneration through suppression of catabolic genes and perhaps proteoglycan production [152].

Biocellular injectates such as whole blood and PRP are extremely irritating immediately upon injection. Regional pain blocks have therefore become an important adjunct in the treatment paradigm with biocellular autografts. If used with inadequate or improperly placed local anesthesia, even under US guidance, these agents produce overwhelming nonlocalized deep somatic pain lasting for up to 10 min which subsides to a tolerable level after about 30 min and which follows a typical primary, secondary, and tertiary curve for collagen maturation with the pain levels inherent therein. Thus, pain subsides over the secondary cellular maturation time frame of 6–8 weeks resulting in a pain-free state. Intra-articular hip injections of PRP with or without bioscaffold, in the presence of significant degenerative changes, when used with local anesthesia under US guidance produce a significant pain that subsides to a preinjection level in about 2 weeks.

Clinical Effectiveness

Multiple publications on RIT include randomized trials [63, 72, 75–77, 153], non-randomized publications, and prospective and retrospective clinical studies as well as case reports [65, 78] and systematic reviews [78]. In one of the systematic reviews of prolotherapy injections for chronic low back pain, Yelland et al. [78] included four randomized high-quality trials with a total of 344 patients. Two of these four studies [72, 76] demonstrated significant differences between the treatment and control group. However, Yelland et al. [78] could not pooled their results because in the study of Ongley

et al. [76], manipulation allegedly confounded independent evaluation of results. And in the other study by Kline et al., there was no significant difference in mean pain and disability scores between the groups [72]. The third study was demonstrated no improvement in either group [77]. The fourth study was the earlier one of Yelland et al. reporting only mean pain and disability scores of 40 patients in each group [75] showed no difference between groups. But in each group, there was more than 50 % improvement maintained for more than 2 years. Therefore, Yelland et al.'s [75] study clearly demonstrated that relatively large volumes of normal saline injected in the low back ligaments are therapeutic and are not a placebo. The conclusions of this systematic review were confusing and unrealistic such as that there was conflicting evidence regarding the efficacy of prolotherapy injections in reducing pain and disability in patients with chronic low back pain or that in the presence of co-interventions, prolotherapy injections were more effective than controlled injections, more so when both injections and co-interventions were controlled concurrently.

Another controlled trial is eliminated from the systematic review because it could not be pooled by Wilkinson [63] who demonstrated that when specific diagnosis is applied, the positive results approach 89 %. There is substantial evidence from non-randomized prospective and retrospective studies as well as case reports that cannot be discussed here due to a limited size of this publication [17–22, 65]. Similar results were demonstrated by Alfredson et al. in peripheral tendinosis [52–55] and Topol et al. in groin strains [79–83].

The growing use of biologic agents deserves a special attention. The clinical translation of MSCs from the lab to the bedside is already taking place; Centeno et al. published early case studies in which positive MRI changes were observed in knees and hip joints after MSC injections [143–145]. They have also noted that the complication rate of expanded MSC injection procedures is no greater than other needle-based interventional techniques [146]. Their submitted publication data on 339 patients demonstrated a safety profile better than surgical techniques such as total knee arthroplasty. They have recently submitted for publication a large case series of 250 knee and hip osteoarthritis patients treated with percutaneous injection of MSCs. Prior to MSC injections, two-thirds of the knee patients were total knee arthroplasty (TKA) candidates, only 6 % of the patients opted for TKA after the injections; additionally, both treated groups reported better relief than an untreated comparative group.

Other authors have described similar safety profiles using more invasive surgical implant techniques. Wakatani published an 11-year prospective study of 45 knees (in 41 patients) treated with autologous bone marrow-derived MSCs, with results indicating both safety and efficacy [147]. Nejadnik recently described a comparison between surgically implanted chondrocytes versus MSCs placed by needle in 72 knees [153]. The MSC-treated knees demonstrated good safety, less donor site morbidity, and better efficacy when compared with an autologous chondrocyte implantation procedure. Haleem has noted that autologous, cultured bone marrow MSCs reimplanted into articular cartilage defects in platelet-rich fibrin demonstrated evidence of healed cartilage in some patients [148].

While very little has been published on intervertebral disc repair in humans, some clinical data is available. Yoshikawa recently published on two patients who were treated with surgically implanted MSCs that showed less vacuum phenomenon on follow-up imaging [142]. The only other human data of which we are aware is produced by Centeno's group from 2005 to 2010, under IRB supervision and now being prepared for publication (unpublished data). Replicating the Sakai study [149] wherein cultured MSCs were placed into the disc produced little measureable results, their experience was similar. However, a third case series performed with changes in culture, injection technique, and diagnostic criteria (changed from degenerative disc disease DDD to chronic disc bulge with lumbar radiculopathy). The last model showed encouraging clinical and imaging results. Presented literature, especially newer publications, does offer convincing evidence of RIT efficacy in carefully selected patients, when specific diagnostic entities are treated and strict diagnostic criteria and injection techniques are applied [52–55, 63, 78–84, 142–148].

Mechanism of Action of Chemical Injectates

Based on literature review [11, 12, 17–22, 49–55, 57, 63–65, 71–104] and the above described pharmacologic properties of the injectates, current understanding of the mechanism of action is complex and multifaceted. Obviously, *phenol- and glycerin*-containing solutions, depending on concentration, produce *temporary neurolysis or neuromodulation* of peripheral nociceptors and provide modulation of antidromic, orthodromic, sympathetic, and axon reflex transmissions. Modulation of sympathetic transmission via nervi vasorum leads to modulation of local hemodynamics in tendons, ligaments, and bone; this in turn decreases blood pressure which leads to pain reduction. Hyper-/hypoosmolar injectates provide the same initial action; purple discoloration of the skin is frequently observed after injection of several adjacent interspinous ligaments.

Conversely, sclerosants act initially on modulation of hemodynamics with subsequent regression of neoneurogenesis. When sclerosant was deposited into pathologic neovascularities ventral to Achilles tendon, restoration of normal longitudinal microcirculation was documented by power Doppler. Chemomodulation of collagen through inflammatory, proliferative, and regenerative/reparative response is induced by the chemical and pharmacologic properties of all injectates and mediated by cytokines and multiple growth factors.

A relatively large volume of osmotically inert or active injectate assumes the role of a space-occupying lesion in a relatively tight, slowly equilibrating, extracellular compartment of the connective tissue. Inert injectates are also used to disrupt adhesions that have been created by the original inflammatory attempts to heal the injury or for hydrodissection of fibrotic bands.

Temporary repetitive stabilization of the painful hypermobile joints, induced by inflammatory response to the injectates, provides a better environment for regeneration and repair of the affected ligaments and tendons.

Compression of cells by relatively large extracellular volume as well as cell expansion or constriction due to osmotic properties of injectate stimulates the release of intracellular growth factors. Cellular and extracellular matrix damage induced by mechanical transection with the needle stimulates inflammatory cascade, governing release of growth factors [11, 12, 17–22, 49–55, 57, 63–65, 71–104].

Indications for regenerative injection therapy are listed in Table 12.2. General contraindications are those that are applicable to all of the injection techniques. A list of general contraindications is presented in Table 12.3.

Table 12.2 Indications for regenerative injection therapy

Cervicogenic headaches	Osteoarthritis, osteoarthrosis/arthritis, spondylolysis, osteochondrosis and spondylolisthesis
Unhealed fractures, pseudoarthrosis	Rheumatoid arthritis with osteoarthritis
Chronic enthesopathies, tendinosis or ligamentosis with small fiber neuropathies and neuralgias after sprains/strains or overuse occupational and postural conditions known as repetitive motion disorders (RMD)	Peripheral nerve and tendon entrapments
Small unhealed painful intersubstance ruptures of muscles ligaments and tendons	Osgood Schlatter disease
Internal disc derangement (cervical, thoracic, lumbar)	Postsurgical cervical, thoracic, and low back pain (with or without instrumentation)
Painful hypermobility and instability of the axial and peripheral joints due to capsular laxity	Other posterior column sources of nociception refractory to steroid injections, nonsteroidal anti-inflammatory therapy (NSAID), and radiofrequency procedures
Vertebral compression fractures exerting stress on adjacent joints and soft tissue	Enhancement of manipulative treatment and physiotherapy

Table 12.3 Contraindications for regenerative injection therapy

General contraindications	Specific contraindications
Allergy to anesthetic solutions	Acute arthritis (septic, gout, rheumatoid, or posttraumatic with hemarthrosis)
Bacterial infection, systemic or localized to the region to be injected	Acute bursitis or tendonitis
Bleeding diathesis secondary to disease or anticoagulants	Acute non-reduced subluxations, dislocations, or fractures
Fear of the procedure or needle phobia	Allergy to injectable solutions or their ingredients such as dextrose (corn), sodium morrhuate (fish), or phenol
Neoplastic lesions involving the musculature and osseous structures	
Recent onset of a progressive neurological deficit including but not limited to severe intractable cephalgia, unilaterally dilated pupil, bladder dysfunction, bowel incontinence, etc.	
Requests for large quantity of sedation and/or narcotics before and after treatment	
Severe exacerbation of pain or lack of improvement after local anesthetic blocks	

Vertebral and Paravertebral Injection Sites and Techniques

Any innervated structure is a potential pain generator. The same nerve usually supplies several structures; therefore, there is a significant overlap of all known pain maps (Figs. 12.1, 12.2, 12.3, 12.4, 12.5, and 12.6). The main question is, "How to navigate in this sea of unknown?" For the purpose of RIT, the following step by step approach is implemented. Patients' "pain and tenderness" is accepted for face value without dismissal or allocation to a distant "proven" source. The *knowledge of clinical anatomy, pain patterns, and pathology guiding the clinical investigation* is based on clinical experiments of many researchers over decades. Diagnostic ultrasound may reveal tendinosis and neovascularities in the tender areas.

Tenderness over posterior column structures is an objective finding, especially in the midline, as is the rebound tenderness in any abdominal quadrant [17, 22, 57, 63–65, 104]. The tender areas are identified by palpation and marked. Confirmation is obtained by needle tapping the bone and local anesthetic block of the tissue at the enthesis keeping the innervation in perspective.

Using palpable landmarks for guidance, experienced practitioners have been safely injecting, with or without fluoroscopic guidance, the following posterior column elements innervated by the dorsal rami: tendons and ligaments enthesis at the spinous process, lamina, posterior ZJ capsule, and thoracolumbar fascia insertions at the transverse process.

Theoretically, 0.5 % lidocaine solution is an effective, initial diagnostic option for pain arising from posterior column elements when utilized in increments of 0.5–1.0 ml injected after each bone contact; in practice, hyperosmolar lidocaine/dextrose in 4:2 or 3:2 dilution is used initially blocking the structures innervated by terminal filaments of the MB with the sequence as follows:

Step A: In the presence of midline pain and tenderness, enthesis of ligaments and tendons at the spinous process

are blocked initially in the midline at the previously marked level(s).

Step B: The blocked area is reexamined about 1 min after each injection for tenderness and movements that provoked pain.

If tenderness remains at the lateral aspects of the spinous processes, injections are carried out to the lateral aspects of their apices, thus continuing on the course of medial branches or dorsal rami. Step B is repeated.

Persistence of paramedial pain is calling for investigative blocks of ZJ capsules (cervical, thoracic, and lumbar) and costotransverse joints. Step B is repeated.

Perseverance of lateral tenderness dictates investigation of the structures innervated by the lateral branches of the dorsal rami, such as the enthesis of iliocostalis or serratus posterior superior/inferior at the ribs, the ventral sheath of thoracolumbar fascia at the lateral aspects of the lumbar transverse processes, or at the iliac crests. Step B is repeated. In this fashion, all potential nociceptors on the course of MB and LB are investigated from their periphery toward their origins. Thus, the differential diagnosis of pain arising from vertebral and paravertebral structures innervated by MB and LB is made based on the results of the blocks (Figs. 12.9, 12.10, and 12.11). Manipulation under local anesthesia can be performed after anesthetic has taken effect, and the musculature is sufficiently relaxed [154]. Pain from the upper cervical synovial joints presents a diagnostic and a therapeutic challenge; therefore, it is a diagnosis of exclusion.

The possibility of serious complications dictates that all intra-articular injections of the axial synovial joints, specifically atlantoaxial and atlantooccipital, ZJ, costovertebral, and intervertebral discs, should be performed only under fluoroscopic guidance by an experienced practitioner [3, 4, 14–16, 25, 58–61, 73, 74]. Conversely, the intra-articular injections of SJ joint are grossly overemphasized [39, 51, 57, 63, 64, 72]. This was recently proven again by Murakami et al. [155].

Fig. 12.11 Drawing demonstrating sites of tendon origins and insertions (enthesis) of the paravertebral musculature in the cervical, thoracic, lumbar, and pelvic regions with parts of the upper and lower extremities. Clinically significant enthesopathies with small fiber neuropathies and neuralgias are common at the locations identified by *dots*. *Dots* also represent most common locations of needle insertion and RIT injections (Note: Not all of the locations are treated in each patient) (Modified from Sinelnikov [31]. Modified and prepared for publication by Tracey James. All rights reserved. No part of this picture may be reproduced or transmitted in any form or by any means without written permission from Felix Linetsky M.D.)

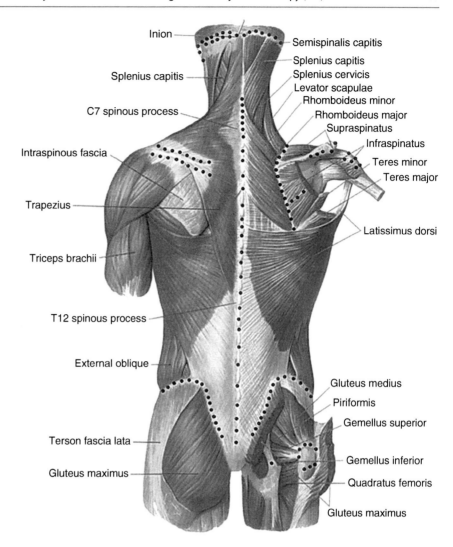

Most commonly injected sites of painful spinal enthesopathies of the posterior column are innervated by the medial (MB) and lateral (LB) branches of the dorsal rami:

- Enthesis of ligaments and tendons at the superior, inferior, and lateral surfaces especially at the apex of the spinous processes
- Enthesis at the occipital bone at and between inferior and superior nuchal lines
- Enthesis at the thoracic and lumbar transverse processes
- Capsular ligaments and periarticular enthesis at the cervical thoracic and lumbar ZJs
- Costotransverse joints and capsules
- Tendons and ligaments at the posteromedial, superior, inferior, and lateral surfaces of the iliac crests and spines
- Posterior tubercles and angles of the ribs
- Multiple other common peripheral enthesopathies are depicted in Figs. 12.10 and 12.11 and described below:
- Proximal and distal portions of the clavicle specifically superior acromioclavicular (AC) ligament and AC joint, sternoclavicular (SC) ligament and joint, etc.

- Greater and lesser humeral tuberosities and medial and lateral epicondyles
- Sternum, xiphoid, and anterior ribs
- Pubic tubercles, superior and inferior rami, and ischial spines, tuberosities, and rami
- Greater and lesser femoral trochanters and medial and lateral femoral epicondyles

Side Effects and Complications of RIT

Several types of statistically rare complications occur with regenerative injection therapy [156]. The most recent statistical data on complications came from a survey of 171 physicians providing RIT in 2006 [157].

Responders to the survey had been providing this treatment for a median of 10 years and described treating a median of 500 patients each, giving a median of 2,000 injections each.

The following complications were reported: 164 spinal headaches, 123 pneumothoraxes, 73 temporary systemic reactions, and 54 temporary nerve damage. Sixty-nine adverse events required hospitalization, among them 46 patients with a pneumothorax and none with the spinal headache. Five cases of permanent nerve damage were reported. Only three surveyors included information on the specific injury: one case of mild to moderate leg pain, one case of persistent numbness in a small area of the gluteal region, and one case of persistent numbness in the quadriceps region [157]. These findings were similar to an earlier survey by Dorman of 450 physicians performing RIT/prolotherapy [158]. At that time, 120 respondents revealed that 495,000 patients received injections. Among them, 29 instances of pneumothorax were reported, two of them requiring chest tube placement. Also, 24 of non-life-threatening allergic reactions were reported [158].

Stipulating that each patient had at least three visits and during each visit received at least ten injections, the occurrence of pneumothorax requiring a chest tube was 1 per 247,500 injections. Thus, self-limited pneumothoraxes were 1 per 18,333, and allergic reactions were 1 per 20,625 injections [158].

In the 1960s, five cases of postinjection arachnoiditis were reported [159]. Two were fatal; one was a direct sequence of arachnoiditis and another was a sequence of incompetent shunt and persistent hydrocephalus with increased intracranial pressure. Of the other three cases, the first one with mild paraparesis recovered after a ventriculo-jugular shunt. The second recovered spontaneously with a mild neurological deficit, and the third patient remained paraplegic.

Three other cases of intrathecal injections known to the first author have not been reported in the literature because of medicolegal issues. Two of them resulted in paraplegia. The first occurred after injection at the thoracic level and the second after a lumbar injection. The third case was performed by an untrained person who injected zinc sulfate solution, which is hardly used in today's practice, at the cranio-cervical level, resulting in immediate onset of severe neurologic deficit, quadriplegia, and subsequent hydrocephalus. One case of self-limiting sterile meningitis after lumbosacral sclerosing injections was reported in 1994. Adjacent endplate fractures associated with intradiscal dextrose injections were recently reported [160].

Postspinal puncture headaches have been reported after lumbosacral injections. Two such cases occurred in the first author's practice during the past 20 years. Both patients recovered after 1 week with bed rest and fluids.

Overall, pneumothorax is the most commonly reported complication. Injections of anterior thoracic synovial joints, such as sternoclavicular, costosternal, and interchondral, may also result in pneumothorax.

Conclusions

Double-blind, placebo-controlled, and retrospective studies clearly indicate the effectiveness of RIT in painful degenerative posttraumatic conditions of fibrous connective tissue.

Literature suggests that degenerative cascade is a multi-etiologic disease process. NSAIDs and steroid preparations have limited use in chronic painful overuse conditions and degenerative painful conditions of ligaments and tendons. Microinterventional regenerative techniques and proper rehabilitation up to 1 year supported with mild opioid analgesics are more appropriate.

Cervical thoracic and lumbar discogenic pain continues to be a therapeutic challenge. Encouraging positive results were published after regenerative injections for lumbar discogenic pain with dextrose-based solutions, methylene blue, and mesenchymal stem cells. The work in this direction continues. It appears that cervical and thoracic discogenic pain may be addressed similarly in the near future.

The future is such that, instead of indirect stimulation of growth factors through inflammatory cascade, specific growth factors or their combinations may be available. The challenge will continue to determining which specific growth factors should be used. The other viable possibility is injection of engineered, type-specific tissue derived from stem-cell research [83, 84, 154]. Some variations of nanotechnology will be also added.

As stated by the late Professor Mooney, "The ideas of regeneration and controlled proliferation are slowly moving from the fringe to the frontier of medical care" [161]. A physician versatile in diagnostic and therapeutic injection techniques may have ample opportunity to implement RIT in the treatment of chronic musculoskeletal pain. More information regarding RIT can be found on linetskymd.com and aarom.org. Full texts of many original articles text books and chapters are available on these websites. The individual training with CME credits is available by the American Academy of Regenerative Orthopedic Medicine (AAROM) at Drs. Linetsky, Centeno, Crane, and Hirsch offices.

Acknowledgments The authors would like to extend their special thanks to Jacqueline Ferreira for invaluable help in the preparation of this manuscript and Tracey James for preparation of the illustrations.

References

1. Linetsky F, Willard F. Use of regenerative injection therapy for low back pain. Pain Clin. 1999;1:27–31.
2. Feinstein B, Langton J, Jameson R, et al. Experiments on pain referred from deep somatic tissues. J Bone Joint Surg Am. 1954;36A:981–96.

3. Dwyer A, Aprill C, Bogduk N. Cervical zygapophyseal joint pain patterns: a clinical evaluation. Spine. 1990;15:458–61.

4. Dreyfuss P, Michaelsen M, Fletcher D. Atlanto-occipital and lateral atlanto-axial joint pain patterns. Spine. 1994;19:1125–31.

5. Dussault RG, Kaplan PA. Facet joint injection: diagnosis and therapy. Appl Radiol. 1994;23:35–39.

6. Fukui S, Ohseto K, Shiotani M. Patterns of pain induced by distending the thoracic zygapophyseal joints. Reg Anesth Pain Med. 1997;22(4):332–336. http://dx.doi.org/10.1016/S1098-7339(97)80007-7

7. Kellgren JH. Observations on referred pain arising from muscle. Clin Sci. 1939;4:35–46.

8. Mooney V, Robertson J. The facet syndrome. Clin Orthop Relat Res. 1976;115:149–156.

9. Hackett G. Ligament and tendon relaxation treated by prolotherapy. 3rd ed. Springfield: Charles C. Thomas; 1958.

10. Kellgren J. On the distribution of pain arising from deep somatic structures with charts of segmental pain areas. Somatic Pain. 1939;4:35–46.

11. Hackett G, Hemwall G, Montgomery G. Ligament and tendon relaxation: treated by prolotherapy. 5th ed. Springfield: Charles C. Thomas; 1991.

12. Simons DG, Travell JG, Simons LS. Myofascial pain and dysfunction: the trigger point manual, vol. 1. Baltimore: Williams & Wilkins; 1991.

13. Bonica J, Loeser J, Chapman C, et al. The management of pain. vol I, 2nd ed. Malvern: Lea & Febiger; 1990; 7:136–139.

14. Dreyfuss P, Tibiletti C, Dreyer S. Thoracic zygapophyseal joint pain patterns: a study in normal volunteers. Spine. 1994;19:807–11.

15. Dussault RG, Kaplan PA, Anderson MW. Fluoroscopy-guided sacroiliac joint injections. Radiology. 2000;214(1):273–7.

16. O'Neill C, Kurgansky M, Derby R, et al. Disc stimulation and patterns of referred pain. Spine. 2002;27:2776–81.

17. Linetsky F, Trescot A, Manchikanti L. Regenerative injection therapy. In: Manchikanti L, Singh V, editors. Interventional techniques in chronic non-spinal pain. Paducah: ASIPP Publishing; 2009. p. 87–98.

18. Biegeleisen H. Varicose veins, related diseases, and sclerotherapy: a guide for practitioners. Fountain Valley: Eden Press; 1994.

19. Linetsky F, Mikulinsky A, Gorfine L. Regenerative injection therapy: history of application in pain management: part I 1930s–1950s. Pain Clin. 2000;2:8–13.

20. Linetsky F, Botwin K, Gorfine L, et al. Position paper of the Florida Academy of Pain Medicine on regenerative injection therapy: effectiveness and appropriate usage. Pain Clin. 2002;4:38–45.

21. Linetsky F, Saberski L, Miguel R, et al. A history of the applications of regenerative injection therapy in pain management: part II 1960s–1980s. Pain Clin. 2001;3:32–6.

22. Linetsky F, Derby R, Saberski L, et al. Pain management with regenerative injection therapy (RIT). In: Boswell M, Cole E, editors. Weiner's Pain management: a practical guide for clinicians. 7th ed. Boca Raton: CRC Press; 2006. p. 939–66.

23. Steindler A, Luck J. Differential diagnosis of pain low in the back: allocation of the source of pain by the procaine hydrochloride method. JAMA. 1938;110:106–13.

24. Haldeman K, Soto-Hall R. The diagnosis and treatment of sacroiliac conditions by the injection of procaine (Novocain). J Bone Joint Surg Am. 1938;3:675–85.

25. Bogduk N. Post-traumatic cervical and lumbar spine zygapophyseal joint pain. In: Evans RW, editor. Neurology and trauma. Philadelphia: WB Saunders; 1996. p. 363–75.

26. Williams P. Gray's anatomy, 38th British edition. Philadelphia: Churchill Livingston, Pearson Professional Limited; 1995.

27. Best T. Basic science of soft tissue. In: Delee J, Drez D, editors. Orthopedic sports medicine principles and practice, vol. 1. Philadelphia: WB Saunders; 1994.

28. Willard F. Gross anatomy of the cervical and thoracic regions: understanding connective tissue stockings and their contents. Presented at the 20th American Association of Orthopedic Medicine annual conference and scientific seminar; a common sense approach to "hidden" pain generators, Orlando, 2003.

29. Yahia H, Newman N. A light and electron microscopic study of spinal ligament innervation. Z Mikrosk Anat Forsch. 1989;102:664–74.

30. Leadbetter W. Cell-matrix response in tendon injury. Clin Sports Med. 1992;11:533–78.

31. Sinelnikov RD. Atlas of anatomy, vol. 1. Moscow: Meditsina; 1972.

32. Leadbetter W. Anti-inflammatory therapy and sport injury: the role of non-steroidal drugs and corticosteroid injections. Clin Sports Med. 1995;14:353–410.

33. Jozsa L, Kannus P. Human tendons, anatomy, physiology, and pathology. Champaign: Human Kinetics; 1997.

34. Cotran R, Vinay K, Collins T, et al. Robbins pathologic basis of disease. Philadelphia: WB Saunders; 1999.

35. Freemont A. Nerve ingrowth into diseased intervertebral disc in chronic back pain. Lancet. 1997;350:178–81.

36. Ashton I, Ashton B, Gibson S, et al. Morphological basis for back pain: the demonstration of nerve fibers and neuropeptides in the lumbar facet joint capsule but not in the ligamentum flavum. J Orthop Res. 1992;10:72–8.

37. Tuzlukov P, Skuba N, Gorbatovskaya N. The morphological characteristics of fibromyalgia syndrome. Arkh Patol. 1993;4:47–50.

38. Nirschl R, Pettrone F. Tennis elbow. The surgical treatment of lateral epicondylitis. J Bone Joint Surg Am. 1979;61(6A):832–9.

39. Fortin J, Vilensky J, Merkel GJ. Can the sacroiliac joint cause sciatica? Pain Physician. 2003;6(3):269–71.

40. Khan KM, Cook JL, Taunton JE, Bonar F. Overuse tendinosis, not tendinitis part 1: a new paradigm for a difficult clinical problem. Phys Sportsmed. 2000;28(5):38–48.

41. Alfredson H, Thorsen K, Lorentzon R. In situ microdialysis in tendon tissue: high levels of glutamate, but not prostaglandin E2 in chronic Achilles tendon pain. Knee Surg Sports Traumatol Arthrosc. 1999;7:378–81.

42. Alfredson H, Ljung BO, Thorsen K, Lorentzon R. In vivo investigation of ECRB tendons with microdialysis technique: no signs of inflammation but high amounts of glutamate in tennis elbow. Acta Orthop Scand. 2000;71(5):475–9.

43. Alfredson H, Forsgren S, Thorsen K, Lorentzon R. In vivo microdialysis and immunohistochemical analyses of tendon tissue demonstrated high amounts of free glutamate and glutamate NMDAR1 receptors, but no signs of inflammation, in Jumper's knee. J Orthop Res. 2001;19:881–6.

44. Alfredson H, Forsgren S, Thorsen K, Fahlström M, Johansson H, Lorentzon R. Glutamate NMDAR1 receptors localised to nerves in human Achilles tendons. Implications for treatment? Knee Surg Sports Traumatol Arthrosc. 2000;9:123–6.

45. Alfredson H, Bjur D, Thorsen K, Lorentzon R. High intratendinous lactate levels in painful chronic Achilles tendinosis. An investigation using microdialysis technique. J Orthop Res. 2002;20:934–8.

46. Bjur D, Alfredson H, Forsgren S. The innervation pattern of the human Achilles tendon: studies of the normal and tendinosis tendon with markers for general and sensory innervation. Cell Tissue Res. 2005;320(1):201–6. Epub 2005 Feb 9.

47. Ljung BO, Forsgren S, Fridén J. Substance-P and Calcitonin gene-related peptide expression at the extensor carpi radialis brevis muscle origin: implications for the aetiology of tennis elbow? J Orthop Res. 1999;17(4):554–9.

48. Ljung BO, Alfredson H, Forsgren S. Neurokinin 1-receptors and sensory neuropeptides in tendon insertions at the medial and lateral epicondyles of the humerus. Studies on tennis elbow and medial epicodylalgia. J Orthop Res. 2004;22:321–7.

49. Liu Y, Tipton C, Matthes R, et al. An in situ study of the influence of a sclerosing solution in rabbit medial collateral ligaments and its junction strength. Connect Tissue Res. 1983;11:95–102.

50. Maynard J, Pedrini V, Pedrini-Mille A, et al. Morphological and biochemical effects of sodium morrhuate on tendons. J Orthop Res. 1985;3:234–48.

51. Klein R, Dorman T, Johnson C. Proliferant injections for low back pain: histologic changes of injected ligaments and objective measurements of lumbar spine mobility before and after treatment. J Neurol Ortho Med Surg. 1989;10·2.

52. Öhberg L, Alfredson H. Ultrasound guided sclerosis of neovessels in painful chronic Achilles tendinosis: pilot study of a new treatment. Br J Sports Med. 2002;36:173–7.

53. Alfredson H, Ohberg L. Neovascularisation in chronic painful patellar tendinosis – promising results after sclerosing neovessels outside the tendon challenge the need for surgery. Knee Surg Sports Traumatol Arthrosc. 2005;13(2):74–80. Epub 2004 Nov 26.

54. Alfredson H, Öhberg L. Sclerosing injections to areas of neovascularisation reduce pain in chronic Achilles tendinopathy: a double-blind randomized controlled trial. Knee Surg Sports Traumatol Arthrosc. 2005;13(4):338–44. Epub 2005 Feb 2. PMID:15688235.

55. Alfredson H, Harstad H, Haugen S, Ohberg L. Sclerosing polidocanol injections to treat chronic painful shoulder impingement syndrome-results of a two-centre collaborative pilot study. Knee Surg Sports Traumatol Arthrosc. 2006;14(12):1321–6. Epub 2006 Oct 7.

56. Willard F. The muscular, ligamentous and neural structure of the low back and its relation to back pain. In: Vleeming A et al., editors. Movement stability and low back pain. New York: Churchill Livingston; 1997. p. 1–35.

57. Linetsky F, Parris W, et al. Regenerative injection therapy. In: Manchikanti L, editor. Low back pain. Paducah: ASIPP Publishing; 2002. p. 519–20.

58. Lord S. Chronic cervical zygapophyseal joint pain after whiplash: a placebo-controlled prevalence study. Spine. 1996;21:1737–45.

59. Barnsley L, Lord S, Walis B, et al. Lack of effect of intra-articular corticosteroids for chronic pain in the cervical zygapophyseal joints. N Engl J Med. 1994;330:1047–50.

60. O'Neill C. Intra-articular dextrose/glucosamine injections for cervical facet syndrome, atlanto-occipital and atlanto-axial joint pain, combined ISIS AAOM approach. Presented at the 20th AAOM annual conference and scientific seminar, Orlando, April 30–May 3, 2003.

61. Stanton-Hicks M. Cervicocranial syndrome: treatment of atlanto-occipital and atlanto-axial joint pain with phenol/glycerin injections. Presented at the 20th AAOM annual conference and scientific seminar, Orlando, April 30–May 3, 2003.

62. Zhang J, Tsuzuki N, Hirabayashi S, et al. Surgical anatomy of the nerves and muscles in the posterior cervical spine. A guide for avoiding inadvertent nerve injuries during the posterior approach. Spine. 2003;28:1379–84.

63. Wilkinson H. Injection therapy for enthesopathies causing axial spine pain and the "failed back syndrome": a single blinded, randomized and cross-over study. Pain Physician. 2005;8:167–74.

64. Wilkinson H. The failed back syndrome etiology and therapy. 2nd ed. New York: Springer; 1992.

65. Kayfetz D, Blumenthal L, Hackett G, et al. Whiplash injury and other ligamentous headache: its management with prolotherapy. Headache. 1963;3:1.

66. Resnick D. Diagnosis of bone and joint disorders, volumes 1–6. 3rd ed. Philadelphia: WB Saunders; 1995.

67. Stark D, Bradley W. Magnetic resonance imaging, volumes 1 and 2. 3rd ed. St. Louis: Mosby; 1999.

68. European Society of Musculoskeletal Radiology. http://www.southstaffordshirepct.nhs.uk/policies/clinical/Clin55_DiagnosticUltrasoundProcedures.pdf. Approved 27 Apr 2009.

http://www.essr.org/html/img/pool/shoulder.pdf; http://www.essr.org/html/img/pool/elbow.pdf; http://radiology.rsna.org/content/252/1/157.full.pdf.

69. McNally E. Ultrasound of the small joints of the hands and feet: current status. Skeletal Radiol. 2008;37(2):99–113. Epub 2007 Aug 22.

70. Linetsky F, Stanton Hicks M, O'Neil C. Prolotherapy. In: Wallace M, Staats P, editors. Pain medicine & management – just the facts. New York: McGraw-Hill; 2004. p. 318–24

71. Linetsky F, Saberski L, Dubin J, et al. Letter to the editor. Re: Yelland MJ, Glasziou PP, Bogduk N, et al. Prolotherapy injections, saline injections, and exercises for chronic low-back pain: a randomized study. Spine, 2003; 29:9–16. Spine. Spine. 2004;29(16):1840–1; author reply 1842–3.

72. Klein R, DeLong W, Mooney V, et al. A randomized, double-blind trial of dextrose-glycerin-phenol injections for chronic, low back pain. J Spinal Disord. 1993;6:23–33.

73. Miller M. Treatment of painful advanced internal lumbar disc derangement with intradiscal injection of hypertonic dextrose. Pain Physician. 2006;9(2):115–21.

74. Klein R, O'Neill C, Mooney V, et al. Biochemical injection treatment for discogenic low back pain: a pilot study. Spine J. 2003;3(3):220–6.

75. Yelland M, Glasziou P, Bogduk N, et al. Prolotherapy injections, saline injections, and exercises for chronic low-back pain: a randomized trial. Spine. 2004;29:9–16.

76. Ongley M, Klein R, Dorman T, et al. A new approach to the treatment of chronic low back pain. Lancet. 1987;2:143–6.

77. Dechow E, Davies R, Carr A, et al. A randomized, double-blind, placebo controlled trial of sclerosing injections in patients with chronic low back pain. Rheumatology. 1999;38:1255–9.

78. Yelland M, Yeo M, Schluter P. Prolotherapy injections for chronic low back pain – results of a pilot comparative study. Australas Musculoskelet Med. 2000;5:20–3.

79. Yelland M, et al. Prolotherapy injections for chronic low back pain: a systematic review. Spine. 2004;19:2126–33.

80. Kon E. Platelet-rich plasma: intra-articular knee injections produced favorable results on degenerative cartilage lesions. Knee Surg Sports Traumatol Arthrosc. 2010;18(4):472–9.

81. Mishra A, et al. Platelet-rich plasma compared with corticosteroid injection for chronic lateral elbow tendinosis. P M R. 2009;1(4):366–70.

82. Topol G, et al. Efficacy of dextrose prolotherapy in elite make kicking-sport athletes with chronic groin pain. Arch Phys Med Rehabil. 2005;86(4):697–702.

83. Topol G, Reeves K. Regenerative injection of elite athletes with career-altering chronic groin pain who fail conservative treatment: a consecutive case series. Am J Phys Med Rehabil. 2008;87:890–902.

84. Kon E, et al. Platelet-rich plasma: new clinical application: a pilot study for treatment of jumper's knee. Injury. 2009;40(6):598–603.

85. Robertson J. Structural alterations in nerve fibers produced by hypotonic and hypertonic solutions. J Biophys Biochem Cytol. 1958;4:349–64.

86. Jewett D, Kind J. Conduction block of monkey dorsal rootlets by water and hypertonic saline solutions. Exp Neurol. 1971;33:225.

87. Barsa et al. Functional and structural changes in the rabbit vagus nerve in vivo following exposure to various hypoosmotic solutions. Anesth Analg. 1982;61(11):912–6.

88. Fink et al. Osmotic swelling effects on neural conduction. Anesthesiology. 1979;51(5):418–23.

89. Hitchcock E, Prandini MN. Hypertonic saline in management of intractable pain. Lancet. 1973;1(7798):310–2.

90. Racz GB, Heavner JE, Trescot A. Percutaneous lysis of epidural adhesions – evidence for safety and efficacy. Pain Pract. 2008;8(4):277–86. Epub 2008 May 23.

91. Westerlund T, et al. The endoneurial response to neurolytic agents is highly dependent on the mode of application. Reg Anesth Pain Med. 1999;24(4):294–302.

92. Westerlund T, Vuorinen V, Roytta M. The effect of combined neurolytic blocking agent 5 % phenol -glycerol in rat sciatic nerve. Acta Neuropathol (Berl). 2003;106:261–70.

93. Bodine-Fowler SC, Allsing S, Botte MJ. Time course of muscle atrophy and recovery following a phenol-induced nerve block. Muscle Nerve. 1996;19:497–504.

94. Birch M, Strong N, Brittain P, et al. Retrobulbar phenol injection in blind painful eyes. Ann Ophthalmol. 1993;257:267–70.

95. Garland DE, Lilling M, Keenan MA. Percutaneous phenol blocks to motor points of spastic forearm muscles in head-injured adults. Arch Phys Med Rehabil. 1984;65:243–5.

96. Viel E, Pellas F, Ripart J, et al. Peripheral neurolytic blocks and spasticity. Ann Fr Anesth Reanim. 2005;24:667–72.

97. Raj P. Practical management of pain. 3rd ed. St. Louis: Mosby Inc.; 2000.

98. Zafonte RD, Munin MC. Phenol and alcohol blocks for the treatment of spasticity. Phys Med Rehabil Clin N Am. 2001;12:817–32.

99. Kirvela O, Nieminen S. Treatment of painful neuromas with neurolytic blockade. Pain. 1990;41:161–5.

100. Wilkinson HA. Trigeminal nerve peripheral branch phenol/glycerol injections for tic douloureux. J Neurosurg. 1999;90:828–32.

101. Robertson D. Transsacral neurolytic nerve block. An alternative approach to intractable perineal pain. Br J Anaesth. 1983;559:873–5.

102. Trescot A. HansenH. Neurolytic agents: pharmacology and clinical applications. In: Manchikanti L, Singh V, editors. Interventional techniques in chronic non-spinal pain. Paducah: ASIPP Publishing; 2009. p. 53–8.

103. Lamer T. Neurolytic peripheral joint injections in severely debilitated patients. Presented at the annual meeting of the Florida Academy of Pain Medicine, Orlando, 30 July 2005.

104. Broadhurst N, Wilk V. Vertebral mid-line pain: pain arising from the interspinous spaces. J Orthop Med. 1996;18:2–4.

105. Kevy S, Jacobson M. Point of care concentration and clinical application of autologous bone marrow derived stem cells. Presented at the Orthopedic Research Society, 52nd annual meeting. 19–22 March 2006.

106. Aust L, Devlin B, Foster S. Yield of human adipose-derived adult stem cells from lipoaspirates. Cytotherapy. 2004;6:7–14.

107. Alexander R. Use of PRP in autologous fat grafting. In: Shiffman M, editor. Autologous fat grafting. Berlin: Springer; 2010. p. 140–67.

108. Crane D, Everts P. Platelet rich plasma matrix grafts. Pract Pain Manag. 2008;8:12–26. http://www.prolotherapy.com/PPM_JanFeb2008_Crane_PRP.pdf

109. Everts P, Knape J, Weibrich G, et al. Platelet-rich plasma and platelet gel: a review. J Extra Corpor Technol. 2006;38:174–87.

110. Alhadlaq A, Mao JJ. Mesenchymal stem cells: isolation and therapeutics. Stem Cells Dev. 2004;13(4):436–48.

111. Barry FP. Mesenchymal stem cell therapy in joint disease. Novartis Found Symp. 2003;249:86–96; discussion 96–102, 170–4, 239–41.

112. Bruder SP, Fink DJ, Caplan AI. Mesenchymal stem cells in bone development, bone repair, and skeletal regeneration therapy. J Cell Biochem. 1994;56(3):283–94.

113. Cha J, Falanga V. Stem cells in cutaneous wound healing. Clin Dermatol. 2007;25(1):73–8.

114. Gangji V, Toungouz M, Hauzeur JP. Stem cell therapy for osteonecrosis of the femoral head. Expert Opin Biol Ther. 2005;5(4):437–42.

115. Becker AJ, Mc CE, Till JE. Cytological demonstration of the clonal nature of spleen colonies derived from transplanted mouse marrow cells. Nature. 1963;197:452–4.

116. Friedenstein AJ, et al. Precursors for fibroblasts in different populations of hematopoietic cells as detected by the in vitro colony assay method. Exp Hematol. 1974;2(2):83–92.

117. Zhou Z, et al. Comparative study on various subpopulations in mesenchymal stem cells of adult bone marrow. Zhongguo Shi Yan Xue Ye Xue Za Zhi. 2005;13(1):54–8.

118. Schauwer CD, et al. Markers of stemness in equine mesenchymal stem cells: a plea for uniformity. Theriogenology. 2011;75(8):1431–43. Epub 2010 Dec 31.

119. Vidal MA, et al. Comparison of chondrogenic potential in equine mesenchymal stromal cells derived from adipose tissue and bone marrow. Vet Surg. 2008;37(8):713–24.

120. Niemeyer P, et al. Comparison of mesenchymal stem cells from bone marrow and adipose tissue for bone regeneration in a critical size defect of the sheep tibia and the influence of platelet-rich plasma. Biomaterials. 2010;31(13):3572–9.

121. Yoshimura H, et al. Comparison of rat mesenchymal stem cells derived from bone marrow, synovium, periosteum, adipose tissue, and muscle. Cell Tissue Res. 2007;327(3):449–62.

122. Frisbie DD, et al. Evaluation of adipose-derived stromal vascular fraction or bone marrow-derived mesenchymal stem cells for treatment of osteoarthritis. J Orthop Res. 2009;27(12):1675–80.

123. Banfi A, et al. Proliferation kinetics and differentiation potential of ex vivo expanded human bone marrow stromal cells: Implications for their use in cell therapy. Exp Hematol. 2000;28(6):707–15.

124. Crisostomo PR, et al. High passage number of stem cells adversely affects stem cell activation and myocardial protection. Shock. 2006;26(6):575–80.

125. Izadpanah R, et al. Long-term in vitro expansion alters the biology of adult mesenchymal stem cells. Cancer Res. 2008;68(11):4229–38.

126. Ladage D, et al. Mesenchymal stem cells induce endothelial activation via paracine mechanisms. Endothelium. 2007;14(2):53–63.

127. Zhou S, et al. Age-related intrinsic changes in human bone-marrow-derived mesenchymal stem cells and their differentiation to osteoblasts. Aging Cell. 2008;7(3):335–43.

128. Broberg K, et al. Polyclonal expansion of cells with trisomy 7 in synovia from patients with osteoarthritis. Cytogenet Cell Genet. 1998;83(1–2):30–4.

129. Izuta Y, et al. Meniscal repair using bone marrow-derived mesenchymal stem cells: experimental study using green fluorescent protein transgenic rats. Knee. 2005;12(3):217–23.

130. Horie M, et al. Intra-articular Injected synovial stem cells differentiate into meniscal cells directly and promote meniscal regeneration without mobilization to distant organs in rat massive meniscal defect. Stem Cells. 2009;27(4):878–87.

131. Yamasaki T, et al. Meniscal regeneration using tissue engineering with a scaffold derived from a rat meniscus and mesenchymal stromal cells derived from rat bone marrow. J Biomed Mater Res A. 2005;75(1):23–30.

132. Brittberg M, et al. Treatment of deep cartilage defects in the knee with autologous chondrocyte transplantation. N Engl J Med. 1994;331(14):889–95.

133. Caplan AI. Mesenchymal stem cells. J Orthop Res. 1991;9(5):641–50.

134. Angele P, et al. Engineering of osteochondral tissue with bone marrow mesenchymal progenitor cells in a derivatized hyaluronan-gelatin composite sponge. Tissue Eng. 1999;5(6):545–54.

135. Buckwalter JA, Mankin HJ. Articular cartilage: degeneration and osteoarthritis, repair, regeneration, and transplantation. Instr Course Lect. 1998;47:487–504.

136. Johnstone B, Yoo JU. Autologous mesenchymal progenitor cells in articular cartilage repair. Clin Orthop Relat Res. 1999;367(Suppl):S156–62.

137. Minas T, Nehrer S. Current concepts in the treatment of articular cartilage defects. Orthopedics. 1997;20(6):525–38.

138. Katakai D. Compressive properties of cartilage-like tissues repaired in vivo with scaffold-free, tissue engineered constructs. Clin Biomech (Bristol, Avon). 2009;24(1):110–6.

139. Fritzell P, Hagg O, Nordwall A. Complications in lumbar fusion surgery for chronic low back pain: comparison of three surgical techniques used in a prospective randomized study. A report from the Swedish Lumbar Spine Study Group. Eur Spine J. 2003;12(2):178–89.

140. Deyo RA. Lumbar spinal fusion. A cohort study of complications, reoperations, and resource use in the Medicare population. Spine. 1993;18(11):463–70.

141. Elias WJ, et al. Complications of posterior lumbar interbody fusion when using a titanium threaded cage device. J Neurosurg. 2000;93(1 Suppl):45–52.

142. Yoshikawa T. Disc regeneration therapy using marrow mesenchymal cell transplantation: a report of two case studies. Spine (Phila Pa 1976). 2010;35(11):E475–80.

143. Centeno CJ, et al. Regeneration of meniscus cartilage in a knee treated with percutaneously implanted autologous mesenchymal stem cells. Med Hypotheses. 2008;71(6):900–8.

144. Centeno CJ, et al. Increased knee cartilage volume in degenerative joint disease using percutaneously implanted, autologous mesenchymal stem cells. Pain Physician. 2008;11(3):343–53.

145. Centeno CJ, et al. Partial regeneration of the human hip via autologous bone marrow nucleated cell transfer: a case study. Pain Physician. 2006;9(3):253–6.

146. Centeno CJ, et al. Safety and complications reporting on the re-implantation of culture-expanded mesenchymal stem cells using autologous platelet lysate technique. Curr Stem Cell Res Ther. 2010;5(1):81–93.

147. Wakitani S, et al. Safety of autologous bone marrow-derived mesenchymal stem cell transplantation for cartilage repair in 41 patients with 45 joints followed for up to 11 years and 5 months. J Tissue Eng Regen Med. 2011;5(2):146–50.

148. Haleem AM, et al. The clinical use of human culture-expanded autologous bone marrow mesenchymal stem cells transplanted on platelet-rich fibrin glue in the treatment of articular cartilage defects: a pilot study and preliminary results. Cartilage. 2010;1(4):253–61.

149. Sakai D, et al. Transplantation of mesenchymal stem cells embedded in Atelocollagen gel to the intervertebral disc: a potential therapeutic model for disc degeneration. Biomaterials. 2003;24(20):3531–41.

150. Richardson SM, et al. Intervertebral disc cell mediated mesenchymal stem cell differentiation. Stem Cells. 2006;24(3):707–16.

151. Risbud MV, et al. Differentiation of mesenchymal stem cells towards a nucleus pulposus-like phenotype in vitro: implications for cell-based transplantation therapy. Spine. 2004;29(23):2627–32.

152. Miyamoto T, et al. Intradiscal transplantation of synovial mesenchymal stem cells prevents intervertebral disc degeneration through suppression of matrix metalloproteinase-related genes in nucleus pulposus cells in rabbits. Arthritis Res Ther. 2010;12(6):R206.

153. Nejadnik H, et al. Autologous bone marrow-derived mesenchymal stem cells versus autologous chondrocyte implantation: an observational cohort study. Am J Sports Med. 2010;38(6):1110–6.

154. Dreyfuss P, Michaelsen M, Horne M. MUJA: manipulation under joint anesthesia/analgesia: a treatment approach for recalcitrant low back pain of synovial joint origin. J Manipulative Physiol Ther. 1995;18:537–46.

155. Murakami E, et al. Effect of periarticular and intraarticular lidocaine injections for sacroiliac joint pain: prospective comparative study. J Orthop Sci. 2007;12(3):274–80.

156. Peng B, Pang X, Wu Y, et al. A randomized placebo-controlled trial of intradiscal ethylene blue injection for the treatment of chronic discogenic low back pain. Pain. 2010;149(1):124–9.

157. Dagenais S, Ogunseitan O, Haldeman S, et al. Side effects and adverse events related to intraligamentous injections of sclerosing solutions (prolotherapy) for back and neck pain: a survey of practitioners. Arch Phys Med Rehabil. 2006;87:909–13.

158. Dorman T. Prolotherapy: a survey. J Orthop Med. 1993;15:49–50.

159. Keplinger J, Bucy P. Paraplegia from treatment with sclerosing agents. JAMA. 1960;173:1333–5.

160. Whitworth M. Endplate fracture associated with intradiscal dextrose injection. Pain Physician. 2002;5:379–84.

161. Mooney V. Prolotherapy at the fringe of medical care, or is it the frontier? Spine J. 2003;3:253–4.

Interdisciplinary Functional Restoration and Pain Programs

13

Steven D. Feinberg, Robert J. Gatchel, Steven Stanos, Rachel Feinberg, and Valerie Johnson-Montieth

Key Points

- An interdisciplinary functional restoration approach to pain management has been empirically shown to be therapeutically and cost-effective.
- The biopsychosocial model of diagnosis and treatment operates on the idea that illness and disability is the result of, and influences, diverse areas of an individual's life, including the biological, psychological, social, environmental, and cultural components of their existence.

- It is important to identify those individuals at risk for delayed recovery and transitioning from an acute pain episode to a chronic pain condition.
- Functional restoration programs emphasize a biopsychosocial approach including different disciplines and anticipating an individual's gradual progression to a normal lifestyle.
- Treatment approaches include medication optimization, normalization of function, education, physical reactivation, cognitive-behavioral therapy, various mind-body techniques to manage chronic pain, and return of new functional activities.

S.D. Feinberg, M.D. (✉)
Feinberg Medical Group, 825 El Camino Real, Palo Alto, CA 94301, USA

Stanford University School of Medicine, Stanford, CA USA

American Pain Solutions, San Diego, CA USA
e-mail: stevenfeinberg@hotmail.com

R.J. Gatchel, Ph.D., ABPP
Department of Psychology, College of Science, The University of Texas at Arlington, 313 Life Science Building, Arlington, TX 76019, USA
e-mail: gatchel@vta.edu

S. Stanos, DO
Department of Physical Medicine and Rehabilitation, Center for Pain Management, Rehabilitation Institute of Chicago, 980 N. Michigan Ave, Suite 800, Chicago, IL 60611, USA

Northwestern University Medical School, Feinberg School of Medicine, Chicago, IL USA
e-mail: sstanos@ric.org

R. Feinberg, PT, DPT
Feinberg Medical Group, 825 El Camino Real, Palo Alto, CA 94301, USA
e-mail: rfeinberg14@gmail.com

V. Johnson-Montieth, B.A., M.A., Ph.D. Candidate
Department of Psychology, University of Texas at Arlington, Arlington, TX USA
e-mail: valerie.johnston@mavs.uta.edu

Overview: Pain Rehabilitation and the Restoration of Function

The major purpose of the present chapter is to provide a review of the currently most therapeutically effective method for managing chronic pain—functional restoration (FR). Before doing so, a brief overview of the rehabilitation process will be provided. Indeed, throughout history, the treatment of chronic pain conditions has been difficult, time consuming, expensive, and, all too often, unsuccessful. Many modes of treatment, both invasive (injections, procedures, surgery, etc.) and noninvasive methods (medications, physical therapy, counseling, applications of heat, ice, transcutaneous electrical stimulation, and many others), have been used by the health-care profession in an attempt to eliminate pain and return these patients to a productive, fulfilling life. All too frequently, though, these attempts resulted in failure. Recently, however, an interdisciplinary FR approach to pain management has been empirically shown to be therapeutically and cost-effective. As will be discussed, the FR approach is based on a fundamental understanding of the individual's unique condition as it relates to impairment, disability, and functional limitation.

It should be noted that the *AMA Guides to the Evaluation of Permanent Impairment*, 5th Edition [1], defines impairment as "a loss, loss of use, or derangement of any body part, organ system, or organ function." The 6th Edition [2] defines impairment as "a significant deviation, loss, or loss of use of any body structure or body function in an individual with a health condition, disorder, or disease." One such impairment can involve the loss or abnormality psychologically, physiologically, or functionally at the level of the organs and body systems. Examples of physiologic impairments include muscle weakness, range-of-motion loss, and restriction or lack of ability to perform activities due to related impairments. These impairments can cause inabilities to function in specific vocations including those of being a worker, spouse, student, or parent. Disability is defined by the AMA Guides 5th Edition as "An alteration of an individual's capacity to meet personal, social, or occupational demands because of an impairment." The AMA Guides 6th Edition defines disability as "activity limitations and/or participation restrictions in an individual with a health condition, disorder, or disease." Finally, the American Physical Therapy Association in the Guide to Physical Therapist Practice, Second Edition [3], describes functioning as an umbrella term for body functions, body structures, activities, and participation, denoting a positive interaction between the individual or patient and contextual factors (i.e., background of the individual's life and current situation). Functional limitation is a deviation from normal behavior involved in performing the activities of daily living (ADLs) and may include problems with transfers, standing, ambulation, running, and stair climbing. A formal model proposed by the International Classification of Functioning, Disability and Health (ICF) [4] integrates the individual components into a biopsychosocial-based model where the term "health condition" is exchanged for "chronic pain" (see Fig. 13.1). Chronic pain is affected by body function, activities, and participation as well as influences from the environment and personal factors.

The World Health Organization (WHO) developed a comprehensive model of disablement, the International Classification of Functioning, Disability and Health (ICF) 2009; this classification is depicted in Table 13.1. The ICF framework is intended to describe and measure health and disability at both the individual and population levels and consists of three key components:

1. Body functions and body structures: physiological functions and body parts, respectively; these can vary from the normal state, in terms of loss or deviations, which are referred to as impairments.
2. Activity: task executions by the individual and activity limitations are difficulties the individual may experience while carrying out such activities.
3. Participation: involvement in life situations and participation restrictions are barriers to experiencing such involvement. These components comprise functioning and disability in the model. In turn, they are related interactively to an individual with a given health condition, disorder, or disease and to environmental factors and personal factors of each specific case.

A patient-centered, "whole-person" approach is necessary to effectively address these important individual concepts. A team-centered treatment approach is utilized, focusing on helping patients achieve individual goals, which enable them to improve physical and psychosocial function, decrease pain, and improve quality of life. By working together, the chronic pain rehabilitation team helps patients achieve better outcomes than those achieved by an individual practitioner or interventions (i.e., surgeries, injections, pharmacotherapy, and psychological therapies) in isolation. Basic treatment goals of early and chronic pain rehabilitation programs focus on functional improvement, improved abilities in performing activities of daily living (ADLs), returning to leisure, sport, and vocational activities and improved pharmacologic management of pain and related affective distress (see Table 13.1).

History of Pain Rehabilitation

Early evidence of a rehabilitation approach to the injured person or worker dates back to the Egyptians under Ramses

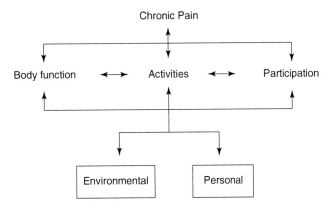

Fig. 13.1 A formal model proposed by the International Classification of Functioning, Disability and Health (ICF) [4] integrates the individual components into a biopsychosocial-based model (Adapted from International Classification of Functioning, Disability and Health (ICF) [4])

Table 13.1 Pain rehabilitation goals

1. Functional improvement
2. Improvement in activities of daily living
3. Relevant psychosocial improvement
4. Rational pharmacologic management (analgesia, mood, and sleep)
5. Return to leisure, sport, work, or other productive activity

From World Health Organization, http://www.who.int/classifications/icf/en/

II, in 1,500 B.C. [5]. Further advances in treating pain seemed to be delayed until many years later, with the birth of the field of anesthesia in the 1840s, the isolation and synthesis of morphine by Serturner in 1806, and the discovery of salicylates in willow bark in the late 1800s [6]. Modern advancements in understanding health and health psychology in the 1950s also shaped a more comprehensive view of the complexities of an individual's pain experience. This led to the view that the experience of pain is a complex phenomenon and multiple models have evolved over time to explain it. Traditionally, the biomedical model explains pain through etiologic factors (e.g., injury) or disease whose pathophysiology results in pain. Over time, it became clear this classic biomedical approach to understanding and treating pain was incomplete. Its exclusive application often resulted in unrealistic expectations on the part of the physician and patient, inadequate pain relief, and excessive disability in those with pain that persists well after the original injury has healed.

George Engel [7] developed a novel theory of health care in which the various areas impacting an individual's disease process are taken into consideration. When developing a health-care plan, Engel posited that there were several factors affecting each individual and his/her disease processes. These factors include (1) biological, (2) sociological, (3) environmental, (4) cultural, and (5) psychological. This became known as the biopsychosocial model [8]. This biopsychosocial model was subsequently successfully applied to the assessment and treatment of chronic pain [9, 10]. In contradiction to the biomedical model, this model recognizes pain is ultimately the result of the pathophysiology, plus the psychological state, cultural background/belief system, and relationship/interactions individuals have with their environment (workplace, home, disability system, and health-care providers). To put it more simply, to treat the pain and the illness, the whole person needs attention.

The modern rehabilitation model evolved after World Wars I and II, with the founding of the fields of physical and occupational therapy as a method to rehabilitate returning soldiers who had been injured in performance of service to their country [11]. The practice of pain rehabilitation increasingly developed during the twentieth century by evolving medical specialties of physical medicine and rehabilitation, anesthesia, psychiatry, and occupational medicine. John Bonica, one of the fathers of pain medicine, championed a more comprehensive biopsychosocial multidisciplinary approach in the United States in 1947. This approach expanded to include a team of clinicians at the University of Washington in the 1960s [12]. Bonica's collaboration with Wilbert Fordyce, a psychologist, incorporated operant conditioning and other behavioral approaches with more specialized, structured, and inpatient multi-week programs. In the

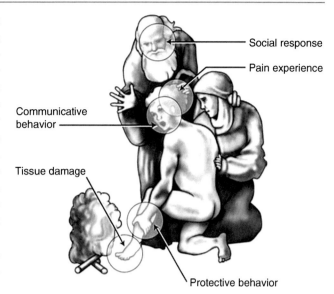

Fig. 13.2 Biopsychomotor response (Modified from Sullivan [15])

1980s, John Loeser formalized a more at structured program the University of Washington. This 3-week long, daily program became a model for interdisciplinary treatment.

An increasingly biopsychosocial approach to pain rehabilitation, facilitated by the merging of behavioral and cognitive fields and subsequent cognitive-behavioral approaches to the assessment and treatment of pain, developed in the 1980s and 1990s [13]. A proliferation of pain treatment facilities was seen between 1980 and 1995. These facilities included the advancement of interventional procedures as treatment for chronic pain [14]. A more recent conceptualization by Sullivan [15], the biopsychomotor model, focuses on behaviors within the pain system incorporating three independent behavioral subsystems: (1) communicative, (2) protective, and (3) social response behaviors. In this model, a pain system is assumed to be only adaptive. The sensory component of the pain system is accompanied by behaviors designed to act on the source, or cause of injury or illness. This may help to explain the wide variability observed in pain behaviors seen across different patients, despite relatively similar levels of reported pain intensity and objective tissue pathology. In this model, a more sensory-based model of pain extends to include behavioral factors: communicative behaviors (i.e., grimacing), protective behaviors (i.e., withdrawing a body part from fire), and social responses (i.e., empathy and solicitous behavior from others). This model, as in the biopsychosocial model, emphasizes dysfunction developing in behavioral systems separate from pain sensation. Subsequent treatments targeting pain behavior likely lead to better clinical outcomes and provide a more pragmatic and inclusive model for the spectrum of pain rehabilitation (see Fig. 13.2).

Table 13.2 The biomedical versus the biopsychosocial model of pain

Biomedical model	Biopsychosocial model
Suitable for acute pain management	Suitable for chronic pain management
Concentrates on physical disease mechanisms	Illness behaviors incur[prating cognitive and emotional responses to pain are acknowledged
Accentuates peripheral perception of pain (nociception)	Understands the role central physiological mechanisms play in the modulation of peripheral nociception or the generation of pain experience in the absence of nociception
Approach to understanding/treating pain is reductionistic	Understanding and treating pain is approached with a multidisciplinary systems perspective
Relies on medical management approaches	Utilizes self-management approaches

Applying a Biopsychosocial Model to Pain Rehabilitation

The biopsychosocial model of diagnosis and treatment operates on the idea that illness and disability is the result of, and influences, diverse areas of an individual's life, including the biological, psychological, social, environmental, and cultural components of their existence. In individuals with chronic pain conditions, the pain continues past the time the initial injury has healed. There are numerous challenges and issues that the patient faces and that must be addressed. These include guarding of the injured area, fear of movement and reinjury, adoption of the sick role along with cultural beliefs about pain, the loss of productivity, a decrease in beneficial leisure activities, the loss of income, and change in the role and responsibilities within the family and the community at large.

There are several factors identifying those individuals at risk for transitioning from an acute pain episode to a chronic pain condition. These factors are (1) unresponsiveness to traditional therapies normally effective for that particular diagnosis, (2) considerable psychosocial factors which negatively influence recovery, (3) unemployment or lengthy absence from work, (4) history of prior delayed recovery or rehabilitation, (5) the employer is not supportive or accommodative of the needs of the individual, and (6) history of childhood abuse: verbal, physical, or mental. Of the previous factors, lost time from work is most predictive of those at risk of encountering delayed recovery [16].

Chronic pain usually starts with an acute pain episode although, in some cases, there is no acute event, but rather the recognition of a pain problem. When a delayed recovery is recognized, the diagnosis and treatment approach should be reconsidered. At this time, psychosocial risk factors should be identified and the patient either treated by the attending physician or specialist using a biopsychosocial approach, or when appropriate, referred to an FR chronic pain program. A treatment plan addressing the presenting symptoms and attendant risk factors delaying recovery can then be developed and implemented. With a diagnosis of delayed recovery, a program focusing on the individual's biomedical condition, not

addressing the complex requirements inherent in delayed recovery, will not be efficacious [9].

Individuals at risk of developing chronic pain conditions, as evidenced by lack of progress toward healing and a return to normalcy, are benefited by a multidisciplinary FR program. Physical and psychological interventions can be employed before disability becomes chronic. Early intervention minimizes long-term treatment costs and the negative physical, psychological, and sociological effects of disability, restoring the individual to an optimal level of functioning [16]. Many times, a purely biomedical model continues to be applied, with a narrow focus on reversing or eliminating nociception, or the "pain generator," and is more focused on a cure than on effective management. The biomedical model ignores or minimizes psychosocial factors, as well as the more complex central changes in the nervous system (i.e., sensitization of tissue, pathways, and neurochemical changes related to affective distress),that, not surprisingly, results in treatment failure (see Table 13.2).

History of Functional Restoration and Work Rehabilitation

Historically, FR is a term that was initially used for a variety of pain rehabilitation programs characterized by objective measure of physical function, intensive graded exercise, and multimodal pain/disability management, with both psychosocial and case management features. The concept of functional restoration was first described in the mid-1980s. Functional restoration programs for chronic pain have strong support in the medical literature going back to the early 1990s. The term "functional restoration" has in recent years become increasing popular with evidence-based medicine support, and it has been adopted as the treatment paradigm of choice for chronic conditions and particularly chronic pain states. Indeed, the effectiveness of functional restoration programs has been independently replicated throughout the world [17]. For patients with more complex or refractory problems, a comprehensive multidisciplinary approach to pain management that is individualized, functionally oriented (not pain-oriented), and goal specific has been found to be the most effective treatment approach [10, 18, 19].

Functional restoration (FR) programs, which are based on a return to work model, evolved along with advancements in occupational medicine, beginning in the 1970s. Prior to this, in the 1920s, programs of habit training, focused on restoring workers affected by disease or injury and later, in 1923, by the incorporation of vocational rehabilitation, were mandated at the federal level by the Vocational Rehabilitation Act. In the 1950s, more objective measures were used to track progress and measure outcomes and served as the starting point for more formal work conditioning and work hardening programs. These innovative programs were championed by Lillian Wegg and Florence Cromwell [20]. Subsequently, in the 1970s, work hardening emerged as a formal industrial management service [21], adopting a similar multidisciplinary approach that was used in the management of chronic pain and disability. Standardized work simulation equipment, assessment, and treatment protocols were incorporated into standard practice in the 1980s, leading to formal accreditation by the Commission on Accreditation of Rehabilitation Facilities (CARF) in the late 1980s and early 1990s.

Recent evidence-based guidelines strongly support the use of interdisciplinary functional restoration-based programs for the treatment of chronic pain, including low back pain [19]. For the treatment of chronic nonradicular low back pain, interdisciplinary functional restoration treatment, including cognitive-behavioral interventions, is supported by high-quality evidence. Within these same evidence-based guidelines, shared decision making for potential surgical intervention for low back pain should include a discussion of interdisciplinary treatment, since interdisciplinary therapy was found to be equally effective in long-term outcome studies [22].

Applying Functional Restoration Approach: Multi- and Interdisciplinary Treatment

Functional restoration is an evidence-based, empirically proven component of multi- and interdisciplinary pain management programs, emphasizing physical activity and psychosocial therapy and anticipating an individual's gradual progression to a normal lifestyle. FR programs emphasize a multidisciplinary, biopsychosocial approach in which physicians, psychologists, occupational and physical therapists, and therapists specializing in other relaxation techniques all work in concert with each other. The ultimate goal is the development and implementation of treatment plans individualized to fit each patient's unique needs. These programs are regarded as the treatment of choice for chronic conditions, particularly chronic pain conditions [23]. Such programs are both therapeutically and cost-effective in treating chronic pain conditions and restoring a patient to a productive lifestyle. Moreover, while FR programs are effective for chronic pain conditions, many believe this type of program would be both cost-effective and efficacious for other chronic conditions as well [24].

Gatchel et al. [25] have delineated the described critical elements of a functional restoration approach, which serves as the foundation for most multi- and interdisciplinary rehabilitation-based programs. These elements include quantification of physical deficits on an ongoing basis; psychosocial and socioeconomic assessment used to individualize and monitor progress; an emphasis on reconditioning of the injured area or body part; generic simulation of work or activity; disability management with cognitive-behavioral approaches; psychopharmacologic management focusing on improving analgesia, sleep, and affective distress; and, in some cases, detoxifying patients from medications (i.e., opioids or benzodiazepines). Individually tailored, these programs initially emphasize moderate physical interventions (i.e., stretching, strengthening, conditioning) and gradually progressing to more active, strenuous therapies with the goal of obtaining maximum rehabilitation and normalization in all facets of a person's lifestyle. This includes return to work, improved socioeconomic factors and self-esteem, and cognitive behavior therapy (CBT) addressing beliefs about pain, the resulting dysfunction, and environmental and socioeconomic factors. Research shows that a chronic pain patient's treatment needs are best addressed by such a multidisciplinary treatment program [26]. However, a biopsychosocial model of health care is not only efficacious in the treatment of chronic pain. Patients presenting with other disease processes are likely to benefit from this type of treatment concept.

Major Components of Functional Restoration

Some confusion has developed with the mixing of terms such as multi- and interdisciplinary models [10]. In the multidisciplinary model, patient care is planned and managed by a team leader, usually a pain specialist (anesthesiologist, physiatrist, neurologist, psychiatrist, or primary care provider), or a psychologist, and often hierarchical, with one or two individuals directing the services of a range of team members, many with individual goals. Treatment may be delivered at different facilities or centers where individual patient progress is not regularly shared between distinct disciplines. In contrast, the more collaborative interdisciplinary model involves team members working together "under one roof" toward a common goal. Team members are able to communicate and consult with other team members on an ongoing basis, facilitated by regular, face-to-face meetings.

The interdisciplinary model provides practical strategies for assessing and treating pain-related deconditioning, psychosocial distress, and socioeconomic factors related to disability. An interdisciplinary team model is characterized by team members working together for a common goal, making collective therapeutic decisions, having face-to-face meetings and patient team conferences, and facilitating communication and consultation. Interdisciplinary teams may be led by a physician (medical director), psychologist, or nurse, and it includes comprehensive assessment incorporating pain medicine, pain psychology, physical functional restoration, and vocational rehabilitation. Physical and occupational therapy assessments are also included in the formal assessment. Interdisciplinary programs are usually housed in one facility, with group goal setting, periodic interdisciplinary team meetings assessing and adjusting treatment progress, program coordination, and discharge planning. The physical aspects of these programs focus primarily on restoring joint mobility, muscle strength, endurance, conditioning, and cardiovascular fitness. The psychological aspects focus on cognitive behavioral strategies for pain management. The coordination of vocational and therapeutic recreation services is an important aspect of care, focusing on aiding patients in their return to work, improving behavioral factors (i.e., coping, catastrophizing, and problem solving) in the workplace, clarifying return to work level of functioning, and, in many cases, providing individual therapy.

In general, formal interdisciplinary programs usually last 3–8 weeks, 4–8 h/day, with tailored group and individual therapies provided in an outpatient setting. Program schedules include individual and group-based therapies. Most importantly, regularly scheduled team conferences help to facilitate progress, troubleshoot patient problems, build consensus, improve communication regarding progress (i.e., complete conference notes and communicate to case managers and referring physicians), adjust goals of therapy, and plan for discharge. Long-term follow-up studies of interdisciplinary treatment programs demonstrate improved return to work rates, pain reduction, and quality of life. In special situations, inpatient functional restoration programs may be indicated. Inpatient pain rehabilitation programs typically consist of more intensive functional rehabilitation and medical care than their outpatient counterparts. They may be appropriate for patients who (1) do not have the minimal functional capacity to participate effectively in an outpatient program, (2) have medical conditions that require more intensive oversight, (3) are receiving large amounts of medications necessitating medication weaning or detoxification, or (4) have complex medical or psychosocial diagnoses that benefit from more intensive observation and/or additional consultation during the rehabilitation process. As with outpatient pain rehabilitation programs, the most effective programs combine intensive, daily biopsychosocial rehabilitation with a functional restoration approach. To again summarize,

the fundamental elements of a functional restoration approach include assessment of the person's dynamic physical, functional, cultural, and psychosocial status. This includes assessment of strength, sensation, range of motion, aerobic capacity, and endurance, as well as measures of what the individual can and cannot do in terms of general activities of daily living, recreational, and work-related activities. Psychosocial strengths and stressors are assessed, including an analysis of the individual's support system, any history of childhood dysfunction or abuse, evidence of mood disorders or psychiatric comorbidity, assessment of education and skills, medication use, any history of substance abuse, presence of litigation, and work incapacity [24]. We will now review the various issues addressed in a comprehensive FR program.

Normalization of Function

Normalization of function is described as the reestablishment of independence and function, while understanding that some physical limitations may be unavoidable. Functional restoration empowers the individual to achieve maximal functional independence, the capacity to regain or maximize activities of daily living, and return to vocational and avocational activities. Depending on the current functional level of the patient, reaching their maximum level of function may take as long as 6 months to a year as they incorporate both a progressive exercise program and active pain management skills into their lifestyle. For physical limitations that are unavoidable, patients should be instructed on assistive devices and modifications for the home, and/or the workplace to allow them to achieve the highest level of function possible.

Education

At the beginning of any treatment, the patient's understanding and belief system of his or her prognosis and treatment must be ascertained. Information from multiple providers can often be misunderstood. Patients are often informed that nothing else can be done for them. Some are given lifting restrictions of no lifting or carrying greater than 10 lb postsurgically, and they continue to adhere to these restrictions for years after the necessity has lapsed. The treating physician and/or physical or occupational therapists, treating in an acute care model, may have informed the patient not to use the body part if it were painful. All of these can leave the patient with incorrect directions on how to best manage chronic pain.

Before the patient considers participating in a functional restoration program, he or she should be informed regarding the differences between functional restoration and other treatment methods. It is not uncommon for the patient to have seen multiple doctors and therapists without any benefit or with a worsening of symptoms. The patient may have little confidence that a functional restoration approach will be more effective than any of the other treatments that they have tried. Therefore, education about diagnosis, prognosis, and expectations concerning treatment and outcome should begin as soon as possible. Explanation of the changes to the patient's body, his or her personal experience, and how this translates to the symptoms they are experiencing is a connection that the provider must make for the patient. The patient must be provided with a confirmation that variability of symptoms and emotions are normal to their condition. The expectations concerning patient effort in the restoration process are emphasized. The active participation of the patient in the setting of treatment goals, his or her personal control of the process, and the success of the treatment are all important aspects contributing to the likelihood of successful completion of the restoration and a return to normalcy. The patient must understand that treatment will provoke discomfort and may be perceived as painful, that they will receive help with managing these symptoms, and that the outcome will be significant improvement in their overall functional level. Education regarding goals based on function, not only pain changes, is important to assist the patient in feeling successful and attaining their goals, as many patients believe that the focus of treatment is to simply reduce their pain level. Finally, the patient must be educated about the negative consequences of inactivity and resting. A significant loss of flexibility, strength, and secondary injury from guarding and abnormal movement are all possible, harmful consequences if the patient does not remain active after functional restoration therapy is complete.

Fear of Reinjury or Movement

Kinesiophobia (the fear of movement and reinjury) commonly obstructs the individual's return to work, a normal home life, and leisure activities after an injury has occurred. Fear related to pain, and subsequent avoidance of activities, has been empirically validated as an important factor in determining the patient's activity levels at 6–12 month post-injury [27]. Typically, patients will push themselves to increase social and physical activities in an attempt to confront and overcome the pain and disability of an injury. This may increase the pain, which increases the fear that an as-yet undiagnosed injury or illness is present. This fear may lead to a maladaptive avoidance response, which leads to lack of exercise and a physical deconditioning; this, in turn, leads to lack of muscle strength and flexibility and an increase in pain and infirmity. The patient must then be reexposed to previously avoided activities and assume a participatory role in the recovery process. Crombez et al. [28] found that "over prediction of pain," a construct closely related to fear-avoidance, was reduced by a gradual, paced, and repeated exposure to the activity individualized to the patient's own fear. Studies have suggested that back pain disability for some patients may be determined more by the fear of pain rather than intensity or other biomedical factors [29]. Treatment to overcome fear-avoidance includes patient education, repeated exposure to activities that have been avoided,

and taking responsibility in an active role to recovery. Patients are educated on how their beliefs and behaviors can lead to a vicious cycle involving catastrophic thoughts, fear, avoidance, disability, and pain. The patient learns the difference between pain and damage, safe positioning, safe activity, and slow progression of exercise. The activity program consists of the fearful activities initially introduced at low levels and then progressed on an individual basis.

Exposure therapy is a type of cognitive behavioral therapy (CBT – see below) and is used to expose an individual to fear-provoking stimuli. The bioinformational theory of fear states that activation of fear association, followed by the availability of new information refuting the fear expectations, is an intrinsic part of fear memory reduction [30]. A therapy used to develop a hierarchy of fear-producing stimuli uses a photograph series of daily activities, using the upper extremities (PHODA-UE), and a series of daily activities involving the lower extremities (PHODA-LE) [31]. In this therapy, patients judge the threat value of the various activities. The therapist then develops individually tailored practice tasks. The patient begins to perform the tasks, beginning with the least fear-inducing tasks, gradually advancing through the hierarchy to the most fear-inducing tasks [24].

Flare-up Management

Flare-ups, the seemingly uncontrolled, overwhelming symptoms of chronic pain, can feel unmanageable. The physical reactions to these flare-ups can include holding the breath, muscle tightening, tightening of chest and stomach muscles, and nausea. Psychological reactions can include fear, anxiety, worry, feelings of being overwhelmed, and anger. As these reactions take place, the pain level increases, incurring further flare-ups. Flare-up management education gives the patient active tools with which to control these symptoms. In the acute model, passive tools such as ice, heat, massage, TENS, rest, and medications are used for pain control. These passive tools are not as effective with chronic pain and often leave the patient dependent on medical providers. Active tools allow for more independence and a feeling of control. Education on ways to prevent flare-ups, and managing current flare-ups, provides the patient with different ways to control his or her pain.

The patient is educated on a variety of tools from all different aspects, including physical, emotional/behavioral, social, cognitive, spiritual, and environmental [32]. Teaching patients how to perform diaphragmatic breathing through pain, using light stretching or exercise, and ways to pace their activity (including setting limits), relaxation techniques, distraction, and visual imagery are some examples of useful tools. The patient is allowed to take multiple breaks during activities, which allows for control of any intensifying symptoms of anxiety, fear, or any other unconstructive response. These breaks are used for deep breathing, relaxation, stretching,

Table 13.3 Pain team shared primary objectives of a cognitive behavioral approach for pain patients

Combat demoralization by assisting patients to change their view of their pain from overwhelming to manageable

Teach patients the coping strategies and techniques to help them to adapt and respond to pain and the resultant problems

Assist patients to reconceptualize themselves as active, resourceful, and competent

Learn the associations between thoughts, feelings, and behaviors, subsequently identify and alter automatic, maladaptive patterns

Utilize more adaptive ways of thinking, feeling, and behaving

Bolster self-confidence and patient's attribution of successful outcomes to their own efforts

Help patients anticipate problems proactively and generate solutions, thereby facilitating maintenance and generalization

Adapted from Sullivan [15]

and/or CBT to help the patients to become calm and relaxed, at which time they are able to resume their activities.

Pacing

Pacing is a tool allowing the patient to change the way they perform, or complete an exercise or activity, successfully increasing strength, tolerance, and function, while managing pain levels. The purpose of pacing and goal setting is regulating daily activities and structuring an increase in tolerance by gradually increasing activity. Pacing activity requires the person to break an activity into active and rest periods. Rest periods are taken before significant increases in pain level occur. It provides structure to the overall activity level, guiding the individual to build an optimum schedule, minimizing pain, and maximizing productivity during the day. Pacing also brings about structure to the day, giving the person a sense of control.

Psychosocial Approaches

Many behavioral and psychosocial variables intensify and aggravate the pain and disability related to chronic pain conditions [26]. These behavioral and psychological variables help maintain the chronic pain condition in some patients. An interdisciplinary approach addresses these variables in an attempt to effectively manage the negative aspects associated with chronic pain. Anxiety, stress, communication skills, ideas about pain, and coping methods are all associated with a patient's ability to successfully or unsuccessfully cope with pain. If patients have negative ideas about themselves and their chronic pain condition, these destructive feelings can spread to their home and families, and they may, in turn, lose the ability to enjoy constructive activities. This reinforces initial negative feelings and causes the patient to become apathetic, depressed, and anxious. The family relationships are negatively modified, responsibility and productivity decrease, and the pain cycle increases with the assimilation of the "sick role." The financial burden that accompanies the loss of productivity and the negative psychosocial and behavioral aspects of the chronic pain condition all contribute to a downward spiral affecting all aspects of a patient's existence [33]. A functional restoration program is designed to recognize all the factors that contribute to an individual's chronic pain

experience and to educate and support the patient to manage and alter those factors successfully. Often, the family is included in some sessions to provide them with a perspective of important pain management techniques that they can help with at home with the patient, as well as to modify any solicitous behaviors they may be providing (as discussed above). The group setting of a functional restoration program increases the feelings of companionship and solidarity with others who are experiencing similar changes. In addition, the use of psychological intervention approaches, such as cognitive behavioral therapy (CBT), and mind-body techniques including biofeedback-assisted relaxation training, hypnosis, deep breathing, and coping skills training can all bring about positive change in a patient's existence [34].

Cognitive Behavioral Therapy (CBT)

Cognitive behavioral therapy (CBT), developed by Aaron Beck, is a form of therapy that combines features of both cognitive therapy and behavioral therapy that assists patients in recognizing, confronting, and changing irrational thoughts (Table 13.3). This type of therapy emphasizes the important role of thoughts and how automatic, but inaccurate thoughts or beliefs in certain situations lead to negative moods, unhealthy behaviors, and attitudes detrimental to the patient and his progression toward a constructive and adaptive lifestyle.

CBT teaches the patients to recognize and replace maladaptive behaviors with healthy, adaptive behaviors. This form of therapy is frequently used on patients with chronic pain and is especially helpful for those who suffer with comorbid psychosocial illnesses, such as depression, anxiety, or somatoform disorders. CBT encompasses a wide variety of treatments, including relaxation, biofeedback, guided imagery, and acquisition of other adaptive coping mechanisms. The treatment plan is easily adapted to the needs of the individual patient. CBT is an important therapeutic component of a multidisciplinary pain clinic program. CBT is an efficacious, cost-effective therapy for chronic pain conditions; however, it does not treat the physiological mechanisms of the pain itself. It does improve the patient's perception of the pain experience, the appraisal of the pain experience, and the subsequent coping mechanisms, as well as the ability to negate the "sick role" that often is adopted by chronic pain patients and the individual's daily functioning [34].

Mind-Body Techniques for Chronic Pain

The mind-body connection uses the power of thoughts and emotions to train the mind to control the body. The techniques include biofeedback and relaxation therapy which commonly includes diaphragmatic breathing, meditation, imagery, and autogenic training.

Biofeedback

A technique in which people are trained to learn how to control certain internal bodily processes, normally occurring involuntarily, such as heart rate, blood pressure, muscle tension, and skin temperature. The results of biofeedback are measured by electromyography (EMG) which measures muscle tension, surface electrodes which measure the galvanic skin response, thermal biofeedback which measures skin temperature, and an electrocardiograph (ECG) which measures heart rate or an electroencephalograph (EEG) which measures brain-wave activity. The patient is taught to use this information to gain control over these involuntary activities. Such biofeedback is used in pain management, assisting the patient in recognizing and controlling factors that aggravate pain. This technique helps the patient learn the connections between emotions and health, improving a patient's awareness toward his or her own body. Through the use of specific instrumentation and computers, physiologic responses are brought closer to conscious awareness and control by their conversion into auditory or visual feedback. With biofeedback, patients are commonly taught to recognize and release tension in their muscles, decrease stress response, control anxiety, slow breathing and heart rate, and raise their skin temperature. Regardless of the specific technique utilized, successful incorporation of relaxation techniques into a patient's treatment plan offers the patient more active self-management tools. The techniques are applicable to daily self-management of chronic pain, as well as during more problematic periods of flare-ups. Formal relaxation training is usually performed by certified relaxation therapist or other allied health professionals, including licensed psychologists, physical, occupational, and/ or recreational therapists.

Relaxation Therapy

The numerous clinical approaches described for biofeedback training apply equally to relaxation therapy and commonly include diaphragmatic breathing, imagery, and autogenic training. The two chief relaxation methods utilized may also be characterized as deep or brief. Deep methods include autogenic training, meditation, and progressive muscle relaxation; brief methods include paced respiration and self-control relaxation. Autogenic training is a common deep

method of relaxation therapy in which the patient imagines being in a peaceful place with pleasant body sensations. Breathing is centered and the pulse is regulated. The patient focuses on his or her body and attempts to make differing parts of the body feel heavy, warm, or cool. Elevated muscle tension has been shown to contribute to chronic musculoskeletal pain [35, 36]. Elevated muscle responses and prolonged muscle tension have also been demonstrated during physical work and stressful situations [37, 38]. A common deep method of relaxation is progressive muscle relaxation. During progressive muscle relaxation training, the patient focuses on contracting and relaxing each of the major muscle groups in attempt to better understand the feeling of tension which can then facilitate subsequent relaxation.

Breathing Techniques: People with chronic pain typically have a dysfunctional breathing pattern, due to living with anxiety, tension, stress, and pain. Abnormal breathing patterns can cause headaches, neck pain, shoulder pain, chest pain, and upper back pain. The body, breath, and mind are linked, and if there are abnormal breath patterns, they are partly due to irregularities in the mind or body. Therefore, if irregularities are eliminated from the physical breath, it has an extremely beneficial effect on the mind as well. When the breath becomes smooth, continuous, slow, and quiet, the mind comes along, also becoming calm and peaceful. The body follows, relaxing much more easily. Diaphragmatic breathing techniques are used in all parts of a functional restoration program to educate and instruct the patient on an effective and active pain management skill. Brief methods are also utilized when the patient senses an acute increase in stress or anxiety. Techniques include self-control meditation (a shortened form of progressive muscle relaxation), paced respiration (the patient breathes slowly and deliberately for a specific time period), and deep breathing (the patient takes a deep breath, holds it for 3–5 s, then slowly releases it). The sequences may be repeated several times to achieve a more relaxed state.

Meditation

Some practitioners consider meditation to be a deep method of relaxation therapy. The ultimate goal is mind-body relaxation and the passive removal of harmful thought processes. Although various forms of meditation are practiced, common forms include mindfulness meditation, transcendental meditation, yoga, and walking meditation. Mindfulness meditation involves the concentration on body sensations and thoughts that occur in the moment. The patient learns to observe these sensations and thoughts without judging them. Yoga and walking meditation are both derived from Zen Buddhism and use controlled breathing and slow, deliberate movements and postures to focus the body and mind. Transcendental meditation involves focusing on a sound or thought and the repetition of a word, mantra, or sound. As with relaxation therapies, meditation may be performed on a daily basis by patients with chronic pain to help maintain a basal level of pain control. It can also be useful in the management of acute and chronic pain "flare-ups."

Guided Imagery

Guided imagery involves the generation-specific mental images with the goal of evoking a general psychophysiological state of relaxation or other specific outcome. The visualizations are initially directed by a practitioner, with the goal of eventual self-guidance. Guided imagery is an essential part of a multi- and interdisciplinary chronic pain management programs. Persistent pain patients typically utilize guided imagery on a daily basis and may need to increase the number of sessions during acute pain "flare-ups."

Physical Medicine Treatments

Physical medicine approaches incorporated into an interdisciplinary program include interventional therapies, passive modalities (i.e., ultrasound, heat, cold), and more active physical therapy interventions including formal physical therapy-directed exercise, aerobic conditioning, strengthening, and stretching. However, the ultimate goal is to teach the patient self-management techniques to decrease and eventually eliminate the reliance upon medical intervention with the ultimate goal of a successful return to work and productivity [24].

Physical Fitness: Aerobic Conditioning, Strengthening, and Stretching

Physical fitness is defined by the American Physical Therapy Association as:

> A dynamic physical state comprising cardiovascular/pulmonary endurance; muscle strength, power, endurance and flexibility; relaxation; and body composition that allows optimal and efficient performance of daily and leisure activities.

Physical activity increases health and fitness, not only to injured body parts, but to the entire person. Exercise has been reported to improve the immune system, cardiovascular system, and digestive functioning; decrease stress levels; improve sleep patterns; and enhance mood. These physically reactivating activities have the benefit of being adaptable to both home and group settings. Physical conditioning encourages socialization in group settings such as health clubs and walking tracks. These activities can also be modified to each individual's physical activity tolerance level. Aerobic activities decrease pain, possibly through endorphin release. These activities also promote increased blood flow to the musculoskeletal system, warming muscle tissue, decreasing stiffness

through joint lubrication, increasing circulation, and improving muscle tissue health. Aerobic conditioning and encouraging physical activity has been shown to reduce disability [39], and it was found that high fear-avoiders, randomized to an exercise class, were over three times more likely at 1 year to report reduced disability, compared to those patients randomized to usual general care (in which patients took part in a back to fitness program which included 8, 1-h sessions over a 4-week period which included low-impact aerobic exercises, strengthening, and stretching) [40].

Stretching exercises allow the individual to successfully learn an important pain management tool and a way for the patient to relearn relaxed, not guarded, movement. Although research on the benefit for stretching for prevention of injury in a healthy individual varies [41], this appears to play an important role in pain management. It is important that the patient learn proper stretching techniques, combined with breathing exercises, to allow for benefit and not pain flares. Patients often report increased pain with stretching due to pushing too hard into muscle resistance and other ROM restrictions. With simple modifications and relaxation techniques, stretching can be a useful and helpful tool. Strengthening and stabilization exercises provide increased muscle tone, muscle strength gains, and normalization of demands placed on the body. Strength and stabilization gains allow decreased mechanical stress on passive structures and a shift toward correct muscle usage patterns. Initially, the strengthening program must focus on exercising in a normal movement pattern and not encouraging a learned abnormal pattern. An exercise program begins at a level that the patient can tolerate with only minimal and sometimes moderate pain flares. The exercise program is carefully balanced, as to avoid excessively aggravating activities involving the affected area, causing a prolonged worsening of symptoms rather than an improvement. This is a challenge to the therapist and the patient, as one must distinguish between fear-avoidance and true harm with activity. The approach is often to find a "happy medium," where activity and exercise (while possibly uncomfortable) are not harmful but helpful. Flare management skills, especially pacing, are used to give the patient the pain control to continue with the program.

The program is then expanded and advanced slowly, in order to allow individuals to successfully complete the activities, encouraging their progression to more strength gains. Some examples of strengthening and stabilization tools include balance exercises, use of a physioball, foam roll, and functional exercise in all three planes of motion. Unlike machine-based exercises, functional exercises and exercises focused on stabilization challenge the patient's body to allow development of the necessary strength to negotiate daily activities. More specialized PT-directed therapy for low back pain treatment may include directional preference assessment (i.e., McKenzie therapy) and neuromobilization. For those with compromised joint function, and comorbid conditions that prevent weight-bearing exercise, aquatic therapy shows benefits in edema control and decrease in stress on affected joints while increasing aerobic capacity, muscle strength, and flexibility [24]. Active therapeutic exercise should be individually assessed and adjusted with an emphasis on ensuring compliance and independence with an agreed upon home program after completion of formal therapy. Other treatments used include Tai Chi, yoga, Feldenkrais, and gait training. Typically, a comprehensive program using a combination of all of these techniques to seek the "best fit" for each patient's needs and physical level is encouraged.

Postural Training

Maintaining correct posture is more than just "standing up straight." It requires finding a balance between the head, trunk, pelvis, and lower extremity, as well as engaging the correct musculature, and maintaining this balance throughout different activities. Factors associated with postural issues include a long history of poor posture leading to an imbalance of muscle length and tone, compensatory postures, disuse syndromes, and prolonged bed rest. Suffering from chronic pain can lead to inactivity, increased down time, and prolonged bed rest, which may lead to loss of muscle strength in the postural and lower extremity musculature. Weak and compromised muscles and muscle groups are common areas of compensatory myofascial pain. Therapy can be directed at these specific areas of impairment. Determining and maintaining the correct posture, with both static and dynamic activities, requires extensive external verbal and tactile cueing, an increased sense of body awareness, and an exercise program focused on correcting the muscular imbalance.

Functional Activities

A functional restoration program focuses on supporting and promoting a patient's ability to return to being a productive member of the community, the ability to enjoy leisure activities, and successfully returning to family responsibilities. Functional activities, such as lifting, carrying, pushing/pulling, hand use and the activities performed in daily living, and leisure activities, are practiced. Treatment begins by helping the individual in assessing their current level of physical abilities in different areas. The patient then performs repetitive functional tasks, while being educated on abnormal or guarding physical movement patterns and correct body mechanics. Flare-up management, appropriate pacing, and gradual development of ability are emphasized. Often, patients are fearful of the specific activities that caused their injury, and overcoming this fear requires extensive education

and instruction. Concurrent education on anatomy, physiology, mechanical stress on the affected structures with different tasks, and that pain does not always signal damage assists the patient in working through their fear. As the patient improves, they are encouraged to assimilate these practices into their home environment, including recreational activities which also increase socialization, exercise, and the utilization of free time [24].

Wellness Therapies

Wellness is defined by the American Physical Therapy Association as "A multidimensional state of being describing the existence of positive health in an individual as exemplified by quality of life and a sense of well-being." Wellness therapies play a significant role in pain management and functional restoration. These techniques are used as flare management techniques, movement therapies, stress management skills, and coping tools. Wellness therapies include a variety of physical and mind-based techniques. Indeed, there are many different forms of mind-body relaxation approaches for pain management, but they all have the underlying purpose of connecting the mind and body through breath, allowing the person to reach a higher state of relaxation. Some techniques commonly used include imagery meditation, mindfulness-based stress reduction, breathing exercises, and progressive muscle relaxation. Movement-based wellness therapies, including Tai Chi and Qigong, provide a way to integrate relaxation into movement. Living with chronic pain can lead to guarding, muscle tension, and abnormal movement patterns. In Tai Chi and Qigong, movements are performed slowly, with deliberate and smooth movement. The focus is on breathing and creating inner stillness—quieting the mind and relaxing the body. This allows the patient to relearn how to move without guarding and tension.

Nutrition Education

As we know, proper nutrition is vital to multiple systems in the body including bone health, reducing the risk of heart disease, and controlling obesity. Diet and nutrition can also play an important role in the management of chronic pain. Certain foods such as those high in fat, sugar, and/or caffeine can intensify the pain response. In addition, some foods act as triggers for certain pain conditions, such as migraine headaches. Nutritional education not only includes the basics of nutrition, foods with anti-inflammatory properties, and the role of supplements but also topics on making smarter choices when dining out, label reading, and easy meals to prepare at home.

Treatment of Secondary Conditions

The potential for individuals suffering from a chronic pain condition to develop secondary conditions is great. Disuse syndromes, abnormal compensatory movement patterns, medications, and depression can cause weight gain and secondary myofascial disorders. These disorders are amenable to treatment. Identification of a compensatory movement pattern during the physical therapy evaluation is important. Initial treatment must focus on renormalizing movement, before strength gains or functional activity increases. It is not uncommon for patients to either show minimal gains or a decrease in current physical function, as they learn how to move in the correct pattern with normal muscle function. Nutrition counseling and education is helpful to combat the weight gain from secondary conditions. Drug, tobacco, and alcohol use are addressed as individuals adapt and adopt a healthier lifestyle. Evaluation of any sexual difficulties, sleep disturbances, or any other difficulties arising from depression, medication use, or the chronic pain syndrome should be addressed and treated [24].

Changes to the Environment

Properly adapting a patient's home and work environment and focusing on ergonomic issues and adaptive equipment in the home and in the workplace can lessen the pain and disability suffered by the chronic pain patient. Although the condition that the individual endures may not change, it is of vital importance that we treat the environment to reduce the dysfunction to a minimum. This is done in order to assure the patient's ability to function successfully, thus ensuring their best possible emotional well-being [24].

Functional Restoration Versus Other Similar Approaches (Continuum of Care)

FR with the biopsychosocial model as its basis has been proven to be the most cost-efficient therapy addressing chronic pain conditions in individuals. Because of the success of these interdisciplinary programs in treating these patients in returning them to home and work activities, there are many "programs" which call themselves interdisciplinary, but are not. These treatment programs are much less effective at treating the myriad of biological, psychological, and societal issues facing the chronic pain patient. It should not be necessary to emphasize that the reputation and outcome data from any treatment program are of vital importance.

Overview of Continuum: Parallel to Integrative Unidisciplinary Programs

Unidisciplinary programs, while incorporating treatment by physicians, psychologists, occupational, and physical therapists, may not be as effective as multidisciplinary programs [42]. Unidisciplinary programs require minimal contact within the treatment providers, usually restricted to progress reports or case histories. This kind of program is minimally effective and only as the initial treatment for patients who have been recently injured, presenting with low levels of disability and no simultaneous existing psychiatric disorders.

Work Conditioning and Work Hardening

These programs are intended for patients who, because of physical limitations, are not yet able to return to work. The American Physical Therapy Association defines "work conditioning" as a rigorous, goal-directed, work-oriented conditioning program intended to recondition musculoskeletal systems (i.e., joint integrity and mobility, muscle functioning). This includes strength and endurance, range of motion, and cardiopulmonary function. The intent of work conditioning is to increase the client's physical ability with the object of returning the individual to work. "Work hardening" is used to restore injured workers suffering from long-term injuries and disabilities, to be able to perform employment activities safely. Work hardening programs use actual or simulated work activities in a highly structured, goal-oriented individualized multidisciplinary program, intended to restore the individual's physical, behavioral, and vocational performance. These programs are geared toward increasing productivity, physical tolerance, and worker behaviors; in addition, ergonomics, job coaching, and transitional work development are also addressed. Such programs are most effective when detailed knowledge of the individual's job requirements is available, along with an in-depth understanding of the patient's physical abilities and specific deficits between his or her abilities and capabilities. An individual focus during therapy allows the gap between the end of physical therapy and the return to the workplace to be successfully bridged [24].

Early Intervention Programs

Early identification and suitable management of patients exhibiting signs of delayed recovery is believed to be an effective method of decreasing the likelihood the patient will develop a chronic pain condition. A restricted but intense early prevention program of physical rehabilitation and education allows a patient to distinguish various obstructions to healing and the eventual return to work. These early intervention programs are helpful for those who show signs of an impeded or delayed recovery and the need for instruction and psychological evaluation and intercession. The early intervention functional restoration programs are similar to the full-time FR programs, but at a lower utilization, duration, and cost than the full-time FR treatment programs. They have been found to be both therapeutically and cost-effective, relative to standard care, for low back pain patients. However, one of the difficulties found with early intervention programs is the fact that insurance companies are reluctant to authorize payment for treatment, in spite of the cost-effectiveness of early functional restoration intervention. However, there is a trend toward the identification of risk factors and early intervention by pain specialists and the willingness of insurers to pay for services [14].

Applying Team Values

Values underlying team decision making in pain rehabilitation has been found to incorporate common decision values shared by team members, workers, and stakeholders. Loisel et al. [43] describes "general values" shared by all that stress the construct that work is therapeutic, pain is multidimensional, and intervention should be graded. These values should, in turn, be shared by team members, the workers, and stakeholders. These values are facilitated by reassurance and the delivering of a single message as a way of more successfully returning a patient to work or previous level of function. These same values can be applied to many barriers presented to the individual patient and stakeholders.

The interdisciplinary team must have a broader view of the disability problem than is typically evidenced in the medical community. Communication between team members and other patient stakeholders (i.e., case manager, adjustor, family members, referring physician) may have some similar, as well as divergent or conflicting, goals. Success of the team may be determined by team values and the decision-making process (see Table 13.4). Curtis initially identified four values important to the rehabilitation team, including altruism, choice, empowerment, equality, and individualism [44]. Subsequently, important values underlying any team decision-making process have been more recently been delineated [43]. Ten common decision values were identified in an observational study of an interdisciplinary team treating injured workers. The ten identified values were divided into four categories: (1) team-related values, (2) stakeholder-related values, (3) worker-related values, and (4) general values influencing the intervention (see Table 13.5).

Table 13.4 Strategies applied by the rehabilitation team to overcome barriers to collaboration

Stakeholders	Strategies applied
Worker	Pain management
	Relaxation
	Education
	Confrontation
	Rational polypharmacy (analgesia, mood, sleep)
Employer	Education
	Asking employers onion on TRW (therapeutic return to work) setting
	Sensitize employer to the support role in relation to the worker
	Asking insurer to use its authority to exert influence on the employer
Insurer	Education
	Sensitize to the issues involved in intervention
	Clarification of the roles and objectives
	Meeting with insurer's case worker before meeting worker or employer to ensure consistency in information delivered
	Acting without interfering
	Choosing convincing information
	Asking for the case worker's support for the intervention
Physician	Inform the physician about the rehabilitation process
	Convincing him/her to take action to facilitate return to work

Adapted from Loisel et al. [43]

Table 13.5 Team-related values for IPC

Team-related values	Comments
Team unity, credibility	Key factors in taking appropriate action and enhancing worker trust
Collaboration with stakeholders	Effective for coordination of care, constraining if it hinders team decisions
Worker's internal motivation	Demonstrated by autonomy and assertiveness
Workers adherence to the program	Worker and team acting as "allies"
Worker's reactivation	Overcome fear of movement and reinjury
Single message	Regarding patient condition, goals, and action of the team
Patient and team member reassurance	While playing down distressing, less helpful information
Graded intervention	Psychological and *physical* progression in order for patient to restore confidence
Pain is multidimensional	Must also be actively controlled
Work is therapeutic	Expose patient/worker to workplace obstacles, positive relationship between worker and employer, and preparing patient for work hardening and conditioning

Adapted from Loisel et al. [43]

References

1. Andersson GBJ, Cocchiarella L, editors. The AMA guides to the evaluation of permanent impairment. 5th ed. Chicago: American Medical Association; 2000.
2. The AMA guides to the evaluation of permanent impairment. 6th ed. Chicago: American Medical Association; 2007.
3. The American Physical Therapy Association. Guide to physical therapist practice. Second edition. American Physical Therapy Association. Phys Ther. 2001;81(1):729–38.
4. International Classification of Functioning, Disability and Health (ICF). http://www.who.int/classifications/icf/en/.
5. Foley BS, Buschbacher RM. Occupational rehabilitation. In: Braddom RL, editor. Physical medicine and rehabilitation. 3rd ed. Philadelphia: Saunders/Elsevier; 2007. p. 1047–54.
6. Zimmerman M. The history of pain concepts and treatment before IASP. In: Merskey H, Loeser J, Dubner R, editors. The paths of pain. Seattle: IASP Press; 1975–2005.
7. Engle GL. The need for a new medical model: a challenge for biomedicine. Science (New Series). 1977;196(4286):129–36.
8. Engel GL. Psychogenic pain and pain-prone patient. Am J Med. 1959;26:899–918.
9. Turk DC, Monarch ES. Biopsychosocial perspective on chronic pain. In: Turk DC, Gatchel RJ, editors. Psychological approaches to pain management: a practitioner's handbook. 2nd ed. New York: Guilford; 2002. p. 3–29.
10. Gatchel RJ, Bruga D. Multi- and interdisciplinary intervention for injured workers with chronic low back pain: invited review. SpineLine. 2005. http://www.spine.org/Pages/Publications/SpineLine/PreviousIssues/2005/sle05sepoct.aspx.
11. Murphy WB, editor. Healing the generations: a history of physical therapy and the American Physical Therapy Association. Alexandria: American Physical Therapy Association; 1995.
12. Bonica JJ. Organization and function of a pain clinic. Northwest Med. 1950;49:593–6.
13. Turk DC. Biopsychosocial perspective on chronic pain. In: Gatchel RJ, Turk DC, editors. Psychological approaches to pain management: a practitioner's handbook. New York: Guilford Press; 1996. p. 33–52.
14. Brena SF. Pain control facilities: patterns of operation and problems of organization in the USA. Clin Anesth. 1985;3:183–95.
15. Sullivan MJ. Toward a biopsychomotor conceptualization of pain. Clin J Pain. 2008;24:281–90.
16. Gatchel RJ, Polatin PB, Noe CE, Gardea MA, Pulliam C, Thompson J. Treatment and cost-effectiveness of early intervention for acute low back pain patients: a one-year prospective study. J Occup Rehabil. 2003;13:1–9.
17. Gatchel R, Okifiji A. Evidence-based scientific data documenting the treatment and cost-effectiveness of comprehensive pain programs for chronic nonmalignant pain. Pain. 2006;7(11):779–93.
18. Flor H, Fyfrich T, Turk DC. Efficacy of multidisciplinary pain treatment centers: a meta-analytic review. Pain. 1992;49(2):221–30.
19. Guzman E. Multidisciplinary rehabilitation for chronic low back pain: systematic review. BMJ. 2001;322:1511–6.
20. Curry R. Understanding patients with chronic pain in work hardening programs. Work programs special interest section newsletter (American Occupational Therapy Association). 1989;3:3.
21. Wegg L. Essentials of work evaluation. Am J Occup Ther. 1960; 14:65–9.
22. Chou R, Loeser JD, Owens DK, Rosenquist RW, Atlas SJ, Baisden J, Carragee EJ, Grabois M, Murphy DR, Resnick DK, Stanos SP, Shaffer WO, Wall EM, American Pain Society Low Back Pain Guideline Panel. Interventional therapies, surgery, and interdisciplinary rehabilitation for low back pain: an evidence-based clinical practice guideline from the American Pain Society. Spine. 2009;34(10):1066–77. doi:10.1097/BRS.0b013e3181a1390d.
23. American College of Occupational and Environmental Medicine. Occupational medicine practice guidelines, chronic pain chapter update. Beverly Farms: Occupational and Environmental Medicine Press; 2008.
24. Feinberg SD, Feinberg RM, Gatchel RJ. Functional restoration and chronic pain management. Crit Rev Phys Rehabil Med. 2008; 20(3):221–35. doi:10.1615/CritRevPhysRehabilMed.v20.i3.30.
25. Gatchel RG, Mayer TG, Hazard RG, et al. Editorial: functional restoration. Pitfalls in evaluating efficacy. Spine. 1992;17:988–94.
26. Turks DC, Swanson K. Efficacy and cost effectiveness treatment of chronic pain: AN analysis and evidence –based synthesis. In: Schatman MF, Campbell A, editors. Chronic pain management guidelines for multidisciplinary program development. New York: Informa Healthcare; 2007. p. 15–38.
27. Siddall PJ, Cousins MJ. Persistent pain: a disease entity. J Pain Manag. 2007;33 suppl 2:s4–10.
28. Crombez G, Vlaeyen W, Heuts P, et al. Pain related fear is more disabling than pain itself: evidence on the role of pain-related fear in chronic back pain disability. Pain. 2005;80:329–39.
29. Vlaeyen J, Linton S. Fear-avoidance and its consequences in chronic musculoskeletal pain: a state of the art. Pain. 2000;85:17–32.
30. de Jong JR, Johan WS, Vlayen JWS, Onghena P, Goossens MEJB, Geilen M, Mulder H. Fear of movement/ (re)injury in chronic back pain education or exposure in vivo as mediator to fear reduction? Clin J Pain. 2005;21:9–17.
31. Jelinek S, Germes D, Leyckes N. The Photograph series of Daily Activities (PHODA); lower extremities [CD-ROM]. The Netherlands: Hogeschool Zuyd, University Maastricht and Institute for Rehabilitation Research; 2003 (iRv).
32. Harden N, Cohen M. Unmet needs in the management of neuropathic pain. J Pain Symptom Manage. 2003;25(5 Suppl 1):s12–7.
33. Bruel S, Chung OY. Psychological and behavioral aspects of complex regional pain syndrome management. Clin J Pain. 2006;22(5):430–7.
34. Gatchel R, Rollings K. Evidence-informed management of chronic low back pain with cognitive behavioral therapy. Spine J. 2008; 8:40–5.
35. McBerth J, Macfarfane G, Bejnamin S, et al. The association between tender points, psychological distress, and adverse childhood experiences: a community-based study. Arthritis Rheum. 1999;42:1397–404.
36. Wheeler A. Myofascial pain disorders: theory to therapy. Drugs. 2004;64:45–62.
37. Sanjsjo I, Melin B, Rissen D, et al. Trapezius muscle activity, neck, and shoulder pain, and subjective experiences during monotonous work in women. Eur J Appl Physiol. 2000;83:235–8.
38. Mork P, Westergaard R. Low-amplitude trapezius activity in work and leisure and the relation to shoulder and neck pain. J Appl Physiol. 2006;100:1142–9.
39. Linton S, van Tulder M. Preventive interventions for back and neck pain problems. Spine. 2001;26:775–87.
40. Klaber J, Carr J, Howarth E. High fear-avoiders of physical activity benefit from an exercise program for patients with back pain. Spine. 2004;29:1167–73.
41. Shrier I. Stretching before exercise; an evidence based approach. Br J Sports Med. 2000;34:324–5.
42. Gatchel RJ, Noe C, Gajarj N, Vakharia A, Polatin PB, Deschner M, Pulliam C. The negative impact on an interdisciplinary pain management program of insurance "treatment carve out" practices. J Workmans Compens. 2001;10:50–63.
43. Loisel P, Falardeau M, Baril R. The values underlying team decision making in work rehabilitation for musculoskeletal disorders. Disabil Rehabil. 2005;27:561–9.
44. Curtis RS. Values and valuing in rehabilitation. J Rehabil. 1998;64:42–7.

Pain and Spirituality

14

Allen R. Dyer and Richard L. Stieg

Key Points
- Pain is a physical symptom, but it is also more than a physical symptom.
- Spirituality (or religion) can be an important source of support and solace in times of difficulty such as facing chronic illness or pain.
- Pain may be seen as a test of faith or endurance.
- Pain and suffering may, for many people, sharpen their sense of meaning and what is important in life.
- Spirituality can be important in the life of physicians as well as in patients.

No one knows where we come from or where we go, but most of us have an intuition that there is a greater dimension that we participate in beyond our present work-----the soul's work

– David Whyte

Introduction

Teaching in the field of pain medicine seems to be dominated by emphasis on pain as a symptom. This is a natural response to the scientism that dominates our medical training, thinking, and practice. The topic of pain and spirituality affords us the opportunity to refocus our attention on the multidimensional aspects of the pain experience, as many have so eloquently done before [1–3]. We introduce our topic by posing several questions: How important is spirituality in the lives of patients? How important is the spirituality in the lives of physicians?

A.R. Dyer, M.D., Ph.D. (✉)
International Medical Corps, 1313 L. Street NW, Suite 220, Washington, DC 20005, USA
e-mail: adyer@internationalmedicalcorps.org

R.L. Stieg, M.D., MHS
1020 15th St., STE 30N, Denver, CO 80202, USA
e-mail: rstieg01@aol.com

What role does spirituality play in health/wellness, recovery from illness, and relief from suffering? How can physicians attend to patients spiritual needs? Can we understand some concepts of spiritual experience in neurophysiological terms? Can such understanding help bridge the gap between the scientific and the spiritual?

Pain and Spirituality

Pain and spirituality are terms that everyone understands, but everyone understands them uniquely. The same words may convey different meanings to different people. "Pain" and "spirituality" are laden with meaning and with ambiguity. In many ways, they are beyond the ability of words to describe. Yet it is language we must use to communicate life's innermost and most personal experiences and their close, ineffable relationship. In order to create a shared understanding that will be important to physicians, no less than patients, we will explore the layers of nuance in pain and spirituality. Especially, the conversation physicians must be prepared to have with their patients depends on some level of mutual understanding and empathy. What is pain? What is spirituality? How do we communicate our experiences of these to others? How do we understand what others intend when they try to communicate their experience to us? Pain is a universal human experience, which in the modern (or postmodern) era may be understood to be either physical or mental/emotion. The dictionary definition reflects this cultural dualism. It tells us that pain is either physical suffering or discomfort (in a particular part of the body) caused by illness or injury or that pain is mental suffering or distress (New Oxford American Dictionary). Body or mind. Either/or. It was not always this way. Aristotle thought of pain as an emotion, like joy. Descartes, who ushered in the idea of a mind-body split, considered pain a sensation. Is physical pain a different experience to emotional pain or different aspects of the same experience? There is an obvious difference between a

T.R. Deer et al. (eds.), *Treatment of Chronic Pain by Integrative Approaches: the AMERICAN ACADEMY of PAIN MEDICINE Textbook on Patient Management*, DOI 10.1007/978-1-4939-1821-8_14,
© American Academy of Pain Medicine 2015

toothache and heartache, but does it make sense to think of unpleasant experience as issuing from separate realms? We might be tempted to say from a medical point of view that pain is a symptom, a problem, something to be treated or eliminated. And often it is. But we would not wish for a world without sensation. We would not wish to eliminate the warning pains that teach a child to pull its hand away from a fire. We would not wish for a world without emotions, the joys that put our sorrows in perspective or vice versa. These are the experiences that make us human, that give life meaning. It is not always fun. It cannot be.

The question of meaning, what we might call the hermeneutics of pain, leads us to the relationship of pain and spirituality. Spirituality, like pain, is richly laden with meaning and ambiguity. For many people, spirituality can be equated with religion. For many people, their faith, their religion, provides a source of meaning and comfort and understanding. It makes life bearable. It may alleviate pain and suffering. In this sense, religion (or spirituality) becomes medically interesting. But for others, religion may be problematic, a source of dogma, discomfort, or divisiveness. So we are led to make distinctions. We look for the clear and distinct idea that so inspired Descartes, but we communicate with languages rich in nuance and ambiguity, that evoke meanings, rather than truncate them.

Religious or Spiritual?

In the latter part of the twentieth century, there has been a trend to distinguish between religion and spirituality. Older (pre-1960s) definitions of "religion" and "spirituality" typically saw the two as interpenetrating, often interchangeable concepts. Most frequently, spirituality was viewed as the intensely internalized aspects of one's espoused religion. Religion has its times of general spiritual intensification. Spirituality was often considered a path or discipline for incorporating religious precepts into one's personal living and consciousness. Spirituality's connection to religion with its theological and ritual dimensions overseen by a priesthood of some kind was considered essential to keep spirituality "within rational bounds" and not spinning out of control. Beginning with the 1970s, articles related to religion and spirituality began to appear with increasing frequency in the psychotherapy literature. Those articles that defined religion and spirituality in mutually exclusive terms tended to value spirituality and be dismissive of religion. Definitions that saw them as overlapping tended to value both [4–6].

In the current phase of intensified interest in spirituality and religion, the option of regarding oneself as "spiritual" but not necessarily "religious" has increased dramatically. "Religion" in many instances is more closely aligned with the political than with the spiritual, while spirituality retains the sense of a personal concern with meaning and transcendence. These concerns may or may not be grounded in institutional beliefs and practices. Whether this concern for the transcendent necessarily involves the sacred is a matter of personal consideration. Being captivated by a sunset, a sports team, or a political campaign is not intrinsically a spiritual experience simply because one feels connected to something larger than oneself. However, if these experiences are imbued with a sense of connection with the sacred, or ultimate reality, or things as they really are, then that would represent a spiritually significant experience. The ordinary activities of everyday life can thus become invested with spiritual meaning as is the case for a Buddhist focusing mindfully on sweeping the steps or eating a raisin, a Jew reciting a prayer while washing his hands, or a Catholic who views preparing a meal as a sacrament. In this sense, both religiousness and spirituality are seen as reflecting "the feelings, thoughts, experiences, and behaviors that arise from a search for the sacred" [4].

What might spirituality be, then, if not an approximate synonym for religious? Spirituality derives from spirits, ghosts, and the rituals that primitive cultures have developed to help cope with the feelings of lost loved ones. We now say more respectfully "traditional cultures," but our euphemism belies the connection with an unrefined, unenlightened, unscientific struggle to make sense and find meaning of a world beyond our control.

Pain and Evil

Evil stands as the antithesis of good, that which is valued. Evil is bad, and pain is disvalued, hence bad, hence evil. Evil is sometimes divided into natural evil, events beyond human control such as tsunamis and earthquakes, and man-made (human-made) evil, the bad things that people do, assaults, murders, and perhaps wars, the activities of sociopaths who act outside the bounds of conscience and civil responsibility. Illness (and pain) defies such classification. While disvalued, they are not necessarily caused unless one believes in an omnipotent being who causes everything. Such a belief challenges faith. Why would an omnipotent being cause suffering? If not as a deserved punishment, it would clearly be an injustice. This apparent contradiction is called theodicy, the vindication of divine goodness and providence in view of the existence of evil. Why would bad things happen to good people? The question is important not only for those who consider themselves religious, but for anyone who experiences suffering and tries to make sense of their experience. It is a conversation doctors should be having with patients, whose insights about their pain experiences offer clues for ways to help relieve their suffering.

The Case of Job

The Hebrew Bible (Old Testament) poses this question is the Book of Job in the context of man's relationship to God. The Hebrew Bible tells the story of a very pious and prosperous man named Job. He had seven sons and three daughters and many possessions. He constantly feared that his sons may have sinned and cursed God in their hearts, so he offered burnt offerings as a pardon for their sins. God asks Satan his opinion of Job, and Satan suggests that he is only pious because he is prosperous. God gives Satan permission to destroy Job's family and his possessions. In spite of these losses, Job remains faithful. "YHVH has given and YHVH has taken away" (Genesis 31:9). Job does not curse God, but he does question him. Satan asks for permission to afflict Job's body as well and causes Job to break out in boils. Still, he does not curse God, even when his wife urges him to do so. Job's three friends, Eliphaz, Bildad, and Zophar, believe that Job must have sinned to incite God's punishment. They believe Job must deserve his suffering because God always rewards good and punishes evil. Job's fourth friend Elihu takes a different view. He argues that Job may not have committed a specific sin for which he is being punished, but that the he is not perfect, and God as creator is such that his motives cannot be questioned by man. Elihu stresses that real repentance entails renouncing moral authority (the knowledge of good and evil), which is God alone. Elihu therefore underscores the inherent arrogance in Job's desire to "make his case" before God, which presupposes that Job possesses a superior moral standard that can be prevailed upon God. Job prays for forgiveness (for himself and his friends), realizing that he cannot understand the ways of God. His wealth is restored twofold; he is given seven more sons and three more daughters and lives to see the fourth generation.

This kind of introspection lies at the heart of one of the most successful disciplines in the treatment of addiction disorders, the 12-Step Programs of Alcoholics Anonymous and related community organizations such as Narcotics Anonymous. Although not widely used, it may have direct applicability to those suffering with chronic pain and other chronic illnesses [7].

Pain and Suffering

David Morris, in his far reaching analysis of pain in our culture, *The Culture of Pain*, has probably gone farther than anyone else in highlighting the tension and contradictions in our modern understanding of pain [8]. He observes that "The secular, scientific spirit of modern medicine has so eclipsed other systems of thought as almost to erase the memory that pain—far from registering its presence mostly in meaningless mental circuits or in some sterile, living death of hysterical numbness – once possessed redemptive and visionary powers. We need to recover this understanding partly because it shows so clearly how pain inhabits a social realm that sprawls well outside the domain of medicine." Suffering is a passive experience. Something bad or unpleasant, like pain or illness, befalls the person. What Morris is suggesting is that the interpretation of that experience may be redemptive in some way, as with the 12-step programs. Understanding this may put suffering into a different context that allows an individual to overcome it, at least conceptually, by active mastery. That taking control may be religious or spiritual or even political in some self-chosen way, a way that modern medicine may have forgotten or dismissed.

The Case of Ivan Ilych

Ivan Ilych was an ordinary man, Tolstoy tells us in his famous story, *The Death of Ivan Ilych*. He had noble qualities. He was cheerful, good-natured, and industrious. After he graduated from law school, his successes led him from one position to another, marriage, children, a nice house, and a life many might find enviable.

It was while decorating his house that he fell from a ladder, a downfall as it were, hurting his side. Pain entered his life, but it subsided. But it was followed by other sensations, a bad taste in his mouth, a pressure in his side where the pain had been. He became worried and preoccupied. He became irritable and withdrew from social activities. He stopped playing cards with his friends. He saw doctors, got prescriptions, more doctors, and more prescriptions. His pain in his side became a constant ache, which consumed his attention. His appearance changed, and this bothered him. It occurred to him that he might be dying, but his family continued to deny this possibility. He doubted his life, the reality of his accomplishments. When he realized that his life had been unalterably changed, he began to scream and he screamed for days. When death finally came, it was anticlimactic. Ivan Ilych, as he was once known, had already been dead for a long time.

Ivan Ilych's pain takes over his life so gradually that it is almost imperceptible. It is only by contrasting what he was with what he became that we appreciate how dramatic the change was. Tolstoy does not tell us exactly what was wrong with poor Ilych. He suggests that it was related temporally to the fall from the ladder, but that it might have been something different. Was it in his mind or his body or should he try to make that distinction? Tolstoy's story presents us with a distinction between the death of a person as a whole and the death of the whole person long before we began to worry about brain death.

The Role of Spirituality in the Lives of Our Patients

Larry Dossey, MD, has reviewed the world literature (more than 2,000 studies) on the role of spirituality and compassion on health stating that roughly half have shown positive statistical significance [9] and that spirituality/religious involvement correlates with decreased health problems and morbidity. He suggests that healing may be more likely to occur only in the hands of dedicated "healing experts." He discusses the famous Harvard study about intercessory prayer [10], noting while the effects of prayer in this study were statistically positive, the study could not be duplicated elsewhere. Dr. Dossey suggests that the difference was the "expertise" and good intentions of those offering the prayer in the Harvard study versus a more scientific experimental design utilizing people with less experience.

For a period of 2 years, thanks to the generosity of the owners of a private rehabilitation center where I carried out my work (RLS), we had as a regular member of the staff an ordained minister who offered both formal and informal spiritual guidance to our patients. Although a Christian minister, she was very much attuned to the spiritual needs of non-Christians and nonpracticing Christians. In addition to receiving voluntary counseling, the patients were given homework and reading assignments to help them get more in touch with their spiritual sides. Those with addiction disorders were also encouraged to actively participate in 12-step community programs. As one of my duties at this center, I conducted exit interviews on hundreds of patients who had completed this multidisciplinary pain treatment. One of my questions was a general one, "What things meant the most to you in your time here at the clinic and what was the least helpful?" Almost invariably, somewhat to my surprise, was the answer that the "minister" had by far been the most helpful. When asked why, responses like "learning to cope" and "experiencing less suffering" were common answers.

Peter Levine, author of *Waking the Tiger, Healing Trauma*, notes the emergence in many patients of spiritual epiphanies as they successfully master significant physical and emotional trauma and suggests a common physiology if healing trauma is done gradually so that suppressed "survival energy" does not emerge rapidly and overwhelm the individual. Gradual therapeutic movement in this direction provides a vital resource for helping people reengage into life after the devastation of trauma. This is a feeling experience, similar to that experienced in virtually every religious tradition, where suffering is understood as a doorway to awakening [11, 12].

The Role of Spirituality in the Working Lives of Physicians

Recent surveys and papers reflect a growing interest among physicians about spiritual issues, including mindfulness, belonging to an organized religion and formal spiritual techniques such as prayer and meditation [13–15]. In order to address those issues, many healthcare professionals have relegated the job to spiritual counselors such as hospital chaplains. We suggest, however, that the spiritual dimension of patient's lives is too important for the physician to ignore. For many pain medicine practitioners that might call for a significant paradigm shift and we would offer a new medical model of treatment to accomplish that. George Engel identified the need for "a new medical model" in 1977 [16]. The model he proposed was a biopsychosocial model intended to expand the bio-reductionistic model then in force. The bio-reductionistic model held that everything you need to know about medicine could be explained by reducing illness to its biological components. That model was extremely successful up to a point. There had been many advances in biomedicine that supported the treat-the-body-as-a-machine approach. Even organs could be replaced intact like the worn out parts of an old automobile. Now, three decades after the publication of Engel's article, we appreciate that the biological model did not explain enough. We realize how mind (and stress) affect the body-machine and how so many of the illnesses people suffer stem from behavioral causes with physiological correlates.

In defense of Engel's originality and insight, I think it could be said that spirituality is implicit in his consideration of the psychosocial. But it must also be recognized that the discussion of spirituality in modern Western thought is strained and uncomfortable. We think it could also be said that a failure to distinguish the spiritual from the religious has impeded a broader consideration of the spiritual.

In opening up the possibility of a conversation about the role of spirituality in health care, we are aware that we would need to consider everything from the array of organized religions to the most unique forms of New Age individualism. And that is precisely the point. Each patient, each person comes to medicine with his or her own unique experience and outlook and needs. And they may find their own unique path to healing. The doctor and healthcare team do not need to share the same experience, but they need to understand the uniqueness of each person's psychosocial and spiritual needs, as well as their own. The team needs to be aware of the impact their own spiritual belief systems have on their interactions with their patients.

Rachel Naomi Remen, MD, has developed a curriculum that is now used in over 30 medical schools in the United States on the subject of medical practice and spirituality [17]. She also offers ongoing retreats for doctors on this same subject who either wish to teach the subject or who have become in some way dispirited themselves and are in need of refreshing [18]. At one of these weeklong seminars, one of the authors (RLS) was introduced to the simple practice of starting each day with yoga and meditation and "remembering to dedicate oneself each day in practice to our patients." In the course of doing this, one becomes more mindful of patients' needs and a better listener. I would submit that this is an informal spiritual practice that, sadly, many healthcare practitioners have abandoned or never even thought about. Indeed, in a series of focus groups held 10 years ago by the National Pain Foundation patient's suffering with chronic pain repeatedly stated that among their greatest needs were healthcare professionals who would listen to them and validate their pain and suffering; something they felt had been sorely missing in their lives. In addition to starting my workday in the manner above, I have also gotten into the habit of setting a quiet place in my office to talk with patients. We both have an easy chair in between which sits a lamp table with a lighted scented candle (which is quickly extinguished for my migraine and chemically sensitive patients), creating a sense of peacefulness and calmness which the patients very much seem to appreciate.

But what of our strong scientific training background? As a society, we value what we can count. We value scientific proof that something is of benefit before it's socially acceptable. Patients, too (even those who consider themselves on a spiritual pathway), may draw strength by having their subjective experiences validated by the tools of science [19].

Is There a Neurophysiologic Basis for Spiritual Experience?

Andrew Newberg, MD, Associate Professor of Radiology and Psychiatry, University of Pennsylvania, discusses the difficulty in matching subjective experiences (which are so variable among individuals and cultures) and objective measures [20]. Neurophysiological changes such as can be measured with functional MRI (fMRI) only capture some of the picture but show that a vast network of brain structures get involved with such practices as prayer and meditation. For example, parietal lobe structures deactivate as practitioners experience a sense of losing themselves while at the same time limbic areas such as the amygdala and hippocampus become active with intense spiritual/emotional experiences. So, too, are there measurable levels in hormones during such experiences.

James Austin, MD, Clinical Professor of Neurology at the University of Missouri-Columbia, is an academic neurologist. Dr. Austin has studied in Delhi, India, and Kyoto, Japan. His highly technical and intellectual discussion in the book *Measuring the Immeasurable* [21] offers the reader more in-depth discussion of the complexities of the science behind our subject. However, all of our growing understanding of the neurophysiology associated with spiritual experience still begs the question of why humans were given this gift of transformative mind.

Putting Spirituality into Everyday Practice

Death, loss suffering, and pain are all part of the human condition. Though we may lament, rail, and complain, we as human beings cannot escape their inevitability. Our challenge is what to do and how to understand in the face of a fate that is almost unbearable and unacceptable. Physicians and healers attending to those who suffer must be mindful of what their patients suffer. As technicians, it would be nice to be able to remove afflictions, and sometimes, this is possible, but more often, it is the task of the healer to help the patient bear what cannot be removed. For each of us, part of the task is coming to comprehend how to live a life that might be less than what we would hope for. That struggle takes time and has been articulated in a number of ways, some of which are illustrated in Table 14.1 [22, 23].

The notion that when faced with a loss or diagnosed with a serious illness, people go through a series of "stages" has become widespread in lay and professional circles [24]. There are no invariant rules, and several nomenclatures illustrate the process. Immediately, people tend to experience some sense of shock, denial, or at least disbelief that such a thing could happen. Almost all descriptors convey some sense of anger, which may be one of the most problematic emotions and difficult to deal with, especially if it is displaced, as it often may be, on the person trying to be helpful and responsive. It may be one of the most difficult things for physicians to deal with. Some sort of sadness, depression, and self-pity may follow, especially if open communication of feelings is not encouraged or tolerated. Eventually, one may come to some sort of acceptance, which does not necessarily mean that everything is alright, but rather that the inevitable reality is acknowledged. For physicians and health professionals, the task faced is how to attend to such suffering. How should one enter into conversation with patients? Are there questions to be asked? Comments to be made? A general rule would be to start with open-ended questions, and LISTEN. Let the person narrate his or her own experience. Avoid judging or being prescriptive. These are challenging and sensitive areas because the basis for empathy is our experience even as we realize that

Table 14.1 Stages of faith and child development [22, 23]

Age group	Fowler's stages of faith	Developmental stages (Erikson and Piaget)	Key attributes
Infancy	Undifferentiated faith	Trust vs. mistrust (Erikson)	Development of basic trust through relationship with parents or primary caregivers; attachment sets the stage for future relationships
		Sensorimotor (Piaget)	Consistency and dependability of caregiving responses and rituals counter feelings of anxiety and mistrust
			Experiences mediated through senses and physical exploration
Early childhood	Intuitive-projective faith	Autonomy vs. shame *followed by* initiative vs. guilt (Erikson)	Literal and concrete thinking
		Preoperational (Piaget)	Imitative, reflects religious beliefs and behaviors of parents/caregivers
			Beginning to develop a sense of right and wrong, drawn to clear-cut representations of good and evil
			May judge things, experiences, or self according to outcome – e.g., viewing illness as a punishment; poor understanding of cause and effect
			Concerned about security, safety, and the power of caregivers to protect
School years	Mythic-literal faith	Industry vs. inferiority (Erikson)	Fairness is an important construct in understanding the world
		Concrete operations (Piaget)	Beginning to take on the stories, beliefs, and observances that symbolize belonging to one's community
			Superstition and magical thinking may be evident, but symbols and concepts remain concrete and literal
			Fuller understanding of cause and effect
			Increasing ability to separate own perspective from that of others
			Beginning to recognize that rewards and punishments do not necessarily correlate to actions ("bad things happen to good people")
Adolescence into young adulthood	Synthetic-conventional faith *followed by* individuative-reflective faith	Identity vs. role confusion (Erikson)	Development of abstract thinking, flexibility of perspective taking
		Formal operations (Piaget)	Sense of identity and "inferiority" are utmost concerns
			Ability to integrate diverse and even contradictory elements into self-identity
			Attachment to beliefs and personal expression of significant people in their lives
			Dependence on others for validation of and clarity about one's identity
			Experience of the world extends beyond the family to school, work, peers, "street society," the media
			Search for identity may include questioning beliefs and practices of family
			Toward end of this stage, critical reflection leads to intentional choices and renewed clarity about personal ideology and belief systems

others may experience and understand things differently, especially in spiritual matters.

Table 14.1 offers a developmental approach, which places Fowler's stages of faith alongside stages of psychological (and physical) development. Table 14.2, stages of grief (words for feelings), indicates some of the feelings people often report in the weeks or months after experiencing a loss or health diagnosis. Table 14.3, the FICA Spiritual History Tool, could be adopted for office use and suggests some widely used approaches to thinking of human development [25]. The stages offer the practitioner self-discipline to minimize assumptions about how someone should behave or respond. Developmental and stage theories help expand the assessment of the patient as an empathic aid to understanding what their world might be like. For example, to say that

Table 14.2 Stages of grief (words for feelings)

Denial	Denial	*Unglaube* (disbelief)
Anger	Anger	*Zorn* (anger)
Bargaining	Accusatory	*Selbstmitleid* (self-pity)
Depression	Self-accusatory	*Traurigkeit* (sadness)
		Gott flehend (pleading with God)
Acceptance	Acceptance	*Anerkennung* (Acknowledgment)

From Kubler-Ross [24]

someone is being "childish" can be harsh and judgmental. To realize that in the face of a threatening illness, even an adult may struggle, and to approach their suffering in a sympathetic and helpful manner may be the best that one can offer.

Table 14.3 The FICA Spiritual History Tool

"How would you like me, your healthcare provider, to address these issues in your healthcare?"
The FICA Spiritual History Tool
F – Faith and Belief
"Do you consider yourself spiritual or religious?" or "Do you have spiritual beliefs that help you cope with stress?" If the patient responds "No," the healthcare provider might ask, "What gives your life meaning?" Sometimes patients respond with answers such as family, career, or nature.
I – Importance
"What importance does your faith or belief have in our life? Have your beliefs influenced how you take care of yourself in this illness? What role do your beliefs play in regaining your health?"
C – Community
"Are you part of a spiritual or religious community? Is this of support to you and how? Is there a group of people you really love or who are important to you?" Communities such as churches, temples, and mosques, or a group of like-minded friends can serve as strong support systems for some patients.
A – Address in Care
The FICA Spiritual History Tool [25]

Ethics, Pain, and Spirituality

Religion and spirituality are for many a main source for ethical values, reasoned and understood. For the health professional, shared ethical norms orient healing activities in a way that patients, clients, or consumers can depend on the person from whom they seek help. The principle of beneficence, respect for autonomy and self-determination, informed consent, confidentiality, and competence are all norms which have governed professional behavior at least since the time of Hippocrates.

One ethical principle demands special attention in the area of religion and spirituality: the respect for boundaries. This is most basically seen in the proscription against sexual activity with patients. Also, it is the basis for the prohibition against entering into a business relationship or other dual relationship. It stems from the recognition that the patient is a different person, not an extension of the professional and not available for the gratification or exploitation of the professional. This can be problematic in the area of dependency relationships, where in fact the patient does need the expertise of the professional. It is ethically incumbent on the professional to recognize that need and not exploit it.

Another boundary that is important for the professional to recognize is the spiritual boundary. If the professional has strong religious beliefs, he or she must be careful not to attempt to impose them – even subtly – on the patient, realizing that we are not in a position to understand the mysteries of the ultimate.

Summary

We hope the preceding discussion will encourage a significant paradigm shift in the world of pain medicine today. Pain is much more than a medical problem, and medical attempts to eliminate or alleviate pain must also account for the complexities of human suffering. Medicine alone does not solve the problem of pain. Our scientific quest to conquer pain only underscores the reality of its complexity and heightens its mystery. The founders of the American Academy of Pain Medicine (formerly the American Academy of Algology) understood and emphasized the multidimensional nature of pain and the strong need for multidisciplinary approaches to its evaluation and treatment. There have been many scientific advances in the subsequent decades since most of which have shifted the focus of attention once again to pain as a symptom, subject to potential eradication by the wonders of our technology and pharmacologic prowess. These advances need to be coupled with a reawakening about the other important dimensions of pain, including the spiritual. There are many roadblocks to doing so [26]. The training of the postmodern twenty-first century pain medicine physician should reemphasize the importance of psychosocial and spiritual treatment if we are to achieve our goal as a truly unique medical specialty.

References

1. Chapman CR, Turner J. Psychological and psychosocial aspects of acute pain. In: Bonica JJ, Loeser JD, Chapman CR, Fordyce WE, editors. The management of pain. 2nd ed. Philadelphia: Lea & Febiger; 1990. p. 122–33.
2. Turk D, Stieg A. Chronic pain: the necessity of interdisciplinary communication. Clin J Pain. 1987;3:163–7.
3. Stieg RL, Williams RC. Chronic pain as a biosociocultural phenomenon, implications for treatment. Semin Neurol. 1983;3:370.
4. Grosch W. Reflections on cancer and spirituality. South Med J. 2011;104(4):249–305.
5. Newberg A, editor. Why God won't go away: brain science and biology of belief. New York: Ballantine Publishing Group; 2001.
6. Rippentrop EA, Altmaier EM, Chen JJ, Found EM, Keffala VJ. The relationship between religion/spirituality and physical health, mental health and pain in a chronic pain population. Pain. 2005;1(16):311–21.

7. Cleveland M, editor. Chronic illness and the 12 steps. A practical approach to spiritual resilience. Center City: Hazelden Publishing; 1999.
8. Morris D, editor. The culture of pain. Berkeley: University of California Press; 1991.
9. Dossey L. Compassion and healing. In: Goldman D, Small G, editors. Measuring the immeasurable. The scientific case for spirituality. Boulder: Sounds True, Inc.; 2008. p. 47–60.
10. Chibnall JT, Jeral JM, Cerullo MA. Experiments in distant intercessory prayer: God, science, and the lesson of Massah. Arch Intern Med. 2001;161:2529–36.
11. Levine P. Trauma and spirituality. In: Goldman D, Small G, editors. Measuring the immeasurable. The scientific case for spirituality. Boulder: Sounds True, Inc.; 2008. p. 85–100.
12. Levine P. Waking the tiger, healing trauma. Berkeley: North Atlantic Press; 1996.
13. Fung G, Fung C. What do prayer studies prove? Christ Today. 2009;53(5):43–4.
14. Büssing A, Michalsen A, Balzat HJ, Grünther RA, Ostermann T, Neugebauer EA, Matthiessen PF. Are spirituality and religiosity resources for patients with chronic pain conditions? Pain Med. 2009;10:327–39.
15. Büssing A, et al. Spirituality, therapeutic self-efficacy and interest in patients. J Explore Sci and Heal. 2009;5(3):150–1.
16. Engel GL. The need for a new medical model: a challenge for biomedicine. Science. 1977;96(4286):129–36.
17. Remen RN, O'Donnell J, Rabow MW. The Healer's art: education in meaning and service. J Cancer Educ. 2008;23:65–7.
18. Remen R. Graduate physician CME curriculum: detoxifying death. The institute for the study of health and illness at Commonweal. http://www.commonwealhealth.org/?s=detoxifying+death
19. Simon T. An introduction to the scientific case for spirituality. In: Goldman D, Small G, editors. Measuring the immeasurable. The scientific case for spirituality. Boulder: Sounds True, Inc; 2008. p. IX–XI.
20. Newberg A. Spirituality, the brain and health. In: Goldman D, Small G, editors. Measuring the immeasurable. The scientific case for spirituality. Boulder: Sounds True, Inc.; 2008. p. 349–72.
21. Austin J. Selfless insight – wisdom: a thalamic meaning. In: Goldman D, Small G, editors. Measuring the immeasurable. The scientific case for spirituality. Boulder: Sounds True, Inc.; 2008. p. 211–30.
22. Erikson EH. Childhood and society. New York: Triad Paladin Press; 1977.
23. Fowler JW, Dell ML. Stages of faith and identity: birth to teens. Child Adolesc Psychiatr Clin N Am. 2004;13(1):17–33.
24. Kubler-Ross E, Kessler D. On grief and grieving: finding the meaning of grief through the 5 stages of loss. New York: Simon and Schuster; 2005.
25. The FICA Spiritual History Tool. The George Washington University Institute for Spirituality and Health. 2012. www.gwish.org. Accessed 23 Jan 2012.
26. Dubois M, et al. Pain medicine position paper. Pain Med. 2009;10(6):972–1000.

Pain Disparity: Assessment and Traditional Medicine

15

September Williams

Key Points
- Pain and other health and health-care disparities are related.
- Pain disparity refers to both unequal distribution of increased pain and decreased effective pain care.
- Pain disparity assessment modifies the standard pain assessment to improve pain care.
- Traditional medicine provides a guide to culturally relevant patient-centered pain management.

Introduction

Millions of people in the world have acute and chronic pain because of (1) ignorance of clinicians, (2) lack of a standardized scientific approach, (3) failure to facilitate adequate treatment of pain by legitimate use of opiates, (4) inadequate balance between use of controlled substances for medical purposes and the prevention of their abuse, and (5) lack of appropriate use of the new non-opiate pharmaceuticals and integrative medicine armamentaria which has expanded over the past decade [1, 2]. Of ten developed countries, World Health Organization (WHO) has estimated that 37 % of adults in these populations have constant pain conditions [3]. Pain is a public health concern because of its prevalence and increasing incidence. In 2010, in the United States, adults with constant pain were conservatively estimated at 16 million [4].

S. Williams, M.D. (✉)
Clinical Medical Ethics, Palliative Care and Film, Ninth Month Consults, 401 Pine Street, Unit D, Mill Valley, CA 94941, USA
e-mail: september.ninthmonth@gmail.com

Pain Disparity

Pain disparity refers to both increased pain and decreased effective pain care. Risk of poor pain care is proportional to the presence of pain itself, particularly when chronic. Pain is an arena of health and health-care disparity because its presence and inadequate management disproportionately affect subgroups of the US and world population (Table 15.1). When groups of people are compared, it may not be possible to clarify causal pathways directly causing differences in health. However, it is well documented that Black and Hispanic peoples are more disadvantaged by health disparities specifically through the mechanism of racism [5]. Racism, how an individual is defined by appearance, is an independent determinant for the quality of health, healthcare, and by corollary pain care [6]. Through racism, ethnic peoples of color are more disadvantaged by health disparities.

Pain Disparity: Oriented Pain Assessment

A given health-care disparity is most easily identified when there is a clear reference point for what is appropriate and reasonable to expect [7]. Palliative medicine literature establishes that it is appropriate and reasonable to expect that most pain can be brought under control by using basic principles of pain management [8]. The best current practice standard of pain medicine is appropriate to expect. However, current best practice pain assessment may not be sufficient for quality care where pain is combined with maximum vulnerability for other unequal health and healthcare.

Controlled chronic pain can be demonstrated by improved patient function, physiologic, emotional, and social comfort. Pain management, falling short of what is reasonable to expect when best practice standards are applied, leads to suspect pain disparity. The pain disparity assessment modifies

Table 15.1 Groups at risk for pain disparity

These vulnerable subgroups include those:
Having English as a second language
Being among ethnic peoples of color
With low income or poor education
Being women or transgender
Old or young
Disabled
Living in the inner city or rural areas
Being veterans from the United States Military
Adapted from Blyth [4]

Table 15.2 Effects of palliative care consultation

Sense of well-being and dignity
Information exchange and communication with the clinician
Respect for the patient treatment preferences
Emotional and spiritual support of patients and their families
Management of distressing symptoms
Choice of care
Access to outpatient, benefits, and services
Adapted from Casarrette et al. [9, pp. 368–381]

the standard pain assessment by considering communication, poverty, health literacy, shared decisional capacity, informed consent, patient concerns about addiction, and unaddressed biopsychosocial needs.

Communication

Pain disparity may be lessened through palliative care consultation. Palliative care consultation enhances communication. The family assessment of treatment at end of life (FATE) was used to compare palliative care consultation with other clinicians managing pain. In one study, care was perceived best with palliative care consults for a variety of reasons (Table 15.2). Effects of palliative care consultation were not race or ethnically related. Improved communication, even for those dying, decreases the negative effect of health-care and health disparities on pain and distressing symptom management across race and ethnic subgroups [9].

Experience and education aside, palliative care consultants may compensate for a key institutional shortcoming of most health-care systems, lost focus on clinician-patient communication under duress of time. Consultants frequently have more dedicated individual time per patient encounter than primary care clinicians. A pain assessment requires patient or proxy interviews exploring loss of function, other distressing symptoms, and pain's relation to them. Emotional, social, psychological, and economic burdens need be explored at the initial evaluation and then re-explored in subsequent encounters. Ultimately, it is the primary care physician who has the long view of a person's chronic pain management failures and successes [10]. Pain consultants assist in prioritizing associated concerns.

Rigorous initial pain assessment should be visible to patients. This, along with continuity of approach in subsequent assessments, provides a shared shorthand for communicating about pain. Pain assessment, like the physical examination, demonstrates to the patient due diligence, a caring and believing clinician. Relevant to communication, the pain assessment can cultivate a working relationship and language between clinician and patient cultures.

Clinician deficit perspectives, associated with deficits in cross cultural or language of communication, may drive poor pain assessment. Patients uncomfortable in the medical culture may present with apparent stoicism, excited expression, or historically appropriate distrust. Observing and responding to these presentations appropriately improve communication.

Poverty

Risk of poverty corresponds with being a person of color in the United States. An analysis of poverty finds nearly a 1:4 ratio of poverty for African Americans, "nonwhite" Hispanic Americans, and Native Americans. This rate is roughly 25 % of the respective populations. In comparison, 13 % of all Americans live in poverty. The highest rates of US poverty are among those living in inner city and rural areas [11]. All ethnic peoples of color are not poor. Nonetheless, most ethnic peoples of color have a disproportionately high risk for chronic pain and pain disparity.

Poorly managed acute pain often leads to persistent pain. Persistent pain can cause loss of function associated with poor employment, decreased educational capacity, and cross generational illiteracy. Clinicians will see pain disparity next to fiscal stress. Pain clinicians need to know that level of fiscal stress relates to medication access, transportation to appointments, basic utilities like telephones, and child care needs while participating in pain therapies. Appropriate social services referrals can diminish some poverty-related effects on poor pain management.

Health Literacy

Limited health literacy is prevalent and associated with low socioeconomic status and poor access to healthcare. Health literacy is defined as the degree to which individuals have the capacity to obtain, process, and understand basic health information and services needed to make appropriate health decisions [12]. Low health literacy is an independent risk factor for health disparities, particularly in older people, who are also disproportionately affected by pain [13]. A pain disparity assessment clarifies a patient's educational level, numerical and reading literacy. Verbal English literacy may mask variable capacity to read and write; particularly in inner-city communities, the elderly and those whose home language is not English. Pain rating scales can serve as an equalizing tool. Commonly, a numerical scale from 1 to 10 is used [14]. Unfortunately, numerical pain scales may be difficult for those with low mathematical, language, and health literacy.

If a patient seems unable to learn the 1–10 scale the clinician should explore that this may herald low health literacy. With this recognition of low health literacy appropriate selection of pain scale can be determined. A common adjustment is to convert the register of the scale to 1–5. The altered scale is multiplied by the clinician to reflect the 1–10 scale. This should be done with notation in the chart. Care should be taken so that other clinicians do not misinterpret a patient report of 5 as moderate pain associated with 5/10, instead of severe pain of 5/5. Each subsequent clinician should follow the same pain assessment scale. Simultaneous notation should be made about patient numerical health literacy.

The numerical pain scale can be substituted with a picture scale in low literacy, cognitive impairment, and children [15]. Picture scale efficacy does not seem as good as the numeric scale. Pictures must be appropriately interpreted in a cultural or age context. For persons with advanced dementia, without speech, or in vegetative states, a pain score can be calculated based on subtle observations of physical distress. Pain interpretation of distress in this population is often best in the hands of caregivers, family, or certified nurse assistants, not the clinician. Whatever pain scale used and therapy anticipated, the pain rating is translated into the language of mild, moderate, or severe pain. This facilitates appropriate initial management, choice of integrative therapies, dose of medication, and procedures.

Shared Decisional Capacity and Informed Consent

Where appropriate, a formal contract should be establish for pain management with patients. When a patient is asked to enter into a pain management contract, there is an extra burden placed on clinicians to assess decisional capacity. Where risk is high, stringency of consent is also high. The two-tiered model of shared decisional capacity may be helpful to gage patient clinician understanding of specific therapies [16]. This tiered approach discloses the risks and benefits of the therapy and considers barriers to explore when understanding of disclosure is blocked. Some of these barriers may be reversible if the clinician and the patient understand their existence (Table 15.3).

Table 15.3 Two-tiered assessment of shared decisional capacity

Tier one: disclosure	Tier two: barriers to disclosure
Patient/proxy is able to express	Clinician considers
Medical indication	Physiological states (anoxia, dementia, aphasia)
Expected outcome with therapy	Drugs (prescription/illicit)
Expected outcome without therapy	Pain
Alternative therapies	Stages of death, dying, or grief
Voluntary acceptance of proposed therapy	Educational differences (language, literacy, integrative medicine integration toward complimentary therapies)
	Institutional chauvinisms (ageism, sexism, genderism, classism, professionalism, colonialism, racism)

Modified from Dula and Williams [16], Emanuel [17]

The WHO stepwise escalation of drug therapy for pain is based on the pain rating scale [18]. Understanding the value of a patient's previous attempts at pain management, integrative or not, determines the validity of stepwise pain recommendations. Beginning at the lowest level of opiate may not be appropriate, often true for cancer pain and those with established reasons for opiate tolerance or addiction. Use of opiates may be precluded by previous pain management history.

Regardless of the therapy, once pain is being treated, there needs to be a follow-up at relatively close interval [19]. This is particularly for those in health-care underserved settings using opiates as part of therapy as time between clinic appointments may be prolonged. Telephone or email is being increasingly used for initial follow-up. Pain left unmanaged pushes the neurological response toward constant pain. Follow-up pain assessment and documentation (PAD) is best when including the four domains: analgesia, activity or function, [20] adverse effects (constipation, respiratory depression, sedation, myoclonus, delirium, urinary retention, drowsiness), and aberrant behaviors [21]. Drug-related aberrant behaviors include drug seeking because of pseudo addiction insufficient analgesia resulting in clock watching, tolerance cycle, or addiction.

Addiction Concerns

The National Institute of Drug Abuse (NIDA), of the National Institutes of Health, recommends assessment of addition potential by screening for cigarettes, alcohol, and illicit drug abuse. The screening involves the ask, advise, assess, assist, and arrange (addiction specialist) approach [22]. Each racial, ethnic, age, and gender group has been explored by NIDA for prevalence of addictive behavior by substance abused.

For instance, in the United States, African Americans and Americans of European descent have the same prevalence of 6 % addictive behavior and illicit drug abuse. NIDA believes, as an example, racial profiling results in statistical over representation of African Americans in the prison system related to drug abuse.

For those with pain and present addiction or risks, an honest plan needs to be made for pain management. The plan requires knowing the person's base opiate use, efficacy of previous therapies, treatment contracts, and commitment by clinicians to arrange substance abuse treatment. Community resources or state medical board opiate monitoring systems should be used to learn the truest history of prescribed opiates. If methadone maintenance for addiction is in place, it should continue at the same dosage and received at the outpatient facility assigned. The usual dose of methadone should not be changed, baring high side effect profile. Additional opiates of choice may be added to the methadone for pain management.

Refusal of appropriate therapy by those without addiction potential may accentuate pain disparity. Pain left unmanaged often results in a persistent pain cycle. In intact communities of color, there seems a burden of responsible people to not want to leave a legacy of weakness by the use of opiates or to avoid tainting the body with drugs.

Pain and Diseases of Health Disparities

Many diseases of health-care disparities have pain as a fellow traveler. Acute pain is related to discrete events, better localized and so is less evasive. The specialty of emergency medicine has been aggressive about research on acute care pain disparity [23]. Advances in pain science may shift a disease's pain category. An example of such a shift is changing the pain classification of rheumatoid arthritis from the chronic pain category to the more accurate recurrent.

Persistent pain is referred to as chronic pain. Persistent pain is more indolent with a source less easily defined than acute pain. Chronic malignant pain includes cancer, HIV/AIDS, amyotrophic lateral sclerosis (ALS), multiple sclerosis, end-stage organ failure, advanced chronic obstructive pulmonary disease, advanced congestive heart failure, and Parkinsonism. Chronic nonmalignant pain encompasses chronic musculoskeletal pain such as spinal pain or low back pain, chronic degenerative arthritis, osteoarthritis, rheumatoid arthritis, myofascial, chronic headache, migraine, and bone pain. Significantly, this group also tends to be frequently ambiguously reported because it has a neuropathic component associated with nerve compression and visceral pain [24].

Persistent pain occurs more frequently in those with health and health-care disparities. When pain is ascribed to an underlying disease, it tends to be more accepted as "real" by a scientifically based medicine system. An example is the validation of pain in HIV/AIDS leading to the realization that pain is the second most reported symptom, just behind fever, in AIDS. For many ethnic peoples of color, the scientific basis for pain is less meaningful than the nonphysical suffering pain causes. The health-care community should be aware that its response to undefined pain ranges from care and compassion to judgmental, sometimes devolving into blaming or inappropriate personalization of responsibility [25].

Choice of Pain Therapies

Clinicians caring for people with persistent pain should carefully review and educate themselves about pain relevant reimbursement coding systems. The complexity of the biopsychosocial issues of pain disparity require more diagnostic and treatment time in individuals with multiple health disparities. Clinical pharmacy specialist, social workers, nurses, and behavioral medicine consultants may need clinician support to access indicated medications and therapies. There is a growing understanding that medications alone are frequently inadequate to decrease persistent pain disparity.

Research supports the effectiveness of self-management programs in pain care. A meta-analysis of 17 self-management education programs for arthritis found that they achieved small but statistically significant reductions in pain ratings and reports of disability [26]. Self-Management occurs with or without clinician involvement through emotional, social, and media influences. Formal clinical assistance likely provides better targeted outcomes. Programs have combined pain self-management with therapy for depression, in cancer pain patients [27]. Convenience of schedule, location, and frequency of programs significantly improves participation rates. An individual's reinforced belief that they can control their own pain is a strong determiner for successful pain management [28].

Emotion and pain are closely tied. Harnessing positive emotions shows improvement in pain. Pain, [29] anxiety, depression, and fear form a vicious cycle one entity feeding on the other [30]. Anger is prominent for those in pain. Anger is often directed at health-care providers, significant others, and insurance companies. Of great concern is that studies show anger more manifest as self-loathing than directed at others [31]. Therapies which improve emotional competency, like cognitive behavioral or group therapy, are important adjuncts in pain management. Expressed emotion is a window to pain perception. Cultural transparency in emotional expression between clinicians and patients is required before appropriate psychological support can be provided.

Traditional Medicine and Patient-Centered Care

Increasingly, pain is considered a disease and not simply a distressing symptom. Disease prevention and management are profoundly influenced by community engagement [32]. Community engagement requires culturally relevant care; those who have the problem may have the solution. Traditional medicine provides a guide to culturally relevant, patient-centered care. Among those at highest risk for healthcare disparities are Native, Hispanic, African, and monolingual non-English-speaking Asian Americans.

The majority of the world's people use traditional medicine as their primary care. Traditional medicine is "the health practices, approaches, knowledge and beliefs incorporating plant, animal and mineral-based medicines, spiritual therapies, manual techniques and exercises, applied singularly or in combination to treat, diagnose, and prevent illnesses or maintain well-being" [33]. When traditional medicine is used by medical systems outside of the culture of its origin, it is called complimentary or alternative medicine. When the former is used in conjunction with allopathic medicine, it is called integrative medicine. Traditional medicine is based on nonscientific systems and knowledge which have evolved over thousands of years. The cultural practitioner of traditional medicine operates from a shamanistic base, traversing both the physical and the spiritual world. Traditional medicine seeks to create care that incorporates whole patient principles and is closely allied with patient-centered care [34]. In traditional medicine, the healing dialog often exists in the arena of spirituality.

Culture is how a group of individuals define themselves. A person's expression, tolerance, and understanding of the meaning of pain are related to culture [35]. Culture tells people how to behave in relationship to pain [36]. Exploration of cultural touchstones provides a means of initiating a cross-cultural exchange between clinicians and patients about pain. A mnemonic for cultural touchstones is family, spirituality, struggles, and icons of culture (FaSSI).

There is rarely a separation between traditional medicine and spirituality. Consciousness raising therapies like meditation, prayer, and yoga are used in all traditional medicine systems. Spiritual assessment tools can clarify personal cultural values and probable acceptance of traditional medicine by a patient [37]. Among these tools is HOPE: what gives hope, organized religion, preferred response to spirituality, effects of spirituality on illness, pain, and suffering. Another similar spiritual assessment is FICA: faith and beliefs, importance of spirituality to life, community of spiritual support, addressing of spirituality by the clinician. More general cultural familiarity can be found through exploring a cultural or individual resonance with screen narratives, books, and arts [38, 39].

There are specific current and historical struggles affecting communities of health disparities. Some of these struggles deteriorate the biopsychosocial-spiritual axis in a way described as a cultural posttraumatic syndrome [40]. This deterioration, when manifest by escalating nonresponse to allopathic pain management, should prompt consideration of traditional or integrative medicine therapy. Cultural icons and associated rituals provide a shorthand for recognizing a person's identification with a culture. The significance of icons to an individual provides a gentle entree to cross culture exchange between patients and clinicians.

Applying FaSSI allows review of Native American, Hispanic, African, and Asian American traditional medicine. The goal is to provide examples of cross-cultural information about traditional medicine important to pain clinicians during epidemic pain disparity.

Native American Traditional Medicine

In the United States, Native Americans include Alaskan Natives. Applying FaSSI allows review of Native American traditional medicine in relationship to Hispanic, African, and Asian Americans. Though in the US Native Americans include Alaskan Natives, it is the people of the lower 48 states who underscore the historic, cultural, and genetic intersections of those most burdened by health disparities.

Family: Extended family is a crucial factor in the life of Native Americans. Kinships are increased through marriage and adoption rituals. Most American Indian households, until recently, consisted of at least three-generation families. This means that a Native American baby boomer was likely in direct contact with elders born at the turn of the last century. Elder generations frequently are more deeply tied to core cultural practices and values. Family is essential in helping people recover from illness, ameliorating pain and suffering. Family extends to ancestors and clan relationships. It is considered important to have family close at hand when one is hospitalized. Strength is drawn from having support of significant individuals to reaffirm identity. Reflection of the role of family in settling suffering and its cousin, grief, is seen in some ancient Native American practices of burying babies in the home of their bereaved parents. Now, modern parents keep the spirits of their babies from wandering too far by making photographs [41].

Spirituality: A medicine man or woman guides the ailing person to approaches which allow rebalancing between self, nature, and the supernatural. Native religion believes that the Great Spirit is manifested by the natural environment and kinship relationships. Symptoms of illness, like pain, are brought to the attention of a medicine person after trying customary local folk remedies, herbs and procedures. These initial treatments usually derive from the natural environment.

If symptoms do not resolve, the person needs both natural and supernatural assistance. The medicine people provide this combined level of care, being both priest and physician. The medicine person uses rituals to communicate with the Great Spirit, through nature or supernatural intermediaries [42]. There are many spiritual healing forms in Native American culture including the medicine wheel, which is a 10,000-year-old tool. Each Native American tribe has a variation. The medicine wheel of the Lakota people is an example.

The Lakota originates from the lands now occupied largely by the Dakota states. The home geography influences the interpretation of the medicine wheel. The medicine wheel is a circle divided into four equal quarters. The spokes of the wheel each represents direction: north, south, east, and west. The center of the wheel represents "self, balance, harmony, and learning." The quarters of the wheel represent parts of the self's natural, spiritual, and emotional universe. It also describes races of people. Each quadrant has a color. The colors of the quadrants are white, yellow, black, and red. Red symbolizes the South, red people, heart, and emotion. Yellow symbolizes yellow people, the East, sun, spiritual, and values. Black represents black people, the West (where the sun sets), the earth, the physical, and the action. White stands for the North, white people, snow, wind, brain, mental, and decisions [43].

The medicine wheel clarifies the direction of imbalance and how to change when in pain or suffering. The medicine man (woman) interprets the map of the wheel. The symptomatic person may be told to shift toward, for instance, the black, which is also toward the physical. This may be the case if one is too ethereal, spiritual, or yellow, bringing the person back down to earth. The imbalance of illness is thought to be physical, emotional, and related to others in the human and spiritual environment. This complicated calculus of the medicine wheel combines observation of the ill person, with treatments prescribed by the medicine person.

Struggle: Diaspora, being separated from homeland and culture, is a common theme of struggle. Loss of the integrity of Native American traditional medicine preceded damage to the psychosocial cultural system of Native Americans. With the formation of the Indian Health Services, traditional medicine was supplanted. Infectious disease incidence went down, rates of disparity states like alcoholism, cirrhosis, suicide, homicide, hypertension, cigarette smoking, and diabetes became disproportionately identified with Native communities.

The Trail of Tears, a major struggle in Native American history, underscores the strength of strong cultures and their healing traditions to survive against the odds. Native Americans were forced from their homelands in the southeastern states by federal troops and driven westward to Oklahoma beginning in 1831. The legal justification for this march was the Indian Relocation Act. Seventeen thousand Choctaw people were among the first relocated, 6,000 of who died before reaching the Oklahoma territory. Members of five major Native Nations of the southeast were in the march. The lands, its sustenance, customs, and families were also disrupted and killed in the process of this march [44].

A Native American baby boomer, in pain, could easily has shared a home with a grandparent who personally knew a family member who marched the Trail of Tears. Three-generational knowledge is easily culturally accessible and lays in the base of the current generation's identity. The Indian Freedom of Religion Act, enabling Native Americans to practice traditional spirituality, was only passed by both houses of congress in 1978. The United Nations Declaration of Rights of Indigenous Peoples was passed in 2007 [45, 46].

Icons and Rituals: There is no stronger icon or sets of healing practices in Native American traditional medicine than the "medicine wheel". Replicas of medicine wheels are seen in many places as adornments on fancy dance costumes, braid ties, painted, or as in tradition, laid out with stone and pigments. Other icons include medicine hoops, smudging, sand painting, replicas of spirit animals, and medicine bags. Jewelry is often considered to carry the blessings of those from whom it was received. The amount of jewelry worn is not simply for adornment but for protection.

Notes for Pain Clinicians: Those caring for Native American people should ascertain the level of a patient identification with traditional culture and traditional medicine. Icons and language style provide clues. A formal spiritual assessment (see HOPE and FICA above) provides an entry point for reviewing cultural beliefs. Consultation with traditional Native American healers may be an appropriate care enhancement particularly in refractory pain and in death and dying. During clinical critical points, care should be taken to not remove cultural icons from a person's body if possible. Maintaining identity is important to healing when in allopathic settings [44]. Clinics serving larger numbers of Native American people may have within the clinic community access to traditional healers with whom a practice relationship can be cultivated.

Mexican Traditional Medicine

Family: Family members, including extended family, are responsible for the health of their loved ones. Family contacts the appropriate traditional practitioner on behalf of the symptomatic person. In Mexican traditional medicine, this person is a curandero (a) or a yerbera (o). The family chooses which practitioners to consult first. It is the family that sees that other routine herbs and activities have not helped prior to consultations. Often, the curandero (a) will not ask the ill person about the problem but will refer questions to the family members of the ill person. The idea of autonomy of the patient, without family inclusion, is anathema. The family is responsible for carrying out the instructions that will facilitate cure [47].

Mexican folk medicine divides illness between hot and cold categories. Like Native American medicine, the goal is to keep the symptomatic person in a balance between the two. Heat from fever and respiratory phloem is treated with heat—to draw the heat from the body. A poultice of stewed tomatoes might be applied. Key family members are taught to prepare and apply the poultice. Many herbs have medicinal functions in Latino cultural medicine. These therapies are often found in the family kitchen. Garlic for anorexia, oregano for dry cough, rose water for fever, linseed for constipation, and aloe vera for burns. Many of these have a scientific basis but that is not what drives people to use traditional healers. The curandero prescribes and teaches family to use these therapies.

Family members are charged by the curandero with specific chants or prayers to be said to God for the patient. There are therapeutic and preventive instructions called remedios (remedies). These are preventive teachings using words or parables that instruct and remind the person to use certain preventive practices. An example is the phrase "consejos sobre la regla, which reminds a woman to not eat spicy foods while menstruating." Menstruating is considered to be hot. Spicy foods are also hot, both together would give a profound imbalance in equilibrium. These are verbal sayings which the culture spreads generation by generation for prevention of illness.

Struggle: In 2006, Hispanic people of the United States were estimated to be 44.3 million. In 2000, the same communities were estimated at 35.6 million [48]. Hispanic is a US government term differentiating those Spanish-speaking people born in the Americas from those European born. Fifty percent of the Hispanic peoples in the United States have linage from Mexico. Before the arrival of Spanish colonialist in the 1500s, Mexican people were the indigenous Native peoples of the southern part of North America, including the land in the lower portion of the United States. In the early 1800s, Mexican people fought for their independence from Spain and won. In the mid-1800s after the United States-Mexico War, the USA seized lands previously owned by Mexico. Mexicans living in the United States, who could not repatriate to Mexico for fiscal reasons, suffered the diasporas effect as many immigrant laborers experience today.

The US-Mexico War, ended in proximity to the Emancipation Proclamation. Work previously done by the exploitation of African slave labor was left undone. This period resulted in economic depression of the United States. In the period from the late 1800s until the 1930s, Mexican workers first became essential to the US infrastructure: building railroads, working in foundries, agriculture, and mining [1]. Having known one another in the Mexican-Spanish colonial period, Mexican Americans again met African Americans in the workplace. From 1880 to 1930, the rate of Mexican American lynching in the United States was 27.4 per 100,000 of population. This statistic is second only to that of the African American community during the same period, an average of 37.1 per 100,000 population [49].

Spiritualism: Mexican traditional medicine, heavily influenced by indigenous Native American medicine, strives for balance and harmony. Spiritualism is used in healing and is the basis for a patient's understanding, not scientific principles. Spiritualism in Hispanic culture is a mixture of Catholicism, indigenous/Native Mexican culture, and African influences. The body and the mind are healed at the same time as the spirit. Prayers and chants are said to appeal to God. They are said by the curandero, the patient, and the family. The prayers are also to provide comfort to the patient and decrease fear and anxiety.

Curanderos direct the symptomatic person's own inner energies toward healing. A curandero may transfer energy to the ill person, for example, by laying on of hands. This exchange supports the ill person until they garner their own energies. The curandero may be exhausted (siento debil) or drained by the exercise while the ailing person will be more at ease. The energy is delivered to the curandero through communication with supernatural intermediaries to God. This approach is mostly used when the illness is thought to be supernatural, in combination with specific physical therapies prescribed by the curandero. The curandero uses ancient spiritual practices and references (Mayan, Aztec, origin) and Catholic rituals and practices (Virgin of Guadeloupe, saints with key domains of influence). Mexican traditional medicine presumes that the body and spirit are always connected. Unnatural agents such as pharmaceuticals or drugs are discouraged. The body and blood must be clean as well as the thoughts pure if the ill person is to heal [50].

Icons: Many instruments in healing ceremonies are associated with Catholicism. They are also used to prevent harm to a person while weakened with illness or in daily life. Amulets, medals, holy water, and blessed herbs may be worn by the sick person. These are reminiscent of the medicine bags often found around the neck of Native American people. Prayers are placed in sacramental urns in front of candles, usually written on paper or tree bark. Statues of the Virgin Mary, the Virgin of Guadeloupe, saints, and crucifixes are icons of respect conferring protection seen in jewelry, homes, and vehicles.

Notes for Pain Clinicians: Asking the question, "Has a curandero's assistance been sought?" may open a field of dialog between a clinician and a Latino patient. Demonstrating a respect for a nonscientific basis for healing may resonate with a patient's core values. Both traditional Mexican and allopathic medicine are often used simultaneously, people know when immediate life threatening illness requires one or the other. Use of a curandero may evidence that a patient's belief system significantly includes the supernatural realm. Clinicians who see people presenting with icons of their culture may want to ask, "What does this mean to you?" Expressing interest in the meaning of icons demonstrates respect for a person's beliefs, important because respect may be under siege for those with persistent pain. Pain clinician awareness of the curandero's treatment, prevention, and education plan may be referenced and incorporated in the clinician's therapeutic approach.

African American Traditional Medicine

Family: It is difficult to separate family and struggle in African American history or in response to pain. At slave ports in the United States, Africans were forbidden to use their language, customs, traditions, and healing practices. Families and tribes were dispersed and sold away from one another, fracturing culture and family. Slave owners often allowed traditional African medicine healers to retain skills as means of maintaining the slave work force; sick slaves could not work. Slave doctors and midwives acting as both healers and spiritual guides became key parts of maintaining the extended families created in the slave quarters [51]. These African-born slave healers hid slave illness from owners. This practice of hiding illness and pain protected members of slave extended families from being sold away from one another, experimented on, or made eunuch [52, 53].

The doctor serving African Americans is at best advantage when considered a member of the extended family. Such clinicians demonstrate more "cool" than other clinicians. That is, they absorb heat, stress, and emotional charge related to illness [54]. The responsibility of family to protect, as in Native American and Mexican communities, is paramount. For African Americans, there is historically safety in numbers. The skills, education, icons, and appearance of African American family members are heterogeneous. Capacity to understand and manipulate complex medical systems is generally thought better with more family participants.

Struggle: For Americans of African descent, there are multiple diaspora, the first being the uprooting from Africa. The second being the profound negative effect of slavery on African American family and cultural retention. The third diaspora relates to African American unity with Native Americans and Mexicans. In the Maroon movement, escaped slaves, again separated from their people, preserved some of the traditional base of African medicine. The basis of African traditional medicine, shared reverence for the earth, similar worship styles, and capacity to move agilely over land, formed relationships between the Maroon and Native Americans. African slaves and Native Americans combined families. The March of Tears included 10–18 % of the five

nations uprooted from the southeast USA to Oklahoma in the early 1800s [55].

Some African slaves were welcomed into Mexico at the time of the March of Tears to avoid their recapture. By 1810, Mexican slavery was abolished by Mexico's second president, who was of African and indigenous Mexican origin. African slaves originally brought to Mexico by Spanish colonialist became principle fighters for Mexican independence [56].

Spirituality: Because of the multiple diaspora, the African origin of African American traditional medicine is less clear than that of Native, Hispanic, or Chinese Americans. Much of the medical knowledge of African American slaves evolved from Yoruba medicine. Traditional Yoruba medicine began with the migration of the East African Yoruba across the trans-African route leading from the mid-Nile river area to the mid-Niger, West African region [57]. Yoruba medicine traditions incorporated and influenced many other African healing traditions en route to the Atlantic. These traditions included Egyptian medicine which became the source of western medicine disseminated through the Mediterranean to the East (Greece) by the Phoenicians. African cultural healing traditions included medicine men who acted as priest and physicians, similar to the Native American and the Mexican traditions.

Yoruba medicine also sees health as harmony with nature and the supernatural. Disease is considered to reflect disharmony [58]. Evidence of the link between spirit and body is reflected in the persistence of medicine dolls use in the Caribbean. The medicine dolls come from Yoruba tradition. Pins are stuck in the doll replicas of the patient. The pins guide supernatural forces to the points of illness. These African healers were trained to use roots, minerals, and plants for solutions drunk or applied to the body. Therapies had a direct relationship to Yoruba gods or forces. The god forces being Okydnare (the self-existent being of one source), Orisha (good forces), and Ashe (nature). Additionally, in Yoruba medicine, the human physical form has a dual potential through the evolution of the human spirit to supernatural.

This duality of the natural and supernatural is not unlike the Christ story reflected in Christianity. Yoruba spirituality likely helped African American culture become tightly linked to Christianity. It has been said that the key feature of African American Christianity is, "African Americans want to be saved and saved by Jesus Christ" [59]. Suffering is related to sharing kindredness with the suffering of Christ before resurrection. Pain is sometimes thought to be a punishment or originating from hard times endured by previous generations [60].

The therapies used in African traditional medicine are similar to those in Native, Mexican, and Chinese medicine. In Yoruba medicine, the natural world is linked to the spiritual world through the seven major Orisha or good forces.

Each Orisha has different capacities corresponding to places on the body and their illnesses. Specific combinations of herbs serve specific Orisha. The African Orisha herbs were replaced by other flora in the Americas with the assistance of Native Americans. African folk medicine remnants are common for self medication of discomfort distressing symptoms include chamomile or ginger for abdominal cramping and garlic, rose hips, lemon, and honey for cough. These therapies originate from distant knowledge of the Orisha.

Okydnare, the self-existent being of one source or life force, may be transferred through the laying on of hands, prayer, and speaking in tongues to a person to relieve pain [61]. Use of drugs alone will likely be less effective among those African Americans with pain disparity inclined to embrace folk or integrative medicine practices. In this case, touch therapies like massage may improve acceptance and effectiveness of medication therapies.

Icons: African Americans may wear symbols of African heritage. It is common for African American college graduates to wear kente cloth sashes with their graduation gowns. Kente cloth is a multicolored silk and cotton woven cloth which originated in eleventh century, West Africa. Different colors and patterns have different meanings. Those used at graduations, mean new beginnings, often have touching pyramid point shapes symbolizing keys. The neck sash itself is a sign of dignity and was original worn by African chiefs.

Styles of hair and clothing often derive from the duo African and African American origin. Children are named to demonstrate African roots. People shake hands with handshakes which communicate kindredness to Africa and a belonging to one another. Frequently the same handshake is recognized by African born, African Americans, and others close to both.

Notes for Pain Clinicians: Intact African American culture is a culture of relationships [62]. As many family members as can fit into the room may be invited by a patient or proxy when clinical information is exchanged. "Dress up" for clinic visits is a sign of the patient's self-worth and respect for the clinician. "Dress up" may mask, or even improve, the level of discomfort a person is feeling while at clinic. Family confirmation of effective pain management while at home should be sought.

Negative side effect experience may cause patient resistance to pain management. These may be patients more comfortable with self-management programs and integrative medicine. In clinical practice, stoicism may present as a result from spiritual beliefs but also from distrust. Formal spiritual assessment (HOPE or FICA) should be done by the pain clinician. Especially for African Americans, the spiritual assessment is an essential part of the pain disparity assessment. Acknowledging the history of previous medical abuses of African Americans can forge an alliance with the patient to try to do better.

Chinese Traditional Medicine

Family: The traditional Chinese household is three generational: parents, the eldest son and his wife, their children, and unmarried sisters of the eldest son. Commonly, the oldest male in the house will control all the family affairs. It is often seen with older Chinese American women, will defer to oldest man in the family in clinical settings. The first born boy is historically considered the most important child in the household. This practice originated because girl children marry and leave the family. When the oldest man in the family dies, it is the oldest son who will replace him. The traditional family structure is still often maintained in rural modern China, Hong Kong, and Taiwan and frequently in some form in Chinese American families. In families observing this hierarchy, clinicians may find themselves conferring with relatively young men about their elders [63]. A savvy translator of the appropriate Chinese language and the region from which the family has come may be needed for pain assessment, informed consent, and pain contracts.

Struggle: Indentured laborers in the Americas increased in direct response to the end of African slavery in the Americas. The best understanding of the contact between Chinese, African slaves, Native American, and Mexican people in the Americas is in chronicles of indentured Chinese laborers' interactions in the Caribbean and especially in Cuba [64]. This forced diaspora continued from the mid-1800s into the 1900s. During the economic depression following the United States Civil War and WWI, Asian indentured workers like Mexican workers was used as scapegoats for lack of jobs. Chinese workers built railroads, farmed, and mined. Chinese Americans were lynched as were African Americans and Mexican Americans.

The Chinese Exclusion Act specifically targeted Chinese immigrants to the United States. Many Chinese people were forced to return to China in the midst of major Chinese upheaval at the rise of World War II. Of the estimated 20 million people that died in Asia as a result of that war, half were estimated to have been killed in China [65]. The battle of Shanghai in the beginning of World War II is embedded in the memory of many American Chinese elders. From 1910 to 1940, Angel Island in the San Francisco Bay was one of the notorious processing and detention centers. Nearly 60,000 Asian people were detained there. The conditions at the detention center lacked sanitation. Infectious disease was rampant. The barracks burned on the island, aiding the movement to repeal the Chinese Exclusion Act.

Spirituality: Confucianism, Taoism, and Buddhism are historically the three major religions of Chinese people. Confucianism is more a way of thinking about the world than a religion. There are many Christian Chinese as well. Chinese Christianity may be an admixture of values from the major religions and the old Chinese religions predating the three majors.

Spiritual understanding is tightly linked to Chinese medicine. Chinese medicine is estimated to be approximately 5,000 years old. It is significant to many Asian cultures because of the patterns of Chinese migration and integration throughout Asia. The Yellow Emperor Huang Ti took a specific interest in Chinese medicine and learned it in a series of dialogs with practitioners. These dialogs were scribed, the exchanges becoming the written text of Chinese medicine, rare in other traditional medicines [66]. Chinese medicine particularly reflects many refined ideas of Taoism.

Taoism is about the balanced relationship between human beings and nature. The law of Tao deals with the opposites of human beings, ideas, and objects. Opposing energies are kept in check by the Yin and Yang. Yin is described as negative, dark, cold, and feminine. Yang is positive, light warm, and masculine. Persistent imbalance results in illness. These opposite pairs exist on the condition of each other. Chinese medicine also places primary emphasis on the balance of Qi (Chi), or vital energy. Opening blocks in these energies utilizing 12 meridians of the body is the basis of acupuncture. Most conditions of disease are believed caused by an imbalance in energy manifested by wrong diet or strong displays of emotional feelings (drama). Harmony can be restored by self-restraint and herbs. Man is also subject to the universal laws of nature manifested as fire, earth, metal, water, and wood [67]. Each of these properties is ascribed to different organs of the body. The body and the mind are always integrated, for better or worse. Every organ also is considered to encompass properties of taste, emotion, sound, odor, season, climate, power, and fortification of other structures of the body.

Dietary therapeutic manipulations are also controlled by the balance of Yin and Yang or Hot and Cold. Hot disease is treated with herbs or foods that are cold and vice versa to restore the balance. Other procedures in Chinese traditional medicine include meditation, martial arts, (Tai Chi chuan and Kung fu), acumassage, acupressure, and moxibustion (burning of artemisia vulgaris or moxa). Moxibustion works somewhat like sage in Native American healing, the latter being significant in cleansing and the Chinese being opening meridians [68]. The choice of type of therapy is dependent on the physical exam of pulses and ways in which the meridians may be altered.

Icons: Closely related to pain issues are rituals and icons around death. The next life can be altered by disrupting the spirit in its transition through drama. The moment of death, like life, must be calm and balanced. Transition of the spirit is facilitated by the icon of Xi Bo during funerals [69]. Xi Bo yellow and silver squares of paper are folded to resemble ancient coins, then floated on water, and lit on fire at the time of a person's funeral. Xi Bo symbolizes money being offered to a person who has died so that they can go on their journey with the protection of wealth. There are restrictions on who may handle Xi Bo. Pregnant women, or those menstruating, cannot touch Xi Bo. These women are thought to have a power to stop the Xi Bo ability to help the dead in crossing into the next life by consumption of the Xi Bo. Use of Xi Bo paper is so common that they are found in Chinese grocery stores.

The most powerful icon in Chinese culture is the mythical dragon. The dragon is made of the parts of other animals: birds, lizards, and so on. The dragon's power derives from the ability to move from one life form to those whose body parts it shares without dying [70].

Notes for Pain Clinicians: Apparent stoicism or restraint in pain expression may result from patient perception of generations of hardship endured as immigrants. In the setting of family and friends, stoicism is not always a pattern; there are cultural reasons why clinicians may have difficulty "seeing" pain expression in Asian patients. Excess dramatic expression is seen to disrupt balance. Showing weakness is culturally unacceptable for many Asian cultures including Chinese. A Chinese patient may refuse an initial pain medication to avoid showing weakness or because of fears of imbalance; subsequent offers may be accepted after sufficient strength is demonstrated through initial refusals [71]. Wholeness is important in life and death. Clinicians should strive to have all the person's physical parts present for the funeral and transition to the next life.

Conclusion

July of 2011, the Academy of Science, through the Institute of Medicine, issued its extensive report, Relieving Pain in America: A blueprint for transforming Prevention, Care, Education and Research [72]. This report affirms the importance of emerging pain science validating a basis for the observed effectiveness of some integrative therapies on pain perception and neuroplasticity [73]. It also identifies pain as an overarching disparity related to most other health-care disparities. Pain disparity oriented additions to the standard pain assessment support integrative medicine.

Pain clinicians committed to expanding their cross-cultural knowledge are better able to address pain disparity. Traditional medicine provides a model for culturally relevant patient-centered approaches to pain care. One third of people in the United States are estimated to use complimentary or alternative medicine [1]. Ethnic peoples of color are disproportionately affected by epidemic pain disparity. The same people rarely are able to access services related to their own cultural traditional medicines: complimentary, alternative, and integrative medicine. Given broader access, integrative medicine with its already firm hand on traditional medicine, is positioned to decrease pain disparity through culturally relevant patient-centered pain care.

References

1. WHO normative guidelines on pain management. 2011. http://www.who.int/medicines/areas/quality_safety/delphi_study_pain_guidelines.pdf. Accessed 5 June 2011.
2. International Association for the Study of pain declaration of Montreal. 2011. http://www.iasp-pain.org/Content/Navigation Menu/Advocacy/DeclarationofMontr233al/default.htm. Accessed 10 Aug 2011.
3. Tsang A, Von Korff S, Lee J, et al. Common chronic pain conditions in developed and developing countries: gender and age differences and comorbidity with depression-anxiety disorders.J Pain. 2008;9:883–9.
4. Blyth FM. The demography of chronic pain: an overview. In: Croft P, Blyth FM, van der Windt D, editors. Chronic pain epidemiology: from aetiology to public health. Oxford: Oxford University Press; 2010. p. 19–27.
5. Bonham V. Race, thnicity and pain treatment: striving to understand the causes and solutions to the disparities in pain treatment. J Law Med Ethics. 2001;29:52–68.
6. Whittle J, et al. Racial differences in the use of invasive cardiovascular procedures in the Department of Veterans Affairs medical system. N Engl J Med. 1993;329:621–7.
7. National healthcare disparities report, 2003 summary AHRQ 2002. 2011. http://www.ahrq.gov/qual/nhdr03/nhdrsum03.htm. Accessed 24 June 2011.
8. Bial A, Levine S. UNIPAC three: assessment and treatment of physical pain associated with life limiting illness. In: Storey CP, Levine S, Shega JW, editors. Hospice and palliative care training for physicians: a self study program: a self study program (UNIPAC). Glenview: American Academy of Hospice and Palliative Medicine; 2008.
9. Casarette D, Pickard A, Baily F, et al. Do palliative consultations improve outcome? In: Meier D, Issacs S, Hughes R, editors. Palliative care: transforming the care of serious illness. San Francisco: Jossey-Bass; 2010. p. 369–81.
10. Bodenheimer T, Grumback K, Berenson R. A lifeline for primary care. N Engl J Med. 2009;360(26):2693–6.
11. DeNavas-Walt C, Proctor D, Smith J. Income poverty and health insurance coverage in the united states. In: US census bureau current population reports 2007. Washington, DC: U.S. Government Printing Office; 2008. p. 235.
12. Nielsen-Bohlman L, Panzer A, Kindig A. What is health literacy. In: Committee on Health Literacy, Institute of Medicine, editor. Health literacy: a prescription to end confusion. Washington, DC: National Academic Press; 2004. p. 31–58.
13. Sadore R, Meta K, Simon E. Limited literacy in older people and disparities in health and health care access. J Am Geriatr Soc. 2006;54:770–6.
14. Quill T, Holloway R, Shah M, et al. Pain management. In: Quill T, editor. Primer of palliative care. 5th ed. Glenview: American Academy of Hospice and Palliative Care; 2010. p. 11–2.
15. Huckenberry MJ, Wilson D. Wong-baker faces pain rating scale. In: Wong's essentials of pediatric nursing. 8th ed. St Louis: Mosby; 2008. p. 12–80.
16. Dula A, Williams S. When race matters. Clin Geri Med. 2005; 21:239–53.
17. Emanuel L, editor. Palliative care II: improving care. Philadelphia: Saunders; 2005.
18. WHO Expert Committee. Cancer pain relief and palliative care: report of a WHO expert committee. Geneva: World Health Organization; 1990. p. 7–21.
19. Osteoarthritis pain relief "only a phone call away?". 2011. http://www.niams.nih.gov/Recovery/chronicles/osteoarthritis_phone_call.asp. Accessed 3 July 2011.
20. Karnofsky and ECOG scores. http://www.aboutcancer.com/karnofsky.htm. Accessed 10 Aug 2011.
21. Emanuel LL, Ferris FD, von Gunten CF, Von Roenn J. EPEC-O: Education in Palliative and End-of-life Care for Oncology. Module 2 © The EPEC Project,™ Chicago, IL, 2005. p.12–14.
22. Passik S, Kirsh K, Whitcomb L, et al. A new tool to assess and document pain outcomes in chronic pain patients receiving opioid therapy. Clin Ther. 2009;26(4):552–6.
23. Screening for drug use in general medical settings resource guide. http://www.nida.nih.gov/nidamed/resguide/resourceguide.pdf. Accessed 3 July 2011.
24. Todd KH. Ethnicity and analgesic practice. Ann Emerg Med. 2000;35:11–6.
25. WHO normative guidelines on pain management. 2011. http://www.who.int/medicines/areas/quality_safety/delphi_study_pain_guidelines.pdf. Accessed 5 June 2011.
26. Pizzo P, Clark M. Summary. In: Institute of Medicine, editor. Reliving pain in America: a blueprint for transforming prevention, care, education and research. Washington, DC: National Academy of Science; 2011. p. S1–16.
27. Warsi A, LaValley MP, Wang PS, Avorn J, Solomon DH. Arthritis self-management education programs. Arthritis Rheumatol. 2003; 48:2207–13.
28. Kroenke K, Spitzer RL, Williams JBW, Löwe B. An ultra-brief screening scale for anxiety and depression: the PHQ-4. Psychosomatic. 2009;50:613–21.
29. Bruce B, Lorig K, Laurent D. Participation in patient self-management programs. Arthritis Care Res. 2007;57(5):851–4.
30. Park S, Sonty N. Positive affect mediates the relationship between pain-related coping efficacy and interference in social functioning. J Pain. 2010;11(12):1267–73.
31. Bair MJ, Wu J, Damush TM, Sutherland JM, Kroenke K. Association of depression and anxiety alone and in combination with chronic musculoskeletal pain in primary care patients. Psychosomataic Med. 2008;70(8):890–7.
32. Okifuji A, Turk D, Curran S. Anger in chronic pain: investigations of anger targets and intensity. J Psychosom Res. 1999;47(1):1–12.
33. Community engagement: definitions and organizing concepts from the literature. In: Principles of community engagement. 2011. http://www.cdc.gov/phppo/pce/. 27 July 2011.
34. World Health Organization. WHO fact sheet no. 134: traditional medicine. 2011. http://www.who.int/mediacentre/factsheets/fs134/en/2008-12-01. Accessed 5 July 2011.
35. Integrative Medicine and Patient-Centered Care. Commissioned for the IOM summit on integrative medicine and the health of the public. 2011. http://www.iom.edu/~/media/Files/Activity%20Files/Quality/IntegrativeMed/Integrative%20Medicine%20and%20Patient%20Centered%20Care.pdf. Accessed 14 July 2011.
36. Wenger AF. Cultural meaning of symptoms. Holist Nurs Pract. 1993;7:22–35.
37. Zborowski M. People in pain. San Francisco: Jossey-Bass; 1969. p. 30–2.
38. Puchalaski CM, Carlson DB. Developing curricula in spirituality in medicine. Acad Med. 1997;73(9):970–4.
39. Colt H, Quadrelli S, Friedman L. Picture of health: medical ethics and the movies. New York: Oxford University Press; 2011. p. 1–560.
40. Azul La Luz W. Hispanios in the valley of death: street-level trauma, cultural-PTSD, overdoses, and suicides in north central New Mexico. 2011. http://repository.unm.edu/handle/1928/10352. Accessed 18 Aug 2011.
41. Defrain J, et al. Stukkbirb: the invisible death. In: Bertman S, editor. Grief and the healing arts. Amityville: Baywood Publishing Company Inc; 1999. p. 427.
42. Joe J, Galerita J, Pino C. Cultural health traditions: American Indian perspective. In: Paxton PP, Branch MF, editors. Safe nursing

care for ethnic peoples of color. New York: Appleton-Century-Crofts; 1976. p. 81–98.

43. Vickers J. Medicine wheels: a mystery in stone. Alberta Past. 1992;8(3):6–7, Winter; 93–4.

44. Katz LK. Liberty among the Indians. In: Black women of the old west. New York: Atheneum; 1995. p. 3–6.

45. The American Indian Religious Freedom Act, Public Law No. 95-341, 92 Stat. 469. 2011. http://www.nativeamericanchurch.net/Native_American_Church/LS-AmericanIndianReligiousFreedomAct.html. Accessed 2 July 2011.

46. Canby JC. American Indian law in a nutshell. New York: West Publishing Company; 1988. p. 339, 340.

47. Rodriquez-Dorsey P. Cultural health traditions: Latino/Chicano perspectives. In: Paxton PP, Branch MF, editors. Providing safe nursing care for ethnic peoples of color by Marie Foster Branch and Phyllis Perry Paxton. New York: Appleton-Century-Crofts; 1976. p. 272.

48. U.S. Census Bureau, population estimates July 1, internet release date February 08, 2008. 2011. http://www.census.gov/population/www/socdemo/hispanic/hispanic_pop_presentation.html. 5 July 2011.

49. Shaw R. Beyond the fields: Cesar Chavez, the UFW, and the struggle for justice in the 21st century. Los Angeles: University of California Press; 2008. p. 1–253.

50. The lynching of persons of Mexican origin or descent in the United States, 1848 to 1928. 2011. http://findarticles.com/p/articles/mi_m2005/is_2_37/ai_111897839/pg_9/. Accessed 1 July 2011.

51. Roman OI. Carrrismatic medicine, folk healing and folk sainthood. Anthropology. 1965;75:1152.

52. Jacques G. Cultural health traditions: a black perspective. In: Paxton PP, Branch MF, editors. Safe nursing care for ethnic peoples of color. New York: Appleton-Century-Crofts; 1976. p. 115–44.

53. Hatch J, Holmes A. Rural and small town African American populations and human rights post industrial society. In: Secundy MG, Dula A, Willimas S, editors. Bioethics research concerns and directions for African Americans. Tuskegee: Tuskegee University, National Center for Bioethics in Research and Health Care; 2000. p. 68–80.

54. Dula A. The need for a dialogue with African Americans. In: Dula A, Goering S, Secund M, Williams S, editors. It just ain't fair: westport. Conn: Praeger; 1994. p. 1–315.

55. Thompson RS. Esthetic of the cool. Afr Art. 1973;2(1):40–67.

56. Katz LK. Black women of the old west. New York: Atheneum; 1995. p. 1–79.

57. Gonzales P, Rodriquez R. African roots stretch deep into Mexico. 1996. http://www.mexconnect.com/articles/1935-african-roots-stretch-deep-into-mexico. 4 July 2011.

58. Karade BI. The handbook of Yoruba religious concepts. York Beech: Samuel Weiser, Inc; 1994. p. 1–23.

59. Lipson GJ, Dibble ST, editors. Culture and clinical care. San Francisco: UCSF Nursing Press; 2005. p. 1–14.

60. When we are asked: spirituality (VHS/DVD). Directed by September Williams. USA 2004. USA. Ninth Month Productions/APPEALproject.RWJ. 98 mins. 2011. http://divinity.duke.edu/initiatives-centers/iceol/resources/appeal#details. 25 July 2011.

61. Cultural diversity: pain beliefs and treatment among Mexican-Americans, African-Americans, Chinese-Americans and Japanese-Americans Alvarado, Anthony pain reliefCultural Diversity: Al. 2011. http://commons.emich.edu/cgi/viewcontent.cgi?article=1126&context=honors. Accessed 1 July 2011.

62. Cultural diversity: pain beliefs and treatment among Mexican-Americans, African-Americans, Chinese-Americans and Japanese-Americans Alvarado, Anthony pain reliefCultural Diversity: Al. 2011. http://commons.emich.edu/cgi/viewcontent.cgi?article=1126&context=honors. Accessed 25 June 2011.

63. When we are asked: race, class, culture (VHS/DVD). Directed by September Williams. USA 2004. USA. Ninth Month Productions/APPEALproject.RWJ. 98 mins. 2011. http://divinity.duke.edu/initiatives-centers/iceol/resources/appeal#details. 25 July 2011.

64. Chinese family life. 2011. http://www.mitchellteachers.org/WorldHistory/AncientChinaCurriculum/ModernChineseFamilyLife. Accessed 5 July 2011.

65. Yun L. The coolie speaks: Chinese indentured laborers and African slaves in Cuba. Philadelphia: Temple University Press; 2008. p. 1–336.

66. Japanese occupation of China. 2011. http://factsanddetails.com/china.php?itemid=59. Accessed 20 July 2011.

67. Veith I. The yellow Emperor's classic of internal medicine, 1949. Berkeley: University of California Press; 1970.

68. Lawson-Wood D, Lawson-Wood J. Five elements of acupuncture and Chinese massage. Health Science Press, Wellingborough: UK; 1973.

69. Chow E. Cultural health traditions: Asian perspectives. In: Paxton PP, Branch MF, editors. Safe nursing care for ethnic peoples of color. New York: Appleton-Century-Crofts; 1976. p. 99–115.

70. A Chinese funeral. 2011. http://www.bearspage.info/h/tra/ch/fun.html. Accessed 20 July 2011.

71. Cultural China traditions, myths and legends. Shanghai News and Press Bureau. http://traditions.cultural-china.com/en/13Traditions991.html. 20 July 2011.

72. Cultural diversity: pain beliefs and treatment among Mexican-Americans, African-Americans, Chinese-Americans and Japanese-Americans Alvarado, Anthony pain reliefCultural Diversity: Al. 2011. http://commons.emich.edu/cgi/viewcontent.cgi?article=1126&context=honors. Accessed 70–79. Accessed 1 July 2011.

73. IOM (Institute of Medicine). Relieving pain in America: a blueprint for transforming prevention, care, education, and research. Washington, DC: The National Academies Press; 2011.

Sleep and Chronic Pain

Nicole K.Y. Tang, Claire E. Goodchild, and Lynn R. Webster

Key Points

- Sleep is essential for well-being, and the lack of it compromises both physical and mental health.
- Complaints of sleep disturbance have been documented in a variety of individuals reporting pain symptoms.
- Common sleep disorders detected in patients reporting pain symptoms include insomnia, periodic limb movement disorder/restless leg syndrome, and obstructive and central sleep apnea.
- Experimental studies have produced evidence indicating a possible reciprocal relationship between pain and sleep, such that pain worsens sleep and sleep deprivation/fragmentation increases pain perception. These findings highlight the importance of addressing sleep disturbance in patients presenting with pain symptoms.
- Pain-related sleep disturbance can be effectively managed using pharmacotherapy (e.g., NSAIDs, opioids, anticonvulsants, antidepressants, hypnotics) and/or psychological therapy (e.g., cognitive behavioral therapy for primary insomnia, pain management program based on cognitive behavioral principles).
- Clinicians should carefully assess the sleep complaints presented by patients with pain symptoms and use the information obtained to devise appropriate treatment plans.

N.K.Y. Tang, D. Phil. (Oxon) (✉)
Arthritis Research UK Primary Care Centre, Keele University, Staffordshire, ST5 5BG, UK
e-mail: n.k.y.tang@cphc.keele.ac.uk

C.E. Goodchild, B.Sc., M.Sc., Ph.D.
Department of Psychology, Institute of Psychiatry, King's College London, De Crespigny Park, Denmark Hill, London SE5 7UB, UK
e-mail: claire.goodchild@kcl.ac.uk

L.R. Webster, M.D.
Lifetree Clinical Research and Pain Clinic, 3838 South 700 East, Suite 200, Salt Lake City, UT 84106, USA
e-mail: lrwebstermd@gmail.com

Introduction

Chronic pain can be unrelenting. Unlike acute pain for which therapies could provide relief, chronic pain can seldom be cured. Persistent pain often impairs functioning [1–3]. It may be surprising but chronic pain patients' quality of life has been found to be lower than those of patients with chronic illnesses (e.g., chronic obstructive pulmonary disease) or life-threatening diseases (e.g., HIV/AIDS) [4]. While some individuals manage to live fulfilling lives despite pain, others suffer both physically and mentally and go on to develop anxiety, depression, and even increased suicidal ideation and behavior [5]. One plausible reason is that, to many chronic pain patients, pain is not the only source of distress and disability. Among the many other concomitant health and emotional problems, sleep (or the lack of it) is a particular area with which most chronic pain patients want help.

Increasingly, chronic pain patients have voiced their concerns over their interrupted sleep. Aside from pain reduction, these patients have repeatedly identified better sleep as one of the most important outcomes desired from new forms of treatment [2, 6]. This is a justified request because we now know that the vast majority of chronic pain patients report problems sleeping and more than half of them have insomnia of a severity that warrants clinical attention [7–9]. We also know that persistent insomnia is linked to many negative consequences, including reduced daytime functioning (e.g., tiredness, poor concentration, memory, and alertness) and increased mood disturbance (e.g., irritability, lethargy) [10]. Consistently, chronic pain patients with sleep complaints tend to experience greater levels of physical and psychosocial disability than those who do not report any difficulty sleeping [11, 12]. Leaders in the field are now recommending that treatments be diversified, such that the focus is not only on reducing/managing pain but also on improving physical and emotional functioning [13, 14]. Given this context, greater understanding of sleep disturbance in chronic pain and the available treatment options will give clinicians the competitive edge to offer services that truly address the patient's needs.

In this chapter, we will briefly review the basics of sleep, revisiting the importance and structure of sleep and describing the types/patterns of sleep disturbance commonly observed in patients with chronic pain. We will then examine the interplay between pain and sleep and provide a brief road map for sleep assessment. Finally, we will review the recent advances in both pharmacological and psychological treatments for insomnia occurring with chronic pain. The advantages and disadvantages of the existing treatment options will be considered, and avenues for future research and treatment development highlighted.

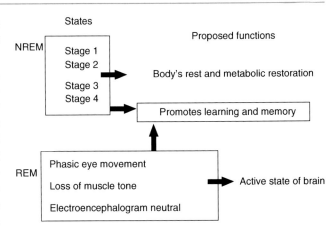

Fig. 16.1 Sleep stages and function

Background: Sleep Basics

Importance of Sleep

Sleep is essential for well-being, and the lack of it compromises both physical and mental health. The exact role of sleep is unknown, but it is believed to be necessary for homeostasis and to impact protein synthesis, cellular growth and proliferation, metabolism, and immune function among other biological processes. The importance of sleep has been demonstrated in animals: serious pathologies and death resulted when sleep in rats was disrupted via mild physical stimulus, perhaps because of interference with thermoregulation [15].

One possible benefit of sleep is that when cerebral energy output is reduced, cell resources engage in protein synthesis, helping to preserve brain structure and function. Studies in rats showed that sleep deprivation causes a reduction in the proliferation of cells [16]. Another possible vital role for sleep is that of providing a needed period of energy conservation [17], perhaps helping to combat the accumulation of free radicals. Sleep deprivation has been linked to oxidative stress, and recovery sleep has been shown to assist in restoring antioxidant balance [18].

Sleep's association with the immune system is apparent in the need for more sleep when one is sick. Animals with infection increase levels of sleep [19], and infection levels increase when they are deprived of sleep [20]. Sleep deprivation also leads to elevated levels of immunity-related, inflammatory cytokines in rats [21]. It is believed that the dysregulation of the immune system wrought by sleep disorders worsens chronic inflammatory conditions such as rheumatoid arthritis (RA) and fibromyalgia (FM) [22].

In humans, cardinal sequelae of sleeplessness include difficulty concentrating, memory lapses, irritability, fatigue, lethargy, and emotional instability. Insomnia is associated with an elevated risk of road and work accidents [23], and longitudinal studies indicate that insomnia heightens the risk of developing depression, anxiety, and substance-related problems [24–32].

Sleep Architecture

Humans experience two main types of sleep: rapid-eye-movement (REM) sleep and non-rapid-eye-movement (NREM) sleep. NREM sleep can be subdivided into four stages: N1 through N4 sleep (Fig. 16.1) [33, 34]. During a typical night's sleep, the sleeper may cycle through these stages four to six times per night with each cycle lasting, on average, 60–90 min [35]. With each subsequent cycle, REM sleep tends to lengthen while the time spent in deep sleep lessens. The light sleep of stage N1 lasts for 5–10 min, progressing to N2, during which body temperature and heart rate decrease. These sleep stages are followed by the deep sleep – or slow wave sleep (SWS) – phases of N3 and N4. During N3 sleep, delta waves alternate with faster waves, while N4 is marked by delta waves almost exclusively. During stage N4 sleep, the sleeper can only be aroused with vigorous stimulation and, if awakened, does not report dreaming. The SWS phases are followed by the REM period, during which dreams usually occur, breathing is rapid and shallow, heart rate and blood pressure rise, the eyes jerk rapidly, and the brain waves return to the levels observed during the wakened state (Fig. 16.1).

The amount of sleep required varies between individuals, and the amount of sleep obtained is influenced by age, environmental demands, and many other biological, psychological, and social factors. There is no clear consensus what constitutes "normal" sleep, but conventionally, sleep is considered disturbed if it is characterized by a long sleep onset latency (SOL; ≥30 min), long duration of awakening after sleep onset (WASO; ≥30 min), short total sleep time (TST; ≤6.5 h), low-quality/nonrefreshing sleep, or a sleep efficiency (SE; the proportion of time in bed asleep) of 85 % or below (Table 16.1).

Table 16.1 Abbreviations of sleep architecture

Sleep architecture	
NREM	*Non-rapid-eye-movement sleep* composed of four distinct stages: N1 and N2 are characterized by lighter sleep, while N3 and N4 are regarded as deeper stages of sleep
REM	*Rapid-eye-movement sleep* follows stage N4 sleep, and dreams usually occur during this period. This phase is characterized by rapid, shallow breathing, raised heart rate and blood pressure, jerky eye movement, and brain wave patterns similar to wakefulness. Also known as paradoxical sleep
SWS	*Slow wave sleep*: stages N3 and N4 of NREM; N4 consists almost entirely of SWS
SOL	*Sleep onset latency*: time taken to fall asleep
WASO	*Wake after sleep onset*: time awake following initial onset of sleep
TWT	*Total wake time*: cumulative amount of time awake
TST	*Total sleep time:* cumulative amount of time sleeping
SE	*Sleep efficiency* expressed as a percentage of time in bed asleep: (total sleep time/total time in bed) × 100 %
SQ	*Sleep quality*: a subjective rating of quality of sleep

Scientific Relevance to Pain Care

Prevalence and Pattern of Sleep Disruption in Chronic Pain

Complaints of sleep disturbance have been documented in a variety of individuals reporting pain symptoms. A large-scale community-based survey investigating the prevalence of sleeping difficulties in multiple European countries found that 23.3 % of participants who reported experiencing pain also reported difficulties sleeping, while only 7.4 % of participants reporting impaired sleep were without pain [36]. In a prospective postal survey of adults in the UK, pain reported at baseline was a significant risk factor for developing insomnia symptoms 1 year later [37]. These findings are consistent with those obtained from the Sleep in America Survey conducted in 2003, indicating that the presence of bodily pain increased the odds of insomnia by approximately twofold in older adults [38].

Sleep disturbance is a common consequence of acute pain; estimates of sleep disturbance experienced during hospitalization postsurgery range between 22 and 61 % [39–41]. In these patients, polysomnography (PSG; an instrument to measure sleep) has indicated frequent awakenings, shorter TST and SE, as well as more frequent transitions between the sleep stages with longer duration of N1 sleep, and reduced SWS and REM sleep [40, 42]. This disturbance is generally short-term, and TST returns to preoperative levels within 1 week of hospitalization for the majority of patients [39–41]. Similarly, nighttime pain in patients hospitalized for burn injuries is associated with frequent awakenings and

reduced sleep quality and TST. Sleep disturbance was reported by 75 % of patients on at least one night during the 5-day study period [43].

Sleep disturbance is also a common problem in cancer and a number of chronic pain conditions, such as RA, osteo-arthritis (OA), FM, headache, and musculoskeletal pain conditions. In a review of cancer-related insomnia, the prevalence of sleep disturbance in this population was estimated between 30 and 50 % post-diagnosis [44]. The insomnia rate only dropped slightly (estimated between 24 and 44 %) when assessed 2–5 years after treatment [44] suggesting insomnia itself is a chronic problem for this population, although cancer pain specifically increases difficulties initiating sleep and frequent awakenings [45].

Confining the focus to chronic noncancer pain, as many as 90 % of the patients attending tertiary pain clinics have complaints with their sleep [7, 8, 11, 46, 47], and approximately 53 % of these patients have insomnia of a severity that warrants clinical attention [9]. Apparently, the pattern of sleep disturbance in these chronic pain patients is largely comparable to that of patients with primary insomnia [48]. Common problems cited by chronic pain patients are initiating sleep and frequent awakenings [7, 8]. Studies using PSG have indicated that chronic pain patients have more micro-arousals, more body movements during sleep, more frequent transitions between the sleep stages with increased N1 and N2 sleep and reduced N3 and N4, frequent awakenings, and lower SE, compared to healthy volunteers [49, 50]. Sleep disruption experienced by these patients is also characterized by reduced spindle activity at N2 sleep [51], an increase in the rate of cyclic alternating pattern (CAP); [52] a lack of heart rate variability reduction [53] and an intrusion of electroencephalographic (EEG) activity in the alpha range (8–13 cps) during NREM sleep [54]. Although alpha-delta sleep was once thought to be a signature of pain-related sleep disturbance [55], there is now conflicting evidence suggesting otherwise [56–59]. It remains open as to whether or not there is a neuro-physiological marker of sleep complaints exclusive to the pain population.

Primary Sleep Disorders Other than Insomnia in Chronic Pain

Sleep disorders other than insomnia, including periodic limb movement (PLMD) and sleep apnea, have a heightened prevalence among patients with chronic pain [60, 61]. PLMD and restless leg syndrome (RLS) are closely related movement disorders that often disturb sleep onset and maintenance. PLMD occurs during sleep with spontaneous movement of the lower extremities. RLS occurs during the day or night and is associated with an unpleasant sensation in the lower extremities somewhat relieved with movement. There is always a strong urge to move with RLS, and it can be the genesis of movement and pain at night. Approximately 80 % of patients with RLS have PLMD [62]. The etiology of PLMD and RLS is not well understood, but some forms appear to be due to a dopaminergic dysfunction. Secondary PLMD and RLS have been associated with iron deficiency, folate deficiency, chronic renal failure, OA, and small-sensory-fiber disease [63]. Pain from OA and dysesthesias from small sensory nerve disease are factors that contribute to sleep disturbances with patients who have PLMD and RLS [64].

Chronic headaches appear to be strongly associated with obstructive sleep apnea (OSA); OSA sufferers are seven times more likely to experience chronic headaches (defined as occurring 15 or more times per month) than people in the general population [65]. The severity of the headaches, which tend to occur in the morning, is directly related to the severity of OSA [66]. A strong association also appears to exist between FM and sleep apnea. The prevalence of FM in a study of 50 patients with sleep apnea was tenfold higher than in the general population [67]. Patients with FM often experience OSA [60], and it is possible that OSA plays an etiologic role in some cases of FM. In one case study, a woman with FM and OSA saw great improvement of her FM symptoms after being treated for OSA with nasal continuous positive airway pressure (CPAP) [68]. However, the current research on the link between primary sleep disorders and chronic pain is thin; the rate and variety of comorbid sleep disorders may have been underdetected and/or underreported.

Sleep-Pain Interaction

We have seen that disturbed sleep and chronic pain frequently go together and that the relationship is often assumed to be bidirectional. There are studies showing that the introduction of nociceptive stimuli during sleep can produce cortical arousal [69–71] and that deprivation of sleep – in particular, REM sleep and SWS – can heighten pain intensity [72–74]. However, as more experimental data accrue, the relationship between sleep and pain emerges to be more complex than originally thought.

On the effect of sleep disturbance on pain, there are confusing findings regarding the relative importance of REM sleep and SWS disruption in pain responses. For example, in one study of healthy pain-free sleepers, the loss of 4 h of sleep associated with REM sleep disruption had a greater hyperalgesic effect than the loss of an equal amount of sleep that was associated with NREM sleep interruption [75]. In another study [72], recovery sleep following SWS interruption, but not REM interruption, increased pain thresholds. Contrary to the previous study [75], this finding suggests that SWS plays a more important role than REM sleep in deter-

mining the pain tolerance levels. Further, in an elegant study designed to tease apart the effect of sleep deprivation from sleep fragmentation, healthy controls who were in the sleep fragmentation condition demonstrated a significant loss of pain inhibition and an increase in spontaneous pain, while sleep deprivation did not produce any effect on pain thresholds. This interesting finding indicates that the lack of sleep continuity, rather than simple sleep restriction, impairs endogenous pain-inhibitory function and increases spontaneous pain [76].

Pain is frequently cited by patients as the cause of their sleep disturbance [8], and consistently, pain intensity ratings have been found to predict sleep disturbance [47, 77]. However, not all studies identify a significant relationship between pain severity and sleep [78], and certainly not every pain patient has problems sleeping. A subset of individuals with high pain intensity manage to have normal sleep or even regard themselves as "good sleepers" [7, 9, 47, 78]. Although there are clinical studies noting pain to be predictive of subsequent poor sleep, the amount of within-subject variance in sleep explained by pain was rather small and often became nonsignificant when other psychological variables (e.g., pain attention, presleep cognitive arousal) were statistically controlled for [79, 80]. In fact, evidence is accruing to suggest that cognitive behavioral factors common in primary insomnia (such as rumination, worry, health- and sleep-related anxiety, poor stimulus control, pre-sleep arousal, and dysfunctional sleep beliefs) may be better predictors of insomnia severity than pain intensity per se [9, 81, 82, 151].

Clinical Practice

Sleep Assessment

When a pain patient is complaining of insomnia, there are various ways to assess the complaint, such that both the subjective distress of the complaint and the objective characteristics of the sleep disturbance are captured. Although there are sophisticated tests and equipment available for the measurement of sleep, most cases of insomnia are primarily diagnosed by clinical evaluation.

A *detailed clinical interview* should include a careful evaluation of the patient's sleep history, medical and psychiatric history, current and past use of substances, and history of treatment for the sleep problem. When asking the patient about the sleep history, it is important to gather information about the (1) typical sleep-wake schedule; (2) past diagnosis of and treatment for sleep/psychiatric disorder(s); (3) nature and onset of the current sleep complaint; (4) frequency, severity, and duration of the sleep problem; and (5) whether or not the sleep problem has daytime consequences or is causing significant distress. This should provide information to establish if the patient meets the basic diagnostic criteria for insomnia – the three most commonly used classification systems are DSM-IV-TR [83], ICD-10 [84], and ICSD-2 [85]. Moreover, it would be helpful for the clinician to ask questions about the following: the patient's occupation (e.g., doing shift work or jobs requiring frequent long haul travel), general lifestyle (e.g., leading a sedentary lifestyle; napping often; consuming excessive alcohol, drugs, caffeine, and/or other stimulants), current and past life stresses that could cause anxiety and depression (e.g., pain, bereavement, divorce, job loss), bedroom environment (e.g., too hot/cold/ bright/noisy, having a bed partner who snores), general beliefs about sleep (e.g., "I must have 8 h of sleep a night!"), sleep practices (e.g., having a pre-sleep wind-down routine; if woken up, staying in bed for hours to try and go back to sleep), and their typical response to a poor night's sleep (e.g., feeling annoyed and frustrated; worried about losing control over sleep; cutting daytime appointments for fear of not being able to function well; going to bed early to catch up on sleep, even when not sleepy). This should help establish the psychophysiological factors precipitating and perpetuating the sleep problems. There are structured interview schedules available to guide and assist the assessment of insomnia and sleep disorders. Examples of these include the structured interview for sleep disorders according to DSM-III-R [86] and the Duke Structured Interview Schedule for the diagnoses of DSM-IV-TR and International Classification of Sleep Disorder, second edition (ICSD-2) [87]. The use of these instruments, however, requires training and practice.

While a thorough clinical interview should form the core of the evaluation, a combination of self-report questionnaires and a sleep diary (with or without actigraphy) can be used to aid the assessment. *Self-report questionnaires* such as the Insomnia Severity Index [88], the Pittsburgh Sleep Quality Index (PSQI) [89], the Mini-Sleep Questionnaire [90], the Uppsala Sleep Inventory [91], the Medical Outcome Study Sleep Questionnaire [92], and the Dysfunctional Beliefs and Attitudes About Sleep Scale [93, 94] have been used to assess sleep difficulties in chronic pain conditions. However, it must be emphasized that most of these questionnaires are designed to measure sleep quality rather than for diagnostic purposes. As such, their scores should be interpreted with caution as they are neither sufficient to establish a differential diagnosis nor to guide the planning of treatment. Moreover, retrospective responses to these sleep questionnaires are often obscured by recall bias and mood state of the individual at the time of assessment [95].

It is good practice to prescribe 2 weeks of *sleep diaries* to obtain a more stable picture of the sleep pattern [10]. Each diary entry is essentially a short questionnaire to be completed immediately after waking to provide information concerning the previous night for sleep onset latency (SOL), frequency and total duration of wake time after sleep onset

(WASO), total sleep time (TST), and sleep efficiency (SE). Depending on the nature of the sleep complaint, sleep diaries may also include reports of sleep quality (SQ), pain, use of medication and substances, daytime sleepiness, and fatigue to provide additional information for assessment and case formulation. Although sleep diaries are generally easy to use and there have been clinical reports suggesting therapeutic benefits associated with regular sleep monitoring, care must be taken to explain to the patient the rationale and procedure of the sleep monitoring so as to enhance adherence.

If appropriate, the use of a sleep diary can be complemented by the use of an *actigraph* (also known as an accelerometer), which is a wristwatch-like device to be worn on the nondominant wrist to measure and record the intensity and duration of physical motion. The rationale behind the use of this technology in sleep research is that frequent and intense movement during the night is indicative of wakefulness. With the aid of an algorithm, data extracted from the actigraph can be used to provide objective estimates of basic sleep parameters, such as SOL, WASO, and TST. The actigraphic measurements of TST, WASO, and SE compare well ($r = 0.49$–0.98) with corresponding sleep parameters recorded by polysomnography [96]. Actigraphy has shown modest agreement ($r = 0.34$–0.44) when compared with subjective reports of sleep given by people with musculoskeletal pain [77]. Actigraphy has also demonstrated a high degree of stability across nights ($r = 0.4$–0.81) [77, 97]. A strong relationship ($r = 0.64$) has also been observed between the actigraph measure of TST and the perceived sleep quality reported by women with FM [98]. However, it should be noted that actigraphy is recommended to establish the sleep-wake pattern over time rather than to generate estimates of sleep parameters as this technology may underestimate SOL and overestimate TST in individuals who manage to lie still over long periods. Kushida et al. [99] recommend that sleep diaries and actigraphy should be used simultaneously to provide more detailed information regarding sleep.

Although *polysomnography (PSG)* is considered the gold standard of sleep measurement [10, 99], it is not recommended for routine sleep assessment. PSG can provide information about the architecture of sleep (see "Sleep Architecture") via three measures: electroencephalography (EEG: measurement of brain waves/electrical activity), electrooculography (EOG: measurement of eye movement), and electromyography (EMG: measurement of facial muscle tension) [100]. Coupled with other electrophysiological measures (e.g., EKG, electrocardiograms, nasal/oral air flow, oxygen desaturation, leg movement), the clinician could extract useful information for the diagnosis of sleep disorders such as sleep apnea, PLMD, and RLS (which are described in "Primary Sleep Disorders Other than Insomnia in Chronic Pain"). However, the use of PSG can be intrusive to the patient's sleep, expensive to conduct, and laborious for the clinician to set up and score the results. These limitations are some of the reasons why PSG is often less accessible to the general public and the duration of sleep study is usually restricted to a short period of time (less than three nights). PSG is not indicated unless the pain patient is suspected of having primary sleep disorders. A sleep study is recommended, however, when a patient is on high-dose opioids (>150 mg), considering the strong association between daily opioid dosage and sleep apnea [101]. A home study is less expensive than in-lab PSGs and, in most cases, is sufficient to diagnose sleep-disordered breathing and to differentiate central sleep apnea from OSA. Patients with sleep apnea must be treated accordingly or have their daily opioid dose decreased, after which a repeat sleep study is recommended.

Managing Sleep Disturbance in Patients with Chronic Pain

Sleep disturbance co-occurring with chronic pain can be managed using pharmacotherapy and/or psychological therapy. The sections below describe these treatment approaches, and Table 16.2 provides a summary of their respective mechanisms, advantages, and disadvantages with a view to informing clinical decisions (Table 16.2).

Pharmacological Treatment

A number of pharmacological treatments are available for patients' sleep disturbances and pain; however, adverse effects are frequent, and patients should be monitored closely for medication-related effects on sleep pathology and pain sensitivity. Pharmacologic treatment options to manage pain include nonsteroidal anti-inflammatory drugs, opioids (morphine, oxycodone, methadone, codeine, fentanyl, buprenorphine, hydromorphone, dextropropoxyphene, and pentazocine), tricyclic antidepressants (amitriptyline), and selective norepinephrine reuptake inhibitors (duloxetine). Options to manage sleep disturbances include hypnotics and related drugs, such as benzodiazepines (BZDs-clonazepam) and nonbenzodiazepines (zolpidem, zaleplon, and eszopiclone) [122, 123]. Patients treated with opioids and BZDs should be cautioned not to take more medication than directed, even if pain is uncontrolled, because unauthorized escalation of doses could be lethal. Opioids and BZD doses should be reduced by approximately 20 % if the patient develops a flu or severe respiratory infection. For nocturnal pain, off-label use of anticonvulsants and antidepressants is less likely than opioids to depress respiration.

Some pharmacologic treatments can impact sleep architecture, sleep restoration, and pain threshold levels. Morphine, for example, has reduced SWS (by 75 %) and REM sleep, while increasing N2 sleep, [124] and in a sepa-

rate study, morphine and methadone increased N2 sleep and significantly decreased N3 and N4 sleep ($p < 0.001$) [125]. In contrast, patients with chronic pain from OA showed significantly lower pain scores from baseline following morphine sulfate as well as increases in TST and SE [126]. Some newer anticonvulsants have been found to have negligible impacts on sleep architecture, and some may even improve it. For instance, gabapentin and pregabalin were found to promote modest increases in SWS without affecting REM sleep in healthy adults [103, 104, 127, 128].

Additional adverse effects must be considered when treating patients pharmacologically. For example, opioids, particularly methadone, have been associated with a high rate (75 %) of sleep-disordered breathing in patients with chronic pain [129]. Concomitant BZD administration was shown to have a significant additive effect on methadone-related central sleep apnea. In another study, the prevalence of central sleep apnea was found to be 30 % in patients undergoing methadone maintenance treatment [130].

Methadone is not the only opioid associated with alarming levels of sleep apnea. There appears to be a dose relationship of all opioids to central sleep apnea. A linear relationship of opioid dose to central sleep apnea has been reported with immediate release and sustained release formulations. Doses of 150 mg morphine equivalence have approximately a 70 % probability of central sleep apnea [101]. Hypoxia due to hypoventilation has also been observed in patients on chronic opioid therapy even without evidence of sleep apnea (Lynn Webster, personal communication).

Tricyclic antidepressants (TCAs), commonly administered for neuropathic pain, concurrently address symptoms of insomnia and depression. A meta-analysis of 61 clinical trials found that TCAs have demonstrated effectiveness for treatment of diabetic neuralgia and postherpetic neuralgia and to some extent for central pain, atypical facial pain, and postoperative pain after breast cancer treatments [131]. Possible adverse effects of TCAs include drowsiness, dry mouth, blurred vision, constipation, urinary retention, and more serious heart-related conditions [131]. Tricyclic antidepressants have been linked to increased risk of suicide attempts [107, 108] and may reduce seizure thresholds in vulnerable individuals [132]. The newer SNRI formulations (e.g., duloxetine, milnacipran, desvenlafaxine) are reported to have much fewer side effects and increased tolerability. This is particularly important to elderly patients who tend to be more sensitive to the side effect profile of many medications.

Benzodiazepines (BZDs) are frequently used to treat sleep disorders, but their efficacy for sleep disturbances complicated by pain is unclear, and more research is needed. Some studies show improved sleep outcomes, including decreased SOL and WASO and increased TST; however, many other studies demonstrate either no effect or heightened levels of pain compared to controls [123]. It should be

Table 16.2 Mechanisms, advantages, and disadvantages of the mainstream pharmacological agents and psychological treatments for chronic pain patients with concomitant insomnia

Treatment	Mechanism	Advantages	Disadvantages
Analgesics (e.g., NSAIDs, opioids)	NSAIDs reduce inflammation and algesia by inhibiting arachidonic acid but have no sedative effect. Inhibition of prostaglandin biosynthesis is through inhibition of COX-1 and COX-2 enzymes. COX-1 activation leads to production of prostacyclin which is cytoprotective. COX-2 is induced in inflammatory cells. The ratio of COX-1 to COX-2 determines the likelihood of adverse effects. Opioids bind to mu, delta, and kappa receptors; effect is to decrease presynaptic calcium flux, which decreases neurotransmitter release. Opioids also increase postsynaptic K+ flux, resulting in hyperpolarization of the neuron, decreasing conductance and transmission. The analgesic and sedative effects of opioids arise from the inhibition of cholinergic, adenosinergic, and GABAergic transmission	The analgesic effects of NSAIDs may reduce nighttime arousal The sedative effects of opioids hasten sleep onset.	Analgesics may increase awakening and alter sleep architecture, suppressing SWS and REM sleep Other side effects include nausea, vomiting, diarrhea, constipation, skin complaints, dry mouth, dizziness, headaches, blurred vision, and fluid retention. The more severe complications are stomach ulcers and kidney/liver failure There is also the risk of addiction with prolonged use of opioids [102]
Anticonvulsants (e.g., gabapentin, pregabalin)	Mechanism is not known but appears to involve activation of the alpha2-delta protein subunit, which decreases Ca+ flux and slows depolarization of neuronal activity of postsynaptic neurons.	Demonstrated efficacy in improving pain and functional measures, including sleep [103] Increase SWS without detrimenting REM sleep [104] Effective in the treatment of RLS and PLMD [105] Pregabalin is thought to be less of a risk for dependence/abuse than other classes of medication [106]	Pain relief happens when optimal dose is achieved. Optimal doses of these drugs vary from individual to individual; careful monitoring and patient titration are required Some patients cannot tolerate these drugs well, particularly those who are on high doses, causing premature drug withdrawals Common adverse effects include dizziness, peripheral edema, somnolence, confusion, headache, dry mouth, and constipation
Tricyclic antidepressants (e.g., amitriptyline, nortriptyline)	Inhibit neuronal uptake of norepinephrine and serotonin into the presynaptic nerve terminals by inhibiting the serotonin and norepinephrine transporters at an approximately 1:8 ratio. They also block postsynaptic sodium, calcium, and potassium channels	Some evidence of pain relief Hasten sleep onset Beneficial for pain patients with concomitant mood problems	Off-label use only; none of the TCAs has been approved by the FDA for treatment of DPNP or any type of pain TCAs alter sleep architecture. Possible side effects include daytime drowsiness, dry mouth, blurred vision, constipation, urinary retention, and heart conditions TCAs may increase the risk of suicide attempt [107, 108] Amitriptyline is a relative contraindication for older patients and patients with any cardiovascular disease [109]
Selective reuptake inhibitors (e.g., duloxetine, venlafaxine, milnacipran, desvenlafaxine)	Prevent serotonin and norepinephrine form being reabsorbed into the presynaptic terminals. Duloxetine differs from venlafaxine in that it is comparatively more noradrenergic. Venlafaxine has a 30-fold higher affinity for serotonin than for norepinephrine, while duloxetine has a tenfold selectivity for serotonin [110]. Approximate potency ratios (5-HT:NE) are 1:10 for duloxetine and 1:30 for venlafaxine	Lack most of the side effects of tricyclic antidepressants and monoamine oxidase inhibitors Duloxetine is approved for the management of neuropathic pain associated with diabetic peripheral neuropathy and FM	Nausea is the most common side effect for most drugs in this class This class of drug is also associated with increased blood pressure and insomnia [110–112] Cytochrome P450 isoenzymes inducers and inhibitors can affect drug levels

(continued)

Table 16.2 (continued)

Treatment	Mechanism	Advantages	Disadvantages
Hypnotics (e.g., clonazepam, zolpidem)	Facilitate GABAergic transmission. BZDs and other hypnotics (non-BZDs) bind to the gamma subunit of the GABA-A receptor, which increases chloride ion conductance and inhibition of the action potentials	Established efficacy for both BZDs and non-BZDs for acute and short-term management	Potential side effects include daytime drowsiness, dizziness, impaired memory, concentration, and psychomotor performance
		Fast-acting	There is the risk of tolerance and dependence with extended use, and rebound insomnia may occur after discontinuation [113]
Pain management programs (multidisciplinary programs in the US)	Treatment delivered by multidisciplinary team. Program content varies but generally includes psychoeducation on pain, relaxation techniques, physical exercises, CT for pain, and behavioral pain and stress management strategies; many programs also offer sleep hygiene education	Moderate treatment effects have been achieved for improved coping and self-efficacy regarding pain [114]	Treatment effects are generally small for reducing pain severity [114]
		The group format encourages social support and facilitates behavioral change [115]	Focus of treatment is largely on rehabilitation. Not enough individual therapy time for complex cases that present with other comorbid anxiety, mood, and sleep problems
			Limited coverage on sleep; only minimal improvements on sleep are detected in graduates of PMPs [116]
			Remission rates in a range of pain and functional outcome measures are between 18 and 33 %, with 1–2 % of the patients reliably deteriorate during the period of treatment [117]
CBT for insomnia	Treatment delivered both individually or in groups by trained psychologists or behavioral sleep medicine specialists. Content varies but generally include psychoeducation on sleep, sleep hygiene, relaxation training, CT for sleep, sleep restriction, stimulus control, paradoxical intention, biofeedback, and imagery training	Highly efficacious and cost-effective; recommended for chronic insomnia [118]	Improved sleep does not necessarily bring about a reduction in pain [119–121]
		Durable treatment has been achieved in core sleep parameters when CBT-I is directly applied to treat pain-related insomnia [119, 120]	Remission rates in individuals with pain-related insomnia are between 16 and 57 % [119–121]
			Further refinement is required to address sleep-interfering processes specific to chronic pain patients [48]
			The initial stage of CBT-I involves cutting down time resting in bed and the introduction of mild sleep deprivation. This may aggravate pain/discomfort for some individuals
			The use of sleep restriction therapy involves getting out of bed and going to another room when woken from sleep. This may be difficult for patients who have restricted mobility

NSAIDs nonsteroidal anti-inflammatory drugs, *COX* cyclooxygenase enzyme, *K+* potassium cation, *GABA* gamma aminobutyric acid, *SWS* slow wave sleep, *REM* rapid eye movement, *Ca+* calcium cation, *RLS* restless leg syndrome, *PLMD* periodic limb movement disorder, *TCAs* tricyclic antidepressants, *FDA* food and drug administration, *DPNP* diabetic peripheral neuropathic pain, *BZDs* benzodiazepines, *CT* cognitive therapy, *PMPs* pain management programs, *CBT-I* cognitive behavioral therapy for insomnia

noted that prolonged use of BZDs has been associated with increased risk of hip fractures in the elderly [133], although some research shows that prior risk factors such as depression and antidepressant use often precede a new BZD prescription in older adults [134]. It appears that newer BZDs and the non-BZDs may offer enhanced safety and greater efficacy as related to sleep outcomes, but data are limited with relation to pain management [123, 135].

Nonpharmacological Treatment

Although pharmacological management of insomnia is commonly used as the first-line treatment for pain-related sleep disturbance, clinical experience tells us that many patients prefer not to have another tablet for sleep, not only because of the adverse effects mentioned above but also for fears of potential drug interaction, tolerance, and dependence. While pharmacotherapy can have a favorable risk-benefit profile in many individuals, evidence in support of its efficacy and safety beyond 6–12 months is currently thin [113]. Long-term hypnotic medication is usually not indicated for the type of insomnia experienced by chronic pain patients, which often is as chronic as the pain itself and requires a different approach of management.

While most cases of insomnia in chronic pain were precipitated by the onset of pain, the relative importance of pain as a maintaining factor decreases as the insomnia persists. Factors perpetuating the insomnia proliferate as the patient develops compensatory strategies to cope with the pain (e.g., resting in pain, inactivity, ruminating about the pain) and the sleep loss (e.g., extending bedtime, daytime naps, drinking large amounts of tea and coffee to stay alert during the day). Similar to what is happening in primary insomnia, these perpetuating factors tend to be cognitive behavioral in nature and are often amenable to psychological treatments grounded on the cognitive behavioral principles. Multidisciplinary pain programs, which are sometimes called pain management programs (PMP), and cognitive behavioral therapy for primary insomnia (CBT-I) are obvious alternatives to pharmacological treatments. These two forms of treatment will be reviewed in this section with a particular focus on their effectiveness for pain-related insomnia.

Pain management programs (PMPs) – frequently referred to as multidisciplinary pain programs in the United States – are usually delivered to groups of patients and cover three main areas. Patients are taught about the physiology, psychology, and function of pain and shown how to utilize relaxation techniques and coping skills. Components of PMPs typically have a strong behavioral focus, encouraging patients to get back in action, pace their activities, set goals, and direct their activities towards achieving those goals. Some PMPs also include cognitive treatment components that focus on identifying and challenging negative thoughts and beliefs about pain and on managing the psychological effects of pain and stress. Although sleep is often discussed in the form of sleep hygiene education in many standard PMPs, it is not normally included as an outcome measure in treatment studies [136]. There are, however, some notable exceptions that have investigated the effect of PMPs on sleep.

A randomized, controlled trial (RCT) conducted by Redondo et al. [137] compared cognitive behavioral therapy (CBT) versus a physical exercise program in 40 women with FM. The CBT comprised eight sessions, each 2.5 h long and 1 week apart, providing information about FM, teaching behavioral techniques for pain management, and advising on sleep and resting. Despite success in improving patients' ability to cope with pain and their daily functioning, sleep did not improve when rated posttreatment or at the 6-month and 1-year follow-up. Similarly, there was no significant improvement in sleep in patients assigned to the physical exercise program.

Gustavsson and von Koch [138] led an RCT comparing a group program of pain and stress management against individual physiotherapy in 37 patients seeking treatment for chronic neck pain. The pain and stress management program involved 7 weekly sessions, each lasting 1.5 h, which taught anatomy, etiology, and physiology concerning neck pain and developing strategies for managing pain and stress, including applied relaxation training. It should be noted that relaxation training is also commonly incorporated in CBT-I; although not specifically instructed to do so, participants in Gustavsson and von Koch's study could have used the relaxation techniques to reduce sleep-interfering somatic and cognitive tension at night. However, those who completed the treatment (*n* = 29; 78 %) reported no significant improvement in their sleep after completing the treatment or at the 20-week follow-up [138].

Becker et al. [139] randomly assigned 189 patients seeking treatment for chronic pain to one of three groups: treatment at a multidisciplinary pain center, treatment from a general practitioner (GP), or a 6-month wait-list group. After 6 months, those patients treated by the multidisciplinary pain team reported a small improvement in their sleep as well as reduced pain intensity and improved psychological well-being. However, the clinical significance of the improvement in sleep was not discussed.

Ashworth et al. [116] investigated the within-group effect of a PMP on unhelpful sleep beliefs as well as sleep quality in 42 chronic pain patients. The PMP was delivered in a group format and consisted of 12 weekly sessions. The Pittsburgh Sleep Quality Index (PSQI) [89] and the Dysfunctional Beliefs and Attitudes about Sleep Questionnaire (DBAS) [93, 94] were administered to evaluate improvements in sleep. No improvements were reported for self-reported TST, estimated SE, or dysfunctional beliefs about sleep. However, patients did report shorter SOL and improved satisfaction with sleep quality, and reduced use of medication and daytime dysfunction. There was no control group in this study, and thus the reported benefits in sleep might have been inflated.

Although these studies can be commended for including sleep as an outcome measure, they (with the exception of Ashworth et al. [116]) mostly relied upon single-item ratings of sleep, and none used more detailed sleep diaries or objective measures of sleep, which are more reliable measures of sleep improvement and are commonplace in sleep research. Based on the findings reported above, it appears that only minimal improvements can be obtained in sleep when the focus of the treatment is on better managing pain. One possible explanation for this is that the insomnia experienced by these pain patients, though triggered by pain, is predominantly perpetuated by factors that are not addressed by individual pain clinicians or multidisciplinary programs.

With the growing understanding of pain-related insomnia as a problem in its own right, colleagues in the field have progressed to use CBT-I to specifically address sleep problems in chronic pain. CBT-I involves teaching patients about the science of sleep and the factors that affect it, collaborating with the patient to improve sleep efficiency using strategies such as sleep restriction (reducing time spent in bed to increase physiological sleep pressure) and stimulus control (reestablishing the association between the bed/bedroom and sleep). Cognitive elements of the therapy address sleep-specific worries and beliefs, especially those that instigate sleep-related anxiety (e.g., "if I can't sleep I won't be able to function tomorrow"), and safety-seeking behaviors (e.g., spending excessive time in bed and napping during the day to make up sleep) that further aggravate the sleep problem.

There is an emerging body of research investigating the effectiveness of *CBT-I for treating pain-related insomnia*, and four RCTs have been published during the past decade involving patients with chronic nonmalignant pain.

Currie et al. [119] conducted the first RCT to examine the effectiveness of CBT-I to treat pain-related insomnia. Sixty patients with chronic musculoskeletal pain were randomly allocated to either CBT-I ($n = 32$) or wait-list control. The CBT-I consisted of 7 weekly 2-h sessions delivered in a group format by six psychology doctorial students/interns with previous training in CBT interventions. The content of the treatment included psychoeducation about sleep and good sleep hygiene, relaxation training, cognitive therapy, sleep restriction therapy, and stimulus control. Sleep, pain, and mood were assessed at baseline, posttreatment, and after 3 months using 2-week sleep diaries, actigraphy, PSQI [89], Multidimensional Pain Inventory Pain Severity Scale (MPI-PS) [140], and Beck Depression Inventory (BDI) [141], respectively. Participants receiving CBT-I reported significantly improved SOL, WASO, and SE as measured by the sleep diaries and greater sleep quality measured by the PSQI posttreatment compared to the control group. Within-group analysis also indicated a significant reduction in movement monitored by actigraphy posttreatment compared to the baseline assessment. These improvements were maintained 3 months posttreatment with 16 % of patients achieving improvements that were clinically as well as statistically significant (SOL and WASO <30 min, SE > 85 %, and PSQI < 6). CBT-I, however, had no significant impact upon pain severity or mood.

Edinger et al. [120] compared CBT-I ($n = 18$) with basic sleep hygiene education ($n = 18$) and usual care ($n = 11$) for treating patients with FM. The CBT-I was delivered by experienced clinical psychologists to patients following an individual format in 6 weekly sessions, the duration of which varied between 15 min and 1 h. The CBT-I consisted of psychoeducation about sleep, sleep restriction therapy, and stimulus control. Sleep was assessed using sleep diaries, actigraphy, and Insomnia Symptom Questionnaire (ISQ) [142]. Pain was assessed using the McGill Pain Questionnaire (MPQ) [143] and the Brief Pain Inventory (BPI) [144] while mood was assessed using the Profile of Mood States (POMS) [145] and the mental health composite score of the Medical Outcomes Survey 36-Item Short-Form Health Survey (SF-36) [146]. Posttreatment patients who received CBT-I reported shorter SOL, longer TST and SE, shorter SOL recorded by actigraphy, and lower ratings on the ISQ (indicating improved sleep) compared to patients receiving usual care, and these differences remained at 6-month follow-up. These improvements in sleep were considered by Edinger et al. [120] to be clinically significant for 57 % of the CBT-I group (TST $\geq$ 6.5 h, TWT < 60 min, and SE $\geq$ 85 %, which is consistent with that defined in the CBT-I literature). Significant improvements were also observed in mood but not in pain.

Jungquist et al. [121] evaluated the impact of CBT-I on sleep disturbance and pain severity and pain interference. Nineteen patients with chronic neck or back pain individually received 8 weekly sessions of CBT-I from a CBT-trained nurse. The sessions lasted between 30 and 60 min and included sleep hygiene education, cognitive therapy, stimulus control, and sleep restriction. Sleep was measured using sleep diaries and the Insomnia Severity Index (ISI) [88]; pain was assessed using the MPI-PS, [140] the Pain Disability Index (PDI) [147], and a daily pain rating; mood was measured using the BDI [141]. Posttreatment patients reported significant improvements compared with controls in their self-reported SOL, WASO, SE, and overall ISI score. These improvements reached clinical significance for 42 % of the group according to the criteria (SOL and WASO < 15 min) of Jungquist and colleagues [121]. However, the improvements in sleep did not translate to significant improvements in pain and mood.

Vitello et al. [148] evaluated the efficacy of CBT-I on sleep disturbance and pain in 23 older adults with OA. The study follows their parent RCT [149], which compared CBT-I with an attention control condition in older adults with insomnia comorbid with a variety of chronic illnesses and found significant group differences posttreatment for sleep (CBT-I showed greater improvements) but not pain, as measured with MPQ [143]. This is a secondary analysis focusing on the within-group effect in a subgroup of OA patients to examine the durability of sleep improvements and to gauge the extent to which improved sleep can reduce pain.

The CBT-I consisted of 8 weekly sessions delivered in a group format by two clinical psychologists, each session lasting 2 h. The sessions involved teaching good sleep hygiene practice, relaxation training, cognitive therapy, stimulus control, and sleep restriction. Outcome measures included 2-week sleep diaries, short-form MPQ [143], and bodily pain subscale of the SF-36 [146], which were taken at baseline, posttreatment, and 1-year posttreatment. Patients who received CBT-I reported improved SOL (effect size = 0.55), WASO (effect size = 0.72), and increased SE (effect size = 0.88) posttreatment compared to baseline.

At 1-year follow-up, all improvements in sleep were maintained, and TST had also increased significantly (effect size = 0.46). Although the focus of the study was to examine the efficacy of CBT-I for reducing pain, only a small improvement was reported on the SF-36 measure (effect size = 0.31) and was not confirmed when measured with the SF-MPQ. Further, the gain on the SF-36 was not maintained when assessed 1-year posttreatment.

It appears that CBT-I originally developed for the treatment of primary insomnia can be successfully applied to treat pain-related insomnia. The pre-posttreatment effects for sleep are encouraging, ranging from 0.55 to 2.15 for SOL, 0.72–1.45 for WASO, 0.21–0.99 for TST, 0.88–2.01 for SE, and 0.76–3.25 for SQ [119–121, 148]. In terms of clinical significance, between 16 and 57 % of the patients achieved remission at posttreatment, and it appears that those treatments that adopted the individual format produced a higher remission rate than those that adopted the group format.

The knowledge that sleep deprivation/fragmentation increases pain perception has raised the hope that improvements in sleep could result in a significant improvement in pain. Unfortunately, the reciprocal relationship between sleep and pain is not as apparent in the therapeutic context as in the experimental setting. The results from the above-reviewed RCTs indicate that sleep improvement does not necessarily bring about a therapeutic effect on mood and pain [119–121]. The only RCT where an improvement in pain was observed reported inconsistent results from the SF-36 pain items and the SF-MPQ, and the result was obtained from a secondary analysis that specifically looked at the within-group change that will provide larger effect sizes than between-group comparisons [150]. Although it is encouraging to know that CBT-I, if well designed and executed, could have some positive impact on a patient's pain complaint, CBT-I per se is not sufficient to provide meaningful pain relief for patients suffering from chronic pain.

Taken together, PMPs incorporating just the sleep hygiene component of CBT-I typically do not produce any major benefit to pain patient's sleep. Although CBT-I directly applied to treat insomnia is efficacious in alleviating sleep disturbance, its therapeutic effect is not strong enough to prompt a discernable reduction in pain intensity or pain-related interference. The respective limitations of PMPs and CBT-I have led us to think that a hybrid form of psychological treatment that combines the most potent treatment components of PMPs and CBT-I to simultaneously address sleep and pain may be able to produce better outcomes. Given the intractable nature of chronic pain and the demonstrated inconsistent relationship between sleep and pain, the focus of such treatment should not be on using sleep to achieve pain reduction. Instead, we think that using better sleep as a means to improve the patient's daytime functioning, activity level, and overall quality of life may be more a meaningful goal.

Future Directions

We have only just begun to understand more about the impact of acute and chronic pain on sleep and the reverse impact of sleep disturbance on pain perception and tolerance. There are still many basic and clinically relevant questions to be answered. More effort will be required to delineate the mechanisms through which sleep and pain interact, both at the physiological and psychological levels. We know from experimental studies that the presentation of painful stimuli could have an arousal effect on healthy volunteers. However, scant evidence suggests that an increase in pain has the same effects on individuals who have already been experiencing pain for some time. As such, it would be important for future research to further examine these pain-sleep interaction pathways using clinical pain patient samples. In characterizing the impact of sleep disturbances on pain responses, recent additions to the literature indicate that the suppression of SWS and REM sleep may have differential effects on pain perception and that it may be sleep disruption, rather than sleep deprivation, that is contributing to the increased pain complaints. Developing an experimental model of sleep fragmentation that closely approximates the intermittent sleep pattern seen in patients with acute or chronic pain may allow future research to better study the impact of sleep disruption in different contexts. And of course, more research is required to understand the elevated rates of several sleep disorders (e.g., RSL, PLMS, OSA) in subgroups of pain patients.

Currently, there are a number of methods available to manage sleep disturbances concomitant to chronic pain. Each has its own advantages and disadvantages, and clinicians need to weigh the risks and benefits of each approach when planning treatment for their patients. Although both pharmacotherapy and nonpharmacotherapy have demonstrated efficacy in reducing insomnia symptoms, neither has consistently demonstrated that improved sleep is associated with a significant reduction in pain. Perhaps, the relationship between sleep and pain is not completely reciprocal in a therapeutic context. Most RCTs investigating the effect of CBT-I on sleep and pain complaints only had a short follow-up duration. Future RCTs with longer follow-up periods should provide an answer if time is what is needed for the effect of improved sleep on pain to be seen. Also, it is unclear what neuromechanisms underpin the transition from acute to persistent insomnia in chronic pain. It would be interesting to see whether the application of CBT-I could reverse some of these biological changes after treatment. Well-designed, longitudinal imaging studies may shed new light on the neuroplasticity of the brain.

Hybrid treatment that incorporates the most potent components of existing pain and sleep treatments to simultaneously address pain and insomnia may be the way forward if the therapy goal is to achieve significant improvement in both pain and sleep domains. Hybrid treatment could be an integration of psychological treatments of different focus (e.g., PMPs + CBT-I) or a combination of both pharmacological and nonpharmacological treatments (e.g., pregabalin plus CBT-I). More research will be needed to inform the design, structure, format, sequence, and duration of such treatment.

Summary and Conclusion

Chronic pain and insomnia are two of the most common forms of health problems in today's society. Each of them is a debilitating health condition in its own right. When both are presented in the same patient, pain and sleep interact to produce a condition that is even more challenging for the patient to self-manage and for health-care professionals to treat. Existing evidence indicates that the standard unidimensional approach of treatment is insufficient. Research and clinical efforts are now focusing on better understanding the pain-sleep interaction and developing more effective strategies to deal with both pain and insomnia symptoms simultaneously. A more integrative treatment approach with diverse clinical targets is likely to be the model of effective pain management in the future.

References

1. Becker N, Bondegaard TA, Olsen AK, et al. Pain epidemiology and health related quality of life in chronic non-malignant pain patients referred to a Danish multidisciplinary pain center. Pain. 1997;73:393–400.
2. Casarett D, Karlawish J, Sankar P, et al. Designing pain research from the patient's perspective: what trial end points are important to patients with chronic pain? Pain Med. 2001;2:309–16.
3. Smith BH, Torrance N, Bennett MI, et al. Health and quality of life associated with chronic pain of predominantly neuropathic origin in the community. Clin J Pain. 2007;23:143–9.
4. Smith MT, Carmody TP, Smith MS. Quality of well-being scale and chronic low back pain. J Clin Psychol Med S. 2000;7:175–84.
5. Tang NKY, Crane C. Suicidality in chronic pain: a review of the prevalence, risk factors and psychological links. Psychol Med. 2006;36:575–86.
6. Turk DC, Dworkin RH, Revicki D, et al. Identifying important outcome domains for chronic pain clinical trials: an IMMPACT survey of people with pain. Pain. 2008;137:276–85.
7. Morin C, Gibson D, Wade J. Self-reported sleep and mood disturbance in chronic pain patients. Clin J Pain. 1998;14:311–4.
8. Smith M, Perlis M, Smith M, et al. Sleep quality and presleep arousal in chronic pain. J Behav Med. 2000;23:1–13.
9. Tang NKY, Wright KJ, Salkovskis PM. Prevalence and correlates of clinical insomnia co-occurring with chronic low back pain. J Sleep Res. 2007;16:85–95.
10. Morin CM, Espie CA. Insomnia: a clinical guide to assessment and treatment. New York: Springer; 2004.
11. McCracken LM, Iverson GL. Disrupted sleep patterns and daily functioning in patients with chronic pain. Pain Res Manag. 2002;7:75–9.
12. Theadom A, Cropley M, Humphrey K. Exploring the role of sleep and coping in quality of life in fibromyalgia. J Psychosom Res. 2007;62:145–51.
13. Dworkin RH, Turk DC, Farrar JT, et al. Core outcome measures for chronic pain clinical trials: IMMPACT recommendations. Pain. 2005;113:9–19.
14. Turk DC, Dworkin RH, McDermott MP, et al. Analyzing multiple endpoints in clinical trials of pain treatments: IMMPACT recommendations. Pain. 2008;139:485–93.
15. Rechtschaffen A, Bergmann B, Everson C, et al. Sleep deprivation in the rat: X integration and discussion of the findings. Sleep. 1989;25:68–87.
16. Guzman-Marýn R, Suntsova N, Stewart D, et al. Sleep deprivation reduces proliferation of cells in the dentate gyrus of the hippocampus in rats. J Physiol. 2003;549:563–71.
17. Schmidek W, Zachariassen K, Hammel H. Total calorimetric measurements in the rat: influences of the sleep-wakefulness cycle and of the environmental temperature. Brain Res. 1983;288:261–71.
18. Everson C, Laatsch C, Hogg N. Antioxidant defense responses to sleep loss and sleep recovery. Am J Physiol Regul Integr Comp Physiol. 2005;288:R374–83.
19. Toth L. Sleep, sleep deprivation and infectious disease: studies in animals. Adv Neuroimmunol. 1995;5:79–92.
20. Everson C. Sustained sleep deprivation impairs host defense. Am J Physiol. 1993;265:R1148–54.
21. Everson C. Clinical assessment of blood leukocytes, serum cytokines, and serum immunoglobulins as responses to sleep deprivation in laboratory rats. Am J Physiol Regul Integr Comp Physiol. 2005;289:R1054–63.
22. Ranjbaran Z, Keefer L, Stepanski E, et al. The relevance of sleep abnormalities to chronic inflammatory conditions. Inflamm Res. 2007;56:51–7.
23. Ohayon MM, Caulet M, Philip P, et al. How sleep and mental disorders are related to complaints of daytime sleepiness. Arch Intern Med. 1997;157:2645–52.
24. Becker PM, Brown WD, Jamieson AO. Impact of insomnia: assessment with the sickness impact profile. Sleep Res. 1991;20:206.
25. Breslau N, Roth T, Rosenthal L, et al. Daytime sleepiness: an epidemiological study of young adults. Am J Public Health. 1997;87:1649–53.
26. Chang PP, Ford DE, Mead LA, et al. Insomnia in young men and subsequent depression. The Johns Hopkins study. Am J Epidemiol. 1997;146:105–14.
27. Ford DE, Kamerow DB. Epidemiologic study of sleep disturbances and psychiatric disorders. An opportunity for prevention? JAMA. 1989;262:1479–84.
28. Mellinger GD, Balter MB, Uhlenhuth EH. Insomnia and its treatment. Prevalence and correlates. Arch Gen Psychiatry. 1985;42:225–32.
29. Neckelmann D, Mykletun A, Dahl AA. Chronic insomnia as a risk factor for developing anxiety and depression. Sleep. 2007;30:873–80.
30. Simon GE, VonKorff M. Prevalence, burden, and treatment of insomnia in primary care. Am J Psychiatry. 1997;154:1417–23.
31. Vollrath M, Wicki W, Angst J. The Zurich study. VIII. Insomnia: association with depression, anxiety, somatic syndromes, and course of insomnia. Eur Arch Psychiatry Neurol Sci. 1989;239:113–24.
32. Weissman MM, Greenwald S, Nino-Murcia G, et al. The morbidity of insomnia uncomplicated by psychiatric disorders. Gen Hosp Psychiatry. 1997;19:245–50.
33. Stickgold R, James L, Hobson J. Visual discrimination learning requires sleep after training. Nat Neurosci. 2000;3:1237–8.
34. Stickgold R, Whidbee D, Schirmer B, et al. Visual discrimination task improvement: a multi-step process occurring during sleep. J Cogn Neurosci. 2000;12:246–54.

35. McCarley R. Neurobiology of REM and NREM sleep. Sleep Med. 2007;8:302–30.

36. Ohayon MM. Relationship between chronic painful physical condition and insomnia. J Psychiatr Res. 2005;39:151–9.

37. Morphy H, Dunn KM, Lewis M, et al. Epidemiology of insomnia: a longitudinal study in a UK population. Sleep. 2007;30:274–80.

38. Foley D, Ancoli-Israel S, Britz P, et al. Sleep disturbances and chronic disease in older adults: results of the 2003 National Sleep Foundation Sleep in America Survey. J Psychosom Res. 2004; 56:497–502.

39. Gabor JY, Cooper AB, Hanly PJ. Sleep disruption in the intensive care unit. Curr Opin Crit Care. 2001;7:21–7.

40. Redeker NS. Sleep in acute care settings: an integrative review. J Nurs Scholarsh. 2000;32:31–8.

41. Rosenberg-Adamsen S, Kehlet H, Dodds C, et al. Postoperative sleep disturbances: mechanisms and clinical implications. Br J Anaesth. 1996;76:552–9.

42. Redeker NS, Hedges C. Sleep during hospitalization and recovery after cardiac surgery. J Cardiovasc Nurs. 2002;17:56–68.

43. Raymond I, Nielsen TA, Lavigne G, et al. Quality of sleep and its daily relationship to pain intensity in hospitalized adult burn patients. Pain. 2001;92:381–8.

44. Savard J, Morin CM. Insomnia in the context of cancer: a review of a neglected problem. J Clin Oncol. 2001;19:895–908.

45. Dorrepaal KL, Aaronson NK, van Dam FS. Pain experience and pain management among hospitalized cancer patients. A clinical study. Cancer. 1989;63:593–8.

46. Atkinson JH, Ancoli-Israel S, Slater MA, et al. Subjective sleep disturbance in chronic back pain. Clin J Pain. 1988;4:225–32.

47. Pilowsky I, Crettenden I, Townley M. Sleep disturbance in pain clinic patients. Pain. 1985;23:27–33.

48. Tang NKY, Goodchild CE, Hester J, Salkovskis PM. Pain-related insomnia: A comparision study of sleep pattern, psychological characteristics and cognitive-behavioural processes. Clinical journal of pain. 2012;428–436.

49. Wittig R, Zorick F, Blumer D, et al. Disturbed sleep in patients complaining of chronic pain. J Nerv Ment Dis. 1982;170:429–31.

50. Hirsch M, Carlander B, Vergé M, et al. Objective and subjective sleep disturbances in patients with rheumatoid arthritis. A reappraisal. Arthritis Rheum. 1994;37:41–9.

51. Landis C, Lentz M, Rothermel J, et al. Decreased sleep spindles and spindle activity in midlife women with fibromyalgia and pain. Sleep. 2004;27:741–50.

52. Rizzi M, Sarzi-Puttini P, Atzeni F, et al. Cyclic alternating pattern: a new marker of sleep alteration in patients with fibromyalgia? J Rheumatol. 2004;31:1193–9.

53. Martinez-Lavin M, Hermosillo AG, Rosas M, et al. Circadian studies of autonomic nervous balance in patients with fibromyalgia: a heart rate variability analysis. Arthritis Rheum. 1998;41:1966–71.

54. Moldofsky H, Scarisbrick P, England R, et al. Musculoskeletal symptoms and non-REM sleep disturbance in patients with "fibrositis syndrome" and healthy subjects. Psychosom Med. 1975;37:341–51.

55. Moldofsky H, Lue F. The relationship of alpha and delta EEG frequencies to pain and mood in 'fibrositis' patients treated with chlorpromazine and L-tryptophan. Electroencephalogr Clin Neurophysiol. 1980;50:71–80.

56. Horne JA, Shackell BS. Alpha-like EEG activity in non-REM sleep and the fibromyalgia (fibrositis) syndrome. Electroencephalogr Clin Neurophysiol. 1991;79:271–6.

57. Pivik RT, Harman K. A reconceptualization of EEG alpha activity as an index of arousal during sleep: all alpha activity is not equal. J Sleep Res. 1995;4:131–7.

58. Rains J, Penzien D. Sleep and chronic pain: challenges to the alpha-EEG sleep pattern as a pain specific sleep anomaly. J Psychosom Res. 2003;54:77–83.

59. Schneider-Helmert D, Whitehouse I, Kumar A, et al. Insomnia and alpha sleep in chronic non-organic pain as compared to primary insomnia. Neuropsychobiology. 2001;43:54–8.

60. Dauvilliers Y, Touchon J. Sleep in fibromyalgia: review of clinical and polysomnographic data. Neurophysiol Clin. 2001;31:18–33.

61. Moldofsky H, Tullis C, Lue F. Sleep related myoclonus in rheumatic pain modulation disorder (fibrositis syndrome). J Rheumatol. 1986;13:614–7.

62. Montplaisir J, Boucher S, Poirier G, et al. Clinical, polysomnographic, and genetic characteristics of restless legs syndrome: a study of 133 patients diagnosed with new standard criteria. Mov Disord. 1997;12:61–5.

63. Sun ER, Chen CA, Ho G, et al. Iron and the restless legs syndrome. Sleep. 1998;21:371–7.

64. Polydefkis M, Allen RP, Hauer P, et al. Subclinical sensory neuropathy in late-onset restless legs syndrome. Neurology. 2000; 55:1115–21.

65. Sand T, Hagen K, Schrader H. Sleep apnea and chronic headache. Cephalalgia. 2003;23:90–5.

66. Loh N, Dinner D, Foldvary N, et al. Do patients with obstructive sleep apnea wake up with headaches? Arch Intern Med. 1999; 159:1765–8.

67. Germanowicz D, Lumertz MS, Martinez D, et al. Sleep disordered breathing concomitant with fibromyalgia syndrome. J Bras Pneumol. 2006;32:333–8.

68. Sepici V, Tosun A, Köktürk O. Obstructive sleep apnea syndrome as an uncommon cause of fibromyalgia: a case report. Rheumatol Int. 2007;28:69–71.

69. Drewes AM, Nielsen KD, Arendt-Nielsen L, et al. The effect of cutaneous and deep pain on the electroencephalogram during sleep – an experimental study. Sleep. 1997;20:632–40.

70. Lavigne G, Zucconi M, Castronovo C, et al. Sleep arousal response to experimental thermal stimulation during sleep in human subjects free of pain and sleep problems. Pain. 2000;84:283–90.

71. Lavigne G, Brousseau M, Kato T, et al. Experimental pain perception remains equally active over all sleep stages. Pain. 2004; 110:646–55.

72. Onen S, Alloui A, Gross A, et al. The effects of total sleep deprivation, selective sleep interruption and sleep recovery on pain tolerance thresholds in healthy subjects. J Sleep Res. 2001; 10:35–42.

73. Moldofsky H, Scarisbrick P. Induction of neurasthenic musculoskeletal pain syndrome by selective sleep stage deprivation. Psychosom Med. 1976;38:35–44.

74. Lentz MJ, Landis CA, Rothermel J, et al. Effects of selective slow wave sleep disruption on musculoskeletal pain and fatigue in middle aged women. J Rheumatol. 1999;26:1586–92.

75. Roehrs T, Hyde M, Blaisdell B, et al. Sleep loss and REM sleep loss are hyperalgesic. Sleep. 2006;29:145–51.

76. Smith MT, Edwards RR, McCann UD, et al. The effects of sleep deprivation on pain inhibition and spontaneous pain in women. Sleep. 2007;30:494–505.

77. Wilson KG, Watson ST, Currie SR. Daily diary and ambulatory activity monitoring of sleep in patients with insomnia associated with chronic musculoskeletal pain. Pain. 1998;75:75–84.

78. Chapman JB, Lehman CL, Elliott J, et al. Sleep quality and the role of sleep medications for veterans with chronic pain. Pain Med. 2006;7:105–14.

79. Affleck G, Urrows S, Tennen H, et al. Sequential daily relations of sleep, pain intensity, and attention to pain among women with fibromyalgia. Pain. 1996;68:363–8.

80. Nicassio PM, Moxham EG, Schuman CE, et al. The contribution of pain, reported sleep quality, and depressive symptoms to fatigue in fibromyalgia. Pain. 2002;100:271–9.

81. Theadom A, Cropley M. Dysfunctional beliefs, stress and sleep disturbance in fibromyalgia. Sleep Med. 2008;9:376–81.

82. Smith MT, Perlis ML, Carmody TP, et al. Presleep cognitions in patients with insomnia secondary to chronic pain. J Behav Med. 2001;24:93–114.

83. American Psychiatric Association. Diagnostic and statistical manual of mental disorders. Text Revision edition. 4th ed. Washington, DC: American Psychiatric Association; 2000.

84. World Health Organization. International statistical classification of diseases and related health problems 10th revision. 2007. http://apps.who.int/classifications/apps/icd/icd10online/. Accessed 16 Sep 2009.

85. American Academy of Sleep Medicine. International classification of sleep disorders: diagnostic and coding manual. 2nd ed. Westchester: American Academy of Sleep Medicine; 2005.

86. Schramm E, Hohagen F, Grasshoff U, et al. Test-retest reliability and validity of the structured interview for sleep disorders according to DSM-III-R. Am J Psychiat. 1993;150:867–72.

87. Edinger JD, Kirby AC, Lineberger MD, et al. DUKE structured interview schedule for DSM-IV-TR and international classification of sleep disorders, second edition (ICSD-2) sleep disorder diagnoses. Durham: Veterans Affairs and Duke University Medical Centers; 2006.

88. Bastien C, Vallières A, Morin CM. Validation of the insomnia severity index as a clinical outcome measure for insomnia research. Sleep Med. 2001;2:297–307.

89. Buysse DJ, Reynolds III CF, Monk TH, et al. The Pittsburgh sleep quality index: a new instrument for psychiatric practice and research. Psychiatry Res. 1989;28:193–213.

90. Zomer J, Peled R, Rubin AHE, et al. Mini sleep questionnaire for screening large populations for excessive daytime sleepiness complaints. In: Koella W, Ruther E, Schulz U, editors. Sleep 1984. Stuttgart: Gustav Fisher Verlag; 1985. p. 467–70.

91. Hetta J, Almqvist M, Agren H, et al. Prevalence of sleep disturbances and related symptoms in a middle-aged Swedish population. In: Koella W, Ruther E, Schulz U, editors. Sleep 1984. Stuttgart: Gustav Fischer Verlag; 1985. p. 373–6.

92. Hays RD, Martin SA, Sesti AM, et al. Psychometric properties of the medical outcomes study sleep measure. Sleep Med. 2005;6:41–4.

93. Morin CM. Insomnia: psychological assessment and management. New York: Guilford Press; 1993.

94. Morin CM. Dysfunctional beliefs and attitudes about sleep: preliminary scale development and description. Behav Ther. 1994;17:163–4.

95. Espie CA. The psychological treatment of insomnia. Chichester: Wiley; 1991.

96. Tyron W. Issues of validity in actigraphic sleep assessment. Sleep. 2004;27:158–65.

97. Lavie P, Epstein R, Tzischinsky O, et al. Actigraphic measurements of sleep in rheumatoid arthritis: comparison of patients with low back pain and healthy controls. J Rheumatol. 1992;19:362–5.

98. Landis CA, Frey CA, Lentz MJ, et al. Self-reported sleep quality and fatigue correlates with actigraphy in midlife women with fibromyalgia. Nurs Res. 2003;52:140–7.

99. Kushida CA, Chang A, Gadkary C, et al. Comparison of actigraphic, polysomnographic, and subjective assessment of sleep parameters in sleep-disordered patients. Sleep Med. 2001; 2:389–96.

100. Lichstein KL, Riedel BW. Behavioral assessment and treatment of insomnia: a review with an emphasis on clinical application. Behav Ther. 1994;25:659–88.

101. Walker J, Farney R, Rhondeau S, et al. Chronic opioid use is a risk factor for the development of central sleep apnea and ataxic breathing. J Clin Sleep Med. 2007;3:455–61.

102. Ballantyne JC, Mao J. Opioid therapy for chronic pain. N Engl J Med. 2003;349:1943–53.

103. Gilron I. Gabapentin and pregabalin for chronic neuropathic and early postsurgical pain: current evidence and future directions. Curr Opin Anaesthesiol. 2007;20:456–72.

104. Legros B, Bazil C. Effects of antiepileptic drugs on sleep architecture: a pilot study. Sleep Med. 2003;4:51–5.

105. Garcia-Borreguero D, Larrosa O, de la Llave Y, et al. Treatment of restless legs syndrome with gabapentin: a double-blind, cross-over study. Neurology. 2002;59:1573–9.

106. Drug Enforcement Administration DoJ. Schedules of controlled substances: placement of pregabalin into schedule V. Final rule. Fed Regist. 2005;70:43633–5.

107. Tiihonen J, Lonnqvist J, Wahlbeck K, et al. Antidepressants and the risk of suicide, attempted suicide, and overall mortality in a nationwide cohort. Arch Gen Psychiatry. 2006;63:1358–67.

108. Perroud N, Uher R, Marusic A, et al. Suicidal ideation during treatment of depression with escitalopram and nortriptyline in genome-based therapeutic drugs for depression (GENDEP): a clinical trial. BMC Med. 2009;7:60.

109. Berger A, Dukes EM, Edelsberg J, et al. Use of tricyclic antidepressants in older patients with painful neuropathies. Eur J Clin Pharmacol. 2006;62:757–64.

110. Bymaster F, Dreshfield-Ahmad L, Threlkeld P, et al. Comparative affinity of duloxetine and venlafaxine for serotonin and norepinephrine transporters in vitro and in vivo, human serotonin receptor subtypes, and other neuronal receptors. Neuropsychopharmacology. 2001;25:871–80.

111. Fava M, Mulroy R, Alpert J, et al. Emergence of adverse events following discontinuation of treatment with extended-release venlafaxine. Am J Psychiatry. 1997;154:1760–2.

112. Thase M. Effects of venlafaxine on blood pressure: a meta-analysis of original data from 3744 depressed patients. J Clin Psychiatry. 1998;59:502–8.

113. Krystal AD. A compendium of placebo-controlled trials of the risks/benefits of pharmacological treatments for insomnia: the empirical basis for U.S. clinical practice. Sleep Med Rev. 2009;13:265–74.

114. Smith MT, Haythornthwaite JA. Cognitive-behavioral treatment for insomnia and pain. In: Lavigne G, Sessle B, Choiniere M, Soja P, editors. Sleep and pain. Seattle: ISAP; 2007. p. 439–57.

115. British Pain Society. Recommended guidelines for pain management programmes for adults. London: British Pain Society; 2007.

116. Ashworth PCH, Burke BL, McCracken L. Does a pain management programme help you sleep better? Clin Psychol Forum. 2008;184:35–40.

117. Morley S, Williams A, Hussain S. Estimating the clinical effectiveness of cognitive behavioural therapy in the clinic: evaluation of a CBT informed pain management programme. Pain. 2008; 137:670–80.

118. Lichstein KL, Wilson NM, Johnson CT. Psychological treatment of secondary insomnia. Psychol Aging. 2000;15:232–40.

119. Currie SR, Wilson KG, Pontefract AJ, et al. Cognitive-behavioral treatment of insomnia secondary to chronic pain. J Consult Clin Psychol. 2000;68:407–16.

120. Edinger JD, Wohlgemuth WK, Krystal AD, et al. Behavioral insomnia therapy for fibromyalgia patients: a randomized clinical trial. Arch Intern Med. 2005;165:2527–35.

121. Jungquist CR, O'Brien C, Matteson-Rusby S, et al. The efficacy of cognitive behavioral therapy for insomnia in patients with chronic pain. Sleep Med. 2010;11:302–9.

122. Nikolaus T, Zeyfang A. Pharmacological treatments for persistent non-malignant pain in older persons. Drugs Aging. 2004;21:19–41.

123. Menefee LA, Cohen MJ, Anderson WR, et al. Sleep disturbance and nonmalignant chronic pain: a comprehensive review of the literature. Pain Med. 2000;1:156–72.

124. Shaw I, Lavigne G, Mayer P, et al. Acute intravenous administration of morphine perturbs sleep architecture in healthy pain-free young adults: a preliminary study. Sleep. 2005;28:677–82.

125. Dimsdale J, Norman D, Dejardin D, et al. The effect of opioids on sleep architecture. J Clin Sleep Med. 2007;3:33–6.

126. Rosenthal M, Moore P, Groves E, et al. Sleep improves when patients with chronic OA pain are managed with morning dosing

of once a day extended-release morphine sulfate (AVINZA): findings from a pilot study. J Opioid Manag. 2007;3:145–54.

127. Foldvary-Schaefer N, De Leon Sanchez I, Karafa M, et al. Gabapentin increases slow-wave sleep in normal adults. Epilepsia. 2002;43:1493–7.

128. Hindmarch I, Dawson J, Stanley N. A double-blind study in healthy volunteers to assess the effects on sleep of pregabalin compared with alprazolam and placebo. Sleep. 2005;28:187–93.

129. Webster L, Choi Y, Desai H, et al. Sleep-disordered breathing and chronic opioid therapy. Pain Med. 2008;9:425–32.

130. Wang D, Teichtahl H, Drummer O, et al. Central sleep apnea in stable methadone maintenance treatment patients. Chest. 2005; 128:1348–56.

131. Saarto T, Wiffen P. Antidepressants for neuropathic pain. Cochrane Database Syst Rev. 2007;CD005454.

132. Haddad PM, Dursun SM. Neurological complications of psychiatric drugs: clinical features and management. Hum Psychopharmacol. 2008;23 Suppl 1:15–26.

133. Chang C, Wu E, Chang I, et al. Benzodiazepine and risk of hip fractures in older people: a nested case-control study in Taiwan. Am J Geriatr Psychiatry. 2008;16:686–92.

134. Bartlett G, Abrahamowicz M, Grad R, et al. Association between risk factors for injurious falls and new benzodiazepine prescribing in elderly persons. BMC Fam Pract. 2009;10:1.

135. Roehrs T, Roth T. Sleep and pain: interaction of two vital functions. Semin Neurol. 2005;25:106–16.

136. Morley S, Eccleston C, Williams A. Systematic review and meta-analysis of randomized controlled trials of cognitive behaviour therapy and behaviour therapy for chronic pain in adults, excluding headache. Pain. 1999;80:1–13.

137. Redondo JR, Justo CM, Moraleda FV, et al. Long-term efficacy of therapy in patients with fibromyalgia: a physical exercise-based program and a cognitive-behavioral approach. Arthritis Rheum. 2004;51:184–92.

138. Gustavsson C, von Koch L. Applied relaxation in the treatment of long-lasting neck pain: a randomized controlled pilot study. J Rehabil Med. 2006;38:100–7.

139. Becker N, Sjogren P, Bech P, et al. Treatment outcome of chronic non-malignant pain patients managed in a Danish multidisciplinary pain centre compared to general practice: a randomised controlled trial. Pain. 2000;84:203–11.

140. Kerns RD, Turk DC, Rudy TE. The West Haven-Yale multidimensional pain inventory (WHYMPI). Pain. 1985;23:345–56.

141. Beck AT, Ward CH, Mendelson MM, et al. An inventory for measuring depression. Arch Gen Psych. 1961;4:561–71.

142. Spielman AJ, Saskin P, Thorpy MJ. Treatment of chronic insomnia by restriction of time in bed. Sleep. 1987;10:45–55.

143. Melzack R. The short-form McGill pain questionnaire. Pain. 1987;30:191–7.

144. Cleeland CS. Measurement of pain by subjective report. In: Chapman CR, Loeser JD, editors. Advances in pain research and therapy, volume 12: issues in pain measurement. New York: Raven; 1989. p. 391–403.

145. McNair DM, Lorr M, Droppleman LF. EDITS manual for the profile of mood states. San Diego: EDITS; 1971.

146. Ware JE, Snow KK, Kosinski M, et al. SF-36 health survey: manual and interpretation guide. Boston: The Health Institute, New England Medical Center; 1993.

147. Tait RC, Pollard CA, Margolis RB, et al. The pain disability index: psychometric and validity data. Arch Phys Med Rehabil. 1987; 68:438–41.

148. Vitello MV, Rybarczyk B, Von Korff M, et al. Cognitive behavioral therapy for insomnia improves sleep and decreases pain in older adults with co-morbid insomnia and osteoarthritis. J Clin Sleep Med. 2009;5:355–62.

149. Rybarczyk B, Stepanski E, Fogg L, et al. A placebo-controlled test of CBT for co-morbid insomnia in older adults. J Consult Clin Psychol. 2005;73:1164–74.

150. Haynes PL. Is CBT-I effective for pain? J Clin Sleep Med. 2009;5:363–4.

151. Tang NKY, Goodchild CE, Sanborn AN, Howard J, Salkovskis PM. Deciphering the temporal link between sleep and pain in a heterogeneous chronic pain patient sample: A multilevel daily process study. Sleep. 2012;5(35):675–68.

Empowerment: A Pain Caregiver's Perspective

Julia Hallisy

Key Points
- Witnessing a loved one in pain is a significant source of fear and anxiety for caregivers, even if they seem to be coping well.
- Caregivers are often expected to assume complicated medical duties without proper training or emotional support.
- There are many reputable sources of information and support for patients and caregivers, and they need to be made aware of appropriate networks.
- The siblings of an ill child may have an especially difficult time adjusting to the changes in their lives, and their unique situation needs to be acknowledged and addressed.
- Caregivers often experience extreme exhaustion and feelings of isolation, and their own interpersonal relationships may suffer – including their relationship with the patient.
- Many caregivers experience a significant loss of control when the patient enters the hospital, and their knowledge and expertise may not be recognized or utilized.

Introduction

Managing a loved one's pain is one of the most difficult and anxiety-provoking responsibilities facing caregivers. Pain management by caregivers requires information, skills, support, and compassion. Too often, caregivers find that they are overwhelmed by this formidable responsibility and unsure of where to turn for help.

J. Hallisy, B.S., D.D.S (✉)
595 Buckingham Way # 305, San Francisco 94132, CA, USA
e-mail: julia@empoweredpatientcoalition.org

In my own case, my late daughter Katherine Hallisy was diagnosed at 5 months of age with bilateral retinoblastoma and faced five recurrences of her cancer before her death in February 2000 at the age of ten. Kate's cancer was aggressive and accompanied by episodes of chronic pain. An above-the-knee amputation led to both physical and unrelenting "phantom" pain. Radiation years earlier to Kate's right orbital area eventually led to a non-operable tumor in her skull and proved to be one of our most formidable pain management challenges. I learned that while each pain experience is personal and subjective, in many ways, it is shared by the entire family and each caregiver.

Pain and Patients

The fear of pain is a major concern for cancer patients [1] and for any individual facing a serious or prolonged illness. It is not just the physical burdens of pain that are problematic. The nonphysical manifestations of pain including anxiety, personality changes, feelings of helplessness, a sense of frustration, sudden anger, and guilt can be devastating for the patient's sense of well-being and for their relationships with those around them.

Patients and their advocates and caregivers are given numerous details about a diagnosis and proposed treatment plan, but may receive little information early on about the "pain control plan." Those facing serious illness and their caregivers need to feel confident that they have been given enough information to assess pain levels, training in how to competently manage pain, and assurances that they will have access to the best resources and pain specialists. Those who are taught to view pain as a normal and often inevitable process will not be blindsided and unprepared if pain becomes a challenging issue. I have had many caregivers express their deep-rooted fear that the patient will experience pain that becomes impossible to control and patients often fear untreatable pain more than death itself. These feelings may be impossible to avoid, but addressing them openly and early in the course of treatment may alleviate a great deal of anxiety for both patients and caregivers.

Pain and Caregivers

Pain is ever changing, difficult to manage, and physically and mentally debilitating for both patients and their caregivers. Acting as a caregiver for a patient with severe or chronic pain is one of the most stressful and demanding roles a person can accept. Research studies confirm that caregivers of cancer patients who are in pain have significantly higher levels of depression and anxiety [2]. Aside from the obvious and understandable levels of fear, being a caregiver thrusts people into physically demanding roles that they are often not trained for or emotionally prepared to handle.

Caregivers are often asked to assume intricate medical duties such as assessing pain levels accurately, administering and monitoring powerful medications, and communicating with teams of highly trained medical personnel including oncologists, pharmacists, and nurse practitioners. In my personal situation, I was given a brief tutorial on drawing blood from Kate's central line, flushing the line with heparin, and changing the dressing around the central line, and then I was expected to assume these duties at home on my own. I was also responsible for watching for signs of infection and blood clots. Even as a health-care professional, I was overwhelmed and fearful that I would make a critical mistake that could jeopardize my daughter's health.

Managing my daughter's central line often meant that I was the one causing her physical and emotional pain. We both knew that the line went directly into a vessel near her heart, and we felt the stress associated with changing the dressing or tugging on the skin. It was impossible to have a dressing change that was painless and that did not cause moments of intense stress. It is even more difficult to deal with the patient's pain when it is your actions that are causing the distress. No matter how many times you tell yourself that you are only doing what must be done, this is a predicament that caregivers are not prepared for and often face alone.

Caregivers may not fully comprehend the true scope of their responsibilities, especially when they lead to emotional dilemmas. Health-care professionals need to provide caregivers specific information about the requirements of their duties, but they must also prepare people for the many psychological components that are a part of tending to the ill.

Seeking Information and Support

When my daughter was diagnosed with cancer in 1989, there were few resources available to find current information about retinoblastoma. I was not familiar with the Internet or medical information search companies, so I went to our local medical school bookstore and looked at pediatric textbooks that contained data and statistics that were outdated and frightening.

Fortunately, patients and their advocates now have access to cutting-edge resources for facts and support when facing illness. There are an ever-growing number of people who are willing to take the time and expend the effort to learn about their symptoms, diagnosis, tests, and medications. There are some physicians who discourage their patients from doing their own research and admonish them to "stay off the Internet." Once a patient shows any interest in seeking their own facts, it would be helpful for professionals to be supportive of these efforts and to guide people to reputable sources of information.

The government offers many sites appropriate for the public, including Healthfinder.gov, MedlinePlus, Agency for Healthcare Research and Quality (AHRQ), and the Centers for Disease Control and Prevention (CDC). Patients can be advised to look for web sites that contain the HONcode which guarantees that the site abides by standards for reliable health information.

Another excellent resource is Planetree Health Resource Centers for information and support. Planetree offers "health links" which is a list of the best sites for health information, and some Planetree centers will conduct a literature search and assemble an information packet on a specific illness for a reasonable fee. This is a good resource for people who do not want to spend time doing research or who aren't savvy with computers. Some Planetree centers offer lecture series and links to online support groups as well.

Choosing a Doctor/Changing Doctors

What I look for in a physician has evolved over the last two decades. When Kate was first diagnosed, her pediatrician gave us a referral to an oncologist, which we accepted without question. I didn't know how to research his background, to ask for any other referrals or second opinions, or to set up a brief meeting to see if he seemed to be a "good fit" for our daughter and our family. I have learned over the years that thought and research is needed before establishing relationship with a physician. Extra care should go into choosing a doctor with whom patients are likely to have a long-term relationship such as internists, oncologists, or pain specialists.

I have now set the bar high, and my requirements for a good doctor-patient relationship must include excellent communication and access, a sense of warmth and compassion, absolute truth and transparency, and a feeling of trust. If any of these are lacking, I know I need to make a change. We had the experience of realizing that we needed to leave the care of Kate's oncologist after 8 years of working together, so I have lived through the thought process and the emotional aspects of changing doctors during a complicated treatment plan.

In 1998, we came to the unexpected and immediate conclusion that we needed to find a new oncologist for Kate. Kate had a bad reaction to one of her three chemotherapy drugs, and the decision was made by all to discontinue the medication. We hoped to continue her regimen with the remaining two drugs, knowing that it was less than ideal. Even though all the tests had shown no cancer anywhere in Kate's body at the time, the tumor board and our oncologist decided to invoke a "futile care" policy and stop all chemotherapy. Our oncologist called me at the end of my work day with no advance warning to inform me that the hospital would be stopping treatment because the cancer "will undoubtedly come back." I was supposed to be comforted by his comment "Don't worry – we will be sure you have lots of pain medicine." I was alone, stunned, and panic stricken, and I had to drive home and break the news to my husband. I had never felt so abandoned by a physician or another human being in my life.

There had been times along the way that we weren't happy with this doctor's level of communication or his demeanor, but we made the mistake of brushing these intuitive feelings aside. Now in my work as a patient advocate, I routinely advise people to heed these internal warning signals and to search for a provider who includes them in thought processes, rationales, and the decision-making process. Patients may come to their physicians with misgivings about a specialist or other provider, and I suggest that doctors listen carefully to the patient's concerns and encourage them to find a new practitioner if they are unhappy in any way.

Pain and Family Caregivers, Including Siblings

Many patients suffering from illness and chronic pain are cared for at home by relatives. While family members may seem like the logical choice to be caregivers, they often face unique challenges and stresses. The services of outside caregivers may be a financial burden, and families often want their loved ones to be cared for in their own familiar home environment.

Children caring for parents have their own families, careers, and other responsibilities in addition to the many hours spent providing care for loved ones. Vacations, hobbies, relationships, and travel plans may all have to be altered or abandoned to make time for the patient. Many caregivers are elderly spouses who may have their own health issues and physical limitations. Many family members are so emotionally involved in the situation that it can become difficult to notice subtle changes in the patient's condition. Certainly, fatigue and worry can impair a family member's ability to assess pain levels and to deliver quality care on a consistent basis.

Other family members are impacted by the experiences of the caregiver, including spouses, friends, coworkers, and siblings who may all notice a decline in the caregiver's attitude, health, and demeanor. Children of caregivers may be adversely affected by the stressful situation their parent is facing, and siblings of an ill child may have an especially difficult time adjusting to the changes and the disruption in their household.

I have had the unfortunate and life-altering experience of being a sibling of a critically ill child and the parent of a daughter facing a life-threatening illness. I watched my parents become consumed with making complex medical treatment decisions when my late sister was diagnosed with a congenital cardiac defect that necessitated a complicated open heart surgery. At 7 years old, I desperately wanted to understand what was happening and I sensed that the problem with her heart posed a risk to her life. When I asked my mother point-blank if my sister could die, she broke down in tears and couldn't form an answer. I wanted to know the truth about the situation, but I immediately knew that I had asked the wrong question.

Siblings see their lives change overnight, and they may feel that they are losing touch with their parents both physically and emotionally. Siblings need and want to know the truth, but they want to ease their parent's burden even more, so they internalize their fears and their questions remain unanswered. Siblings often tell me that they felt removed from their sibling's illness and that they had to find their own ways of dealing with the stress of seeing their brother or sister in pain. Ten years after their sister's death, my own two sons react very differently to the memory of Kate's experience with cancer. My younger son who was six at the time remembers more of Kate's exuberant personality and the fun things they did together like playing games on her bed. My older son who was twelve at the time says he "prefers not to think about" the doctors, hospitals, and the episodes of extreme pain he witnessed. His sister's illness and the resulting consequences still make him angry and frustrated. He was just old enough to have the memory of the suffering leave a permanent imprint on his psyche. Editor's note: I would highly recommend eye movement desensitization and reprocessing (EMDR) for the caregiver's older son, even this far removed in time. This process clears out long-term potentiation in the brain and is the most potent and very fast treatment for PTSD symptoms. It is a good tool, but also requires a good therapist to do it successfully. There is an EMDR Guild which lists all certified practitioners in her area.

My sons did not assume medical duties, but they ministered to their sister by being her legs when she was healing from her amputation, watching movies and playing games at her bedside and sharing stories about school and friends to keep her updated on the outside world. Brothers and sisters often play important roles in the life of their sibling, but may do so with the great burden of mystery and worry. Parents naturally want to protect their other children from the hardships of illness which is why it is important for professionals to be prepared to offer guidance or referrals long before siblings have sequestered their emotions or are struggling to cope with a new and stressful family dynamic.

Challenges to Caregivers' Relationships

The stresses to interpersonal relationships often begin so subtly that it can be difficult to realize that they are happening. Friendships, marriages, parental roles, and coworker relationships can all suffer when a person takes on caregiving responsibilities. Being a care provider often demands every free moment and can leave people with little or no time for maintaining or sustaining relationships.

The stress-filled environment of pain control duties can make a person short-tempered, lonely, and defensive. It becomes too easy for the caregiver to feel isolated and overwhelmed and to think that "no one understands" [3]. Caregivers often stop allocating time for themselves and their relationships and may even come to view them as unnecessary intrusions into their duties. Again, medical professionals can caution people about this phenomenon right from the beginning and encourage people to nourish their personal relationships. The reality is that small steps may be in order and caregivers may need to choose one or two people that they will work at staying in contact with. Caregivers can also ask a few people to commit to reaching out and making regular contact with them, which takes the responsibility off their shoulders.

Caregivers need to realize that they will experience an ever-changing range of emotions and communicate to their loved ones that they should expect a wide variance in their demeanor. Conversations with friends or relatives can run the gamut from stoic and forced to prolonged venting sessions about the challenges facing the caregiver. Naturally, some friends will find these conversations difficult, and they will struggle to find the right words of support. In time, the calls and visits may dwindle. Professionals can encourage caregivers to be open and honest about their feelings and to tell people right up front that they are having a bad day or that they just need someone to listen when they want to talk about their problems. Some friends and family will be better at certain roles than others, so caregivers should try to establish a small group of "go-to" people who can help them through these ups and downs.

It's important for caregivers to be reminded to take the time to nurture their relationship with the patient. Caregivers who are feeling isolated and exhausted will not be able to hide these emotions from the patient, who will share in the deleterious effects on their relationship and worry that they are pushing their loved one to the breaking point. It is important for caregivers to remember what their relationship with the patient was like before illness intervened and to try to have moments every day when they set their role as a caregiver aside and interact with the patient as simply a friend, spouse, or child.

Professionals should have current information available for caregivers about new social networking and communication models such as CarePages.com, CaringBridge.org, or LotsaHelpingHands.com. Caregivers and patients can provide online updates for friends and family to stay informed about the patient's condition and about any ways that they may be able to contribute and assist. These sites have the capability to set up meal delivery schedules, blogs, photos, message boards, and monetary donations. These sites are powerful tools for caregivers to stay connected to their supporters and to feel like they are keeping people updated without taking precious time away from the patient.

Caregivers must be told up front that they need to work at becoming accustomed to asking for help from those around them and that a strong and capable caregiver recognizes that they will occasionally need assistance. We must update the definition of a good caregiver from someone who takes on a superhuman role all on their own to someone who is strong enough to realize that they cannot possibly be 100% every hour of every day.

Caring for the Caregiver

Just as each illness has a unique progression and path, each caregiver faces challenges that can be difficult and life-altering. Caregivers may routinely face ongoing stress, sleep deprivation, lack of exercise, compromised nutrition, and insomnia. On a much more serious level, caregivers may struggle with debilitating depression, alcohol or substance abuse, impaired job performance, fears about financial issues, a sense of isolation, and posttraumatic stress disorder.

Caregivers may comprehend that they have to take care of themselves, but making this a reality can feel next to impossible. We were told that many marriages do not survive the serious illness of a child. Apparently, even our marriage was hanging in a life-or-death balance, which was another concern to add to our ever-growing list. While I appreciated the admonishment to take care of my marriage (and still value it to this day), I would like to see caregivers receive specific ideas for keeping their relationships on the right track. Simple suggestions such as taking 15 min each day to talk or simply be alone together, keeping a notebook or journal to share thoughts, sending text messages, or choosing an upbeat song as your inspiration and listening to it together can make a big difference. I would like to see providers consult with therapists to compile lists of small steps to maintain friendships and marriages to distribute to caregivers and then follow up at visits to see if they are taking time away from their duties to care for themselves.

Providers should ask if the caregiver has formed a "caregiving plan" to help cope with the realities and the responsibilities of the situation. The doctor should remind the caregiver that providing care to the patient could go on much longer than anticipated and that additional caregivers may be needed at some point. Caregivers need to find out if any friends or family members are able to help, how any costs will be managed, and if any public or private resources or assistance are available to them.

I would advise caregiver's right from the beginning to think about their "support team" and to choose one or two small things they will do for themselves each day. Professionals can weave this thought process into the initial conversations to stress the importance of caring for the caregiver. A support team can help provide nutritious meals or make trips to the grocery store, they can sit with a loved one while the caregiver walks around the block for 15 min, and they can watch for signs of fatigue and depression that the care provider may not recognize.

It can quickly become difficult to respond to every inquiry or to thank every person who shows kindness. It quickly becomes a time management challenge and yet another source of stress. In time, it just seems easier to have calls go straight to voice mail or to ignore requests for updates. The evolution of Internet updates and patient information web sites is important because friends and family can be updated regularly by one entry, and patients and caregivers can feel good about their ability to communicate and stay connected to others. The above mentioned CarePages, CaringBridge, or LotsaHelpingHands are excellent resources for sharing information with others. In addition, social media such as Facebook and Twitter are excellent means of disseminating and sharing information on a large scale.

Caring for a person experiencing symptoms of pain may lead to feelings of loneliness and isolation. Some friends and visitors will not be able to sustain a relationship in the face of such basic human suffering. It is often just as distressing for visitors to see the toll the disease is taking on the patient as it is for the caregiver. Caregivers may unconsciously begin to isolate themselves from outsiders if they become overwhelmed by the time and energy required to provide constant updates on the patient's condition, if they fear assessment of their skills, or if they feel that others, including their doctors, are making judgments about their decisions.

The Power of Human Touch

It is common for the home environment to develop an institutional feel because it can function like a mini hospital. And just like what happens in a hospital, the caregiver may be in and out of the patient's room dozens of times a day to check on the person, to bring meals, or to administer medications. The caregiver may be so busy with duties that they do not recognize the physical disconnect that is developing between them and the patient.

Studies have shown that the human touch can relieve stress and may even diminish the perception of pain [4].

Touching, hugging, stroking, and even massage therapy send a powerful message to the patient that they are not "damaged" or frightening to others. Humans crave touch – especially as a means of comfort and solace. Studies also show that interacting with and petting animals can lower a patient's blood pressure and relieve stress simply from the beneficial effects of touch [5]. Caregivers should be reminded to utilize massage, acupressure, holding hands, stroking the forehead, or spending time with pets as a means of relieving stress for both themselves and the patient and as a potentially powerful tool to alleviate pain.

Assessing Pain Levels

Evaluating and responding to the patient's pain is a formidable task. In reality, only the patient truly knows what level their pain is at, but caregivers are always on alert and watching for the subtle signals that the patient is uncomfortable. The patient's tone of voice, anxiety level, facial expressions, sighing, and restlessness can all be signs of escalating pain. It is important that caregivers realize that pain is now considered the "fifth vital sign" and that it is just as important to monitor and treat pain symptoms as it is fever or high blood pressure.

If the patient is able, it is always a good idea to involve the individual in assessing the amount of pain. Instead of announcing "I'm going to give you more pain medication," the caregiver can say "I'm noticing that you are frowning and you seem restless. Are you having any pain?" This way, the patient will not receive a dose of pain medication that they may not need, and they will retain a sense of control over their pain management.

When pain medication is being given through a pain pump, caregivers face additional challenges. Caregivers are always instructed not to press the button for the patient, but sometimes by the time a patient wakes up from a narcotic-induced sleep, they are already in significant pain. Should the caregiver press the button? Not press the button? These are the types of real-life dilemmas that caregivers face many times a day and ones that take their toll on their confidence and challenge their sense of morality. Practitioners can help by acknowledging that caregivers may run into ambiguous situations and that they should feel comfortable bringing up these conflicts and asking for help. It will help caregivers to be reminded that each person and each situation is unique and that commonly accepted rules may need to be adjusted.

Caregivers should be informed that when possible, they should include the patient in assessing pain levels and watch for trends or patterns in the signs that precede an episode of pain. The patient will feel less helpless, and the caregiver will become more skilled at recognizing the sometimes subtle indicators of distress. Caregivers need to know that sometimes the rules may need to be changed along the way and that they should never feel that they are doing something wrong or feel the need to be secretive or to hide their pain control decisions from providers.

Administering Pain Medications

Caregivers develop a respect and appreciation for the power of narcotic drugs to relieve pain, but at the same time they have a deep sense of fear and anxiety associated with these powerful medications. When you are administering pain medications, the sense of total responsibility and accountability can be overwhelming. Caregivers routinely fear noxious side effects, oversedation, reduced respirations, and addiction.

What caregivers may fear even more is running low on pain medications (especially on weekends or over holidays), the phenomenon of "breakthrough" pain, and pain control in the middle of the night when they feel particularly alone and vulnerable. Establishing procedures to address these valid concerns will make the task of administering medications much easier for caregivers. Caregivers need to establish a written system or log to monitor pain medication amounts so that they don't run low. Caregivers need to know that breakthrough pain is a common occurrence and that a plan for handling this special pain situation must be in place long before it happens. Caregivers must have an efficient and reliable method to contact a professional during the day, nights, weekends, and holidays if they encounter a problem.

All caregivers should be advised to have a medication log that they use to keep a record of all medications, dosages, times given, and any side effects or other observations. Caregivers need to be instructed to document potentially important observations. Was there breakthrough pain and additional medication needed? Was the patient overly anxious at any time? Were there any new side effects? Is the patient having regular bowel movements and are they being noted? Medication administration records are a vital tool in hospitals, and we need to reinforce this procedure to caregivers. A written record will reduce the stress of trying to rely on memory and worries about overdosage of medication and will facilitate communication with physicians and other providers. Caregivers need to know that administering medications for pain control is an important job and that written notes will make this task easier for them.

Caregivers must be encouraged to keep these logs, and professionals can underscore their importance by asking that they bring them to office visits or have them available during phone consultations. The most efficient system would involve professionals dispensing these forms in their offices or via computer download. Examples of Internet sites that can be of assistance in this effort are www.mymedicineschedule.com and www. PartnersAgainstPain.com. MyMedicineSchedule.com is a free

web site that allows patients to "build personalized medication schedules," and the site can even send e-mail reminders to refill prescriptions. PartnersAgainstPain.com offers "pain diary" forms, medication schedules, and pain assessment charts. This type of computer technology is an efficient means of helping caregivers manage medication delivery schedules.

Record keeping is a proven method for reducing errors, monitoring patient progress, and communicating effectively. I would like to see patients and caregivers benefit from these advantages and feel a sense of control and empowerment when managing complex drug regimens at home.

Side Effects and the Fear of Addiction

The side effects of strong pain medications are alarming for caregivers. Nausea, vomiting, loss of appetite, weakness, weight loss, constipation, changes in personality, delirium, night terrors, and oversedation cause caregivers great concern on a daily basis. It can seem like a full-time job to entice a person who has no appetite to eat enough food to keep themselves nourished. Nausea and vomiting are uncomfortable and lead to an almost immediate loss of appetite, weight loss, and weakness. Constipation can be an extremely challenging problem and always carries a risk of infection and bowel obstruction. Bad dreams, a complete change in personality, delirium, and sedation can change the patient into someone who is almost unrecognizable to the caregiver. Caregivers discover quickly how much is at stake and realize how little room there is for error.

The fear of the patient becoming addicted to narcotics is a common and ongoing worry for caregivers. The fact is that many chronic pain patients will become addicted to narcotics at some point in their course of treatment [6]. When I expressed my concerns about my daughter's reliance on narcotics, I was told by our first oncologist "Don't worry about it." Telling a patient or a concerned caregiver not to worry is pointless and ineffective. In hindsight, I would have preferred to hear "Of course dependence is always a concern, but for right now our primary goal is to manage the pain. Addiction, if it happens, can be dealt with later."

This response acknowledges the fear and focuses on the task at hand. Simply telling a caregiver not to worry will only compound the anxiety because the message they will hear is "Your loved one is desperately ill and will likely never come off of narcotics." Even if this is the reality and even if the caregiver is fully aware of the poor prognosis, they will continue to experience stress about addiction. Providers need to educate caregivers about the phenomenon of tolerance and explain that it is normal to experience an increase in the amounts of pain medication over time. When a caregiver is stressed about an increase in dose, they should be reminded of the fact that those experiencing real and ongoing pain will likely need more medication over time [7].

It is important for providers to address side effects, tolerance, and addiction early in the treatment plan and to assure caregivers that they are valid concerns. Ideally, the patient or caregiver express a fear or concern, they are encouraged to voice their questions, the provider answers inquiries both truthfully and with compassion, any fears are acknowledged, and a clear plan is formed to assist the caregiver in dealing with their immediate challenges.

When Pain Escalates

It may be an inevitable part of disease progression to have steadily increasing pain levels. Escalating pain is worrisome to the caregiver, frightening for the patient, and more difficult to manage. Increasing the dose of pain medicine may be medically indicated, but it often causes great angst for both patients and caregivers.

Changing the amount of pain medication mandates a discussion with the physician and patients, and caregivers may have an underlying fear that they are giving the impression that they are giving up or are becoming resigned to the inevitable. Care providers are always concerned that the patient may not be completely honest about escalating pain levels because they don't want to worry the caregiver. Patients may not want to experience more sedation or other side effects. As patients sense that their prognosis is becoming more guarded, they often want to "be in the moment" and alert enough to interact with loved ones.

Physicians may become frustrated by or question the patient's or the caregiver's resistance to using more medications, but when you take the above fears into account, it becomes easy to understand conflict at this stage. Doctors must be prepared to address these fears and to have the potentially difficult conversations with both patients and caregivers. This is a time for compassionate truth and honesty. I always appreciated our oncologist's candor when he told us that my daughter's escalating pain concerned him and that he was going to order a scan or a blood test to check for disease progression. My fear was acknowledged and out in the open, and I was actively taking steps to address the underlying cause.

A doctor who senses reticence to pain medications can simply confront the issue head on and ask "Does increasing the pain medication make you worry that the illness is progressing?" or "Tell me what worries you about the pain medications we are using." This will address the issue directly and take the pressure off the patient and the caregiver who may be struggling to voice their concerns. Doctors should acknowledge that escalating pain levels cause real fear, that it is a fear that the doctor sees in many patients, and that it could indeed be an indication that the patient has moved into a new phase of their illness. Facing and sharing fears diffuse their ability

to run rampant and cause feelings of helplessness. It has been my experience that patients have more fear about the topics their doctors leave unspoken.

Losing Control in the Hospital

Pain management in the hospital setting can be more challenging and anxiety-provoking. The caregiver is no longer at the helm of the ship and may feel a profound loss of control. Patients are rarely as comfortable or relaxed in the hospital as they are at home, and levels of pain medications may need to be increased as an inpatient. Both patients and caregivers will experience disruptions in their daily routine, sleep deprivation, and increased stress levels while hospitalized.

When my daughter was hospitalized, we continued to utilize her regular programmable pain pump, but I no longer had the ability to administer immediate "bolus" injections like I did at home. Kate would have to ask for additional medication, the nurse would have to find a second nurse to confirm the dose, and then the key to unlock the narcotics drawer had to be tracked down in order to retrieve the medication. Often, there would only be one nurse on the floor, especially during meal times. The delivery of much-needed pain medication was delayed by many minutes, which allowed Kate's pain to escalate to a point that the additional dose was not always adequate to completely eliminate her pain. This was a problem we completely avoided at home, but the policies and procedures of a hospital can be a hindrance to efficient and timely pain relief. It seemed surreal to have to watch my child needlessly suffer when we were in a major medical center surrounded by staff and medications.

It was always much more effective to have a pharmacist available to consult at the bedside and to have access to staff members who were trained in pain relief. It is vital for someone to keep a close watch on the dosing schedule and to anticipate the need for additional medications. Providers should take the time to ask the patient and the caregiver what their normal schedule and routine is like and, hopefully, a medication log is being used at home that can be shared with the hospital staff. The caregiver needs to be involved because they are the expert on the patient's daily needs, and the staff should let caregivers know that they need their input and assistance. I would like to see doctors and hospitals routinely acknowledge the efforts and their expertise of caregivers and use this resource for everyone's benefit.

End-of-Life Pain Issues

Once a patient's medical condition progresses to the point that active treatment is not indicated, the need for excellent pain relief is more essential than ever.

Caregivers are just as dedicated and focused on providing pain control at the end of life, but it may cause an increased amount of fear and anxiety.

If hospice care is initiated, the caregiver may experience a loss of control and they may feel that they are losing touch with the patient's regular physician. The hospice team members will be making decisions and guiding pain control methods which may make the caregiver feel confused and even abandoned by the doctor. It would be ideal for the patient and the caregiver to know that they can call on the original doctor for support and brief consultations. Caregivers will feel much more comforted by a person that they know, and the physician can reinforce the hospice pain management plan.

Another pressing concern will be the issue of respiratory depression and overdose. The end of life may require greater amounts of pain control medications [8]. The patient's pain may not only be due to the progression of their illness, but from bed sores, weight loss, dehydration, or agitation. Caregivers experience great anxiety about administering a potentially lethal amount of medication. It is a stressful conundrum – you want to see a loved one out of pain, but you don't want to feel responsible for hastening their death. These moments are the ones that can leave a family in peace or cause regrets and angst for years.

When a physician is informed that one of his or her patients has passed, it would be ideal to send a card or a note to express their condolences about the patient's death and to acknowledge the hard work and dedication of the caregiver.

Conclusion

Pain control issues are only one of the many challenges facing caregivers, but they are often the most difficult. Practitioners play a major role in assisting and supporting caregivers, and they have the power to transform the caregiving experience with information, education, and compassion. Perhaps the most important goal is to acknowledge that caregiving is a difficult job each and every day, but that it is also one of the most rewarding and selfless actions a person can take.

I never heard a doctor or nurse simply state that caring for a terminally ill child was an excruciatingly difficult task, but that it is also a calling to which I had been chosen. It would have made a remarkable difference for Kate's providers to tell me that they had all the confidence in the world in my abilities and that we were doing a wonderful job as a family caring for our daughter and sister. Caregivers need to hear the words.

References

1. Miaskowski C, Kragness L, Dibble S, Wallhagen M. Differences in mood states, health status, and caregiver strain between family caregivers of oncology outpatients with cancer-related pain. J Pain Symptom Manage. 1997;13(3):138–47.
2. Porter LS, Keefe FJ, McBride CM, Pollack K, Fish L, Garst J. Perceptions of patients' self-efficacy for managing pain and lung cancer symptoms: correspondence between patients and family caregivers. Pain. 2002;98:169–78.
3. http://www.thefamilycaregiver.org/connecting_caregivers/the_caregiver_story_project.cfm. Accessed 1 Sep 2009.
4. Carlson K, Eisenstat SA, Ziporyn T. The new Harvard guide to women's health. Cambridge: Belknap Press (Harvard University Press); 2004. 27.
5. Barker SB. Therapeutic aspects of the human-companion animal interaction. Psychiatr Times. 1999;16(2):45.
6. Streltzer J, Johansen L. Prescription drug dependence and evolving beliefs about chronic pain management. Am J Psychiatry. 2006;163: 594–8.
7. Kissin I, Bright CA, Bradley Jr EL. Can Inflammatory pain prevent the development of acute tolerance to alfentanil? Anesth Analg. 2001;92:1296–300.
8. Ward SE, Berry PE, Misiewicz H. Concerns about analgesics among patients and family caregivers in a hospice setting. Res Nurs Health. 1996;19:205–11.

Patient and Caregiver's Perspective

18

Heidi J. Stokes

Key Points

- Each patient is unique and multidimensional. Chronic pain invades all areas of our lives—physical, emotional, spiritual, and financial.
- Pain is abstract. No words, symbols, or a smiley face chart can begin to explain it.
- Living with chronic pain is a "life"—but not the life anyone dreamed of or desires.
- Patients living with chronic pain have trouble discerning "emergency pain" from chronic pain.
- Doctors excel at providing heroic medicine, but often get bored and frustrated when dealing with patients with chronic pain.
- Americans are led to believe that there is a pill or procedure to fix everything.
- A compassionate, competent, doctor is a rich blessing to patients and to the world.

Introduction

When Dr. Albert Ray asked if I would be willing to write a textbook chapter about pain from a patient's perspective, I said "Yes" without hesitation. While I have no degree in medicine, I have been a lifelong academic in the study of chronic pain.

My scholarship began at the age of 17 when a baffling series of health crises led to a diagnosis of systemic lupus erythematosus in my senior year of high school. It marked the beginning of intense, personal research into my disease and the world of pain it brought along with it. While it was never the field of study I would have voluntarily chosen, it has been a rich education, nonetheless.

H.J. Stokes (✉)
3504 44th Ave South, Minneapolis, MN 55406, USA
e-mail: heidi@aaronstokes.com

Dr. Ray and I met through the *National Pain Foundation.* I had been honored by that organization at their *Triumph Dinner* in San Francisco where I received the 2008 *Triumph Award,* given to an individual living with pain who has made a significant difference in the lives of others. It was a wonderful honor, a Cinderella moment in my life, and I believe such a dinner and award marked a sea change in the way chronic pain is acknowledged and addressed.

First, it indicates a general consensus that chronic pain is real, even though it can't be captured, photographed, or pinned down. And it shows that we are seeing chronic pain as its own category, not treating it as something that tags along with rheumatoid arthritis, lupus, Temporomandibular Joint Dysfunction (TMJ) and Physician Assistant (PA), neurological disorders, and the rest. Chronic pain can stand on its own, regardless of its origins.

The *Triumph Award* says to me that we are not just physical beings, not just systems. That we are complex individuals and attention must be paid not just to our bodies but also our minds, spirit, and emotions. Our illness is not our identity. Its failure to leave the body isn't a failure on the part of the "patient," doctor, or medical community.

The award also recognized that as a person living with chronic pain, you can look at the life you have today and accept it, even embrace it. You can refuse to give in. You can abandon your fear, cherish the moment, and embrace your life. Of course, it is not the life you wanted, but it is life nonetheless. I owe a huge debt of gratitude to the doctors and everyone in the medical community who pulled me through and saved my life.

I love a challenge, and I certainly got one. Sometimes, that challenge is getting up in the morning. But with pain and fatigue, you have to manage. You go to work, you cook dinner for your family, you may run a company (as I do with my husband), you hang onto your integrity, and you do the best you can. And then you do more.

I believe the *Triumph Award* legitimized living with chronic pain.

T.R. Deer et al. (eds.), *Treatment of Chronic Pain by Integrative Approaches: the AMERICAN ACADEMY of PAIN MEDICINE Textbook on Patient Management*, DOI 10.1007/978-1-4939-1821-8_18,
© American Academy of Pain Medicine 2015

I'm saying this because the reality of pain is not sharable. There is no Vulcan mind meld. I can tell you my pain, but you can't measure it, and you may not even believe me. You may think I'm there for the drugs. You may think I am a big baby. It happens all the time.

Smiley Faces Pain Chart

We seem stuck in preschool when dealing with pain. In doctor's offices right now, we are still pointing at numbered emoticons—round smiley faces that turn to frowns and then tears—to rate our pain level. You don't know how badly I wanted to have a pain tolerance test—hook my skull up to electrodes and put my hand in a vice—so we could both know what my pain tolerance is and what my pain level means. So I will be believed, perhaps even respected, for what I am battling daily.

My pain began as result of a rampaging immune system that attacked my blood, liver, brain, heart, lungs, and kidneys: systemic lupus erythematosus. A teenager alone in a hospital room far away from family and friends, I asked a doctor how long I had to live. He said if the disease continued to progress—4 years. I believed him. My own godmother lost her daughter at age 14 to lupus. Back in 1977, lupus patients with blood, heart, liver, brain, muscle, and joint involvement didn't live long after their initial diagnosis. Perhaps the fact that it took most patients-years to get an accurate diagnosis contributed to that high mortality. In fact, my doctors had to do an about-face from searching for an infectious agent or parasite, to looking at lupus.

Lupus is like a roller coaster. In the first year, I kept track of the times I was in the hospital—seven. After that, it wasn't quite as important. I've had joint pain and swelling, fever, enlarged spleen, hepatitis, encephalitis, pleurisy, pericarditis, myocarditis, nephritis, and gastritis—a long, long list. At this point, I haven't been in a hospital in years.

A New Source of Pain

But if the crushing fatigue and body aches and pains of lupus were not enough, a rare reaction to the drug Compozine took things to a much higher number on the smiley face chart.

While hospitalized at age 22, this time for gastritis, an injection of Compozine triggered violent spasms in my jaw, face, and mouth. My eyebrows froze in a freakish look of surprise. I couldn't speak, and my tongue became ridged and pointy. Then my jaw started sliding back and forth with such force that it dislocated. I was terrified. When the nurse came into my room, she took one look at me and ran out of the room yelling. Looking at myself in the mirror, I thought, hey, maybe I'm actually *possessed*. Maybe that's what this has been about from the beginning!

The nurse came back with a doctor, not a priest, and gave me a shot of Benadryl. The news spread across the hospital about my reaction, and in moments my room was crowded with nurses, doctors, and orderlies all wanting to take a peek at the spectacle. They had heard of this reaction, but no one had witnessed it firsthand. I felt like I was in the zoo. After the shot, the nurse did tell me what was going on. She said I had a rare drug reaction and I would get better. About 8 h later, the whole ordeal repeated. My jaw started to skate back and forth, and this time I heard snaps and pops. After more Benadryl brought things back to normal, my jaw remained permanently locked shut. I now drank my meals through a straw, and suffered agonizing headaches, before eventually receiving bilateral jaw implants.

The good news was the surgery was successful. After 2 weeks, I could open my mouth, and after about 6 months I could even eat pizza! While I could not move my jaw from side to side, I could finally open and close my mouth. The bad news was that the surgery triggered a severe lupus flare leaving me so ill that for a time, I was dependent on a walker. Things went very well with the implants, until they were recalled by the FDA. They were discovered to be causing severe bone erosion. The FDA ordered the removal of all implants, with no alternatives waiting in the wings. I had the implants for 9 years, and after the first year adjustment period, I was satisfied with them. Then they pulled them out, leaving me with my current bone-on-bone arrangement. I can open my mouth wide enough for a White Castle slider, but not a hotdog. I haven't bitten into an apple in 25 years. The headaches are horrible. On the smiley face chart, the face would be wrinkled and cursing. A visit to the dentist is a torture—let's not even go there.

In those early years of disease and pain, I was a novelty. Lupus wasn't that common, and I was visited, poked, and prodded by many physicians. My case was unique and interesting. Doctors love the heroic aspects of their profession: saving a life, pulling you away from death's grip, and placing you back, once again, into the living.

I found doctors were extremely attentive when the bells and beeps were going off and organs and body systems were compromised. But after the heroics are over, and you are no longer sick enough to be in the hospital (but not well enough to really participate in your own life), you, as a patient, become less important, perhaps even dull. Pretty soon, it's just "hang on and I'll see you in 6 weeks."

Eventually, I realized there is no magic wand, no heroic trek to find the source for healing. Life isn't a television drama where the mysterious disease process that has you by the throat is discovered and pounced on by a genius team of attractive experts with a diagnosis and cure found within the hour, even accounting for commercials. This was a hard lesson to learn as an optimistic Midwestern American who grew up (with television) in the most technologically advanced and wealthy country in the world.

In the first years, I honestly believed the doctors were holding out on me that they did not care that I was living in a deeply compromised and often hopeless state. Or maybe they didn't believe the fact that I was suffering? It was a strange time. Well-meaning people suggested diets, vitamins, coffee enemas, and such. I had a religious person suggest that I must have unrepented sin in my life. This almost-dying thing, this pain, was my fault. I was being punished, and I needed to atone, or confess . . ., something. I remember asking this person why she was wearing glasses. Perhaps, it was only a minor sin. I did, however, play it safe that night and prayed an extra long prayer listing anything and everything I could think of that might have played a role.

But my faith has been a strong lifeline for me. Even though I have a wonderful husband, son, parents, sister, and dear friends, faith has kept me centered. "Faith is something that we hope for and certain of what we do not see." One day I will be well, if not in this world, the next.

But now, back to Earth. Let me tell you a little more about how a person reacts to being ill and in chronic pain.

This Can't Be Happening

I decided at some point in this lingering three-way relationship between me, pain, and my doctor that the problem must be in a failure to fully communicate with my doctor. I believed the problem was a lack of clarity. I would go to my appointment with a detailed list of questions and carefully detailed symptoms. I expected that one day, soon my doctor would comprehend my situation, slap his forehead, and say, "Yes! But of course! You need to take *this* medication! It is all too clear!"

Then would follow the perfect prescription for a pain-free life.

But during the visit, I would realize this wasn't going to happen. I would feel the golf ball-sized lump in my throat, and I would blink very carefully so the tears wouldn't flow down my cheeks. If the doctor was male, as he often was, I also needed to be very careful not to make him think I was some sort of out-of-control emotional woman, a lingering stereotype.

I would leave the doctor's office devastated—without hope.

How can I live this way? How am I going to get back into my life and complete my plans? How on Earth can anyone live like this? But I did, and years continued to pass. Holding out for hope of a cure or relief was difficult. The very doctor that changed my life pulled me out of the woods and kept me out of the hospital—ultimately became unhelpful. At one time, I wanted to kiss his feet; now I wanted to kick him in the shin. I was too upset and too controlled to have a heart to heart with him. I hoped and believed he would help me—that

he would understand—and the blood tests would reveal something new. Perhaps, I would be placed on some sort of new treatment.

Of course that didn't happen. I waited, and waited, and I felt myself putting my life on hold. My real identity had nothing to do with illness or pain. I was an extrovert, an athlete, a musician (percussionist), an artist, a friend, a daughter, and a sister. I was Annie Oakley in my high school production of *Annie Get Your Gun*. "Anything you can do, I can do better!"

Lupus made my life, that "real life," stop. My high school friends didn't know how to relate to me because we no longer had anything in common. They were in school with dances and homecoming, and I was being tutored at home in my pj's, my face a huge moon from prednisone, my hair falling out. Besides a concoction to make the pain and fatigue manageable, I needed a book, a manual, some sort of leg up on this situation.

Pain and illness are such great disappointments, both to you and those around you. You want so much to go back to that lovely "old you." That healthy 16-year-old with her whole life ahead of her. Her future? Limitless. You are waiting, waiting for it as the years go by, and then you realize, this is it. I must give her up. I must redefine my life. I must even redefine joy.

Sometimes, I just sit in my office with an ice pack on my head and a heating pad on my neck, and everyone knows I do. I just make sure I take the ice pack off before I see clients. And I have to be aware that pain is often conveyed in my voice and is interpreted as irritation. I must make a special effort in maintaining my voice and carriage. I can be abrupt without knowing it. I become annoyed with people who can't immediately get to the point.

If I can't control my pain or manage it, everything, and I mean everything, becomes compromised. I'm more prone to mistakes. Concentration can be difficult. When you wake up in the morning really achy and sore, you don't feel you can just pop out of bed and start moving. It feels like it's going to kill you. You may panic knowing you have a full day ahead and you can hardly crawl out of bed. You can always think of tomorrow, like the song in *Annie*. It will be better tomorrow.

So, I wake up every day to some level of chronic pain and fatigue. It is part of my life, and I know now there is no perfect prescription. The doctors have only so many weapons at their disposal. You break a bone, you get a cast. You come down with strep throat, you get penicillin. But chronic pain and fatigue are still murky and not particularly intellectually stimulating for either the doctor or patient.

Yes, there are a host of drugs out there, but none of them can totally erase discomfort and all have their side effects. Opiates work to ease pain and bring sleep and can give you a few hours of reprieve, but they begin to lose their effectiveness, and doctors are increasingly fearful of prescribing them.

Today, I treat pain with a combination of ice packs, heat, breathing, stretching, and water exercise with deep muscle Botox injections—which are godsend—muscle relaxants and drugs used to treat diabetic neuropathy. I have a fairly wide range of other medications to manage lupus. It is a long and boring list.

Different Types of Pain

But there is still a lesson that I have had trouble absorbing during this education, one that began after I had been living with pain for years. Just when I thought I was managing my illness very well—that I really knew what I was doing—I found I had more learning to do.

It was because I had become so used to pain that I found myself in serious trouble. The lesson involved the difference between acute pain, get to the doctor pain, and chronic pain. As an example, one day at work, I felt something wet trickling down my neck, it was blood. After a hasty urgent care visit, it was determined I had ruptured my eardrum. I was referred to an ear, nose, and throat specialist who read me the riot act.

"Didn't it hurt?"

"Yes, it hurt like heck."

"Why didn't you come in? You could have damaged hearing in that ear!"

"I just thought it was jaw pain."

He sent me to a new age counselor who talked about how we need to be in touch with our bodies. Whatever, I supposed I did learn a few tips.

It was a little more serious when I was giving birth to my son. Labor had been going on for hours, and I had entered a new pain level. Agony.

"I've never been in this kind of pain in my life," I told the nurse flatly.

"Yes," she said.

Only when the fetal monitor showed my son's heart stuttering and stopping did I get an immediate C-section. Things were not going well in the natural birth department.

"Why didn't you say anything?!" the nurse asked me the following day.

I said, "I did! I told you I had never had that kind of pain before".

She said, "Yes, you told me. However, you were articulate, and should have been screaming!"

"Not being a baby" could have cost me my baby. Even today, I don't regard myself as an expert on distinguishing acute pain from chronic pain. This is one of my husband's greatest fears. He is sure that one day I will have a heart attack or stroke and I will not know it is an emergency. I will think it is just a new addition to the same old, same old world of chronic pain. I agree it is a concern.

My Prescription for Doctors

During the years that it took me to become an award-winning "scholar" of pain, I have had the opportunity to observe many, many doctors. Today, I am able to distill those countless hours and conversations to help you know how your patients see you and what they need from you. Here it goes.

Even before you enter the exam room, stop, read the chart, and collect your thoughts. When you step in, take the time to make eye contact and maybe smile (it's zero on Wong-Baker chart if you need a reference). I honestly find that a simple smile has a major effect on reducing anxiety.

The appointment is only 15 min in your back-to-back schedule, but it holds an entirely different level of importance for us. We have been waiting weeks for these few minutes. We have taken time off work, battled traffic, searched for a parking place, and waited, reading old magazines, in your waiting room. Then we sit in a little exam room all by ourselves, maybe in a less than flattering robe, waiting for your entrance and eventual verdict.

We have come prepared, maybe we've even rehearsed what we would like to say to you, but when you come in and smile, actually see us and acknowledge the situation, angst can dissolve, and a real connection can take place.

Like it or not you've become a major figure in our lives, and our contact with you sometimes feels like our lifeline—it all comes down to those few minutes. There we are, something is wrong with us, and we feel miserably vulnerable. It's awful!

When I talk to you, for goodness' sakes look at me. I know you are rushed and the pressure is extreme, but we need you to be attentive. I want to know that you comprehend my situation and recognize the compromised life I have to live. I don't want sympathy, but a little compassion can go a long way. Be honest and open, and don't be afraid to say, "I am not sure," or "I don't know." Do say, "I am willing to do my best to help you out."

Discuss possible treatments; let us know that there are other approaches or options, even if it is something we might not like. Sometimes simple things are lifesavers. For years, I didn't know ice took down inflammation. I just thought it numbed the pain, and I don't like to be cold. Once, when I was getting a cortisone shot in my shoulder, the PA told me what movements to avoid and what movements would be easy and helpful. It was a surprise, like the ice, and so simple. I wish I had known years before.

There are a lot of resources out there online and a lot of goofy ranters. If you know of a book, a web site, or a support group that you respect, please write it down for us. And if we are taking too much of your time that day, see if you can arrange a follow-up visit or let the nurse know that we need to schedule a longer visit next time.

In my years of study, I have seen arrogant doctors that have no business working with patients. I have also seen doctors who began the healing process as soon as they came through the door, simply through their very presence.

You are in a healing profession. You are giving service. Remember the oath you took to do no harm. Poor interactions can seriously jeopardize the therapeutic relationship that we need to get better, or even just stay the course.

If you are the go-to doctor for my disease, but you don't listen to me or extend any hope, you are going to be giving me only half of what I need. If you can't make headway with a patient, please suggest another doctor for a second opinion. I understand there are difficult, irate, and demanding patients. But you have the home court advantage when they are sitting in your office, possibly in a flimsy hospital gown, wondering if their backside is showing.

Believe me, these people are feeling helpless and isolated. They probably don't know the terminology. They are in your world, not theirs, and everything is new. It's not just the patient that needs you; our families, employers, and friends all depend on you to help patch us together, so we can participate in life and community again. A good, kind, competent doctor is one of the richest, deepest, life-changing blessings a patient can have. Wow, what a gift you can be to this world.

Take a Vacation?

And last, here is something you might not think about. Your patient is likely under financial stress. It costs a fortune to have a chronic illness. Relaxing vacations? Not likely. Help with the housework? I wish. Weekly massage? Forget it. I don't even want to see a parking meter or a pay ramp when I come to see you.

As for taking time off work, that's the source of our health insurance. No work, no insurance. We may have taken off a day without pay to see you or used another vacation day for our illness. The inconvenience is extraordinary.

Note that the burdens of chronic pain are also financial. Your patients have mortgage payments, car payments, and staggering medical bills. They live with the same stresses you and others have, but must perform under constant duress, and often with frightening uncertainty about their futures. For instance, I have to run a business AND be a wife and mother. That's at least two full-time jobs while living with chronic pain.

I hope this story, from a nonacademic is helpful in your work with patients. If revealing my life with pain helps a new generation of doctors empathize and better treat tomorrow's patients, then my struggle is worth something.

It's been 33 years since those first terrifying and lonely days of early diagnosis—I'm still here! I have learned, and grown, and taken responsibility for my new life. I have found excellent doctors, and we have developed ways to understand and productively work with each other. We are even starting to adequately rate pain by not only viewing its level, but also measuring how it affects our day-to-day life.

It has been quite an education, and I am honored to be able to pass along what I have learned.

I will always be grateful to those doctors who have stuck by me through thick and thin and problem-solved my various needs with diligence, care, expertise, and sometimes even a sense of humor. You are a gift to my family and me: Dr. James Reinersten, Dr. Eric Schned, Dr. John Schousboe, Dr. James Swift, and Dr. Tom Hainlen.

Pain Medicine in Older Adults: How Should It Differ?

Debra K. Weiner, Jordan F. Karp, Cheryl D. Bernstein, and Natalia E. Morone

Key Points

- Degenerative skeletal disease is a normal part of aging; imaging should not be used to guide care in the majority of older adults with chronic pain.
- Pain is common, but it is not a normal part of aging; the majority of older adults are motivated to get better, and their pain and associated disability should be treated as aggressively as in younger patients.
- The older adult with chronic pain should not be treated as a chronologically older version of a younger patient with chronic pain; they should be treated as an older adult first and a patient with pain second.
- Successful pain management for the older adult requires differentiating the patient's weak link(s) from their treatment target(s).
- Non-pharmacological pain management strategies should be prioritized for older adults in an effort to limit medication-associated toxicities that are more common and dangerous than those experienced by younger patients.
- All older adults should undergo formal screening of their cognitive function; the older adult with dementia requires an approach to pain evaluation and management that is distinct from that used for cognitively intact patients.
- Primum non nocere: Opioid analgesics and pain itself can both cause harm (e.g., falls, cognitive dysfunction); the potential risks associated with treatment must be weighed against the risks of no treatment.

D.K. Weiner, M.D. (✉)
Geriatric Research Education and Clinical Center, VA Pittsburgh Healthcare System, Pittsburgh, PA, USA

University of Pittsburgh School of Medicine, 3471 Fifth Ave., Suite 500, Pittsburgh, PA 15213, USA

Department of Medicine, Psychiatry and Anesthesiology, University of Pittsburgh School of Medicine, 3471 Fifth Ave., Suite 500, Pittsburgh, PA 15213, USA
e-mail: dweiner@pitt.edu

J.F. Karp, M.D.
University of Pittsburgh School of Medicine, Pittsburgh, PA, USA

Department of Psychiatry, University of Pittsburgh Medical Center, 3811 O'Hara Street, Pittsburgh, PA 15213, USA
e-mail: karpjf@upmc.edu

C.D. Bernstein, M.D.
Department of Anesthesiology, University of Pittsburgh School of Medicine, Pittsburgh, PA 15213, USA

5750 Centre Avenue, Suite 400, Pittsburgh, PA 15206, USA
e-mail: berncd@upmc.edu

N.E. Morone, M.D., M.S.
Department of Medicine, University of Pittsburgh School of Medicine, 230 McKee Place, Suite 600, Pittsburgh, PA 15213, USA

Geriatric Research Education and Clinical Center, VA Pittsburgh Healthcare System, Pittsburgh, PA, USA
e-mail: moronene@upmc.edu

Introduction

Older adults (commonly defined as those $\geq$ age 65) are not simply a chronologically older version of younger patients. Homeostenosis, that is, progressive restriction of an aging organism's capacity to respond to stress because of diminution of its biological, psychological, and social reserves, underlies the distinction of old from young [1]. As pain is a stressor that commonly accompanies aging, the provision of safe, clinically effective, and cost-effective pain care to older adults requires awareness of these specific aging-related changes [2]. The main goals of this chapter are to (1) educate the pain practitioner in basic principles of aging needed to guide the evaluation and treatment of older adults, (2) provide clinical case examples to illustrate the advantages of treatment that is guided by these principles as compared with traditional pain care and why traditional pain care may actually harm these patients, and (3) offer specific therapeutic guidelines for the treatment of nociceptive, neuropathic, and widespread pain in older patients.

Background

America is aging at a rapid pace. In 2000, approximately 35 million people (12.4 % of the total population) were ≥ age 65, and in 2050, this number is anticipated to rise to an estimated 86.7 million (20.6 % of the total population) [3]. Those ≥ age 85 represent the most rapidly growing segment of the population. Of all chronic health conditions that limit activity and heighten the risk of disability in older adults (e.g., dementia, diabetes mellitus, cardiovascular disease), painful musculoskeletal disorders such as arthritis and low back pain are the most common [4]. Pain practitioners are, therefore, ideally positioned to impact the lives of older adults in a profound way.

Scientific Foundation

The purpose of this section is to present scientific data that negate commonly held beliefs about older adults that have lead to the undertreatment of pain in this vulnerable population.

Myth #1
Pain is a normal part of aging.

Reality #1
Although degenerative skeletal disease is a normal part of aging, chronic pain is not. Additionally, chronic pain can lead to serious health consequences for older adults.

Discussion: While pain is common in older adults, it is not normal. A key principle of aging is as follows: *Many findings that are abnormal in younger patients are common in older people and may not be responsible for a particular symptom* [5]. Using low back pain (LBP) as an example, data demonstrate clearly that degenerative disease of the lumbar spine is nearly ubiquitous in those age 65 and older [6–8] and that magnetic resonance imaging (MRI) evidence of moderate to severe lumbar spinal stenosis occurs not uncommonly in those who are asymptomatic [9]. Although large epidemiological studies that focus exclusively on older adults are lacking, existing data suggest that fewer than half of these individuals experience LBP and an estimated 14 % experience associated functional decline [10]. Degenerative disease of the appendicular skeleton also is common. For example, asymptomatic hip osteoarthritis occurs in over half of older women [11].

Further, older adults with chronic noncancer pain may experience numerous adverse consequences such as impaired physical function, depression and anxiety, social isolation, sleep and appetite disturbance, impaired neuropsychological performance, an increased burden of medical comorbidity, and excessive utilization of health care resources [10, 12–23]. Community-dwelling older adults with chronic pain also have significantly worse self-rated health (a powerful predictor of morbidity and mortality) than those without pain [24], suggesting that unrelieved pain may be associated with enhanced mortality.

Myth #2
Older adults do not feel pain as much as younger patients; thus, conditions associated with pain in younger patients may not be associated with pain in older adults. Thus, pain treatment does not need to be aggressive in these individuals.

Reality #2
Laboratory data do not support diminished ability of older adults to perceive pain. Some data point to their diminished ability to regulate (through top-down inhibition) peripheral nociceptive stimuli, and this suggests that practitioners may need to provide even more aggressive analgesia to older adults.

Discussion: Histopathological and biochemical studies indicate decreased density of myelinated and unmyelinated peripheral nerve fibers [25–27], and an increased number of degenerated fibers are associated with aging [28]. Selective age-related impairment of myelinated nociceptive fiber function also has been demonstrated [29, 30].

Additional evidence points to age-associated central changes in significant neurotransmitters. In the dorsal horn of the rat, progressive age-related loss of serotonergic and noradrenergic neurons has been demonstrated [31, 32]. There is a decline in the concentration and turnover of catecholamines, gamma-aminobutyric acid (GABA), and opioid receptors [33–35] in the limbic system and a lower density of serotonin receptors [36]. Aging-associated biochemical changes are also evident in the cerebral cortex in general [37–44] and in the prefrontal cortex in particular [45]. Thus, older adults may have an inadequate quantity of key pain-modulating neurochemicals.

Laboratory studies of pain threshold and tolerance have been performed exclusively on healthy individuals. The application of these data to patients in pain is unknown. Somatosensory thresholds for non-noxious stimuli in healthy older adults increase with age, while results associated with noxious stimuli have been variable and dependent upon the type of stimulus applied [30]. One of the most carefully designed studies comparing pain threshold and tolerance to pressure, heat, and ischemic stimuli in young and old humans demonstrated no significant age-associated differences in response to heat or pressure and significantly lower tolerance and threshold to ischemic stimuli in old versus young [46].

Age differences in temporal summation (i.e., enhancement of perceived pain intensity when noxious stimuli are delivered repetitively above a critical rate), a correlate of wind up in animals, also have been examined in the laboratory, with findings summarized as follows: (1) Older adults appear to have enhanced temporal summation to heat but not pressure as compared with younger individuals [47]. (2) Older adults have enhanced temporal summation in response to electrical stimulation compared to younger adults [48]. These findings suggest that older adults may have reduced capacity to downregulate their nervous system response to pain after an initial period of sensitization [49].

Myth #3

As with younger chronic pain patients, treatment of psychological dysfunction (e.g., depression, anxiety, poor coping skills) is the most important aspect of chronic pain treatment for older adults.

Reality #3

For the majority of older adults with chronic pain, identifying and treating the numerous physical pain contributors (i.e., the appropriate treatment targets) holds the key to optimizing symptomatic relief. The law of parsimony (Occam's razor) *should not* guide treatment, and the "weakest link" may not be the treatment target.

Discussion: Although older adults with chronic pain tend to have more physical limitations than younger patients, in general, they are more psychologically robust, with better coping skills and mental health, less fear avoidance, and a greater sense of life control [50]. While large population-based studies have not been performed, preliminary data indicate an estimated one in three older adults with chronic nonmalignant pain seen in a tertiary referral center's interdisciplinary pain clinic has a high burden of psychological dysfunction [17]. For these individuals, the practitioner should consider prescribing interdisciplinary pain rehabilitation that includes psychological treatment. Two-thirds of the older adults in this sample did not have high levels of psychological dysfunction and would not, therefore, require such treatment.

Our research and clinical experience suggests that for the majority of older adults with chronic pain who do not have significant psychological dysfunction, ascertaining the numerous biological/physical contributors to the patient's pain syndrome and their pain-associated functional limitations holds the key to prescribing effective treatment. More often than not, the older adult with chronic pain has numerous contributors to pain, even when the patient reports pain at a single site. A related key principle of aging is as follows: *Because many homeostatic mechanisms are often compromised concurrently, there are usually multiple abnormalities amenable to treatment and small improvements in each may yield dramatic benefits overall* [5]. We recently published a case series of older adults with postherpetic pain and comorbid myofascial pain [51]. These patients had been treated with numerous neuropathic pain medications that resulted in side effects and/or suboptimal pain relief. Significant symptomatic improvement occurred only after the myofascial component of their pain was treated.

Another example of multiple pathologic contributors to single-site pain is chronic low back pain. We have demonstrated that 82% of older adults with chronic low back pain have multiple potential sources of pain including myofascial pain (95.5 %), sacroiliac joint pain (83.6 %), hip disease (24 %), and fibromyalgia syndrome (19.3 %) [52]. Further, while 25 % of these individuals reported neurogenic claudication, 50 % of them also had other spinal/leg pathology that might have accounted for their low back and leg pain.

These data should be considered in the context of studies that have demonstrated substantial rates of failed back surgery syndrome in those who undergo decompressive laminectomy for the treatment of lumbar spinal stenosis [53, 54]. The effect on low back/leg pain is unknown of addressing associated pathology (e.g., fibromyalgia, hip joint arthritis) instead of or in addition to surgically treating the degenerative lumbar disease. Until the answer to this question is ascertained, the most clinically effective and cost-effective treatment(s) for these patients will remain elusive.

A related key principle of aging is as follows: *Presentation of a new disease depends on the organ system made most vulnerable by previous changes, and because the most vulnerable organ system ("weakest link") often differs from the one newly diseased, presentation is often atypical* [5]. Consider, for example, the hospitalized older adult who develops acute confusion (i.e., delirium). The most common causes of delirium in hospitalized older adults are adverse drug reactions and infections [55]. Rational evaluation and treatment of these patients is guided by a search for potentially offensive medications and/or infections such as a urinary tract infection or pneumonia. Unless there are focal neurological findings, brain imaging is not indicated because while the brain is the "weakest link," it is not the treatment target. Similarly, for older adults with low back pain, the lumbar spine may be the weakest link and successful treatment might lie in identifying and treating conditions outside of the spine itself. An illustrative case is presented later in this chapter (Case 1 below).

Myth #4

Treating pain in older adults will reduce the risk of disability.

Reality #4

While quality of life can be improved by treating pain in older adults, effective strategies to reduce the risk of disability are elusive. Preliminary data indicate that brain-targeted as opposed to body-targeted treatment may represent the "missing link." Additional research in this area is needed.

Discussion: While treating pain is essential for improving quality of life and diminishing its interference with performance of daily activities [23], treating pain as a physical symptom does not appear to reduce the risk of future dependent living status, that is, disability. Large studies examining the efficacy of physical therapy for the treatment of chronic low back pain (CLBP) in older adults have not been performed. Preliminary evidence suggests that lumbar spine-focused physical therapy for these patients does not improve pain or physical function [56, 57]. Those who undergo decompressive laminectomy for lumbar spinal stenosis experience less pain, but not significantly improved function [58].

We have gathered several sets of data that support the potential role of the brain in generating pain-related disability in older adults with CLBP. Specifically, evidence supports the following: (1) Neuropsychological performance mediates the relationship between pain and physical function [13]. We have shown in older adults with CLBP that the modest relationship between pain severity and disability is no longer significant when neuropsychological performance (NP) is statistically controlled (i.e., after NP is removed from the relationship). This implies either that NP mediates the relationship between pain and disability or that NP and disability share common pathways in the brain. (2) Older adults with CLBP, as compared with older adults who are pain-free, have structural brain changes in the middle corpus callosum, middle cingulate white matter, and gray matter of the posterior parietal cortex as well as impaired attention and mental flexibility [59]. (3) Older adults with CLBP that is self-reported as being disabling have more severe changes in brain morphology than older adults with CLBP that is not disabling, and the duration of chronic pain is associated with the severity of changes in brain morphology [60]. The exact cause of the brain changes and the extent to which these changes are reversible or modifiable is not known. (4) Mindfulness meditation, a treatment directed at altering the brain's perception of/reaction to pain, reduces pain's interference with performing daily activities [61]. Additional research in this area may be at the cutting edge of developing treatments that not only reduce pain but reduce the risk of disability for older adults with CLBP. Given the suboptimal outcomes associated with lumbar spine-focused treatments, such research is critically needed.

Myth #5

Opioids should be used with extreme caution if at all in older adults.

Reality #5

Opioids and pain itself are associated with multiple potential deleterious effects. If opioids are prescribed, the adage "start low and go slow" should guide treatment. Meticulous, ongoing follow-up is the only way to answer, "Do the benefits of opioids outweigh their risks?"

Discussion: As with all medications, risks and benefits must be balanced. Opioids may result in a number of deleterious side effects in older patients. As noted in the introduction to this chapter, as people age, there is progressive restriction in their physiological reserve capacity (i.e., homeostenosis). This can take many forms that include decline in neuropsychological performance [62], sarcopenia and reduced mobility [63, 64], changes in analgesic pharmacokinetics and pharmacodynamics [65], and social isolation. When opioids are used, therefore, the practitioner must be vigilant for side effects for which older adults may be at increased risk such as falls, hip fracture, and delirium. And because older adults have enhanced pharmacodynamic sensitivity to opioids [66, 67], the patient and his caregiver must be educated about these risks, even when low doses are prescribed.

That being said, risks associated with opioids must be balanced with the risks associated with pain itself. As summarized in Table 19.1, many of the deleterious effects associated with opioids are identical to those associated with pain. Older adults with chronic low back pain have more impaired balance [68] and, therefore, a greater risk of falls than those who are pain-free. While delirium is a potential side effect of opioids, it is also a potential side effect of pain, especially for hospitalized older adults or those in nursing homes. A study of 541 older adults who underwent hip fracture repair demonstrated that better pain control on higher doses of intravenous morphine was associated with a lower risk of postoperative delirium [69]. Others have shown that cancer patients who require long-term opioids may experience improved neuropsychological performance as a result of more effective pain management [70, 71].

Myth #6

Treatment of pain in older adults with dementia should be guided by the same basic principles as for those who are cognitively intact.

Reality #6

Older adults with dementia are not simply a cognitively impaired version of those who are cognitively intact. An evidence base to guide treatment of pain in older adults with

Table 19.1 Opioids in older adults: balancing risks and benefits

Symptom/side effect	Associated with opioids	Associated with pain	Management/monitoring approach
Depression	X	X	Consider treating depression as first step and observe effect on pain
Anxiety	X	X	Consider treating anxiety as first step and observe effect on pain
Agitation	X	X	Consider referral to psychiatry to determine cause and most appropriate treatment of agitation
Mobility difficulty/falls	X	X	Falls risk should always be screened in the older adult with chronic pain. If balance impairment is evident, an assistive device should be recommended along with referral to physical therapy for instruction in proper use. If opioids are considered, education regarding the risk of falls is essential for all older adults. If opioids are considered for the older adult with baseline mobility impairment, the practitioner must refer to physical therapy in an effort to optimize balance *prior* to prescribing opioids
Delirium	X	X	Patients with dementia have a heightened risk of delirium with opioids and with pain. A cognitive function screen should be considered an essential vital sign for older adults
Constipation	X		Discussion about starting a stimulant laxative at the first sign of constipation should occur at the time that the opioid is prescribed
Urinary retention	X		Especially important to educate the older male with benign prostatic hypertrophy and baseline voiding symptoms about this risk
Respiratory depression	X		More common in high doses
Sleep disturbance	X	X	Although nocturnal pain may prompt prescription of an opioid at bedtime, patients should be educated about their potential deleterious impact on sleep
Diminished appetite	X	X	As with other symptoms, the patient should ascertain the relative risks and benefits
Increased utilization of health care resources	?	X	Our clinical experience suggests that drug-seeking behavior is unusual in older adults in the absence of poorly treated pain

dementia is lacking; there is no substitute for thoughtful implementation and critical observation of empirical interventions.

Discussion: Just as aging is associated with extreme heterogeneity in the deterioration of biological, psychological, and social reserves as well as physical function, so too is dementia a heterogeneous process. The most common form of dementia is Alzheimer's disease (AD) and the vast majority of data regarding pain, and dementia applies to this condition.

A number of studies that have been done with pain-free older adults in the laboratory highlight that those with Alzheimer's disease have altered pain processing as compared with cognitively intact individuals. Functional brain imaging suggests that those with AD experience enhanced attention to painful stimuli as compared to those without AD [72]. Others have demonstrated that AD patients self-report pain intensity of acute stimuli (e.g., pressure, venipuncture) similar to that of cognitively intact individuals, but that their facial expressions associated with these stimuli are more exaggerated and nonspecific [73, 74]. Data also suggest that other behavioral manifestations of pain, such as guarding, bracing, and rubbing, also may be nonspecific in those with AD [75], that is, these "pain" behaviors may be an expression of the disordered movement that occurs in association with dementia, even in the absence of

pain. Additional research in this area is clearly needed so that pain can be accurately detected in patients who have dementia and others with communication impairment.

Evidence also suggests that older adults with dementia may have blunted treatment expectancy [76]. It has been well-established in the pain literature that treatment expectancy is synergistic with pharmacodynamic analgesic efficacy [77, 78]. That is, the absence of belief in treatment efficacy negatively impacts treatment outcomes, even in those who are cognitively intact. If, in fact, patients with dementia have reduced treatment expectancy, these individuals may require larger analgesic doses to achieve desirable treatment outcomes. The reader should be aware that controlled studies of this hypothesis have never been undertaken and are needed. Until scientific evidence exists, the practitioner should be aware of the differences in pain processing between older adults with and without dementia and approach treatment prescribing accordingly.

Application to Clinical Practice

The key to optimizing treatment outcomes for older adults with chronic pain is to start with comprehensive assessment. The purpose of this assessment is threefold: (1) to identify all

Table 19.2 History and physical examination for the older adult with persistent pain: the essentials

History [79]

Answers to the following questions will help to ascertain the older adult's pain signature and, therefore, key treatment outcomes.

1. How strong is your pain (right now, worst/average over past week)?
2. How many days over the past week have you been unable to do what you would like to do because of your pain?
3. Over the past week, how often has pain interfered with your ability to take care of yourself, for example, with bathing, eating, dressing, and going to the toilet?
4. Over the past week, how often has pain interfered with your ability to take care of your home-related chores such as going grocery shopping, preparing meals, paying bills, and driving?
5. How often do you participate in pleasurable activities such as hobbies, socializing with friends, and travel? Over the past week, how often has pain interfered with these activities?
6. How often do you do some type of exercise? Over the past week, how often has pain interfered with your ability to exercise?
7. Does pain interfere with your ability to think clearly?
8. Does pain interfere with your appetite? Have you lost weight?
9. Does pain interfere with your sleep? How often over the past week?
10. Has pain interfered with your energy, mood, personality, or relationships with other people?
11. Over the past week, how often have you taken pain medications?
12. How would you rate your health at the present time? Excellent, good, fair, poor, or bad?

Past history/review of systems: This portion of the history will identify key medical, psychological, and social comorbidities that may impact treatment response.

Medical comorbidities	Relationship to treatment
Constipation	If present at baseline, a stimulant laxative should be prescribed (e.g., senna) at the same time that an opioid is started
Lower extremity edema	May be exacerbated by a nonsteroidal anti-inflammatory drug
Hypertension Congestive heart failure Peptic ulcer disease Renal insufficiency	Gabapentin and pregabalin can contribute to lower extremity edema Renal insufficiency should be kept in mind when dosing various analgesics (see Tables 19.4 and 19.5)
Obesity	Some medications may contribute to weight gain, such as gabapentin, pregabalin, and tricyclic antidepressants
Sleep disturbance	While pain may disrupt sleep, opioids are also associated with disruption in sleep architecture
Difficulty walking/falls	While pain itself can contribute to weakness, difficulty walking, and falls, older adults can have mobility difficulty independent of pain. In these individuals, care must be taken to avoid medications that can themselves contribute to mobility impairment, for example, opioids, pregabalin, gabapentin, and tricyclic antidepressants
Memory loss	As noted in the text, pain itself can cause decrements in multiple domains of neuropsychological performance. With effective pain treatment, memory may improve. Practitioners must be aware, however, that many pain medications may contribute to confusion, for example, opioids, pregabalin, gabapentin, tricyclic antidepressants, and others (see Tables 19.4 and 19.5)
Psychological factors	
Depression Anxiety	Untreated depression and/or anxiety can impair top-down inhibition; thus, the older adult with comorbid depression and/or anxiety must be treated for these disorders as part of pain treatment
Coping skills	Poor coping skills (e.g., tendency to catastrophize) can inhibit the efficacy of pain treatment. While most cognitively intact older adults seem to cope well with chronic pain, the minority who do not should be referred for cognitive behavioral therapy as a part of pain treatment
Self-efficacy Confidence in mobility Fear of movement	Physical therapy reduces fear avoidance beliefs (i.e., fear of moving because of concerns about exacerbating pain) in older adults [57]. Older adults with a history of falls may exhibit fear of falling, may have low confidence in mobility, and may have low self-efficacy (i.e., lack of confidence in their ability to engage in certain behaviors to affect desired outcomes). For these individuals, referral to a pain psychologist and physical therapist should be part of pain treatment
Treatment expectancy	Treatment expectancy must be established at the outset of pain evaluation. Patients who believe that treatment will work will likely improve (i.e., placebo effect). Those who believe that treatment will not work will likely not improve (i.e., nocebo effect)
Social factors	
Social/caregiver support	Social isolation can interfere with the older adult's ability to distract themselves from their pain and, therefore, intensify their pain experience. This may be especially problematic for the older adult with dementia.
Financial status	The practitioner should always consider the older adult's financial resources when prescribing treatments.

(continued)

Table 19.2 (continued)

Medical comorbidities	Relationship to treatment

Physical examination

1. Vital signs
   (a) Cognitive function
   Mini-Cog [92, 93]: Examiner gives the patient three unrelated words to remember. Then, she/he gives the patient a blank piece of paper and asks them to draw a clock with the hands pointing to a specific time. Then, the patient is asked to recall the three words. Patients who are able to recall all three words have a low likelihood of dementia. Those who recall zero words have a high likelihood of dementia. For those who recall 1–2 words, the examiner should assess the accuracy of the clock-drawing test. If there are gross errors, the patient should be referred for evaluation of possible dementia.
   (b) Mobility
   (c) Traditional vital signs

2. Functional performance
   (a) Balance
   Modified postural stress test ([94]; see Fig. 19.4): Examiner stands behind the patient with hands on sides of pelvis and states, "I am going to pull you backwards gently and try to throw you off balance…Do not let me…Are you ready?" Then, the examiner pulls the patient toward himself gently. If the patient is able to resist easily, try pulling a little more forcefully and observe response. The older adult whose balance is easily perturbed has decreased postural control and may be at heightened risk for falls.
   (b) Basic functional tasks – chair rise, ability to pick up object from floor, ability to place hands behind neck and waist (movements needed for dressing), and manual dexterity (e.g., ability to button and unbutton clothing, tie shoes)

3. Comprehensive identification of pain comorbidities
   (a) Knee/hip arthritis in patients with low back pain
   (b) Shoulder disease in those with neck/upper back pain
   (c) Myofascial pain in all patients, including those with neuropathic pain [51]

4. Comprehensive routine physical examination

treatment targets, (2) to establish the patient's unique pain signature that should be used to determine the efficacy of treatment, and (3) to identify key comorbidities that could constrain various treatment options. Table 19.2 outlines the essential components of a comprehensive history [79] and physical examination for the older adult with chronic pain that is designed to address each of these three goals.

Below is a series of real cases that actualize how to integrate principles of aging into the practice of pain medicine and illustrate how to comprehensively identify treatment targets, establish the older adult's pain signature (i.e., the way(s) that the patient manifests pain such as reduced appetite, difficulty walking, and confusion) [79], and identify potentially limiting comorbidities.

Case 1

An 82-year-old woman presented with low back pain for many years that had started insidiously and had lead to increasing functional limitations. She reported 7–8/10 sharp/burning daily pain that she experienced bilaterally, below the waist, and was worsened by standing, lifting, walking, and bending. There were no red flags. She had undergone numerous treatments without benefit including acupuncture, chiropractic, traction, physical therapy, aqua therapy, multiple epidural corticosteroid injections, and inpatient pain rehabilitation. She took prn naproxen for pain relief. Musculoskeletal examination revealed mild kyphoscoliosis, tenderness to pal-

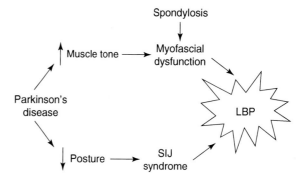

Fig. 19.1 Synthesis of Case 1. For details, see text. *LBP* low back pain, *SIJ* sacroiliac joint

pation of both sacroiliac regions, and bilateral piriformis taut bands and trigger points. Neurological examination revealed symmetrical reflexes, 5/5 strength throughout, shortened stride length, and an anxious affect. The initial working diagnoses were (1) sacroiliac joint syndrome, (2) myofascial pain, and (3) anxiety for which physical therapy, sacroiliac joint injections, and gabapentin were prescribed.

One month later, she had experienced no pain reduction or functional improvement. A more detailed history uncovered the development over the past year of change in her voice (softening), handwriting (smaller), posture (increased forward flexion), and facial expression (less animated). A more detailed physical examination uncovered mild cogwheeling of her right arm. A neurology consultation was obtained to address the possibility of Parkinson's disease. The consultant felt that there were "no full-blown Parkinsonian signs or symptoms," but the presence of her masked facies, diminished blink, minimal asymmetrical cog-wheeling, Myerson's sign, and tendency to retropulse prompted a trial of levodopa/carbidopa 25/100 bid.

One month later, the patient reported average 4/10 pain (~50 % reduction from baseline), improved posture, and balance as well as walking capacity and flexibility.

Discussion: The synthesis of this case is presented in Fig. 19.1. The treatment targets for this patient were her Parkinson's disease and her myofascial pain. Her pain signature was comprised primarily of decreased physical function. Her impaired gait was also the primary comorbidity of concern. This placed her at heightened risk of falls. Had opioids been prescribed, the practitioner would have had to be especially vigilant for worsening mobility. Prior to prescribing such medications, the patient would have had to be educated about the risk of falls and hip fracture.

This case highlights the fact that PD is not infrequently associated with pain. Forty to fifty percent of patients with PD have pain that is not explained by other obviously painful disorders [80, 81]. Fifteen percent have pain as their presenting symptom (e.g., unilateral shoulder pain) [82]. Twenty-five percent have pain that precedes motor symptoms [83]. Patients may report muscle cramps or tightness, typically in the neck, paraspinal, or calf muscles; painful dystonias; joint pain; neuropathic pain; or less commonly, generalized pain [84]. Oral and genital pain syndromes that are similar to symptoms occurring in patients with tardive dystonia and akathisia from neuroleptics also have been described in patients with PD [85, 86]. The underlying pathogenesis of pain in PD can be central, peripheral, or mixed. Sensory thresholds to experimentally delivered painful stimuli are reduced in PD [87]. Unlike peripherally generated pain, such as that experienced by our patient, central PD pain that is associated with abnormal nociceptive input processing is not affected by dopamine administration [88].

Perhaps most importantly, this case illustrates that successful treatment of the older adult with low back pain requires identifying the proper treatment targets (Parkinson's disease [PD]) rather than simply treating the weak link (axial spondylosis). Had this patient elected to go forward with spinal surgery, the likely outcome, as compared with the actual outcome, is depicted in Fig. 19.2. In this figure, the "existing approach" represents common practice and the "proposed approach" is what we recommend.

Case 2

An 82-year-old woman presented with low back pain and right leg pain for two years with documented central canal stenosis on MRI. She had worked full time in a dress shop

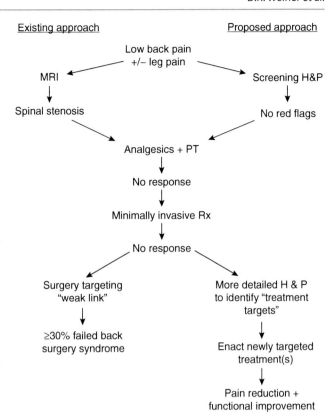

Fig. 19.2 A comparison of two approaches for the management of older adults with low back +/− leg pain. The approach commonly used (existing approach) focuses on imaging to direct treatment. Because the predictive value of abnormal imaging has not been critically examined in older adults and because abnormalities occur commonly, with or without pain, this approach frequently results in failed treatment. The proposed approach relies on a comprehensive history and physical examination to guide treatment that often targets multiple pain contributors. *H&P* history and physical examination, *MRI* magnetic resonance imaging, *PT* physical therapy

and was forced to retire 2 years ago because the company was downsizing. She said that her pain started at that time and had gotten progressively more severe. Her pain was made worse by prolonged standing or walking, and she was having increasing difficulty performing heavy housework. Her pain was made better with rest and heat application. She denied fever, chills, weight loss, and change in her bowels or bladder function. She reported poor balance and multiple near falls at home. She lived alone. She was becoming increasingly fearful of leaving her home. Medications at the time of presentation, all of which had been prescribed to treat her pain and pain-associated anxiety, included gabapentin, oxycodone CR, celecoxib, tramadol/acetaminophen, olanzapine, escitalopram, and lorazepam. Physical examination revealed poor balance, dementia (memory problems and very impaired clock-drawing test) [89], kyphoscoliosis, and tenderness of the right sacroiliac joint/lumbar paraspinal musculature/tensor fasciae latae/iliotibial band. Because of extreme guarding behavior, strength testing was invalid.

Fig. 19.3 Synthesis of Case 2. For details, see text

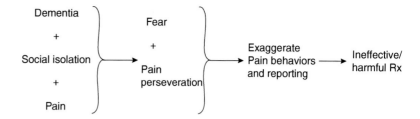

Because of polypharmacy, high falls risk, and social isolation, the patient was admitted to a nursing home for detoxification. All of her medications were discontinued with the exception of regularly scheduled acetaminophen and prn tramadol. She reported minimal pain and her balance improved markedly. It was recommended that her family strongly consider placing her in an assisted living facility. They chose to seek other opinions from pain practitioners. Immediately following discharge, the patient's pain complaints escalated and multiple other pain regimens were attempted including a morphine pump trial, all of which failed. She was eventually placed in an assisted living facility where she did well.

Discussion: The synthesis of this case is presented in Fig. 19.3. As noted earlier in this chapter, to prescribe effective treatment, the practitioner must differentiate the weak link from the treatment target(s). In this case, chronic pain was the weak link and fear/social isolation the treatment targets. Her pain signature consisted of pain perseveration and significant utilization of health care resources. The main potentially treatment-limiting comorbidities were her dementia and balance frailty.

One of the first discussions that we have with patients in chronic pain revolves around treatment expectations. Specifically, patients with chronic pain need to understand that it is realistic to expect partial but not complete pain relief. Treatment of the older adult with dementia is complicated by the fact that information provided in treatment counseling sessions may not be remembered and ongoing reinforcement may be necessary. Such reinforcement is often successful when the patient has an involved and supportive caregiver (and one who does not catastrophize about the patient's pain) and health care providers who are willing to communicate a consistent message. In this patient's case, inconsistent messages were delivered (i.e., although it was clear that the patient's fear and social isolation in the setting of dementia were primarily responsible for her suffering, the patient's family insisted that her pain was responsible and more aggressive pain treatment was sought).

While many patients with dementia can report pain reliably [90, 91], the meaning of these reports must be ascertained in order to prescribe effective treatment. Is the patient's pain reporting a manifestation of perseveration (that occurs not uncommonly in patients with dementia)? Or, is

the patient's pain reporting a more general signal of distress? Or, is the patient's pain reporting an indication of pain-related suffering? If there is pain-related suffering, then pain-specific treatment must be implemented. In the case of our patient, her pain reporting appeared to be a manifestation of both perseveration and a more general signal of distress (i.e., anxiety surrounding social isolation and dementia). Thus, while treatment did involve analgesics, providing a supportive environment was the primary therapeutic element.

This case highlights the need to screen for dementia at the time of the initial history and physical examination. One of the most efficient and effective screening tools is the Mini-Cog, described in Table 19.2 [92, 93]. It takes no more than 2–3 min to perform. If this testing uncovers the possibility of dementia, the patient should be referred to a geriatrician for further evaluation. Older adults with and without dementia often have mobility difficulty and a risk of falling; thus, a balance screen should also be included as part of the baseline assessment. A modified postural stress test [94] can readily be done in the office and is described in Table 19.2 and shown in Fig. 19.4. If this test reveals poor balance, a referral to physical therapy should precede any intervention that could further impair balance (e.g., opioid prescription).

Case 3

An 85-year-old man with advanced Alzheimer's disease presented, along with his wife of 60 years and their daughter, for treatment recommendations to address "persistent reporting of pain" in his lower back. His primary care provider was concerned because the patient's pain ratings had not changed despite numerous analgesic prescriptions. Most recently, he had been prescribed fentanyl that had been titrated to a dosage of 100 mcg/72 h and resulted in hospitalization because the patient became semicomatose. When the dosage was decreased to 50 mcg/72 h, his mental status returned to baseline and he continued to report pain so a pain clinic consult was requested.

At the time of the evaluation, he was sitting in a wheelchair, appeared very comfortable, smiled throughout most of the interview, and had no pain complaints. His history was unreliable because of advanced dementia. His wife reported that the patient had low back pain for many years. She was asked, "Do you think your husband is suffering from his pain,

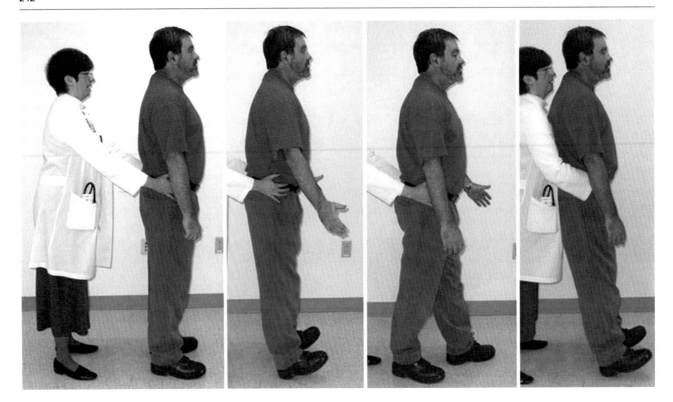

Fig. 19.4 Modified postural stress test. The highest level postural response (i.e., associated with the best balance) is shown on the far left, where there is no obvious movement in response to attempted perturbation. The lowest level "timber response" is shown on the right, where the patient makes no effort to recover upright stance. This response is highly unusual and typically indicates severe supratentorial dysfunction. The middle two photographs depict intermediary responses.

Fig. 19.5 Synthesis of Case 3. For details, see text

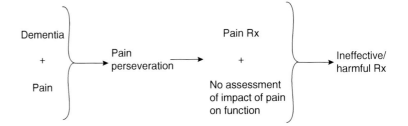

or is he just talking about it?" Without hesitation, she replied, "Oh…he's just talking about it." Together, we decided that the most appropriate treatment would include tapering him off the fentanyl and have him participate in a local day care program for socialization and distraction. His family was educated about the fact that patients with chronic low back pain cannot be made pain-free and that the main goal of treatment is preservation and/or improvement in function to the extent possible. She understood and fully supported the plan.

Discussion: The synthesis of this case is presented in Fig. 19.5 and reinforces the complexities of pain evaluation and management in older adults with dementia. In this patient, chronic pain was the weak link and pain perseveration the treatment target. Pain perseveration was also the major

component of his pain signature. The main potentially treatment-limiting comorbidity was his dementia (i.e., increased risk of falls and/or delirium with opioids). As opposed to the patient in *Case 2* whose pain reporting reflected pain perseveration as a general signal of distress, this patient's pain reporting was a simple representation of pain perseveration that was treated with distraction. Often, this type of perseveration behavior in older adults with dementia is more a problem for the caregiver (i.e., it is stressful to observe the perceived suffering of a loved one, contributing to caregiver burden) than for the patient, and treatment strategies should keep this in mind.

This case also highlights the importance of patient-centered or patient/caregiver-centered decision making. In busy office practices, it may be difficult to take the extra time required to engage in these discussions. Not doing so, however, may lead to unnecessary morbidity, as was the case with this patient.

Case 4

A 67-year-old man presented with low back and left leg pain for 10 months. He had injured his back nearly 50 years earlier associated with heavy lifting. He was treated conservatively and his pain abated within 1–2 months. Ten months ago, he experienced the insidious onset of sharp/burning pain in his left lower back with occasional radiation to the left leg (lateral aspect) that was getting progressively more severe. He reported occasional weakness and numbness of the left leg and progressively more restricted walking tolerance. At the time of presentation, he ambulated with a walking stick and could go one-half block before he had to stop because of pain. He reported multiple falls because his leg "gave way." His pain was worsened by lying prone and trying to straighten his leg while lying supine. It was made better by lying on his side and assuming a fetal position. He denied fever, chills, or change in his bowels/bladder.

A lumbar MRI performed 2 months following the onset of his pain revealed diffuse lumbar spondylosis and moderate central canal stenosis. Treatment had included (1) physical therapy for lumbar spinal stenosis that resulted in no improvement in his pain or function; (2) tramadol that was ineffective; (3) gabapentin that caused nausea, vomiting, and a 15-lb weight loss; and (4) hydrocodone/acetaminophen that was associated with moderate pain relief. Spinal surgery was recommended, but he declined. His only significant medical comorbidity was hypertension.

Notable on physical examination was blood pressure 178/96, ¾ in. leg length discrepancy, mild scoliosis, mild left piriformis tenderness, and an antalgic gait with favoring of the left leg. His gait was slow but steady when performed with his walking stick. Examination of the left hip revealed <15° painful internal rotation. Right hip exam was normal. Neurological exam revealed symmetrical lower extremity reflexes and 5/5 strength throughout with the exception of the left hip flexors and left quadriceps that were 4/5. When the patient was lying supine and asked to raise his left leg, he did so by picking it up with his hands. Hip x-rays revealed marked joint space narrowing of the superior and inferior aspects on the left and no abnormalities on the right. Based on these findings, he was instructed to continue regularly scheduled hydrocodone/acetaminophen and he was referred to physical therapy specifically directed toward the left hip. If these strategies are ineffective, he will be referred for intra-articular hip injection. If he is refractory to all noninvasive and minimally invasive treatments, he will be referred for consideration of a total hip replacement.

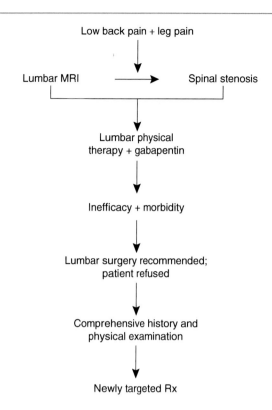

Fig. 19.6 Synthesis of Case 4. For details, see text. *MRI* magnetic resonance imaging

Discussion: The synthesis of this case is shown in Fig. 19.6. The treatment target was his hip osteoarthritis. His pain signature consisted of severe self-reported pain and difficulty walking. His significant comorbidities included hypertension and difficulty walking/falls. Because his symptoms were initially attributed to the lumbar spine, he underwent an unnecessary lumbar MRI and was prescribed medications that resulted in significant adverse events, physical therapy that was ineffective, and a referral for spinal surgery that would likely not have relieved the "pain generator."

This case is presented to highlight the important contribution of hip osteoarthritis to low back pain. The hip-spine syndrome was first described in 1983 and refers to symptoms that exist in the setting of concurrent degenerative pathology in the hip and spine [95]. Three types of hip-spine syndrome were postulated: (1) *simple* when history and physical examination clearly indicate whether the hip or the spine is the primary source of pain; (2) *complex*, when both the hip and the spine are responsible for pain; these cases are said to require ancillary investigations such as nerve root infiltration and intra-articular blocks of the hip joint to disentangle the primary source of pain; and (3) *secondary*, when altered hip function (e.g., flexion deformity with advanced OA) directly changes spinal biomechanics that cause low back pain. The contribution of hip OA to CLBP also is supported by more recent data. Specifically, total hip replacement surgery for patients with severe hip pain and advanced OA on x-ray

Table 19.3 Differentiation of lumbosacral from hip-generated low back/leg pain

Feature	Lumbosacral	Hip	Comments
Pain location	Above pelvis; if comorbid spinal stenosis, pain may involve buttocks and/or legs	Most common referral patterns are buttocks, groin, and thigh	If sacroiliac joint syndrome (SIJS) complicates hip disease, SI pain can coexist with buttocks/groin/thigh pain
Leg pain	Present if comorbid spinal stenosis or knee/hip disease	Often	Radiculopathy pain typically extends the entire leg. Although hip pain can be referred to the lower leg and/or foot, most commonly it involves the buttocks, groin, and thigh
Groin pain	Absent	Often	SI pain can be referred to the groin, so if SIJS complicates lumbosacral pathology, groin pain can occur
Movements that aggravate pain	Spinal extension	Leg extension Hip internal rotation	If comorbid SIJS, side lying and/or flexion may worsen pain
Movements that alleviate pain	Spinal flexion	Hip flexion Hip external rotation	If spine and hip disease co-occur, response to movement patterns may be atypical
Posture	Spinal flexion	Leans forward, with flexion at the hip	When spine or hip disease is mild, there may be no obvious postural abnormalities
Associated symptoms	Paresthesias, radiculopathic pain, lower extremity weakness	Lower extremity weakness	If spine and hip disease co-occur, symptoms can overlap
X-ray findings	Poor predictive validity for pain	Poor predictive validity for pain	Degenerative disease of the lumbar spine exists in > 90 % of older adults without low back pain [8], and spinal stenosis is not uncommon in older adults [9]
			53 % of women with radiographic hip OA report no pain [11]. A definitive diagnosis of hip osteoarthritis should be based on ACR criteria [99]

reduces low back pain and improves overall spine function [96]. In patients with low back pain, diminished hip range of motion predicts poor outcomes following spinal manipulation [97] and after lumbar percutaneous electrical nerve stimulation (unpublished data). Preliminary data suggest that patients with self-reported hip OA respond less favorably to decompressive laminectomy for the treatment of lumbar spinal stenosis (LSS) than those without hip OA [98].

It is likely that many older adults have hip-spine syndrome that is both complex and secondary in which both the hip and spine are pain generators, but altered hip function causes abnormal spinal biomechanics and low back pain, that is, altered hip function adds insult to injury. Although severe hip flexion deformity may be absent, we hypothesize that underlying lumbar spondylosis makes the lower back vulnerable and, therefore, more modest alterations in hip function may be needed to cause low back pain. So, the lumbar spine is the weak link and the hip is the treatment target. Well-controlled studies are needed to test this hypothesis. Until definitive answers are available, practitioners must approach the older adult with low back and/or leg pain using a broad perspective to avoid unnecessary "diagnostics" and misguided/potentially harmful treatments. Table 19.3 highlights key history and physical examination differences between pain generated by lumbosacral degeneration and that associated with hip OA. It should be noted that hip x-rays alone cannot be used to make a diagnosis of clinically mean-

ingful hip OA. Fewer than 50 % of patients with radiographic evidence of hip OA report pain [11]. A definitive diagnosis of hip OA should be based on a combination of clinical examination and x-ray findings [99, 100]. Thus, careful examination of the hip should be a routine part of evaluating all older adults who present with low back and/or leg pain.

Treatment Guidelines

The overarching goal of treatment for the older adult with chronic pain is to optimize function and quality of life while minimizing the potential for adverse effects associated with treatment. To accomplish this goal, an integrative stepped-care approach that combines non-pharmacological and pharmacological modalities is recommended. Specific recommendations for treating older adults with nociceptive pain, neuropathic pain, and widespread pain are provided below.

Nociceptive Pain

Figure 19.7 depicts an integrative stepped-care approach for the treatment of nociceptive pain. Topical preparations, cognitive behavioral therapy, interdisciplinary pain treatment, and complementary and alternative modalities (CAM) may

Fig. 19.7 Stepped-care approach for the treatment of nociceptive pain. *CAM* complementary and alternative medicine, *NSAIDs* nonsteroidal anti-inflammatory drugs (Reprinted from: Weiner and Cayea [178], with permission from Debra Weiner and IASP Press)

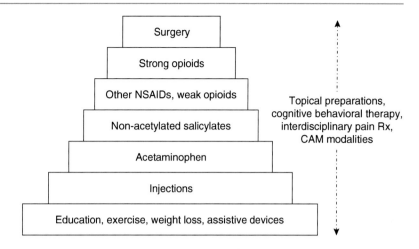

be used at any step, either alone or in combination. The individual steps shown in Fig. 19.7 are arranged from treatments associated with relatively low risk (step 1) to those associated with high risk (step 7).

At the foundation of treatment are education, weight loss, exercise, and other physical therapy approaches (including assistive devices). Sometimes, these approaches are alone sufficient to accomplish desired outcomes. For the older adult with fibromyalgia who is capable of participating in aerobic exercise, no further treatment may be needed. For the patient with kyphosis related to vertebral compression fractures and associated lumbar strain, a four-wheeled walker often is very effective for reducing pain and improving mobility. Education should be targeted at ensuring realistic treatment expectations (i.e., pain reduction but not elimination and improved function despite the persistence of pain) and quelling any pain-associated fears (e.g., becoming crippled and/or losing independence because of pain, having cancer associated with pain).

To avoid risks associated with systemic medication, injections should be considered for the older adult with pain in one or two joints, for example, knee osteoarthritis (OA). Trigger point injections can be an effective adjunct for treating myofascial pain syndromes [101]. There is no strong evidence to guide the prescription of spinal injections for older adults with chronic low back pain (CLBP). In general, injection therapies should be viewed as a tool to enhance compliance with rehabilitation efforts, which represent the mainstay of nociceptive pain treatment. For older adults with diabetes mellitus, patients should be instructed to monitor their blood sugar carefully following corticosteroid injections.

Systemic pharmacologic treatment of mild to moderate nociceptive pain should start with regularly scheduled acetaminophen because of its relatively safe side effect profile and few drug-drug or drug-disease interactions. Acetaminophen exerts its analgesic effect by weak, reversible, nonspecific cyclooxygenase inhibition, and, therefore, prostaglandin synthesis. It has no anti-inflammatory or anti-platelet effect and uncommonly causes gastrointestinal (GI)

bleeding or nephrotoxicity [65]. An overdose of 10 g can cause liver failure and death. Hepatic injury can occur with lower doses when the patient drinks alcohol heavily or is taking hepatic enzyme inducing medications (e.g., rifampin, carbamazepine, phenytoin, phenobarbital). Preexisting liver disease, malnourishment, fasting, or dehydration can also increase the risk of liver injury. Table 19.4 provides dosing guidelines, pharmacokinetics, key drug-drug and drug-disease interactions, and important adverse effects associated with acetaminophen and other medications used for nociceptive pain. To avoid breakthrough pain, it is important to dose analgesics around the clock [102].

When acetaminophen does not provide adequate analgesia or when an anti-inflammatory effect is needed, a nonacetylated salicylate such as salicylsalicylic acid should be considered [103]. As with all nonsteroidal anti-inflammatory drugs (NSAIDs), these drugs primarily promote analgesia via reversible inhibition of cyclooxygenase-2 that in turn blocks prostaglandin-associated sensitization of peripheral nociceptors [104]. Nonacetylated salicylates have a superior safety profile compared with other NSAIDs. They rarely cause GI bleeding. This is of particular clinical importance as adults over the age of 60 have a 3–4 % risk of bleeding while taking NSAIDs as compared to 1 % of the general population [65]. The nonacetylated salicylates also do not interfere with platelet function. Since many older adults are taking a daily aspirin for underlying diabetes or coronary artery disease, this latter benefit is also clinically relevant. These drugs can be combined with opioids if needed.

If a nonacetylated salicylate fails to relieve pain adequately, traditional NSAIDs or weak opioids can be considered. Because of the serious adverse events associated with NSAIDs, we advise that they be used only for brief periods in the setting of inflammatory disorders (e.g., a 7-day course of ibuprofen for an acute flare of gout or pseudogout). NSAIDs cause gastrointestinal bleeding, ulceration, and perforation. Additionally, because of renal prostaglandin inhibition with associated renal artery vasodilatation, NSAIDs promote fluid

Table 19.4 Oral analgesics for nociceptive pain

Medication class	Medication	Recommended dosing	Pharmacokinetics	Key drug-drug interactions	Key drug-disease interactions	Important adverse effects
Other analgesic	Acetaminophen	325–1,000 mg q 4–6 h Maximum daily dose 4,000 mg	Metabolized via glucuronidation Clearance may be reduced in frail older adults	Hepatic injury can occur with modest doses when concomitant use of hepatic enzyme inducing medications (e.g., rifampin, carbamazepine, phenytoin, phenobarbital).	None	Hepatic necrosis with acute 10 g ingestion or chronic use of >4 g/day. Increased toxicity from chronic use occurs with heavy alcohol use, malnourishment, pre-exiting liver disease – decrease maximum daily dose to 2 g Nephrotoxicity (dose dependent)
Non-acetylated salicylates	Salsalate	500–750 mg bid Maximum dose 3,000 mg/day	Metabolized by hydrolysis to salicylate; also metabolized via glucuronidation	No significant drug-drug interactions	See other NSAIDs below	Does not interfere with platelet function; GI bleeding rare
Other NSAIDs	Ibuprofen Naproxen	400 mg tid-qid 250–500 mg bid	CYP2C9/19 CYP2C9 and CYP1A2; clearance significantly reduced with advanced age	Concomitant use of NSAIDs with diuretics and antihypertensives may decrease their effectiveness. Use with corticosteroids and/or warfarin increases the risk of peptic ulcer disease. Increases concentration of lithium and methotrexate	Use NSAIDs with caution in patients with chronic renal failure, heart failure, hypertension, and peptic ulcer disease history	Risk of GI bleeding increased in persons $\geq$ 60 years. Cognitive impairment possible with higher doses. These NSAIDs should be reserved for short-term use in the older adult.
Cyclooxygenase (COX-2) inhibitor	Celecoxib	100 mg bid	CYP2C9/19	Same as NSAIDs above	Same as NSAIDs above	Because of relatively long half-life, naproxen should not be first choice for older adults. COX-2 inhibitor has less GI toxicity, but similar renal toxicity to other NSAIDS. Given long half-life and perhaps greater cardiac toxicity make it not a preferred agent for older adults.
Weak opioids	Codeine Hydrocodone	15–30 mg q 4–6 h 5–10 mg q 4–6 h (alone or in combination with acetaminophen)	Prodrug metabolized by CYP2D6 CYP2D6;not studied in older adults	Few clinically significant drug-drug interactions. Quinidine can inhibit the analgesic effect of codeine.	For all opioids, increased risk of falls in patients with dysmobility. May worsen or precipitate urinary retention when BPH present. Increased risk of delirium in those with dementia Codeine has active renal metabolites that can accumulate with advancing age and renal insufficiency.	Because of increased sensitivity to opioids older adults at greater risk for sedation, nausea, vomiting, constipation, urinary retention, respiratory depression, and cognitive impairment.

		Dosing	Metabolism	Drug interactions	Precautions	Side effects/notes
Opiate receptor agonist/SNRI	Tramadol	Initiate at 25 mg qd. Increase by 25–50 mg daily in divided doses every 3–7 days as tolerated to max dose of 100 mg Four times a day (QID). Renal dosing 100 mg Twice a day (BID).	Prodrug metabolized by CYP2D4, 2B6 and 2D6.	Sedative medications and other opioids. Risk of serotonin syndrome in combination with SSRI and triptans. Seizure risk with MAOI. Rare reports of interaction with warfarin and digoxin. Quinidine can inhibit the analgesic effect.	Seizure disorder (avoid if history of seizures).	Seizures and orthostatic hypotension. Other side effects similar to traditional opioids including sedation, confusion, respiratory depression.
					Adjust dose with renal insufficiency; maximum dose 100 mg bid.	
Strong opioids	Oxycodone (short and long-acting)	Start with 5 mg (short acting) q 4–6 h; after 7 days, determine dose requirements, then convert to long acting.	CYP2D6	As above	As above Oxycodone and morphine have active renal metabolites that can accumulate with advancing age and renal insufficiency.	As above Stong opioids to avoid in older adults: pentazocine, meperidine.
	Morphine (short and long-acting)	Start with 2.5 mg q 4 h and titrate by 2.5 mg increments q 7 days. Convert to long acting after dosing requirements determined.	Large first pass effect and high hepatic extraction ratio results in higher serum levels and decreased clearance; glucuronidation to active renally cleared metabolites.			
	Hydromorphone	Start with 2 mg q 4 h. Increase after 7 days if needed.	Glucuronidation; not studied in older adults			Dose of opioid required (for weak, strong, and tramadol) can be reduced by combining with a non-opioid agent such as acetaminophen.
	Fentanyl transdermal	Start with 12 mcg patch q 72 h. If ineffective after 1 week, increase to 25 mcg. 48 h dosing interval may be required.	CYP3A4			Constipation is very common with all opioids, but not universal; a stimulant laxative (e.g., senna) should be prescribed if needed.
	Methadone	Start with 1 mg q 12–24 h (po, buccal, sc). Titrate ≥ q 7d.	CYP3A4; not studied in older adults	Phentyoin can increase clearance		Fentanyl patch, methadone and other sustained-release opioids should be avoided in those who are opioid-naïve.
						EKG should be obtained and monitored in those on methadone, as may be associated with prolonged QT interval.

retention and may worsen or precipitate congestive heart failure, hypertension, and renal injury; cognitive dysfunction also may occur [65]. Although an NSAID can be combined with misoprostol or a proton-pump inhibitor to reduce the risk of gastrointestinal bleeding, we avoid the chronic use of NSAIDs in older adults whenever possible.

Recommended weak opioids include codeine and hydrocodone. The latter is more potent than codeine (10 mg of hydrocodone is equivalent to 60–80 mg of codeine). Like all opioids, they work by binding to mu receptors in the central nervous system. Their half-life is prolonged in patients with chronic kidney disease. Generally, older adults have an increased pharmacodynamic sensitivity to opioids [66, 105] and are more likely to experience the adverse effects of constipation, sedation, nausea, urinary retention, and cognitive impairment [106]. They are also more at risk for falling, especially if they have preexisting mobility impairment [107]. Because constipation with chronic opioid use is very common, practitioners should anticipate this and advise use of a stimulant laxative such as senna to patients at the first sign of constipation (e.g., 2–3 days without a bowel movement).

While opioids may be required at night, sleep quality may be affected by their nighttime use. Opioids both suppress rapid eye movement (REM) sleep and reduce total time spent in stage 4 (e.g., slow wave or "deep") sleep [108–110]. If sedation or daytime fatigue develops, initiation of methylphenidate (usually at starting doses of 2.5 mg daily or twice daily) can be considered, although large, well-controlled trials are lacking. The novel wake-promoting agents – modafinil and armodafinil – are treatment options for fatigue associated with chronic pain and the sedation commonly encountered with opioid pharmacotherapy. These agents may have safer side effect profiles than central nervous system stimulants, but care must be taken when prescribing for older adults because of potential cardiovascular and elimination concerns. Our recommendations, based on clinical experience, are to initiate treatment with half the recommended starting dose (50 mg/day for modafinil; 25–50 mg/day for armodafinil). Close attention should be paid to increases in blood pressure and heart rate with all of these agents.

Opioids also can cause hypogonadism because they bind to hypothalamic receptors and limit the production of gonadotropin-releasing hormones [111–117]. Estrogen and testosterone production is secondarily reduced resulting in hypogonadism [118–124]. While opioid-induced hypogonadism occurs in both sexes, it is more commonly recognized in men. The symptoms of hypogonadism in older adults include impotence in men and diminished libido in both men and women. Symptomatic improvement is seen after hormone supplementation [125]. Rat studies indicate that low testosterone is associated with increased pain sensitivity [126]. Preliminary evidence also suggests that hypogonadism may limit the anti-nociceptive properties of opioids

[127]. At this time, there are no human studies demonstrating the effect of hypogonadism on pain sensitivity.

Tramadol is a weak mu opioid receptor agonist and blocks the reuptake of norepinephrine and serotonin. It has a similar side effect profile as the typical opioids. Tramadol should be used cautiously or not at all in patients taking other serotonergic medications because of its potential to contribute to serotonin syndrome. Typically used in neuropathic pain, this drug is described in more detail below.

If weak opioids are ineffective, a strong opioid should be considered. Among older adults, oxycodone, the combination of oxycodone/acetaminophen, and morphine are all used commonly. Long-acting preparations of oxycodone and morphine are appropriate in equianalgesic doses for long-term use. Alternative agents such as hydromorphone and fentanyl also can be considered. Although methadone has a long and variable half-life, it can be a very effective analgesic [128]. Meperidine and pentazocine should not be prescribed in the older adult because of enhanced toxicity. For the patient who benefits from opioids but has limiting side effects, an intrathecal opioid pump might be considered.

While many complementary and alternative modalities are not covered by third-party payers, the evidence base for their efficacy in older adults is growing. Data indicate that lumbar percutaneous electrical nerve stimulation is effective for the treatment of chronic low back pain (CLBP), although the minimally effective dose of electrical stimulation has not been determined [56, 57]. Preliminary data indicate that mindfulness meditation reduces pain interference with daily activities in older adults with CLBP [61]. Periosteal stimulation has short-term benefits in reducing pain and improving function in older adults with chronic knee pain and advanced osteoarthritis [129]. Tai Chi and hypnosis may help improve osteoarthritis-associated pain and functional limitations [130, 131]. Given the toxicities associated with pharmacological management of chronic pain in older adults, additional research is needed to expand the scope of proven complementary and alternative modalities that have a favorable risk profile [132].

Practitioners should be aware that vitamin D deficiency is not uncommon in older adults and can contribute to pain, wasting, weakness, and gait instability/falls [133, 134]. Over the years, the recommended serum vitamin D level has varied. Recent studies suggest that 25-OH vitamin D levels between 30–32 ng/mL are optimal to prevent fractures and secondary hyperparathyroidism [135–140]. For patients with vitamin D levels below 20 ng/mL, we recommend supplementation with 50,000 IU once weekly for 3 months and then serum levels should be rechecked. If the level is normal, the patient should be placed on 1,000 IU daily for maintenance. If the vitamin D level is between 20 and 30 ng/mL, patients may be supplemented with 1,000 IU daily. Other studies recommend more aggressive vitamin D supplementation with 50,000 IU biweekly for 3 months in patients with

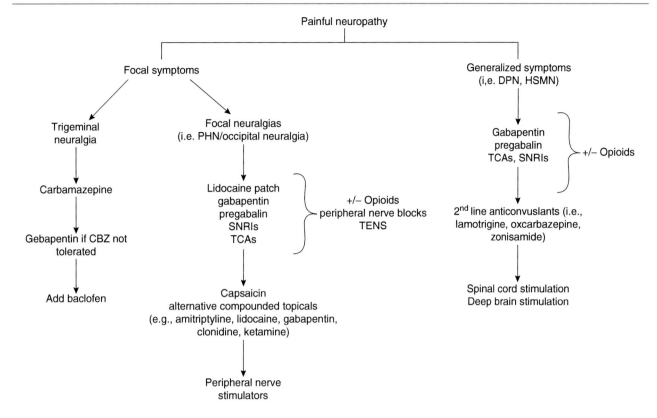

Fig. 19.8 Algorithmic approach for the treatment of painful neuropathy. *CBZ* carbamazepine, *DPN* diabetic peripheral neuropathy, *HSMN* hereditary sensory/motor neuropathy, *PHN* postherpetic neuralgia, *SNRI* serotonin/norepinephrine reuptake inhibitor, *TENS* transcutaneous electrical nerve stimulation, *TCA* tricyclic antidepressant

levels below 10 ng/mL. Supplementation with 50,000 IU once weekly for 3 months is recommended for those with levels between 10 and 32 ng/mL [135].

Vitamin D supplementation is well tolerated in older adults and may have considerable benefits. Vitamin D and calcium supplementation may reduce hip and non-vertebral fractures and fall risk [141–143]. A recent study of statin-associated myalgia demonstrated symptomatic improvement after vitamin D supplementation in deficient patients [144]. Other studies have demonstrated improvement of nonspecific muscle pain after vitamin D supplementation in deficient patients [145]. In one case series, chronic back pain and failed back surgery syndrome improved after vitamin D supplementation [146], although studies have had conflicting results. Despite contradictory data on the relationship between vitamin D levels and fibromyalgia pain [147], we routinely measure vitamin D levels in these patients and supplement if insufficient levels are found.

Neuropathic Pain

An algorithmic approach to the treatment of neuropathic pain is depicted in Fig. 19.8. Monotherapy with an antidepressant or anticonvulsant is the standard-of-care first-line approach for generalized neuropathic pain. For severe pain, an opioid alone or combined with another drug may be necessary. Topical preparations and peripheral nerve blockade are effective for localized symptoms and may be combined with systemic treatments. Those with intractable symptoms may benefit from interventional treatments such as spinal cord and peripheral nerve stimulation.

Table 19.5 contains guidelines for dosing, pharmacokinetics, key drug-drug and drug-disease interactions, and important adverse effects associated with medications used to treat neuropathic pain. Gabapentin and pregabalin have no significant end-organ toxicities and are safe for long-term use in older adults. When initiating and/or titrating these medications, practitioners must be vigilant for the development of sedation, confusion, and/or gait unsteadiness. Starting with a low dose and titrating, these medications slowly can help to avoid these side effects. Weight gain and peripheral edema also occur not uncommonly.

Secondary tricyclic antidepressants (TCAs) are well studied for the treatment of neuropathic pain and provide effective analgesia at approximately 30–50 % of the antidepressant dose [148]. In general, caution should be exercised when prescribing this class of medications for older adults.

Table 19.5 Oral analgesics for neuropathic pain

Medication class	Medication	Recommended dosing	Pharmacokinetics	Key drug-drug interactions	Key drug-disease interactions	Important adverse effects
Anticonvulsants	Gabapentin	Initiate at 100 mg nightly. Increase by 100 mg weekly. Renal dosing: CLcr 30–59 mg/min, titrate to 600 mg bid CLcr 15–29 mg/min, titrate to 300 mg bid CLcr < 15 mg/min, titrate to 300 mg qd Supplemental dosing after dialysis	Renal elimination. Nonlinear pharmacokinetics. Plasma concentration increases disproportionately to dose	Other CNS/sedative medications	Dementia, ataxia	Confusion, dizziness, somnolence, peripheral edema, weight gain. Withdrawal syndrome with abrupt discontinuation
	Pregabalin	Initiate at 25–50 mg nightly. Increase by 25–50 mg weekly up to 100 mg BID. Max dose 300 mg Once a day (QD) Renal dosing: CLcr 30–60 mg/min adjust dose to 150–300 mg QD. CLcr 15–30 mg/min adjust dose to 75–150 mg QD. CLcr <15 mg/min adjust dose to 25–50 QD Supplement dose after dialysis	Renal elimination. Linear pharmacokinetics (plasma concentration is dose proportionate)	Other CNS/sedative medications	Dementia, ataxia	Confusion, dizziness, somnolence, peripheral edema, weight gain
	Carbamazepine	Initiate at 50 mg nightly. Increase by 50 mg every week up to 100 mg BID. Target dose 200–600 mg QD. Max dose 1,200 mg QD. Adjust dose for serum levels (4–12 mg/L). Patients on multiple CNS medications may have toxicity at lower serum levels.	Metabolized by CYP450 3A4; induces CYP450	CYP3A4 inhibitors increase serum CBZ levels. CYP3A4 inducers decrease serum CBZ levels CBZ induces hepatic activity and can lower concentration of numerous drugs		Slurred speech, gait instability, poor coordination; Syndrome of Inappropriate Antidiuretic Hormone Secretion (SIADH); rare severe reactions: Stevens-Johnson syndrome, aplastic anemia, hepatotoxicity, drug-induced lupus Monitor LFTs, CBC, and serum sodium after initiation and during treatment.
TCAs	Nortriptyline Desipramine	10 mg at night. Increase by 10 mg weekly. Max dose 50 mg at night	Metabolized by CYP2D6	CYP2D6 inhibitors increase serum levels. CYP2D6 inducers decrease serum levels Other CNS/sedative medications	Myocardial infarction and bundle branch block; seizures; narrow-angle glaucoma, prostatic hypertrophy; dementia, falls	Arrhythmia, prolongation of QT interval and conduction block. Severe cases may lead to torsades de pointes. EKG prior to use in older adults. Orthostatic hypotension, sedation, confusion, constipation, urinary retention, SIADH

			Metabolism	Drug interactions	Contraindications	Adverse effects
Dual reuptake inhibitors (SNRIs)	Venlafaxine	Initiate at 37.5 mg daily. Increase by 37.5 mg weekly up to 150 mg daily. Max dose 225 mg daily	Metabolized by CYP2D6	Contraindicated within 14 days of MAOI use. May precipitate serotonin syndrome when combined with triptans, tramadol, and other antidepressants.	HTN and uncontrolled narrow-angle glaucoma. Precipitation of mania in bipolar disorder	Sedation/falls, insomnia, nausea, xerostomia, and constipation. Abrupt discontinuation may result in withdrawal syndrome.
	Duloxetine	Initiate at 20–30 mg daily. Increase to 60 mg after 1 week. Max dose 60 mg. Not recommended in ESRD or with CLcr < 30 mL/min.	Metabolized by CYP1A2 and CYP2D6	CYP2D6 inhibitors; contraindicated within 14 days of MAOI use	HTN, uncontrolled narrow-angle glaucoma, and seizure disorder. Precipitation of mania in patients with bipolar disorder	Nausea, dry mouth, sedation/falls, urinary retention, and constipation. Abrupt discontinuation may result in withdrawal syndrome and low risk of hepatotoxicity, but contraindicated with hepatic disease and heavy alcohol
				May precipitate serotonin syndrome when combined with triptans, tramadol, and other antidepressants.		
Topical agents	Lidocaine patch 5 %	1–3 patches topically 12 h on 12 h off. Only 3 ± 2 % of lidocaine patch absorbed. 95 % lidocaine remains in patch form	Hepatically metabolized	Use with caution in patients taking class I antiarrhythmics (tocainamide and mexiletine).	Severe hepatic disease and non-intact skin	Site reactions. Symptoms of lidocaine toxicity are rare and include nausea, nervousness, tinnitus, metallic taste, confusion, and tremor. Toxicity seen with serum lidocaine levels of >5 mcg/mL. Serum levels with lidocaine patch typically 0.13 mcg/mL
			Unknown if lidocaine is metabolized in the skin. Negligible serum metabolite levels after topical application, that is, minimal systemic absorption			
	Capsaicin	Apply thin layer to affected area QID	Cutaneous action. Maximum effect noted after 4–6 weeks of use	None known	Irritation on non-intact skin	Skin reactions and burning. Avoid contact with eyes and sensitive skin areas. Respiratory irritation/cough if inhaled
Muscle relaxants	Baclofen	Initiate at 5 mg nightly. Increase by 5 mg every week as tolerated. Max dose 10 mg TID. Dose adjustment with renal insufficiency	Minimal metabolism; 85 % excreted unchanged in liver and feces	CNS depressants	Ataxia, renal disease, dementia, and seizures	Not recommended for older adults. Confusion, nausea, and sedation Abrupt withdrawal syndrome with hallucinations, seizures, muscle rigidity, and high fever. If severe, may lead to rhabdomyolysis, multi-organ system failure, and death
Opioid analgesics						See Table 19.4

CBC complete blood count, *CBZ* Carbamazepine, *CLcr* creatinine clearance, *CNS* central nervous system, *CYP* Cytochrome P450, *EKG* electrocardiogram, *ESRD* end-stage renal disease, *HTN* hypertension, *LFTs* liver function tests, *MAOI* monoamine oxidase inhibitor, *NSAID* nonsteroidal anti-inflammatory drug

Amitriptyline has the greatest anticholinergic potential and is contraindicated in older adults. If the practitioner wishes to prescribe a TCA, desipramine and nortriptyline are preferred agents. TCAs in general are contraindicated in patients with a history of myocardial infarction, QT prolongation, and/or bundle branch block, and a screening EKG should always be obtained prior to initiating them in older adults [149]. They also are contraindicated in patients with untreated narrow-angle glaucoma because of their potential to exacerbate this condition. Other commonly encountered anticholinergic side effects include sedation, confusion, dizziness, xerostomia, constipation, gait unsteadiness/falls, and urinary retention [107, 150]. For older adults with medical comorbidities that themselves contribute to these symptoms (e.g., urinary hesitancy in the older male with prostatism, poor cognitive function in the patient with dementia, gait unsteadiness typically related to multiple factors), an alternative to TCAs should be considered.

The newer serotonin and norepinephrine reuptake inhibitor (SNRI) antidepressants, duloxetine and venlafaxine, and o-desmethylvenlafaxine are effective for neuropathic pain and have fewer side effects than the TCAs [151, 152]. Duloxetine is Food and Drug Administration (FDA) approved for painful diabetic neuropathy. It is contraindicated for patients with uncontrolled narrow-angle glaucoma and should ordinarily not be prescribed to patients with substantial alcohol use or evidence of chronic liver disease. Nausea (especially during induction or dose escalations) and orthostatic hypotension are not uncommon adverse drug reactions. Venlafaxine, o-desmethylvenlafaxine, and duloxetine, in addition to causing orthostatic hypotension [153], can cause sustained elevations in blood pressure, may lower seizure threshold in patients with a history of seizure, and increase the risk of abnormal bleeding, especially when co-prescribed with NSAIDs, aspirin, or other drugs that affect coagulation.

If monotherapy with a first-line anticonvulsant or antidepressant provides suboptimal analgesia, these medications may be combined. Combining modest doses of gabapentin and morphine is more effective than larger doses of either drug alone [154]. Second-line anticonvulsants, lamotrigine, oxcarbazepine, and zonisamide, are effective for some types of neuropathic pain including painful diabetic polyneuropathy [155, 156].

Opioid analgesics are first-line options for moderate to severe nerve pain [157]. Traditional opioids as well as methadone, a long-acting opioid and N-Methyl-D-aspartic acid (NMDA) antagonist, are effective. Tramadol, a weak mu-receptor agonist with serotonin and norepinephrine reuptake blockade, also is effective for neuropathic pain [158, 159]. Serotonin syndrome may occur when tramadol is combined with other serotonergic medications (e.g., triptans, various antidepressants). Tramadol also lowers the seizure threshold and increases the risk of seizure in patients taking serotonin reuptake inhibitors, tricyclic antidepressants and other tricyclic compounds (e.g., cyclobenzaprine), and other opioids. At therapeutic doses, tramadol has no effect on heart rate, left-ventricular function, or cardiac index, although orthostatic hypotension has been observed.

While tramadol is currently approved for the treatment of moderate to moderately severe chronic pain in adults, a newer compound, tapentadol, is approved for the treatment of moderate to severe acute pain in adults [160]. The analgesic efficacy of tapentadol is thought to occur via mu-receptor agonism and norepinephrine reuptake blockade. The side effect profile of tapentadol is similar to tramadol, but given its recent release, it has not been as extensively used with older adults. The potential side effects associated with opioids are numerous and described earlier in this chapter.

Focal nerve pain is often amenable to treatment with peripheral nerve blockade, topical treatments, and transcutaneous electrical stimulation. Depending on the older adult's risk profile, these treatments may be chosen as first line for those with localized pain. Peripheral nerve blocks with local anesthetics and steroid are used to treat ilioinguinal, occipital, and postherpetic neuralgia. Complications from these interventions are rare and include bleeding and infection. The lidocaine patch and other compounded topical medications (e.g., gabapentin, clonidine, amitriptyline, ketamine either alone or combined) may be beneficial. Capsaicin relieves painful symptoms but may itself be painful and requires 4–6 weeks of use before taking effect.

As noted earlier in this chapter, treatment of comorbid myofascial pain (MP) in older adults with focal nerve pain may result in dramatic pain reduction, as evidenced by our clinical experience with a number of older adults who presented with refractory postherpetic neuralgia [51]. In these patients, pain reduction related to successful non-pharmacological treatment of MP afforded significant dose reduction or complete discontinuation of opioids.

Neuropathic pain secondary to trigeminal neuralgia (TN) is unique and may respond to treatment with carbamazepine (CBZ). Compared to other anticonvulsants, however, CBZ may be less well tolerated [161]. The risk of serious dermatologic reactions (e.g., Stevens-Johnson syndrome), aplastic anemia and agranulocytosis, and hyponatremia must be weighed prior to initiating treatment with CBZ. Gabapentin, while less effective for TN, is a reasonable alternative for those older adults who do not tolerate CBZ. Baclofen, a muscle relaxant, is effective for TN and may be combined with CBZ or gabapentin [162], but muscle relaxants generally should be avoided in older adults as highlighted in the 2012 [163].

Multidisciplinary pain treatment combining physical therapy, occupational therapy, and psychology may be beneficial for those with refractory symptoms. As for patients with nociceptive pain, those with neuropathic pain who benefit from opioids but have limiting side effects, an intrathecal opioid pump might be considered. Spinal cord or peripheral nerve stimulation is a final resort for those who fail systemic, topical, and other non-pharmacological treatments [164, 165]. Motor cortex stimulation may treat severe neuropathic pain involving the face or as a result of intracerebral pathology (i.e., stroke) [166]. A psychological evaluation is required prior to these invasive procedures.

Widespread Pain

Fibromyalgia (FMS) syndrome, the classical condition defined by widespread musculoskeletal pain from which older adults suffer, affects 7 % of community-dwelling women aged 60–79 [167]. Diagnosis requires a history of pain in at least three of four body quadrants lasting at least 3 months and pain with palpation (using 4 kgf) at 11 or more of 18 specific points on the body [168]. Morning stiffness, fatigue, nonrestorative sleep, neuropsychiatric disturbances (e.g., impaired memory, depression), paresthesias, and irritable bowel and bladder symptoms commonly accompany FMS. Depression and/or anxiety should be screened routinely, given their common co-occurrence in FMS and their potential for interfering with analgesic efficacy and treatment adherence.

The first step in treating the older adult with FMS is education. This is especially relevant for older adults and their caregivers who may be puzzled and frightened by the presence of widespread pain; it may be interpreted as a life-threatening condition. A patient-centered care model should be adopted so that the patient, physician, and caregiver collaborate in developing a personalized treatment plan. After providing education, evidence-based non-pharmacological and pharmacological treatments should be implemented.

To date, there have been no non-pharmacological or pharmacological treatment studies of FMS restricted to older adults. Although pharmacological approaches are an important mode of treatment, there is no evidence to support long-term benefit and they should never be used without proven non-pharmacological approaches such as cognitive behavioral therapy and aerobic exercise [169]. When depression or anxiety is comorbid, an antidepressant should be utilized. Low-dose tricyclic antidepressants such as nortriptyline or desipramine improve both sleep quality and symptoms on the global assessment scale and lead to improvement in tender point score, pain, and fatigue [170]. Because of the anticholinergic and cardiac side effects noted above, it may be difficult to increase the dose of tricyclics to a level with antidepressant efficacy. Fluoxetine alone or in combination with amitriptyline also has beneficial effects [171]. We do not, however, recommend the use of either fluoxetine or amitriptyline in older adults. Fluoxetine has a long half-life,

and as noted earlier in this chapter, amitriptyline is more sedating than other tricyclics and has the highest anticholinergic burden. Symptom improvement was not observed in a randomized, double-blind, placebo-controlled study of citalopram [172].

If depression or anxiety is comorbid with FMS and nortriptyline or desipramine is contraindicated, a serotonin norepinephrine reuptake inhibitor such as duloxetine or milnacipran would be suitable. In a 3-month study, compared to placebo, treatment with duloxetine (60 mg twice daily) resulted in more improvement on the Fibromyalgia Impact Questionnaire (FIQ) and a number of other outcomes, independent of its effect on mood [173]. Milnacipran, twice daily, improved pain and other outcome measures in 125 patients with FMS over 12 weeks [174]. Duloxetine is not recommended for patients with end-stage renal disease (ESRD) or severe renal impairment (estimated creatinine clearance <30 mL/min). Milnacipran should not be used in patients with ESRD, and in those with creatinine clearance of 5–29 mL/min, the dose should be reduced by 50 %.

Pregabalin, discussed in the section on neuropathic pain, is one of three FDA-approved medications (duloxetine and milnacipran are the other two) for the treatment of FMS. Because of its anxiolytic properties, if symptoms or anxiety are prominent (and depression is not present), pregabalin may be a good first-line medication. Its molecular precursor, gabapentin, has proven efficacious in the treatment of FMS in mixed age adults [175].

Tramadol, discussed in the section on nociceptive pain, has efficacy in FMS for reducing pain and improving physical function [176]. Tramadol also has been found to be effective in treating the pain of osteoarthritis [177], a disorder that frequently coexists with FMS in older adults.

Cyclobenzaprine has strong efficacy evidence for reducing pain in FMS [169], but because of its strong anticholinergic potential, decreased clearance in older adults, and potential to disrupt cardiac conduction, it should be used cautiously [178].

Future Directions

The field of pain and aging is in its infancy, having originated because of an obvious societal need rather than a distinct body of knowledge. To optimize the treatment of the burgeoning population of older adults, numerous questions must be answered: (1) What drives functional decline in older adults with chronic pain? How should future treatment be targeted to most effectively ameliorate this decline? (2) What is the efficacy and safety of pharmacological and non-pharmacological treatments for older adults? Studies must be designed that include adequate numbers of older adults to provide a meaningful answer to this question. (3) How should our health care resources be funneled to optimize benefits and decrease risks? Until health care policy changes, how can we improve the training of students and health care providers to evaluate and manage pain in older adults in a clinically effective and cost-effective way?

Summary/Conclusions

Older adults with chronic pain should be thought of and cared for as older adults first and as pain patients second. Their management often requires the cooperation of an interdisciplinary team rather than a pain physician in isolation. Until an adequate evidence base exists to direct the treatment of these patients, care should proceed carefully and comprehensively.

References

1. Becker PM, Cohen HJ. The functional approach to the care of the elderly: a conceptual framework. J Am Geriatr Soc. 1984;32:923.
2. Karp JF, Shega JW, Morone NE, Weiner DK. Advances in understanding the mechanisms and management of persistent pain in older adults. Br J Anaesth. 2008;101(1):111–20.
3. US Bureau of the Census. 1997. Aging in the United States – past, present, and future. http://www.census.gov/ipc/prod/97agewc.pdf. Accessed on 1st Jan 2010.
4. Centers for Disease Control and Prevention. 2008. Health, United States, 2008. http://www.cdc.gov/nchs/data/hus/hus08.pdf. Accessed on 1st Jan 2010.
5. Resnick NM, Marcantonio ER. How should clinical care of the aged differ? Lancet. 1997;350:1157–8.
6. Boden SD, Davis DO, Dina TS, Patronas NJ, Wiesel SW. Abnormal magnetic-resonance scans of the lumbar spine in asymptomatic subjects – a prospective investigation. J Bone Joint Surg Am. 1990;72(3):403–8.
7. Weiner DK, Distell B, Studenski S, Martinez S, Lomasney L, Bongiorni D. Does radiographic osteoarthritis correlate with flexibility of the lumbar spine? J Am Geriatr Soc. 1994;42:257–63.
8. Hicks GE, Morone N, Weiner DK. Degenerative lumbar disc and facet disease in older adults: prevalence and clinical correlates. Spine. 2009;34(12):1301–6.
9. Jarvik JJ, Hollingworth W, Heagerty P, Haynor DR, Deyo RA. The longitudinal assessment of imaging and disability of the back (LAIDBack) study: baseline data. Spine. 2001;26(10):1158–66.
10. Reid MC, Williams CS, Gill TM. Back pain and decline in lower extremity physical function among community-dwelling older persons. J Gerontol Med Sci. 2005;60A(6):793–7.
11. Lane NE, Nevitt MC, Hochberg MC, Hung Y-Y, Palermo L. Progression of radiographic hip osteoarthritis over eight years in a community sample of elderly white women. Arthritis Rheum. 2004;50(5):1477–86.
12. Bosley BN, Weiner DK, Rudy TE, Granieri E. Is chronic nonmalignant pain associated with decreased appetite in older adults? Preliminary evidence. J Am Geriatr Soc. 2004;52:247–51.
13. Weiner DK, Rudy TE, Morrow L, Slaboda J, Lieber SJ. The relationship between pain, neuropsychological performance, and physical function in community-dwelling older adults with chronic low back pain. Pain Med. 2006;7(1):60–70.
14. Karp JF, Reynolds CF, Butters MA, Dew MA, Mazumdar S, Begley AE, et al. The relationship between pain and mental flexibility in older adult pain clinic patients. Pain Med. 2006;7:444–52.
15. Rudy TE, Weiner DK, Lieber SJ, Slaboda J, Boston JR. The impact of chronic low back pain on older adults: a comparative study of patients and controls. Pain. 2007;13:293–301.
16. Carey TS, Evans A, Hadler N, Kalsbeek W, McLaughlin C, Fryer J. Care-seeking among individuals with chronic low back pain. Spine. 1995;20(3):312–7.
17. Weiner DK, Rudy TE, Gaur S. Are all older adults with persistent pain created equal? Preliminary evidence for a multiaxial taxonomy. Pain Res Manag. 2001;6(3):133–41.
18. Williamson GM, Schulz R. Pain, activity restriction, and symptoms of depression among community-residing adults. J Gerontol. 1992;47:367–72.
19. Williams AK, Schulz R. Association of pain and physical dependency with depression in physically ill middle-aged and elderly. Phys Ther. 1988;68(8):1226–30.
20. Casten RJ, Parmelee PA, Kleban MH, Lawton MP, Katz IR. The relationships among anxiety, depression, and pain in a geriatric institutionalized sample. Pain. 1995;61:271–6.
21. Gentili A, Weiner DK, Kuchibhatla M, Edinger JD. Factors that disturb sleep in nursing home residents. Aging Clin Exp Res. 1997;9:207–13.
22. Wilson KG, Watson ST, Currie SR. Daily diary and ambulatory activity monitoring of sleep in patients with insomnia associated with chronic musculoskeletal pain. Pain. 1998;75:75–84.
23. Weiner DK, Haggerty CL, Kritchevsky SB, Harris T, Simonsick EM, Nevitt M, et al. How does low back pain impact physical function in independent, well-functioning older adults? Evidence from the Health ABC cohort and implications for the future. Pain Med. 2003;4(4):311–20.
24. Reyes-Gibby CC, Aday L, Cleeland C. Impact of pain on self-rated health in the community-dwelling older adults. Pain. 2002;95(1–2):75–82.
25. O'Sullivan DJ, Swallow M. The fibre size and content of the radial and sural nerves. J Neurol Neurosurg Psychiatry. 1968;31:464–70.
26. Ochoa J, Mair WG. The normal sural nerve in man. II. Changes in the axons and Schwann cells due to aging. Acta Neuropathol. 1969;13:217–39.
27. Rafalowska J, Drac H, Rosinska K. Histological and electrophysiological changes of the lower motor neuron with aging. Pol Med Sci Hist Bull. 1976;15:271–80.
28. Drac H, Babiuch M, Wisniewska W. Morphological and biochemical changes in peripheral nerves with aging. Neuropatol Pol. 1991;29:49–67.
29. Chakour MC, Gibson SJ, Bradbeer M, Helme RD. The effect of age on A delta- and C-fibre thermal pain perception. Pain. 1996;64:143–52.
30. Gibson SJ, Farrell M. A review of age differences in the neurophysiology of nociception and the perceptual experience of pain. Clin J Pain. 2004;20:227–39.
31. Iwata K, Fukuoka T, Kondo E, et al. Plastic changes in nociceptive transmission of the rat spinal cord with advancing age. J Neurophysiol. 2002;87:1086–93.
32. Ko ML, King MA, Gordon TL, Crisp T. The effects of aging on spinal neurochemistry in the rat. Brain Res Bull. 1997;42:95–8.
33. Amenta F, Zaccheo D, Collier WL. Neurotransmitters, neuroreceptors and aging. Mech Ageing Dev. 1991;61:249–73.
34. Barili P, De Carolis G, Zaccheo D, Amenta F. Sensitivity to ageing of the limbic dopaminergic system: a review. Mech Ageing Dev. 1998;106:57–92.
35. Spokes EG. An analysis of factors influencing measurements of dopamine, noradrenaline, glutamate decarboxylase and choline

acetylase in human post-mortem brain tissue. Brain. 1979;102: 333–46.

36. Kakiuchi T, Nishiyama S, Sato K, Ohba H, Nakanishi S, Tsukada H. Age-related reduction of [11C]MDL100,907 binding to central 5-HT(2A) receptors: PET study in the conscious monkey brain. Brain Res. 2000;883:135–42.

37. DeKosky ST, Scheff SW, Markesbery WR. Laminar organization of cholinergic circuits in human frontal cortex in Alzheimer's disease and aging. Neurology. 1985;35:1425–31.

38. Grote SS, Moses SG, Robins E, Hudgens RW, Croninger AB. A study of selected catecholamine metabolizing enzymes: a comparison of depressive suicides and alcoholic suicides with controls. J Neurochem. 1974;23:791–802.

39. McGeer E, McGeer P. Neurotransmitter metabolism in the ageing brain. In: Terry R, Gershon S, editors. Neurobiology of aging. New York: Raven; 1976. p. 389–401.

40. Robinson D. Changes in MAO and monoamines with human development. Fed Proc. 1975;34:103–7.

41. Rogers J, Bloom F. Neurotransmitter metabolism and function in the aging nervous system. In: Finch CE, Schneider EL, editors. Handbook of the biology of aging. New York: Van Nostrand Reinhold; 1985. p. 645–62.

42. White P, Hiley CR, Goodhardt MJ, et al. Neocortical cholinergic neurons in elderly people. Lancet. 1977;1:668–71.

43. Wong DF, Wagner HNJ, Dannals RF, et al. Effects of age on dopamine and serotonin receptors measured by positron tomography in the living human brain. Science. 1984;226:1393–6.

44. Marcusson JO, Morgan DG, Winblad B, Finch CE. Serotonin-2 binding sites in human frontal cortex and hippocampus. Selective loss of S-2A sites with age. Brain Res. 1984;311:51–6.

45. Grachev ID, Swarnkar A, Szeverenyi NM, Ramachandran TS, Apkarian AV. Aging alters the multichemical networking profile of the human brain: an in vivo (1)H-MRS study of young versus middle-aged subjects. J Neurochem. 2001;77:292–303.

46. Edwards RR, Fillingim RB. Age-associated differences in responses to noxious stimuli. J Gerontol A Biol Sci Med Sci. 2001;56:M180–5.

47. Lautenbacher S, Kunz M, Strate P, Nielsen J, Arendt-Nielsen L. Age effects on pain thresholds, temporal summation and spatial summation of heat and pressure pain. Pain. 2005;115:410–8.

48. Farrell M, Gibson S. Age interacts with stimulus frequency in the temporal summation of pain. Pain Med. 2007;8:514–20.

49. Gagliese L. What do experimental pain models tell us about aging and clinical pain? Pain Med. 2007;8:475–7.

50. Wittink HM, Rogers WH, Lipman AG, McCarberg BH, Ashburn MA, Oderda GM, et al. Older and younger adults in pain management programs in the United States: differences and similarities. Pain Med. 2006;7(2):151–63.

51. Weiner DK, Schmader KE. Postherpetic pain: more than sensory neuralgia? Pain Med. 2006;7:243–9.

52. Weiner DK, Sakamoto S, Perera S, Breuer P. Chronic low back pain in older adults: prevalence, reliability, and validity of physical examination findings. J Am Geriatr Soc. 2006;54:11–20.

53. Ciol MA, Deyo RA, Howell E, Kreif S. An assessment of surgery for spinal stenosis: time trends, geographic variations, complications, and reoperations. J Am Geriatr Soc. 1996;44:285–90.

54. Cloyd JM, Acosta FLJ, Ames CP. Complications and outcomes of lumbar spine surgery in elderly people: a review of the literature. J Am Geriatr Soc. 2008;56:1318–27.

55. Inouye SK. Delirium in older persons. N Engl J Med. 2006; 354(11):1157–65.

56. Weiner DK, Rudy TE, Glick RM, Boston JR, Lieber SJ, Morrow L, et al. Efficacy of percutaneous electrical nerve stimulation (PENS) for the treatment of chronic low back pain in older adults. J Am Geriatr Soc. 2003;51:599–608.

57. Weiner DK, Perera S, Rudy TE, Glick RM, Shenoy S, Delitto A. Efficacy of percutaneous electrical nerve stimulation and therapeutic exercise for older adults with chronic low back pain: a randomized controlled trial. Pain. 2008;140:344–57.

58. Weinstein JN, Tosteson TD, Lurie JD, Tosteson ANA, Blood E, Hanscom B, et al. Surgical versus nonsurgical therapy for lumbar spinal stenosis. N Engl J Med. 2008;358:794–810.

59. Buckalew N, Haut M, Morrow LA, Weiner DK. Chronic pain is associated with brain volume loss in older adults: preliminary evidence. Pain Med. 2008;9(2):240–8.

60. Buckalew N, Haut MW, Morrow L, Perera S, Weiner D. Brain morphology differences in older adults with disabling chronic low back pain. J Am Geriatr Soc. 2009;57(4):S58.

61. Morone NE, Greco CM, Weiner DK. Mindfulness meditation for the treatment of chronic low back pain in older adults: a randomized controlled pilot study. Pain. 2008;134:310–9.

62. Ratcliff G, Dodge H, Birzescu M, Ganguli M. Tracking cognitive function over time: ten-year longitudinal data from a community-based study. Appl Neuropsychol. 2003;10(2):76–88.

63. Rolland Y, Czerwinski S, AbellanvanKan G, Morley JE, Cesari M, Onder G, et al. Sarcopenia: its assessment, etiology, pathogenesis, consequences and future perspectives. J Nutr Health Aging. 2008;12:433–50.

64. Ferrucci L, Guralnik JM, Simonsick E, Salive ME, Corti C, Langlois J. Progressive versus catastrophic disability: a longitudinal view of the disablement process. J Gerontol Ser A Biol Sci Med Sci. 1996;51(3):M123–30.

65. Hanlon JT, Guay DRP, Ives TJ. Oral analgesics: efficacy, mechanism of action, pharmacokinetics, adverse effects, drug interactions and practical recommendations for use in older adults. In: Gibson SJ, Weiner DK, editors. Pain in older persons, progress in pain research and management. Seattle: IASP Press; 2005.

66. Kaiko RF. Age and morphine analgesia in cancer patients with postoperative pain. Clin Pharmacol Ther. 1980;28:823–6.

67. Kaiko RF, Wallenstein SL, Rogers AG, et al. Narcotics in the elderly. Med Clin North Am. 1982;66:1079–89.

68. Hicks GE, Simonsick EM, Harris TB, Newman AB, Weiner DK, Nevitt MA, et al. Cross-sectional associations between trunk muscle composition, back pain and physical function in the Health ABC study. J Gerontol Med Sci. 2005;60A(7):882–7.

69. Morrison RS, Magaziner J, Gilbert M, Koval KJ, McLaughlin MA, Orosz G, et al. Relationship between pain and opioid analgesics on the development of delirium following hip fracture. J Gerontol Med Sci. 2003;58(1):76–81.

70. Tassain V, Attal N, Fletcher D, Brasseur L, Degieux P, Chauvin M, et al. Long term effects of oral sustained release morphine on neuropsychological performance in patients with chronic non-cancer pain. Pain. 2003;104:389–400.

71. Jamison RN, Schein JR, Vallow S, Ascher S, Vorsanger GJ, Katz NP. Neuropsychological effects of long-term opioid use in chronic pain patients. J Pain Symptom Manage. 2003;26(4):913–21.

72. Cole LJ, Farrell MJ, Duff EP, Barber JB, Egan GF, Gibson SJ. Pain sensitivity and fMRI pain-related brain activity in Alzheimer's disease. Brain. 2006;129:2957–65.

73. Porter FL, Malhotra KM, Wolf CM, Morris JC, Smith MC. Dementia and response to pain in the elderly. Pain. 1996;68:413–21.

74. Kunz M, Scharmann S, Hemmeter U, Schepelmann K, Lautenbacher S. The facial expression of pain in patients with dementia. Pain. 2007;133:221–8.

75. Shega JW, Rudy T, Keefe FJ, Perri LC, Mengin OT, Weiner DK. Validity of pain behaviors in persons with mild to moderate cognitive impairment. J Am Geriatr Soc. 2008;56:1631–7.

76. Benedetti F, Arduino C, Costa S, Vighetti S, Tarenzi L, Rainero I, et al. Loss of expectancy-related mechanisms in Alzheimer's disease makes analgesic therapies less effective. Pain. 2006;121:133–44.

77. Benedetti F. What do you expect from this treatment? Changing our mind about clinical trials. Pain. 2007;128:193–4.

78. Finiss DG, Benedetti F. Mechanisms of the placebo response and their impact on clinical trials and clinical practice. Pain. 2005; 114:3–6.

79. Weiner DK, Herr K. Comprehensive assessment & interdisciplinary treatment planning: an integrative overview. In: Weiner DK, Herr K, Rudy TE, editors. Persistent pain in older adults: an interdisciplinary guide for treatment. New York: Springer Publishing Company; 2002. p. 18–57.

80. Goetz CG, Tanner CM, Levy M, Wilson RS, Garron DC. Pain in Parkinson's disease. Mov Disord. 1986;1(1):45–9.

81. Witjas T, Kaphan E, Azulay JP, Blin O, Ceccaldi M, Pouget J, et al. Nonmotor fluctuations in Parkinson's disease – frequent and disabling. Neurology. 2002;59:408–13.

82. O'Sullivan SS, Williams DR, Gallagher DA, Massey LA, Silveira-Moriyama L, Lees AJ. Nonmotor symptoms as presenting complaints in Parkinson's disease: a clinicopathological study. Mov Disord. 2008;1(1):101–6.

83. Wolters EC. Variability in the clinical expression of Parkinson's disease. J Neurol Sci. 2008;266:197–203.

84. Truong DD, Bhidayasiri R, Wolters E. Management of non-motor symptoms in advanced Parkinson's disease. J Neurol Sci. 2008; 266:216–28.

85. Ford B, Greene P, Fahn S. Oral and genital tardive pain syndromes. Neurology. 1994;44:2115–9.

86. Ford B, Louis ED, Greene P, Fahn S. Oral and genital pain syndromes in Parkinson's disease. Mov Disord. 1996;11:421–6.

87. Djaldetti R, Shifrin A, Rogowski Z, Sprecher E, Melamed E, Yarnitsky D. Quantitative measurement of pain sensation in patients with Parkinson disease. Neurology. 2004;62:2171–5.

88. Tinazzi M, Del Vesco C, Defazio G, Fincati E, Smania N, Moretto G, et al. Abnormal processing of the nociceptive input in Parkinson's disease: a study with CO_2 laser evoked potentials. Pain. 2008;136:117–24.

89. Tuokko H, Hadjistavropoulos T, Miller JA, Beattie BL. The clock test: a sensitive measure to differentiate normal elderly from those with Alzheimer disease. J Am Geriatr Soc. 1992;40:579–84.

90. Weiner DK, Peterson B, Logue P, Keefe FJ. Predictors of pain self-report in nursing home residents. Aging Clin Exp Res. 1998;10:411–20.

91. Chibnall J, Tait R. Pain assessment in cognitively impaired and unimpaired older adults: a comparison of four scales. Pain. 2001;92:173–86.

92. Borson S, Scanlan J, Brush M, Vitaliano P, Dokmak A. The Mini-Cog: a cognitive vital signs measure for dementia screening in multi-lingual elderly. Int J Geriatr Psychiatry. 2000;15:1021–7.

93. Scanlan J, Borson S. The Mini-Cog: receiver operating characteristics with expert and naïve raters. Int J Geriatr Psychiatry. 2001;16:216–22.

94. Wolfson LI, Whipple R, Amerman P, Kleinberg A. Stressing the postural response. A quantitative method for testing balance. J Am Geriatr Soc. 1986;34:845–50.

95. Offierski CM, Macnab MB. Hip-spine syndrome. Spine. 1983;8(3):316–21.

96. Ben-Galim P, Ben-Galim T, Rand N, Haim A, Hipp J, Dekel S, et al. Hip-Spine syndrome: the effect of total hip replacement surgery on low back pain in severe osteoarthritis of the hip. Spine. 2007;32(19):2099–102.

97. Fritz JM, Whitman JM, Flynn TW, Wainner RS, Childs JD. Factors related to the inability of individuals with low back pain to improve with a spinal manipulation. Phys Ther. 2004;84(2):173–90.

98. Airaksinen O, Herno A, Turunen V, Saari T, Suomlainen O. Surgical outcome of 438 patient treated surgically for lumbar spinal stenosis. Spine. 1997;22(19):2278–82.

99. Altman R, Alarcon G, Appelrouth D, et al. The American College of Rheumatology criteria for the classification and reporting of osteoarthritis of the hip. Arthritis Rheum. 1991;34(5):505–14.

100. Lane NE. Osteoarthritis of the hip. N Engl J Med. 2007;357: 1413–21.

101. Borg-Stein J. Treatment of fibromyalgia, myofascial pain, and related disorders. Phys Med Rehabil Clin N Am. 2006;17: 491–510.

102. Weiner DK. Office management of chronic pain in the elderly. Am J Med. 2007;120(4):306–15.

103. AGS Panel on Persistent Pain in Older Persons. The management of persistent pain in older persons. J Am Geriatr Soc. 2002;50(6 suppl):S205–24104.

104. Nikolaus T, Zeyfang A. Pharmacological treatments for persistent non-malignant pain in older persons. Drugs Aging. 2004;21: 19–41.

105. Bellville JW, Forrest Jr WH, Miller E, Brown Jr BW. Influence of age on pain relief from analgesics. A study of postoperative patients. JAMA. 1971;217(13):1835–41.

106. Weiner DK, Hanlon JT. Pain in nursing home residents – management strategies. Drugs Aging. 2001;18(1):13–29.

107. Weiner DK, Hanlon JT, Studenski SA. Effects of central nervous system polypharmacy on falls liability in community-dwelling elderly. Gerontology. 1998;44:217–21.

108. Kay DC, Pickworth WB, Neider GL. Morphine-like insomnia from heroin in nondependent human addicts. Br J Clin Pharmacol. 1981;11(2):159–69.

109. Shaw IR, et al. Acute intravenous administration of morphine perturbs sleep architecture in healthy pain-free adults: a preliminary study. Sleep. 2005;28(6):677–82.

110. Walder B, Tramer MR, Blois R. The effects of two single doses of tramadol on sleep: a randomized, cross-over trial in healthy volunteers. Eur J Anaesthesiol. 2001;18(1):36–42.

111. Katz N, Mazer NA. The impact of opioids on the endocrine system. Clin J Pain. 2009;25:170–5.

112. Cicero T. Effects of exogenous and endogenous opiates on the hypothalamic-pituitary-gonadal axis in the male. Fed Proc. 1980;39:2551–4.

113. Drolet G, Dumont EC, Gosselin I, et al. Role of endogenous opioid system in the regulation of the stress response. Prog Neuropsychopharmacol Biol Psychiatry. 2001;25:729–41.

114. Genazzani AR, Genazzani AD, Volpogni C, et al. Opioid control of gonadotropin secretion in humans. Hum Reprod. 1993;8:151–3.

115. Grossman A, Moult PJ, Gaillard RC, et al. The opioid control of LH and FSH release: effects of a met-enkephalin analogue and naloxone. Clin Endocrinol. 1981;14:41–7.

116. Jordan D, Tafini JAM, Ries C, et al. Evidence for multiple opioid receptors in the human posterior pituitary. J Neuroendocrinol. 1996;8:883–7.

117. Veldhuis JD, Rogol AD, Samojlik E, et al. Role of endogenous opiates in the expression of negative feedback actions of androgen and estrogen on pulsatile properties of luteinizing hormone secretion in man. J Clin Invest. 1984;74:47–55.

118. Cicero TJ, Bell RD, Wiest WG, et al. Function of the male sex organs in heroin and methadone users. N Engl J Med. 1975;292:882–7.

119. Abs R, Verhelst J, Maeyaert J, et al. Endocrine consequences of long-term intrathecal administration of opioids. J Clin Endocrinol Metab. 2000;85:2215–22.

120. Finch PM, Roberts LJ, Price L, et al. Hypogonadism in patients treated with intrathecal morphine. Clin J Pain. 2000;16:251–4.

121. Paice JA, Penn RD. Amenorrhea associated with intraspinal morphine. J Pain Symptom Manage. 1995;10:582–3.

122. Winkelmuller M, Winkelmuller W. Long-term effects of continuous intrathecal opioid treatment in chronic pain of nonmalignant etiology. J Neurosurg. 1996;85:458–67.

123. Daniell HW. DHEAS deficiency during consumption of sustained-action prescribed opioids: evidence for opioid-induced inhibition of adrenal androgen production. J Pain. 2006;7:901–7.

124. Daniell HW. Hypogonadism in men consuming sustained-action oral opioids. J Pain. 2002;3:377–84.

125. Daniell HW, Lentz R, Mazer NA. Open-label pilot study of testosterone patch therapy in men with opioid induced androgen deficiency (OPIAD). J Pain. 2006;7:200–10.

126. Forman LJ, Tingle V, Estilow S, et al. The response to analgesia testing is affected by gonadal steroids in the rat. Life Sci. 1989;45:447–54.

127. Stoffel EC, Ulibarri CM, Folk JE, et al. Gonadal hormone modulation of mu, kappa, and delta opioid antinociception in male and female rats. J Pain. 2005;6(4):261–74.

128. Gallagher R. Methadone: an effective, safe drug of first choice for pain management in frail older adults. Pain Med. 2009;10(2): 319–26.

129. Weiner DK, Rudy TE, Morone N, Glick R, Kwoh CK. Efficacy of periosteal stimulation therapy for the treatment of osteoarthritis-associated chronic knee pain: an initial controlled clinical trial. J Am Geriatr Soc. 2007;55:1541–7.

130. Gay MC, Philippot P, Luminet O. Differential effectiveness of psychological interventions for reducing osteoarthritis pain: a comparison of Erickson hypnosis and Jacobson relaxation. Eur J Pain. 2002;6:1–16.

131. Song R, Lee E, Lam P, Bae S. Effects of tai chi exercise on pain, balance, muscle strength, and perceived difficulties in physical functioning in older women with osteoarthritis: a randomized clinical trial. J Rheumatol. 2003;30:2039–44.

132. Morone NE, Greco CM. Mind-body interventions for chronic pain in older adults: a structured review. Pain Med. 2007;8(4):359–75.

133. Holick MF. Vitamin D deficiency. N Engl J Med. 2007;357: 266–81.

134. van der Wielen RP, Lowik MR, van den Berg H, et al. Serum vitamin D concentrations among elderly people in Europe. Lancet. 1995;346:207–10.

135. Khazai N, Judd SE, Tangpricha V. Calcium and vitamin D skeletal and extraskeletal health. Curr Rheumatol Rep. 2008;10:110–7.

136. Heaney RP, Dowell MS, Hale CA, et al. Calcium absorption varies within the reference range for serum 25-hydroxyvitamin D. J Am Coll Nutr. 2003;22:142–6.

137. Chapuy MC, Arlot ME, Duboeuf F, et al. Vitamin D3 and calcium to prevent hip fractures in elderly women. N Engl J Med. 1992;327:1637–42.

138. Chapuy MC, Pamphile R, Paris E, et al. Combined calcium and vitamin D3 supplementation in elderly women: confirmation of reversal of secondary hypoparathyroidism and hip fracture risk: the Decalyos II study. Osteoporos Int. 2002;13:257–64.

139. Trivedi DP, Doll R, Khaw KT. Effect of four monthly oral vitamin D3 (cholecalciferol) supplementation on fractures and mortality in men and women living in the community: randomised double blind controlled trial. Br Med J. 2003;326:469.

140. Dawson-Hughes B, Harris SS, Krall EA, et al. Effect of calcium and vitamin D supplementation on bone density in men and women 65 years of age or older. N Engl J Med. 1997;337:670–6.

141. Bischoff-Ferrari HA, Dawson-Hughes B, Willett WC, et al. Effect of vitamin D on falls: a meta-analysis. JAMA. 2004;291: 1999–2006.

142. Bischoff-Ferrari HA, Dietrich T, Orav EJ, et al. Higher 25-hydroxyvitamin D concentrations are associated with better lower-extremity function in both active and inactive persons aged > or =60y. Am J Clin Nutr. 2004;80:752–8.

143. Boonen S, Lips P, Bouillon R, et al. Need for additional calcium to reduce the risk of hip fracture with vitamin D supplementation: evidence from a comparative meta-analysis of randomized controlled trials. J Clin Endocrinol Metab. 2007;92:1415–23.

144. Ahmed W, Khan N, Glueck CJ, et al. Low serum 25 (OH) vitamin D levels (<32ng/ml) are associated with reversible myositis-myalgia in statin-treated patients. Transl Res. 2009;153:11–6.

145. Badsha H, Daher M, Ooi Kong K. Myalgias or non-specific muscle pain in Arab or Indo-Pakistani patients may indicate vitamin D deficiency. Clin Rheumatol. 2009;28:971–3.

146. Schwalfenberg G. Improvement of chronic back pain or failed back surgery with vitamin D repletion: a case series. J Am Board Fam Med. 2009;22:69–74.

147. Tandeter H, Grynbaum M, Zuili I, et al. Serum 25-OH vitamin D levels in patients with fibromyalgia. Isr Med Assoc J. 2009;11: 339–42.

148. Collins SL, Moore RA, McQuay HJ, et al. Antidepressants and anticonvulsants for diabetic neuropathy and postherpetic neuralgia: a quantitative systematic review. J Pain Symptom Manage. 2000;47:449–58.

149. Roose SP, Laghrissi-Thode F, Kennedy JS, et al. Comparison of paroxetine and nortriptyline in depressed patients with ischemic heart disease. J Am Med Assoc. 1998;279:287–91.

150. Dworkin RH, Backonja M, Rowbotham MC, et al. Advances in neuropathic pain: diagnosis, mechanisms, and treatment recommendations. Arch Neurol. 2003;60:1524–34.

151. Goldstein DJ, Lu Y, Detke MJ, Lee TC, Iyengar S. Duloxetine vs. placebo in patients with painful diabetic neuropathy. Pain. 2005;116(1–2):109–18.

152. Sindrup SH, Bach FW, Madsen C, Gram LF, Jensen TS. Venlafaxine versus imipramine in painful polyneuropathy: a randomized, controlled trial. Neurology. 2003;60:1284–9.

153. Johnson EM, et al. Cardiovascular changes associated with venlafaxine in the treatment of late-life depression. Am J Geriatr Psychiatry. 2006;14(9):796–802.

154. Gilron I, Bailey JM, Tu D, Holden RR, Weaver DF, Houlden RL. Morphine, gabapentin, or their combination for neuropathic pain. N Engl J Med. 2005;352:1324–34.

155. Guay DR. Oxcarbazepine, topiramate, zonisamide, and levetiracetam: potential use in neuropathic pain. Am J Geriatr Pharmacother. 2003;1:18–37.

156. Eisenberg E, Lurie Y, Braker C, et al. Lamotrigine reduces painful diabetic neuropathy: a randomized, controlled study. Neurology. 2003;60:1508–14.

157. Eisenberg E, McNicol ED, Carr DB. Efficacy and safety of opioid agonists in the treatment of neuropathic pain of nonmalignant origin. J Am Med Assoc. 2005;293:3043–52.

158. Sindrup SH, Andersen G, Madsen C, et al. Tramadol relieves pain and allodynia in polyneuropathy: a randomised, double-blind, controlled trial. Pain. 1999;83:85–90.

159. Boureau F, Legallicier P, Kabir-Ahmadi M. Tramadol in postherpetic neuralgia: a randomized, double-blind, placebo-controlled trial. Pain. 2003;104:323–31.

160. Hartrick C, et al. Efficacy and tolerability of tapentadol immediate release and oxycodone HCl immediate release in patients awaiting primary joint replacement surgery for end-stage joint disease: a 10-day, phase III, randomized double-blind, active- and placebo-controlled study. Clin Ther. 2009;31(2):260–71.

161. Rowan AJ, et al. New onset geriatric epilepsy: a randomized study of gabapentin, lamotrigine, and carbamazepine. Neurology. 2005; 64(11):1868–73.

162. He L, Wu B, Zhou M. Non-antiepileptic drugs for trigeminal neuralgia. Cochrane Database Syst Rev. 2006;3:(CD004029).

163. The American Geriatrics Society 2012 Beers Criteria Update Expert Panel. American Geriatrics Society updated Beers criteria for potentially inappropriate medication use in older adults. J Am Geriatr Soc 2012;60:616–631.

164. North RB, Wetzel FT. Spinal cord stimulation for chronic pain of spinal origin - a valuable long-term solution. Spine. 2002;27: 2584–91.

165. Stajanovic MP. Stimulation methods for neuropathic pain. Curr Pain Headache Rep. 2001;5:130–7.

166. Saitoh Y, Yoshimine T. Stimulation of primary motor cortex for intractable deafferentation pain. Acta Neurochir Suppl. 2007;97:51–6.

167. Wolfe F, Ross K, Anderson J, Russell IJ, Hebert L. The prevalence and characteristics of fibromyalgia in the general population. Arthritis Rheum. 1995;38:19–28.

168. Wolfe F, Smythe HA, Yunus MB, Bennett RM, Bombardier C, Goldenberg DL, et al. The American College of Rheumatology 1990 criteria for the classification of fibromyalgia-report of the multicenter criteria committee. Arthritis Rheum. 1990;33:160–72.

169. Goldenberg DL, Burckhardt C, Crofford L. Management of fibromyalgia syndrome. J Am Med Assoc. 2004;292(19):2388–95.

170. Carette S, McCain GA, Bell DA, Fam AG. Evaluation of amitriptyline in primary fibrositis. A double-blind, placebo-controlled study. Arthritis Rheum. 1986;29(5):655–9.

171. Goldenberg D, Mayskiy M, Mossey C, et al. A randomized, double-blind crossover trial of fluoxetine and amitriptyline in the treatment of fibromyalgia. Arthritis Rheum. 1996;39(11):1852–9.

172. Norregaard J, Volkmann H, Danneskiold-Samsoe B. A randomized controlled trial of citalopram in the treatment of fibromyalgia. Pain. 1995;61(3):445–9.

173. Arnold LM, Lu Y, Crofford LJ, Wohlreich M, Detke MJ, Iyengar S, et al. A double-blind, multicenter trial comparing duloxetine with placebo in the treatment of fibromyalgia patients with or without major depressive disorder. Arthritis Rheum. 2004; 50(9):2974–84.

174. Gendreau R, Mease P, Rao S, Kranzler J, Clauw D. Milnacipran: a potential new treatment of fibromyalgia. Arthritis Rheum. 2003;48:S616.

175. Arnold L, Goldenberg D, Stanford S, Lalonde J, Sandhu H, Keck P, et al. Gabapentin in the treatment of fibromyalgia: a randomized, double-blind, placebo-controlled, multicenter trial. Arthritis Rheum. 2007;56(4):1336–44.

176. Bennett RM, Kamin M, Karim R, Rosenthal N. Tramadol and acetaminophen combination tablets in the treatment of fibromyalgia pain: a double-blind, randomized, placebo-controlled study. Am J Med. 2003;114(7):537–45.

177. Katz W. Pharmacology and clinical experience with tramadol in osteoarthritis. Drugs. 1996;52(3):39–47.

178. Weiner DK, Cayea D. Low back pain and its contributors in older adults: a practical approach to evaluation and treatment. In: Pain in older persons, progress in pain research and management, vol. 35. Seattle: IASP Press; 2005. p. 332.

Pain Medicine and Primary Care: The Evolution of a Population-Based Approach to Chronic Pain as a Public Health Problem

20

Rollin M. Gallagher

Key Points

- The concept of pain as a major public health problem has been gaining traction, fueled by societal awareness of three intersecting health crises: *first*, pain's contribution to rising health-care costs affecting the competiveness of American business; *second*, hundreds of thousands of American troops returning home with chronic pain and comorbidities such as PTSD (post-traumatic stress disorder); TBI (traumatic brain injury); CARF [no expansion needed]; JCAHO (Joint Commission for the Accreditation of Health Care Organizations); ACGME (Accreditation Council for Graduate Medical Education); VHA (Veterans Health Administration); TENS (transcutaneous electrical nerve stimulation) substance abuse, and suicide risk; and *third*, a growing epidemic of prescription analgesic drug abuse.
- "The pain medicine and primary care community rehabilitation model" (PMPCCRM) is proposed as a performance-based system of integrated, biopsychosocial, interdisciplinary, patient-centered team care in primary care offices closely supported by interdisciplinary pain medicine specialty clinics.
- The PMPCCRM is adopted as the stepped care model in two major capitated health-care systems that rely on cost-effective outcomes, the Department of Veteran Affairs and Department of Defense; however, the goals of PMPCCRM will only be achieved with adequate training to an appropriate level of competency for all clinicians in the system, including both primary care providers and pain medicine specialists.

Introduction

This chapter outlines our progress in establishing chronic pain as a public health problem and in developing a population-based approach to pain management that relies heavily on an informed and skilled primary care sector in the medical home model. Other AAPM book chapters deal with the causes and complexities of different pain conditions and their treatments. This chapter will focus on gains that have been made in structuring models of care that improve primary care treatment and elevate the critically important role that primary care providers play in managing chronic pain.

In 1999, I wrote the following "Conclusion" in a paper for the *Medical Clinics of North America*: "Primary care and pain medicine: A community solution to the public health problem of chronic pain" [1]:

This paper presents commonly accepted evidence that defines chronic pain as a public health problem crying out for a reorganization of the manner in which our health care system manages pain. I have endeavored to present some of the conceptual, administrative and communication factors that may contribute to sustaining the present system of ineffective care. I have described several different but common models of care and why they have been ineffective. Finally, I have introduced the rationale for a new model of care that would remediate some of these problems. This model emphasizes the critical role of two new players in the specialized medical care of pain who relate closely to the functional restoration roles of physical therapists and behavioral specialists. The two new players are the informed *primary care physician* in a community practice, and the *pain medicine specialist* (Fig. 20.1).

Informed *community primary care physicians* contribute their expertise in longitudinal, comprehensive management combined with their more intimate knowledge of health, family

R.M. Gallagher, M.D., M.P.H (✉)
Department of Psychiatry, Anesthesiology and Critical Care,
University of Pennsylvania Perelman School of Medicine,
Philadelphia, PA, USA

Pain Policy Research and Primary Care,
Penn Pain Medicine Center, Philadelphia, PA, USA

Pain Management, Philadelphia Veterans Health System,
Philadelphia, PA, USA
e-mail: rgallagh@mail.med.upenn.edu

Fig. 20.1 The pain medicine and
primary care community
rehabilitation model (PMPCCR)

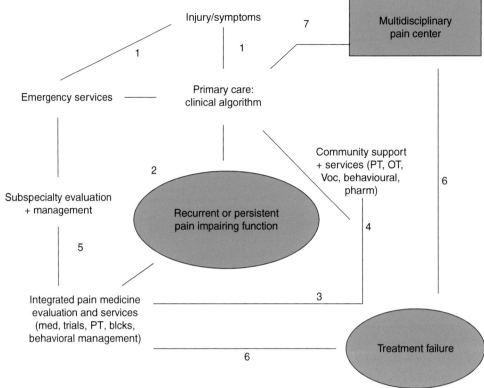

and other psychosocial factors and community resources that might importantly influence the outcome of pain treatment. *Pain medicine specialists* may have initial training and practice experience in a traditional specialty (e.g., anesthesiologist, psychiatrist, neurologist, neurosurgeon, physiatrist) but are now defined by having been board certified by credentialing and examination in the new specialty of pain medicine. The pain medicine specialist provides consultative support to the network of primary care physicians, physical therapists, and behavioral clinicians in the community centers, introduces new cost-effective technology rapidly into the system, and organizes and monitors the cost-effective and timely functioning of a complimentary network of needed sub-specialty services in the tertiary setting.

This model can be built gradually by selective practice collaborations with like-minded practitioners over time and will be supported by the insurance industry who already recognize the need for such a system, by health care system administrators who recognize the competitive advantages of such a system, and by regulators and certifying bodies, such as CARF, that recognize the value of such a system of care. Critical to success will be access to consistent information about the performance of the system, specifically the outcomes of patients as measured most importantly by function and costs, and the professionals' adherence to the processes enhancing quality care that is cost-effective. To demonstrate cost-effectiveness, the system will need to utilize uniform measures of outcomes used nationally to establish performance against accepted benchmarks of quality and cost-effectiveness. Support for such a model can be solicited from health industry constituents such as insurers, managed care companies, and state and federal agencies, and from health care systems such as hospital networks, particularly those with capitated risk. The challenge for these entities will be to identify and support key leaders and practitioners possibly outside traditional specialty structures, who have the necessary commitment to developing such a model.

My editorial in *Clinical Journal of Pain*, then the official journal of the American Academy of Pain Medicine, followed shortly: "The pain medicine and primary care community rehabilitation model: Monitored care for pain disorders in multiple settings" [2]. Both of these papers called for a population-based approach to pain management.

This chapter will review our progress in adopting this population-based approach. I will particularly emphasize some of the structural changes in medicine that are encouraging, even in some cases mandating, the pain medicine and primary care community rehabilitation model and the centrality of a well-trained and rewarded primary care sector for the chronic disease management of pain. I will also marshal some of the emerging evidence that is accumulating to support these changes.

The Decade of Pain Control and Research

Where have we come since 1999? Over the ensuing decade, progress was slow. Our health-care system continued to expand in costs and size without any indication that quality was improving and with considerable data demonstrating deterioration in many sectors and a widening of disparities in health care. Much was written about chronic pain's role in the health economy and its contribution to its costs and disparities. Although certain sectors of American health care (e.g., the Veterans Health System followed by JCAHO) promoted evaluating pain systematically, and the United States Congress declared the "Decade of Pain Control and Research," 2001–2010 [3, 4], the medical establishment made little progress in addressing the deficits in research funding and training and the organizational factors in the health system that perpetuated the public health problem of pain [5, 6].

During the early part of the decade, concerted efforts by the American Pain Foundation joined by the Pain Care Coalition (American Academy of Pain Medicine, American Pain Society, American Headache Association) led to a bill (the so-called Rogers Bill named after its sponsor in Congress, Rep. Bill Rogers from Michigan) to establish a Pain Institute at NIH and more funding for research. Congressional support for this bill was tepid however. The AAPM and American Board of Pain Medicine made applications to the ACGME to establish expanded training for pain medicine specialists but was turned down on two occasions by a negative vote by ABMS members of the review committee – although other non-ABMS members voted for expanding training. Finally, beginning in 2008, the concept of pain as a major public health problem began gaining traction in a wider sector of American society, fueled by three intersecting societal crises. *First*, pain was demonstrated to contribute to the problem of rising health-care costs and its effects on the competiveness of American business and America's economy [7]. *Second*, hundreds of thousands of American troops were returning home from Iraq and Afghanistan for care in the military and veteran health systems with chronic pain, many with comorbidities such as PTSD and post-concussive syndrome, and as substance abuse and suicide rates rose in this population, pain was discovered to be a driving factor [8–10]. *Third,* emerging data demonstrating a growing epidemic of prescription analgesic drug abuse [11, 12] was brought to American consciousness by the national press. Meanwhile, the American Pain Foundation led the development of the Pain Forum, a consortium of professional, patient-centered, and industry organizations, and the Pain Care Coalition expanded to include a powerful partner, the American Society of Anesthesiology. Together, these groups successfully helped marshal three bills through congress: the Veterans Pain Care Act (2008) [13], the Military Pain Care Act (2009) [14], and the inclusion of the provisions of the original NIH Rogers Bill in the national health-care bill for health-care reform (2011) [15]. With the passage of these bills, which require a yearly progress report to congress, rapid transformative changes are occurring in pain management and research in the veterans and military health systems and in NIH. The former two systems, which are capitated and deliver care to a population of patients under a fixed budget, are most relevant to a discussion of the immediate changes that are needed in the health-care system. The NIH, which has long overlooked funding for the naturalistic, health systems, and combination trials demanded by the public health problem of pain [16], much less the development of new treatments, is most relevant in the long run for promoting research that improves the evidence basis for pain management.

Evolving Models of Primary Care for Pain

The *VA Health Administration* (VHS) has instituted a progression of activities, consistent with the PMPCCR model, leading to the publication and dissemination of a Directive, written by this author and Robert Kerns, National Program Director for Pain Management. The Directive outlines a new standard of care for pain for the entire VA [17], Stepped Pain Care [18] Rosenberger et al. Federal Practitioner (2011), which directs that a biopsychosocial model of patient-centered chronic pain care be provided seamlessly and collaboratively in primary care, secondary care, and tertiary care with movement between sectors depending on complexity, treatment refractoriness, comorbidities, and risk. The model is consistent with the medical home model in the national health act in that it emphasizes routine primary care screening for pain and comprehensive assessment, case management by interdisciplinary teams, shared decision-making with patients and their families, and patient self-management. System support for primary care is provided by pharmacy through medication and opioid management, by behavioral health with screening and management of mental health comorbidities, and by evidence-based guidelines and clinical algorithms, as in Fig. 20.2. The evidence basis for this model is emerging from clinical trials and cohort studies in primary care systems, most notably in the VHA, in which specific primary care enhancements improve outcomes in primary care practices managing pain [19–25].

To promote this transformation in all 153 VHA medical facilities and their related outpatient clinics, the VHA's national pain management office is supported by the National Pain Management Strategy Coordinating Committee (NPMSCC), consisting of representatives from several other program offices (e.g., anesthesia, education, mental health, neurology, nursing, primary care, PM&R, research, and quality improvement), and a National Pain Leadership Group consisting of VISN (regional) and facility "points-of-contact," which discuss implementation progress in monthly meetings. National and regional workshops for "pain champions" in each primary care setting are being held in conjunction with transformation of VA care to primary care Pain Aligned Care Teams (PACT) in the medical home model. National workgroups have identified core "competencies" for VHA primary care providers in pain management, as listed in Table 20.1. To provide for the needs of the huge population requiring pain management, these competencies will necessarily be extended considerably to encompass many office-based procedures and interventions as improved training proceeds in primary care, both in postgraduate medical education and continuing education.

Fig. 20.2 Stepped model of care, Veterans Health System

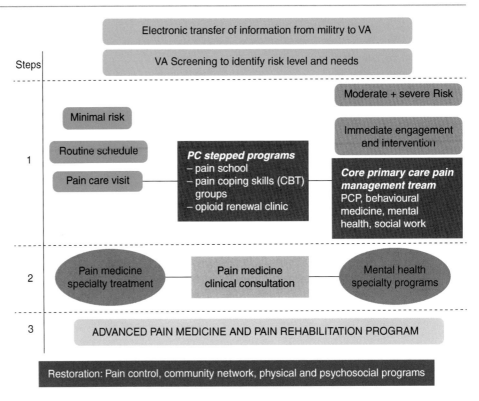

One innovative contribution of the academic and private sector to post-training continuing education is academic detailing, as established by the University of New Mexico's ECHO model of using videoconferencing technology to train providers while they care for patients with complex chronic pain that is beyond the scope of their initial training. In the model of a resident case conference, interdisciplinary teams of clinicians (pain medicine specialists, psychologists, psychiatrists, social workers, and physical therapists) use videoconferencing links to supervise simultaneously several providers whose patients have difficulty accessing specialty pain care due to one or more factors such as distance, transportation, and illness severity. Evaluation of the impact of this model on the outcomes of patients with hepatitis C has shown outcomes equivalent to direct specialty care [26]. Although patient outcomes for pain specialty supervision are not yet published, supervised providers exhibit high satisfaction, confidence in pain care, and the growing capacity to manage chronic pain complexity independently of the specialty team. Providers must attend weekly 2-h conferences for a year and present to and follow with the pain team at least ten cases over that year before sufficient knowledge and skill transfer is achieved so they can approximate pain medicine practice at a specialist level. The ECHO concept has been adopted for trial in six different regions of the VHA in what is now called the Specialty Care Access Network or SCAN-ECHO, and each site is now actively providing such telehealth supervision with plans to link to direct telehealth patient care. The end result will be primary care providers with direct pain

management training in a preceptorship model similar to residency training. To support such a successful postgraduate medical education intervention, credentialing organizations are now challenged to find an acceptable way to test and credentialing such providers in primary care pain medicine.

The Department of Defense (DoD), led by the Army Surgeon General and guided by the Defense and Veterans Pain Management Initiative (DVPMI), in 2009 chartered the Army Pain Task Force, including pain experts from the VA, Navy, and Air Force. The task force intensively studied the problem of pain management in the military over a 6-month period, making dozens of site visits to "best practices" as well as holding three retreats, and published a 163-page report [27] which thoroughly outlined the deficiencies in care and made over 100 recommendations for transforming pain care in the military. Key among the recommendations was adoption of the stepped care model for providing uniform standards for pain care in the military and in the VA. Subsequently, the VA-DoD Health Executive Council (HEC), codirected by the Under Secretaries for Health of both the VA and the DoD, chartered a Pain Management Working Group (PMWG). The PMWG, cochaired by this author, is charged with helping establish a single system of continuous, collaborative, and effective pain care, research, and education for the VA and DoD. The Defense and Veterans Center for Integrated Pain Management (DVCIPM) is a newly functional office chartered under the lead of the army to help operationalize the work of the HEC-PMWG. Projects underway include PASTOR, a standardized pain assessment to be used in all chronic pain encounters, no matter the setting but particularly in primary care, to assist providers in real-time clinical decision-making. The assessments will generate both cross-sectional reports for primary care providers at time of initial assessment as well as longitudinal reports on clinical outcomes. All data will be entered in a data registry and used to establish the benchmarks needed for health-care administrators to address planning and policy, consistent with the PMPCCR model as outlined in the beginning of this chapter. The HEC-PMWG hopes to coordinate DoD and VHA activities in at least two rapidly developing programs, the assessment and data registry project, PASTOR, and the SCAN-ECHO postgraduate training project.

Changes in the "Medical Establishment"

Finally, led by the American Medical Association (AMA), other organizations outside the VA and military have called for changes based on wide recognition of pain medicine training deficiencies for all physicians, particularly primary on who fall the largest burden of care [28–30]. Through the concerted efforts of the AMA's Pain and Palliative Medicine Specialty Section Council (PPMSSC), under the direction of its chairman, Philipp M. Lippe, MD, FACS, the AMA hosted the first national summit on Pain Medicine in 2009. The entire process and its outcomes are described in a 2010 paper in *Pain Medicine* [31]. The process began with the adoption of Resolution 321 (A-08) at an AMA Annual House of Delegates meeting in June 2008. Resolution 321 (A-08) states, in part, that "….the AMA encourages relevant specialties to collaborate in studying: (1) the scope and practice and body of knowledge encompassed by the field of Pain Medicine; (2) the adequacy of undergraduate, graduate, and post graduate education in the principles and practices of the field of Pain Medicine, considering the current and anticipated medical need for the delivery of quality pain care; and (3) appropriate training and credentialing criteria for this multi-disciplinary field of medical practice." Over several months, representatives from all clinical specialties in the AMA convened in a modified Delphi process with representatives of the VA, the military, and major pain organizations. Their task was to identify the most pressing issues affecting the care of pain. The top five issues that emerged from this process are outlined in Tables 20.1 and 20.2.

A retreat was held the day prior to the annual midyear meeting of the AMA in Houston, Texas, in November 2009. Participants thoroughly considered the problem in an open, transparent forum. For the most part, they did not defending turf or position but honestly attempted to understand the problem and agree on the best approach for the benefit of medicine and the population. For the first time, pain medicine specialists, surgeons, internists, family physicians, psy-

Table 20.1 Topics of the First National Pain Medicine Summit, American Medical Association (AMA), November 2009

1. What should all physicians know about pain medicine (i.e., where is the line drawn between primary care pain medicine competency and specialty pain medicine competency)?
2. How should pain medicine be taught?
3. What are the parameters that define the field of pain medicine?
4. What mechanisms do we need to establish the competency of a physician who wishes to practice pain medicine?
5. What are the barriers that prevent patients from receiving adequate pain care, other than the absence of competent pain medicine physicians?

Table 20.2 Pain management core competencies, primary care

1. Conduct comprehensive pain assessment
2. Negotiate behaviorally specific and feasible goals
3. Know/use common metrics for measuring function
4. Optimize patient communication
   (a) How to provide reassurance
   (b) How to foster pain self-management
5. Conduct routine physical/neurological examinations
6. Judiciously use diagnostic tests/procedures and secondary consultation
7. Assess psychiatric/behavioral comorbidities
8. Know accepted clinical practice guidelines
9. Use rational, algorithmic-based polypharmacy
10. Manage opioids safely and effectively
Additional competencies
11. Provide office-based procedures (potentially guided by ultrasound)
    Trigger point injections
    Joint injections
    Peripheral nerve blocks
12. Provide brief or sustaining psychotherapeutic enhancements
    Cognitive reframing
    Motivational interviewing
    Problem-solving
    Supportive patient and family counseling
    Goal-oriented, patient-centered pain management planning
    Relaxation training and meditation
    Weight and food management
13. Supervise/prescribe physical therapies
    Exercise regimens (McKenzie; Krause)
    Ice and stretch
    Neuromodulation (TENS, inferential stimulator)

chiatrists, and others, most in leadership positions in medical schools, the AMA, community practice, and various large organizations, contributed their ideas openly and constructively. The meeting imparted a general sense of a medical community of interest and intent. Regarding education of primary care providers, one of the workgroups, charged with answering the Delphi process-generated question, "What should all physicians know about Pain Medicine (i.e., where is the line drawn between primary care Pain Medicine competency and specialty Pain Medicine competency)?" recommended the following five "next steps" [32]: (1) The AAPM should collaborate with the Association of American Medical Colleges about standards for undergraduate education. (2) Each medical specialty should establish specific pain medicine competencies through ACGME. (3) The American Board of Medical Specialties should recognize pain medicine as a primary specialty to ensure adequacy and consistency of pain medicine specialty training/certification nationally and to assure uniform and reliable education for students in medical schools. (4) The Council on Medical Education of the AMA should resolve to develop a specific educational package on competencies for pain medicine. (5) Gaps in pain care in the ACGME programs should be filled by surveying the Association Program Specialty Directors of ACGME to determine what is currently being taught and what needs to be taught about pain medicine in their programs. The survey could be developed from core competency standards for primary care, perhaps adopting the VA's competencies, as outlined in Table 20.1. Efforts for a follow-up summit to assess progress are underway.

Passage of the National Health Reform Act of 2010 that included the language of the original Rogers Bill required that the NIH attends to pain research and education and charter an Institute of Medicine (IOM) Committee to study and make recommendations for a widespread societal approach to addressing the problem of chronic pain. Since then, NIH has established several working groups to address deficiencies in education and research in pain management [33]. The IOM recently convened the recommended committee and completed a report, "Relieving Pain in America: A Blueprint for Transforming Prevention, Care, Education, and Research," that comprehensively reviewed the public health burden of pain, collated and summarized the literature outlining clinical deficits and needs, and commented on the relevant needed research [34]. The IOM report cogently compiled and summarized an incredible breadth and depth of information supporting the need for a population approach such as presented by the PMPCCR model and the education and training required to establish such a model. However, strikingly absent from the report were specific suggestions for reform of education and training of physicians, which presents the most salient challenge if society is to effectively address the public health problem of pain as the IOM report outlined in such detail. The AMA report went much further. A demand for AAMC-mandated reform of medical student education, ACGME-mandated reform of primary care residency and pain fellowship training as outlined in the AMA Summit Report, would drive the system toward a PMPCCR model and real system change. Causes of this reluctance may reflect the membership of the IOM Committee, which largely represented traditional specialty, research, and patient advocacy interests. Tellingly, there was no representation on the panel from internal medicine or family practice, the specialties that bear the largest burden of pain, whereas there were three psychologists, two ethicists, and one writer.

The Future

The management of pain can no longer be put on medicine's back burner. Society now demands change. Medicine's guild-like structures support the tribal identities that perpetuate fragmented pain care. Doctors would like to continue lucrative practices that focus on technically difficult procedures that are highly reimbursed. These identities and structures are threatened by a new model of integrated and patient-centric team care based in primary care offices and closely supported by the well-trained pain medicine specialist. Thoughtful, biopsychosocial chronic disease management is professionally rewarding if a provider is sufficiently trained and supported because it is effective. There is no greater pleasure than relieving suffering and restoring meaningful life. However, if one has to close practice because reimbursement favors only procedures completed, not outcomes, then change will not occur. Society must make the changes – medicine will not.

How different care will be allocated among primary care and specialty care remains to be determined. There will be two polarities in this determination; either may evolve, or some combination depending on circumstances. Both scenarios emphasize the importance of the primary care provider. In the first scenario, pain medicine specialists will acquire much more specialty training in biopsychosocial pain medicine, encompassing all the training needed for managing complex chronic pain. Primary care providers will continue to enlarge the scope of their practices in pain management but leave complexity and risk management cases to the specialists. In the second scenario, primary care physicians will become subspecialists in pain medicine, with an extra year or more of training much like they do in palliative care, cardiology, and pulmonology, and will care for the vast majority of patients with chronic pain at both the primary and secondary levels of care. They will adopt many of the roles and techniques now practiced in pain medicine specialty care. Pain medicine specialists will manage only the technically complex case requiring special, expensive equipment and training and practiced in tertiary care centers. The collaborative models of care that evolve in these two scenarios will be determined by a complex interaction of health economics, medical politics, and medical science. Hopefully, the patient's and society's mutual best interests will be served by measurement based choices in health care that will drive the ultimate model that emerges.

Fig. 20.3 Disease management in a population of patients in pain [6]

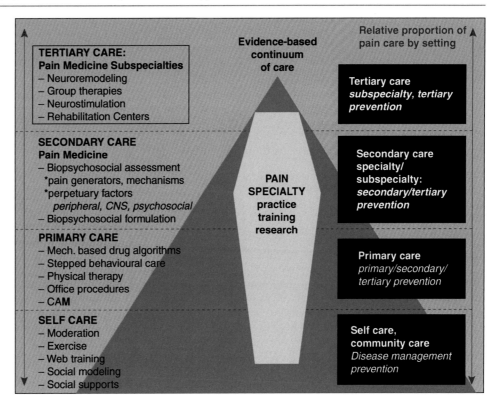

Several specific self-care and primary care enhancement models have already been examined. Davies, Quintner, and colleagues describe how a state in Australia implemented a publicly funded self-management program that greatly reduced the need for primary care and pain specialty care visits and reduced wait times for specialty pain care [35]. Wiedemer et al. describe how a structured opioid management program run by pharmacists in a veterans hospital's primary care clinic reduced aberrant behavior and identified patients with substance use disorders needing referral to addiction treatment [23]. Dobscha and colleagues, in a controlled clinical trial, showed that enhancing primary care of pain with telephone-assisted consultation and support for emotional responses to pain, such as depression, improved patient outcomes and costs over "treatment as usual" condition [36]. Kroenke, Bair, and colleagues implemented a stepped care approach in primary care that demonstrated clinical efficacy for chronic pain with comorbid depression [37].

Who knows whether the primary care subspecialty model, pain medicine specialty model, or some hybrid, depending on local/regional conditions, will dominate the future of pain management. Society and its inevitable reinforcement of efficiency will assure that the PMPCCR model will prevail ultimately. In any case, the optimal result will be the engagement of patient and provider within a seamless continuum of pain management within a health system and society that maximizes pain control, function, and overall quality of life. The widespread use of e-health supported by interactive technologies will engage patient in active,

positive, neuromodulatory behavioral and emotional self-management strategies. These strategies will be culturally socialized within a supportive family, workplace, and community milieu that provides for self-actualization and productivity that enhances self-esteem, rather than destroying it. These strategies will be a foundation of a person-in-pain's biopsychosocial medical pain management, rather than an adjunct to a series of procedures, medications, and other biomedical interventions or outside the clinical milieu altogether. Patients will learn new coping skills that are transferable to other challenges and settings in their life course.

When entering the health system, access to an evidence-based stepped model of care will marshal resources appropriate to the level of need to achieve shared patient-centered goals. A population-based allocation of resources will achieve efficiencies and effectiveness unheard of in today's confusing, inefficient medical environment. Figure 20.3 depicts such a population-based system of care, with the majority of care being self-care using evidence-based methods of primary prevention such as weight control and exercise – much like cardiovascular care relies on self-management of diet and exercise to reduce risk of CV disease. Once pain symptoms ensue, then a seamless stepped model, relying on a healthy foundation of self-management, will begin in primary care. Biopsychosocial outcomes will be continuously monitored so that there are no barriers to pain specialty treatment and "chronification" does not progress to "maldynia" and its attendant costs to patient, family, and society [38].

References

1. Gallagher RM. Pain medicine and primary care: a community solution to pain as a public health problem. Med Clin North Am. 1999;83(5):555–85.
2. Gallagher RM. The pain medicine and primary care community rehabilitation model: monitored care for pain disorders in multiple settings. Clin J Pain. 1999;15(1):1–3.
3. Lippe PM. The decade of pain control and research. Pain Med. 2000;1(4):286.
4. Loeser J. The decade of pain control and research. APS Bull. 2003;13(3). http://www.ampainsoc.org/library/bulletin/may03/article1.htm. Accessed 29 Aug 2011.
5. Gallagher RM. The AMA in health care reform: a "flexner report" to improve pain medicine training and practice. Pain Med. 2010;11(10):1437–9.
6. Dubois M, Gallagher RM, Lippe P. Pain medicine position paper. Pain Med. 2009;10(6):972–1000.
7. Stewart WF, Ricci JA, Chee E, Morganstein D, Lipton R. Lost productive time and cost due to common pain conditions in the US workforce. JAMA. 2003;290(18):2443–54.
8. Gironda RJ, Clark ME, Massengale JP, Walker RL. Pain among veterans of operations enduring freedom and Iraqi freedom. Pain Med. 2006;7(4):339–43.
9. Kerns RD, Dobscha SK. Pain among veterans returning from deployment in Iraq and Afghanistan: update on the Veterans Health Administration Pain Research Program. Pain Med. 2009;10(7):1161–4.
10. Lew HL, Otis JD, Tun C, Kerns RD, Clark ME, Cifu DX. Prevalence of chronic pain, posttraumatic stress disorder, and persistent post-concussive symptoms in OIF/OEF Veterans: polytrauma clinical triad. J Rehabil Res Dev. 2009;46(6):697–702.
11. Gilson AM, Kreis PG. The burden of the nonmedical use of prescription opioid analgesics. Pain Med. 2009;10(S2):S89–100.
12. Birnbaum HG, White AG, Schiller M, Waldman T, Cleveland JM, Roland CL. Societal costs of prescription opioid abuse, dependence, and misuse in the United States. Pain Med. 2011;12(4):657–67.
13. Section 501 of Veterans' Mental Health and Other Care Improvements Act of 2008, Public Law 110-387. 2008. http://www.gpo.gov/fdsys/pkg/PLAW-110publ387/pdf/PLAW-110publ387.pdf. Accessed 10 Oct 2008.
14. Section 711 of National Defense Authorization Act for FY 2010, Public Law 111-84. 2009. http://www.gpo.gov/fdsys/pkg/PLAW-111publ84/pdf/PLAW-111publ84.pdf.Accessed 28 Oct 2009.
15. Section 4305 of Patient Protection and Affordable Care Act, Public law 111-148. 2010. http://www.gpo.gov/fdsys/pkg/PLAW-111publ148/pdf/PLAW-111publ148.pdf. Accessed 23 Mar 2010.
16. Rathmell JP, Carr DB. The scientific method, evidence-based medicine, and rational use of interventional pain treatments. [editorial] (Comment on Merrill DG. Hoffman's glasses: evidence-based medicine and the search for quality in the literature of interventional pain medicine. Reg Anesth Pain Med. 2003;28:547–580) Reg Anesth Pain Med. 2003;28:498–501.
17. VHA DIRECTIVE 2009-053, Pain management. 2011. http://www1.va.gov/vhapublications/viewpublication.asp?Pub_ID=2238. Accessed 23 Aug 2011.
18. Rosenberger PH, Philip EJ, Lee A, Kerns RD. The VHA's national pain management strategy: implementing the stepped care model. Fed Pract. 2011;28(8):39–42.
19. Dobscha SK, Corson K, Perrin NA, Hanson GC, Leibowitz RQ, Doak MN, Dickinson KC, Sullivan MD, Gerrity MS. Collaborative care for chronic pain in primary care: a cluster-randomized trial. JAMA. 2009;301(12):1242–52.
20. Kroenke K, Bair MJ, Damush TM, Wu J, Hoke S, Sutherland J, Tu W. Optimized antidepressant therapy and pain self-management in primary care patients with depression and musculoskeletal pain: a randomized controlled trial. J Am Med Assoc. 2009;301(20):2099–110.
21. Lin EHB, Katon W, Von Korff M, et al. Effect of improving depression care on pain and functional outcomes among older adults with arthritis: a randomized controlled trial. JAMA. 2003;290(18):2428–9.
22. Ahles TA, Wasson JH, Seville JL, et al. A controlled trial of methods for managing pain in primary care patients with or without co-occurring psychosocial problems. Ann Fam Med. 2006;4(4):341–50.
23. Wiedemer N, Harden P, Arndt R, Gallagher RM. The opioid renewal clinic, a primary care, managed approach to opioid therapy in chronic pain patients at risk for substance. Pain Med. 2007;8(7):573–84.
24. Trafton J, Martine S, Michel M, Lewis E, Wang D, Combs A, Scales N, Tu S, Goldstein MK. Evaluation of the acceptability and usability of a decision support system to encourage safe and effective use of opioid therapy for chronic, noncancer pain by primary care providers. Pain Med. 2010;11(4):575–85.
25. Bair M. Overcoming fears, frustrations, and competing demands: an effective integration of pain medicine and primary care to treat complex pain patients. Pain Med. 2007;8(7):544–5.
26. Arora S, Thornton K, Murata G, Derning P, et al. Outcomes of treatment for hepatitis C virus infection by primary care providers. N Engl J Med. 2011;364:2199–207.
27. Office of the Army Surgeon General, Pain Management Task Force Final report: providing a standardized DoD and VHA vision and approach to pain management to optimize the care for warriors and their families. http://www.armymedicine.army.mil/prr/pain_management.html. Accessed 29 Aug 2011.
28. Gallagher R. Physician variability in pain management: are the JCAHO standards enough? Pain Med. 2003;4(1):1–3.
29. Corrigan C, Desnick L, Marshall S, Bentov N, Rosenblatt RA. What can we learn from first-year medical students' perceptions of pain in the primary care setting? Pain Med. 2011;12(8):1216–22.
30. Norris TE. Chronic pain, medical students, and primary care commentary on "what can we learn from first-year medical students' perception of pain in the primary care setting". Pain Med. 2011;12(8):1137–8.
31. Lippe PM, Brock C, David J, Crossno R, Gitlow S. The first national pain medicine summit – final summary report. Pain Med. 2010;11:1447–68.
32. Gallagher R. What should all physicians know about pain medicine? Workgroup report. The first national pain medicine summit – final summary report. Pain Med. 2010;11:1450–2.
33. Reid MC, Bennett DA, Chen WG, et al. Improving the pharmacologic management of pain in older adults: identifying the research gaps and methods to address them. Pain Med. 2011;12(9):1336–57. doi:10.1111/j.1526-4637.2011.01211.x. Epub 2011 Aug 11.
34. Institute of Medicine. Relieving pain in America: a blueprint for transforming prevention, care, education, and research. 2011. http://www.iom.edu/Reports/2011/Relieving-Pain-in-America-A-Blueprint-for-Transforming-Prevention-Care-Education-Research.aspx. Accessed 29 Aug 2011.
35. Davies S, Quinter J, Parsons R, Parkitny L, Knight P, Forrester E, Roberts M, Graham C, Visser E, Antill T, Packer T, Schug SA. Preclinic group education sessions reduce waiting times and costs at public pain medicine units. Pain Med. 2011;12(1):59–71.
36. Dobscha SK, Corson K, Flores JA, Tansill EC, Gerrity MS. Veterans affairs primary care clinicians' attitudes toward chronic pain and correlates of opioid prescribing rates. Pain Med. 2008;9(5):564–71.
37. Kroenke K, Bair MJ, Damush TM, Wu J, Hoke S, Sutherland J, Tu W. Optimized antidepressant therapy and pain self-management in primary care patients with depression and musculoskeletal pain: a randomized controlled trial. JAMA. 2009;301(20):2099–110.
38. Gallagher RM. Chronification to maldynia: biopsychosocial failure of pain homeostasis. Pain Med. 2011;12(7):993–5.

Pain Care Beyond the Medical Practice Office: Utilizing Patient Advocacy, Education, and Support Organizations

William Rowe

Key Points
- There are numerous, credible pain patient education, support, and advocacy organizations.
- The medical practitioner has little time or experience to provide some of the critical assistance elements for their patients.
- Pain patient education, support, and advocacy organizations can provide helpful support and education for pain patients that make a critical difference in their ability to successfully manage their pain.
- Medical practitioners should include referrals to these organizations as standard treatment recommendations.

Why Utilize Patient Education and Advocacy Organizations?

Living with chronic pain is a total-person experience. Chronic pain affects all aspects of an individual's life. The physical effects are clear—pain, sleep deprivation, and curtailed capacity to function. The emotional effects should also be clear—in most cases depression, sense of loss, fear and anxiety, frustration, and diminished hope and confidence. The social effects should also be clear—diminished social activities and contacts, strained marital, family and work relationships, and withdrawal. The effects on work and career should also be obvious—diminished capacity to perform, diminished ability to achieve career goals, possible loss, or end of work life.

These effects in turn contribute to spiraling the individual into a mixed state of pain, fear, withdrawal, anger, anxiety, frustration, hopelessness, and defeat. How does the medical

W. Rowe, M.A. (✉)
American Pain Foundation, 201 N. Charles Street, Suite 710, Baltimore 21201 MD, USA
e-mail: wrowe@painfoundation.org

practitioner deal with all of that in the 10, 15, or 20 min of the periodic office visit? Most people living with chronic pain need a great deal more than what can be provided in the typical office visit. The days and weeks are long when living with pain, and the need for information and support is continuous beyond the medical office visit. The physical-psychosocial impact of pain is well documented [1].

In addition referring to other practitioners who offer complementary therapies, one resource, often not utilized by medical practitioners, is encouraging patients to check out and connect to the multitude of helpful, credible patient education and support organizations. There are many organizations that provide comprehensive information and various support services. Some are defined by a particular pain disease, and some are general about pain in all of its forms. Most have comprehensive websites with information and resources that can assist the person with pain to manage their pain. They all also serve the very important function of connecting the person with pain to others who are living with pain. A common experience of people living with pain is isolation and a sense of being alone and the only person living this pain experience. These patient support sites offer a community of people and an inventory of information and resources to ameliorate the isolation.

There are many potential benefits for people with pain who consult and utilize patient education and support organizations. A short list would include:
- Access to comprehensive, helpful information about their pain condition and treatment options for their pain
- Access to credible, practical, and tested tools for improving your well-being and reducing pain
- Breaking the sense of isolation and connecting individuals to others who immediately understand their challenges
- Presenting links to a multitude of organizations and resources that can be specific to an individual's needs
- Presenting information about key pain advocacy issues and offering instruction and ways to become better personal advocates and advocates for improved pain policy

- Presenting credible and useful information to help people with pain to better communicate with their health-care providers, with family members, and with one's social and work networks
- Presenting information about the latest and future treatment options for pain
- Presenting a general message of hope and confidence that people are listening and working to improve pain care

These benefits are tangible, measurable benefits for people living with pain. Promoting patients to connect to credible patient advocacy, education, and support organizations offers the practitioner an active and helpful complement to the medical services that take place in the office and relieves the practitioner from the challenging and time-consuming burden of being the only source of expertise and consolation. Investigating these resources presents opportunities for patients to take charge of their pain, to become informed, connected, and empowered to take actions to improve their lives.

Patient Organizations and Resources

There are many patient organizations that provide credible information and helpful resources and services for people living with pain. Some focus on specific diseases, and some are about pain and its variety of causes and manifestations. The leading national organizations providing information and support for people with pain are the *American Pain Foundation (APF)* (www.painfoundation.org) and the *American Chronic Pain Association* (www.theacpa.org). Each offers a variety of resources that are web-based and some print and personal resources. In 2010, a third national pain organization, the *National Pain Foundation*, gifted its web and program resources to the American Pain Foundation enhancing the breadth of content of the APF.

A short list of organizations that focus on a particular pain condition includes the *Reflex Sympathetic Dystrophy Syndrome Association* (www.rsdsa.org) which focuses on what is now referred to as complex regional pain syndrome, *TNA The Facial Pain Association* (www.fpa-support.org) which focuses on facial pain conditions such as trigeminal neuralgia, *Lupus Foundation of America* (www.lupus.org), *The Neuropathy Association* (www.neuropathy.org), the *National Vulvodynia Association* (www.nva.org), *Ehlers-Danlos National Foundation* (www.ednf.org), the *Interstitial Cystitis Association* (www.ichelp.org), the *National Headache Foundation* (www.headaches.org), and the *National Fibromyalgia and Chronic Pain Association* (www.fmcpaware.org).

In order to illustrate how a national pain patient organization might be helpful to a person with pain and a helpful supplement to the practitioner's work, consider a scenario where Jane Doe has just visited her doctor with complaints of debilitating low back pain and a long-term, persistent, generalized pain in her shoulders, neck, and upper back. She explains that her shoulder and neck pains have been preventing her from engaging in many of her usual activities and cutting her off from friends. After a thorough history and exam, her doctor diagnosed severe muscle strain in her lower back and possibly a fibromyalgia condition. He recommends customary treatment choices for both conditions and that she consult the resources about back pain and fibromyalgia at the APF website, www.painfoundation.org. He explains in a few minutes his diagnoses offering basic information about muscular strain and fibromyalgia and encourages her to "read-up" on these conditions on the website.

That evening Jane opens up the website of the APF and sees the homepage:

Jane notices a couple of paths to follow: (a) Click on the "Learn About Pain" button; (b) Click on the "PainAid—Support" button. She starts her search with "Learn About Pain" and sees that there is section on "Pain Conditions" where "Fibromyalgia" and "Back Pain" are listed. A search on each of these paths uncovers pages and pages of information about these conditions including Tip Sheets, Fact Sheets, Handbooks, archived webinars, treatment information and self-help resources, interviews with experts, FAQs and links to professionally moderated chat rooms on fibromyalgia and back pain, patient stories, and comprehensive lists of resources including books, websites, and articles. Following the PainAid path, she discovers a list of regularly scheduled professionally moderated Live Chats and a large list of Discussion Boards including a topic section on Fibromyalgia and another on Back Pain.

Jane's first visit to the APF site is more exploratory where she finds topics, skim reads various sections, and makes mental notes for her return. Her initial impressions include a major sense of relief after reading descriptions of "fibromyalgia" and "muscle strain back pain" that provide her a strong sense that the diagnoses were correct. She also was immediately gratified to read the words of others who are experiencing similar pains and limitations confirming that she was not imagining her pains and not "crazy or weak" because she felt those pains. The words she read from others were exact descriptions of what she was experiencing. The quick read of information about treatments also confirmed that the recommendations from her physician were appropriate and standard for the pains she experienced.

After several days of exploring, reading deeper, and viewing webinars on the subjects, Jane felt very informed and equipped to take charge of her pains. She followed her doctor's instructions with confidence and added some treatment activities including gentle stretching and guided relaxation techniques to her self-care. She participated in chats and discussion boards and shared her experiences and learned from the experiences of others. In a brief time, her low back muscle pain ended, and she learned to manage her fibromyalgia pain.

After a few months Jane engaged in some of the advocacy opportunities outlined on the website and felt encouraged that her advocacy was contributing to better care for others who might be in the early stages of addressing their chronic pain.

The information and support that Jane received was vital to her understanding her pain, vital to her commitment to her treatment regimen, vital to her confidence and optimism, and a major contributor to the successful management of her pain. This story is representative of many who utilize the assistance of patient information and support organizations. The list presented earlier is only a small representation of the type and number of organizations available for pain patient support. Patient information, support, and advocacy organizations are a useful supplement to the advice and medical decision making that goes on in the medical office.

Reference

1. Fine PG. Long term consequences of chronic pain: mounting evidence for pain as a neurological disease and parallels with other chronic disease states. Pain Med. 2011;12:996–1004.

Neonatal Pain

Celeste Johnston, Marsha Campbell-Yeo, Ananda Fernandes, and Manon Ranger

Key Points

- Excessive exposure to painful invasive procedures is part of the experience of hospitalized neonates.
- Pain is not treated in more than half of invasive procedures in neonates.
- Assessment of pain in neonates requires a multidimensional approach that also accounts for gestational age
- Although effective for postoperative pain, analgesics, including opiates, topical agents, and nonsteroidal anti-inflammatory agents, are not appropriate for minor procedural pain in neonates.
- Non-pharmacological approaches to pain management have proven to be effective for minor procedural pain.

Introduction

Pain in infants was essentially ignored up until the 1980s. The few reports that did exist were small observational studies [1–4]. In 1987, the first randomized trial on pain in neonates was published in the *Lancet,* in which it was reported that the standard for anesthesia for neonates undergoing repair of patent ductus arteriosus was inadequate and that infants who received an opiate-based anesthetic over the usual nitrous oxide had fewer postoperative complications [5]. At the time

C. Johnston, R.N., D.E. (✉) • M. Ranger, R.N., Ph.D.
School of Nursing, McGill University, 3506 University Street, Wilson Hall, Montreal, QC H3A 2A7, Canada
e-mail: dceleste.johnston@mcgill.ca

M. Campbell-Yeo, R.N., M.N., Ph.D.
Department of Maternal Newborn Program, IWK Health Care, 5850/5980 University Ave., 9700, Halifax, NS B3K 6R8, Canada

A. Fernandes, M.S.N., Ph.D.
Coimbra School of Nursing, Coimbra, Lisbon, Portugal

that article appeared, there was an increased interest in the issue of pain in infants, but there were several challenges in order to proceed. The first challenge was how to assess pain in a uniformly nonverbal population, especially given that most definitions of pain included self-report [6]. The second challenge was to determine which analgesics were effective for which conditions with considerations for safety in this vulnerable population. As will be reported below, there was a need for alternate non-pharmacological approaches to pain control, and thus, studies were required to test which ones were effective for pain, particularly procedural pain.

Infants undergoing surgery now typically receive adequate anesthesia and analgesia due to the pioneering study mentioned above [5] as well as subsequent studies on the effects of surgical pain on neonates [7, 8]. Guidelines on the treatment of surgical pain in neonates suggest opiates for major surgery, and this is usually followed [9, 10]. Now, attention has moved to common procedural pain management [11].

Infants who are hospitalized in neonatal intensive care units are subjected to numerous procedures as part of necessary monitoring and therapeutic interventions. Many of these procedures involve tissue damage, such as heel lance, intravenous line insertions, lumbar punctures, or have been considered to be painful although typically not tissue damaging per se, such as endotracheal intubation or suctioning of in situ endotracheal tubes. Estimates of procedural pain range from 10 per day to 5 per week, with approximately half receiving no pain management strategies [9, 10, 12, 13]. This high exposure to untreated procedural pain at a time of increased developmental plasticity is not inconsequential [14–16]. There is peripheral hypersensitivity [17], behavioral blunting [18, 19], altered cortisol response [20], and altered thermal sensitivity into childhood [21–24].

The challenges of measuring pain in this population, of using pharmacological interventions and of alternate interventions, are being met to some extent. The current state of knowledge on these topics will be presented in this chapter with a conclusion regarding the remaining unmet challenges.

T.R. Deer et al. (eds.), *Treatment of Chronic Pain by Integrative Approaches: the AMERICAN ACADEMY of PAIN MEDICINE Textbook on Patient Management*, DOI 10.1007/978-1-4939-1821-8_22,
© American Academy of Pain Medicine 2015

Pain Assessment

An accurate pain evaluation is an essential step to its management. Although it is well recognized, researched, and has been incorporated into best practice clinical guidelines, this task remains challenging in critically ill infants. Through the recognition that preterm infants feel pain, tremendous advancements in this field have been made and have prompted the development of various unidimensional and multidimensional pain assessment measures [25, 26]. Behaviors identified as being reliable proxy indicators for pain evaluation, such as facial expressions and cry, are not without their limits. As critically ill preterm and term neonates may have limited neurological development and energy to construct a proper observable response to pain, it is not uncommon for these fragile babies to not display any detectable cues of such suffering [27, 28]. With the fast progress of neuroimaging techniques, research focus has shifted to measurement of cortical activity related to noxious events, perhaps providing clinical researchers opportunities to explore the use of associated signals to identify and better understand the pain process. Nonetheless, to date, behavioral displays caused by pain remain the best available means to evaluate the infantile forms of self-report and should be used as "surrogate" measures in clinical practice [6].

Behavioral and Physiological Responses

For National Institute for the Humanities (NICU) practitioners, decoding the subtle infantile expressions of pain remains challenging. This critical task requires a certain level of experience, skill in pain evaluation, and adequate time and patience to regularly observe for expressions of pain. The complex nature of this subjective experience does not aid this matter. To aid clinicians, numerous behavioral or composite pain assessment instruments have been developed, some with more solid psychometric properties than others. These scales predominantly include (1) behavioral signs: facial actions, cry, and body motions; and (2) physiological indicators: heart rate, respiratory rate, arterial oxygen saturation, and blood pressure [29]. Among these, facial expressions have been recognized to be the most stable, sensitive, and reliable proxy measures of pain [4, 13, 30]. Out of the ten facial actions first described in the important work by Grunau and Craig [i.e., Neonatal Facial Coding System (NFCS)] [31], three most frequent and typical expressions have been identified: brow bulge, eye squeeze, and nasolabial furrow [29, 32]. These facial displays have been included in many observational pain scales used to assess infant's pain.

According to neurological developmental principles, "excitability" precedes the capacity of the infant to self-regulate a response, and a vigorous behavioral reaction to a stimulus may reflect neurological maturity [33]. Thus, the absence of observational reactions to a noxious stimulus in a preterm neonate is an indicator of immaturity rather than no pain perception [34]. Moreover, in response to a noxious stimulation, a complex disposition at the spinal or brainstem level is required to enable an infant to display a visible facial expression; this requiring a coordinated motor neuron activity27. Reports of blunted behavioral cues of pain in preterm infants despite cerebral hemodynamic changes have stressed the importance of relying on other means of pain assessment indicators in populations with limited observable behavioral displays [28, 35, 36]. Slater et al. [28] described facial expression latency following a heel-lance procedure in preterm infants and reported that only 64 % of their sample displayed observable facial expression. Moreover, a significant effect of postmenstrual age upon the latency of pain behavior was shown.

Even though more than 40 pain assessment tools are available, no single instrument has demonstrated superiority over the others for use across varied painful conditions or clinical situations. Thus, no specific measure has been set as the "gold standard" for pain assessment of infants in research and clinical practice [37].

Of all of the pain measures developed for use in preterm and term neonates, the Premature Infant Pain Profile (PIPP) is perhaps the most well-known and clinically used multidimensional assessment instrument [38]. As such, it has been reported as being one of the most valid and reliable infant acute pain measure available. In a recent review evaluating their instrument, 13 years after its initial development, the authors were able to index 62 studies that reported having used the PIPP, thus contributing to its validation over the years [32]. Aside from being well established and having solid psychometric features, the particularity of the PIPP is that it includes two contextual variables, behavioral state and gestational age (GA), which have been shown to contribute to the pain response [30, 31, 39, 40]. Other examples of scales that take into account one of these factors are the multidimensional Neonatal Pain, Agitation, and Sedation Scale (N-PASS) [41] and the behavioral Neonatal Infant Pain Scale (NIPS) [42]. As mentioned previously, many acute pain assessment instruments have been developed with varying levels of psychometric testing; some having gone through only very basic testing. Following is a list of those that have published data, two are multidimensional (1, 2) and three behavioral (3–5) instruments: (1) Crying, Requires Increased oxygen, Increased vital signs, Expression, Sleeplessness (CRIES) [43]; (2) *Douleur aiguë du nouveau-né* (DAN) [44]; (3) Scale for Use in Newborn (SUN) [45]; (4) Pain Assessment in Neonates scale (PAIN) [46]; and (5) Behavioral of Indicators of Infant Pain (BIIP) which includes two hand actions [47]. The multidimensional tool Distress Scale for Ventilated Newborn Infants (DSVNI) [48] is the first of its kind to focus specifically on ventilated newborn

Table 22.1 Summary of neonatal pain scales

Type/context pain	Measurement scale	Validated age group
Procedural pain	CRIES	32 weeks–2 months
	DAN	Preterm–3 months
	PIPP	28 weeks–1 months
	NIPS	Premature–6 weeks
	N-PASS	Premature–3 months
	PAIN	26–47 weeks
	SUN	24–40 weeks
	BIIP	23–32 weeks
	DSVNI	37–40 weeks
Postoperative pain	CRIES	As above
	PIPP	
	N-PASS	
Prolonged pain	EDIN	Preterm–9 months

infants. The only scale developed to evaluate prolonged pain in preterm and term neonates until age of 6 to 9 months is the *Échelle de douleur et d'inconfort du nouveau-né* (EDIN) [49]. For a more comprehensive review of the various pain assessment tools developed for use in preterm and term infants, refer to review manuscripts (Table 22.1) [26, 50, 51].

To evaluate pain in critically ill infants, health-care professionals often rely upon unstable and nonspecific physiological indicators such as heart rate, arterial oxygen saturation, respiratory rate, and blood pressure. These parameters could be viewed as more "objective" or quantifiable than other more qualitative behavioral indicators. However, relying on physiological markers can lead to misinterpretation of pain intensity since they have been shown to decrease the internal consistency of many multidimensional pain assessment instruments, are not well correlated to behavioral indicators, and are not specific to the pain response [30, 52, 53]. Other physiological indicators lacking specificity that have been studied to assess stress and pain in neonates are cortisol level from saliva samples [54], skin conductance (palmar sweating) [55–58], and biomarkers such as analysis of heart rate variability [59].

In a sample of 149 infants undergoing an acute painful procedure, Stevens and others examined the factor structure of 19 pain indicators, both physiological and behavioral [29]. Facial actions accounted for a greater proportion of the variance (close to 40 %) with oxygen saturation, heart rate, cry, and heart rate variability accounting for lesser, but important, contributions of 8–26 % of the additional explained variance. As many physiological cues and some behavioral cues, such as crying, are not specific to pain, researchers and clinicians are faced with the difficult task of discriminating between these to decide whether they are truly indicative of pain and not of other similarly manifested states, such as agitation, distress, anxiety, stress, or hunger.

Cortical Responses

As discussed previously, in addition to manifesting related states (i.e., stress, hunger, agitation, etc.) that can be difficult to distinguish from pain expressions, the fragile and immature condition of critically ill infants may lessen their capability to organize and exhibit perceived pain as a recognizable response. Consequently, clinical researchers have explored the use of associated signals to identify pain. The search for a more objective, specific, and sensitive means of measuring pain in this population is inspiring researchers to develop clinically applicable tools. Neuroimaging techniques are becoming more common in pain research; understanding the strengths and limitations of these approaches is important for professionals considering their application for the study and clinical management of pain in neonates. Although we may be far from clinically applicable instruments, promising results have been reported for the use of noninvasive electroencephalography (EEG) [36, 60, 61] and neuroimaging techniques to measure sensory input processing, such as in studies of somatosensory cortical activation [62]. As such, these novel approaches to measuring pain are beginning to provide validation for observational methods [27].

It has been demonstrated with near-infrared spectroscopy (NIRS) that cerebral hemodynamic changes (presumably due to cortical activation) occur in response to stressful and/or painful stimuli in term and preterm newborn infants [63–65]. NIRS is a noninvasive technique that detects subtle changes in the brain (or tissue) concentration of oxygenated and deoxygenated hemoglobin, which are inferred to reflect changes in cerebral metabolism and perfusion. An additional feature of NIRS, as compared to magnetic resonance imaging (MRI) and positron-emission tomography (PET) devices, is its portability directly to the bedside of these fragile patients which allows for continuous signal recording capable of capturing responses to intermittent stimuli.

The study of hemodynamic changes to assess the functional activation in the brain is based on the assumption that a given stimulus will induce a neuronal response which in turn triggers local vasodilation with an increase in cerebral blood volume (CBV) and cerebral blood flow (CBF) [66]. There have been significant advances in this field in the last decade; however, understanding of how blood flow, metabolism, and neuronal activity interact to affect the NIRS signals remains incomplete. Establishing validity of the NIRS measures has also proven difficult because few alternative technologies exist to serve as a gold standard 67. NIRS technology is sensitive to various factors that may confound results. Conditions related to critical illness that may result in metabolic somatosensory changes could confound pain-related activation measurement using NIRS. Patient movement can cause artifacts and disruptions in data collection.

Although NIRS has excellent temporal resolution, it has poor spatial resolution when compared to other functional and structural imaging techniques such as MRI [67]. Therefore, it remains difficult to accurately identify the exact region that is sampled by the NIR light [68]. However, conducting multichannel functional NIRS trials allows for a more accurate mapping of cortical areas and improved discrimination [69] but remains difficult in preterm and term neonates to conduct due to their extremely small heads.

Although our understanding of the multidimensional experience of pain has advanced over the last century, many avenues remain unexplored. NIRS has potential as a noninvasive portable technique for assessing pain evoked cerebral activation in critically ill infants. However, given the complexity of NIRS technology, the paucity of research supporting its use in pain measurement in critically ill infants, and the need for tight control of many confounding factors as well as artifacts, more studies are clearly needed. At this stage, it is perhaps best to consider this neurodiagnostic technique, as well as others previously enumerated, solely as research tools that will improve our understanding of pain perception, increase the psychometric features of currently available pain assessment instruments, and perhaps assess the efficacy of pharmacological and non-pharmacological treatments.

Pharmacological Treatment of Procedural Pain

The most common drugs used to treat neonatal pain include topical and local anesthetics, acetaminophen, and opiates [70]. There are several difficulties with providing pharmacological treatments for procedural pain including safety concerns, insufficient data on specific neonatal pharmacokinetic and pharmacodynamics, difficulty in pain assessment, and lack of long-term neurodevelopmental follow-up. In addition, large variation in reported efficacy for procedural pain attenuation has limited their use in this population.

Topical Anesthetics

Topical anesthetics have been reasonably well researched in this population primarily related to several assumed benefits including noninvasive method of administration, lack of systemic effects, and potential for effectiveness. In an early review paper, Taddio and colleagues [71] evaluated the use of lidocaine–prilocaine cream (EMLA®, Astra Pharma) compared to placebo in treating pain from heel lance, venipuncture, arterial puncture, lumbar puncture, percutaneous venous catheter placement, and circumcision in preterm and term infants. Nine randomized controlled trials (RCTs) were included. Unfortunately, for the most commonly performed procedure in the NICU, heel lance for blood procurement, EMLA was not shown to be beneficial. Similarly, in two later studies examining the effect of tetracaine 4 % gel (Ametop®, Smith & Nephew), on the pain of heel lance in both preterm and term newborns, no reduction in pain scores or duration of crying was noted between the groups [72, 73]. It has been postulated that variation in perfusion and skin thickness of an infant's heel may contribute to this ineffectiveness [74].

Similarly, the use of topical anesthetic has not been shown to be effective in diminishing pain associated with the insertion of intravenous lines or peripherally inserted central catheters (PICC) [75–77]. Some evidence was provided for the use of EMLA in relieving pain during venipuncture; however, results remain inconclusive. There have been five clinical trials examining the effect of topical anesthetic (EMLA and tetracaine 4 %) for pain associated with venipuncture [76, 78–81]. Results show that the application of local anesthetic could decrease the duration of cry but increase the procedure time [79], as well as being dose (0.5 vs. 1 ml) [78] and application time dependent (30 vs. 60 min) [76, 80].

There are no known contradictions to using preemptive local or topical anesthetics for lumbar puncture in neonates, and their use has been associated with increased success in obtaining cerebral spinal fluid (CFS) [82] and potential benefits related to a reduction in pain score and physiological stability [83]. In a randomized trial comparing the effect of lidocaine–prilocaine (EMLA) (1 g over 60–90 min) compared to placebo for 60 infants undergoing a lumbar puncture, infant in the intervention group had lower mean HR at needle insertion ($P = 0.001$) and needle withdrawal ($P < 0.001$) and lower total behavioral score again at insertion ($P < 0.004$) and needle withdrawal ($P < 0.001$) [84].

Currently, the most widely utilized local anesthetic for injection is lidocaine hydrochloride 1 %. It is effective as an adjuvant pain relieving strategy for lumbar puncture, chest tube insertion, and circumcision [85–89].

The use of EMLA to relieve pain caused by a frequently performed procedure in neonates, circumcision, has been shown to be more effective than placebo, as indicated by changes in physiological and behavioral pain indicators [86], and these findings were similar to a later Cochrane systematic review [71]. In another Cochrane review regarding pain relief for circumcision that included 35 trials involving 1,997 full-term and preterm infants, when compared to placebo, dorsal penile nerve block (DPNB), EMLA, and sweet taste all reduced pain response [90]. Of the six trials ($n = 190$) specifically examining EMLA compared to placebo, infants receiving EMLA demonstrated significantly lower facial action scores, decreased time crying, and lower heart rate. However, when EMLA and sweet taste were compared with DPNB, crying and elevation in heart rate were lowest in the DPNB group. Despite the large number of trials, small sample sizes, lack of blinding, large variations in practice, and little use of age appropriate validated pain tools limited the author's ability to make concise recommendations. The authors concluded that topical anesthetic in conjunction with DPNB as well as other pain relieving strategies could be safely implemented as part of routine practice related to circumcision.

Acetaminophen

Acetaminophen is one of the most commonly used analgesics for both mild ongoing pain and intermittent medical procedures [91]. Interestingly, despite its widespread use, there is limited evidence regarding its efficacy related to procedural pain alleviation in newborns [92–95]. Even at very high oral doses (40 mg/kg), it did not diminish the pain associated with heel lance [96]. The widespread use of prophylactic acetaminophen prior to immunization has been recently refuted, although its administration for local pain or swelling postinjections is still supported [97, 98].

The efficacy of intravenous acetaminophen has been better studied, and it appears to be beneficial for the relief of postoperative pain and act as an opioid sparing agent [99–101]. Its use for intermittent procedure pain has not been reported.

Opioids

Although opioids continue to be the mainstay in the neonatal intensive care unit (NICU) for the treatment of ongoing painful conditions such as necrotizing enterocolitis, operative procedures, and postoperative care, their use for more common single procedures performed in the NICU has been less promising [91]. Systemic administered drugs, specifically opioids, are highly sensitive to development [102, 103] and have significantly slower clearance in neonates [104–108]. Morphine and fentanyl are the predominate opioids used in hospitalized newborns with morphine being the most studied.

There have been conflicting reports regarding the efficacy and safety of intermittent and continuous intravenous infusions morphine for routine medical procedures and the stress associated with mechanical ventilation. Morphine does not appear to be beneficial for some of the commonly performed procedures in the NICU such as tracheal suctioning [109] or heel lance [110]. Validated pain scores were not significantly different for 42 preterm infants, mean GA at birth of 27 weeks, randomized to receive a loading dose, and continuous infusion of morphine or placebo during heel lance over three time points [110]. Conversely, in an earlier study conducted by Anand [111], procedural pain (endotracheal suctioning)

response was found to be much lower in the infants receiving morphine compared to placebo. Similarly in a much larger trial, pain scores in response to endotracheal suctioning were lower with morphine [112]. However, the incidence of longer duration of mechanical ventilation, hypotension, and severe intraventricular hemorrhage was higher in infants receiving more frequent intermittent doses of morphine regardless of assigned group.

In a systematic review of 13 RCTs examining the effectiveness of opioid analgesia in reducing the pain experienced from mechanical ventilation, the authors concluded that there was insufficient data to support the routine use of opioids in mechanically ventilated newborns [113]. The broad range of opioid dose and variation in type of analgesia in the trials also contributed to the findings. Of note, pain scores were significantly lower in four of the trials, and the authors did recommend that opioids should be used cautiously and in combination with well-validated pain scoring measures to evaluate their effectiveness. The authors also reported a higher incidence of hypotension and poorer neurodevelopmental outcome associated with midazolam compared to morphine. Therefore, if sedation is required, morphine appears to be a safer choice than midazolam.

There do appear to be some acutely painful conditions that warrant the use of morphine. Intravenous morphine was found to be more advantageous than topical application of tetracaine for the management of pain associated with insertion of a central venous catheter in neonates [75]. Remifentanil, a fast-acting opioid, has also been found to be analgesic for the insertion of a PICC. When compared to placebo, a 0.03 mcg/kg infusion of remifentanil significantly lowered the pain score of very preterm neonates undergoing insertion of a PICC. Mean pain scores [NIPS and PIPP] at skin preparation T1 and needle insertion T2 were significantly different to baseline T0 and recovery T3. No improvement was noted with respect to the number of attempts needed to successfully perform the procedure [114].

There is increasing consensus that opioids with rapid onset in combination with anticholinergics and muscle relaxants should be used for all infants undergoing elective intubation [115, 116]. In a review of nine trials, Shah [117] reported that the use of premedication was associated with a reduction in physiological pain indicators and intubation times. The most common and preferred agents reported were fentanyl, atropine, and rocuronium, although differences in medication and dosages were common across sites [118]. Morphine's slower onset of peak effect could contribute to its lack of efficacy [119]. Results from studies examining two synthetic agents, alfentanil and remifentanil, are promising [120, 121]. Ongoing research to determine the optimal dosage, administration route, and combination of medications as well as the long-term neurodevelopmental effects are warranted [118].

Alternate Strategies for the Treatment of Procedural Pain

Given the frequency of painful procedures in neonatal intensive care units and the difficulties with pharmacological management, the use of alternate or non-pharmacological strategies alone or as adjuvant management is highly recommended.

Alternate and non-pharmacological interventions that have been studied to relieve procedural pain in infants may be categorized in two main groups according to their nature. The earliest group of interventions studied focused on offering pleasant sensorial stimuli or manipulation of the infant's environmental boundaries such as oro-tactile stimulation as in the case of nonnutritive sucking (NNS), oro-gustatory stimulation by sweet solutions, containment and facilitated tucking, and vestibular stimulation, while investigation of the second group of interventions centered on maternal proximity such as breastfeeding and skin-to-skin (SSC) contact came later.

The exact mechanisms underlying the comforting effect of these interventions remains unclear, but it has been postulated that they involve both opioid and non-opioid-mediated systems, namely, the oxytocinergic system. Although there are scant data in neonates regarding endogenous descending, inhibitory mechanisms, the engagement of mechanisms that release endorphins is well established in adults [122, 123] There is a suggestion from the animal literature that the endogenous system is not well developed prior to 32 weeks postconception, but it is likely that it is well developed enough in neonates after 32 weeks, and possibly earlier, to provide some comfort [15, 124].

Oro-Tactile Stimulation by NNS

Sucking movements start in uterus around 12–14 weeks postconceptional age (PCA) [125], the sucking reflex develops around the 17th week postconception, and regular sucking activity is found in fetuses of 27–28 weeks PCA. NNS is stimulated in neonates by placing a pacifier in the infant's mouth.

Based on its effect in reducing fussing and crying in preterm infants in neonatal care [126], several studies have looked at NNS, comparing it to other interventions or no intervention in order to determine whether it decreases the responses of neonates to painful procedures. NNS has been found to reduce the increase in heart rate [127]; reduce crying time in term and preterm neonates [127–132], even in those who are intubated and ventilated [133]; and reduce pain scores [129, 131, 134–139].

Compared to swaddling, NNS after heel lance interrupted crying earlier (23.2 s vs. 58.7) and promoted a faster decline in heart rate although infants spent more time in an alert state (59 % of the time vs. 22 %, $P < 0.01$) [140]. Compared to rocking, heart rate was also significantly reduced by NNS,

but these infants slept more in the rocking group [128]. Compared to sucrose, glucose, and sucrose with pacifier, the median pain scores of term infants who received NNS for venipuncture was significantly lower (2) than that of infants who received sweet solutions (5). Although the scores with sucrose and pacifier (1) were the lowest, they were not significantly different from NNS alone ($P = 0.06$) [136].

Adding other interventions to NNS appears to be beneficial. In a crossover trial, pacifier alone was compared to pacifier plus music therapy, music therapy alone, and no intervention during and after heel lance [139]. All three interventions improved the pain response, compared to no intervention, but NNS combined with music was associated with the lowest NIPS scores and the highest transcutaneous oxygen saturation (TcPaO$_2$) levels, while music therapy alone produced the lowest heart rate. Regarding the synergistic effect of simultaneously using NNS and sweet solutions, while adding a pacifier to sucrose or glucose seems to enhance the effect of sweet solutions used alone [130, 131], adding sucrose or glucose to a pacifier seems to provide no additional benefit than using a pacifier alone [134–138].

Including pacifier with glucose in a combined intervention named sensorial saturation (SS) that includes, besides taste, sight, touch, voice, and smell has shown to be more efficacious than glucose with pacifier in reducing the pain scores of term newborns during heel lance [137].

Oro-Gustatory Stimulation by Sweet Taste

The capacity of infants to distinguish between flavors, namely, sucrose, quinine, and corn oil has been demonstrated [141], and the calming effects of sweet taste have been known for a long time. Animal studies reinforce the evidence from studies in human infants that sucrose, glucose, and fructose but not lactose have a calming and pain-reducing effect, increasing the latency to withdraw from a heated surface in rat pups [142]. A recently updated Cochrane systematic review including 44 studies concluded that sucrose is efficacious and safe to use in single and repeated heel lances and should be considered for venipuncture since it significantly reduces pain behaviors and composite measures [143]. The authors of this review state that for other procedures such as eye examination for retinopathy of prematurity, bladder catheterization, nasogastric tube insertion, circumcision, and subcutaneous injections, further studies are required due to conflicting evidence and that the use of sucrose in extremely low birth weight and unstable and/or ventilated neonates needs to be addressed.

The recommended dose is a small volume of 0.05–0.5 ml of a 24 % sucrose solution for preterm neonates and 1–2 ml, administered 2 min prior to the painful procedure, for term neonates [143]. Concentrations of sucrose have varied from 12 to 50 %, but a ceiling effect seems to be reached at 25 %

[144]. The most common method of administration is via syringe or dropper placing the solution on the anterior surface of the infants' tongue, but a pacifier dipped in a sucrose solution may also be used and is estimated to deliver approximately 0.1 ml [134]. The repeated use of sucrose for heel lance seems to not reduce its efficacy [144, 145]. Regarding concerns about long-term effects, one study has found a poorer neurobehavioral development in neonates younger than 31 weeks PCA [146]. However, a secondary analysis of the same data showed that increased risk occurred in neonates who had more than ten doses of sucrose in 24 h [147]. A subsequent study has found that infants who had procedural pain consistently managed by sucrose and pacifier in the first 28 days of life had no difference in adverse events or clinical outcomes such as intraventricular hemorrhage compared to infants who received no sucrose [148].

Glucose is another well-studied source of sweet taste. Its efficacy in a volume range of 0.3–2 ml of a 30 % solution has been shown for heel lance [149] and venipuncture [136, 150, 151], both in term [149, 150] and preterm [151] infants, as well as for subcutaneous injections in very preterm neonates (25–32 weeks GA) [152].

Comparisons between similar volumes and concentrations of sucrose and glucose show similar effects in reducing pain scores [126, 153–155], and both sucrose [156] and glucose [157] compare favorably to a topical anesthetic cream for venipuncture in full-term newborns.

Favoring Behavioral Organization Through Swaddling or Containment

Wrapping young infants in a cloth is part of the traditional way of care in many cultures [158]. An extensive systematic review of 78 studies evaluating the effects of swaddling, four of which examining pain control, concluded that it reduces crying, physiologic distress, and motor activity; increases sleep; and improves neuromuscular development in preterm infants [158]. Regarding pain control during heel lance, neonates over 30 weeks PCA returned to their baseline facial activity, heart rate, and arterial oxygen saturation levels more quickly [158]. A meta-analysis of four unpublished studies conducted in Thailand also supported the efficacy of swaddling, with moderate to large mean effect sizes in full-term babies during heel lance [159].

Containment or facilitated tucking by holding the infant in a side lying position, arms and legs flexed near the trunk [160], also has been shown to reduce behavioral signs of distress of very low birth weight infants during heel lance [161], endotracheal suctioning [162], and pharyngeal suctioning [163]. Facilitated tucking seems to be more efficacious than water or oxycodone in reducing pain scores during pharyngeal suctioning and heel lance in very low birth weight infants and was equivalent to 0.2 ml of 24 % glucose but presents less short-term adverse effects, such as desaturation and/or bradycardia, than oral glucose [164]. In addition, in two studies, facilitated tucking was performed by parents, offering them an opportunity to participate in alleviating their infants' distress [163, 164].

Vestibular Stimulation

Rocking has also been a traditional way to calm infants and promote sleep. When compared to the use of a pacifier after heel lance in term infants, while both interventions reduced crying and can therefore be considered efficacious, rocking promoted arousal levels more than pacifiers, which promoted sleep [128]. A more recent trial compared rocking, expressed breast milk, 20 % sucrose, water, NNS, and massage in term, stable neonates [165]. Neonates were rocked by lifting the baby's head off the cot on the palm of the hand but not the body and making rocking movements in a gentle, rhythmic manner during and up till 2 min after heel lance. Like infants in the NNS group, infants who received rocking cried less and had lower pain scores at 2 and 4 min after the painful procedure, while infants in the sucrose group had a reduced pain score only at 30 sec [165]. Another trial in preterm infants during heel lance compared simulated rocking (infants in supine or side lying position on an oscillating air mattress), sucrose, usual incubator care with no intervention, and a combination of simulated rocking and sucrose [166, 167]. Simulated rocking combined with sucrose decreased facial expression by 40 % and so did sucrose alone, while simulated rocking was no better than incubator care, suggesting that the pain-reducing effect was related to the sucrose administration.

Auditory Stimulation

Human fetuses' capacity of perceiving sound at different frequencies and responding to them develops from 19 weeks of GA to term [167]. Their ability to learn and remember auditory stimuli from the intrauterine environment as early as 22 weeks GA has been put into evidence by conditioning studies [168]. It was demonstrated that infants as young as 3 days preferred their mothers' voice to the voice of another female [169], and exposure to familiar sounds has been associated to improved physiological stability [170]. The soothing effects of familiar sounds during painful procedures have been evaluated in a few trials. Maternal heart rate, Japanese drum with identical rhythm, and no sound were offered to 131 full-term infants who underwent heel lance [171]. Infants exposed to maternal heart beat had reduced facial response and crying, as well as lower levels of salivary cortisol. Following an identical rationale, 20 preterm infants 32–36 weeks were exposed to recorded and filtered maternal "sing-song" voice or to no voice during a heel-lance procedure in a randomized crossover design [172]. No significant differences were found in pain scores between conditions, and the authors conclude that maternal voice alone, without other components of maternal presence, may not be enough to reduce pain response.

The effects of music to reduce pain have also been examined. A recent systematic review of RCTs of music for medical indications in the neonatal period found six studies that looked at painful procedures, three for circumcision and three for heel lance [173]. Only one of the studies on circumcision [174] had high-methodological quality and showed a lower pain score, lower heart rate increase, and higher arterial oxygen saturation levels, while the other two studies found no significant differences between groups. For heel lance, three trials were included but considered to have poor methodological quality [173]. One crossover trial with 27 infants 28 weeks GA or more found a significant decrease in heart rate and pain scores and an improvement in arterial oxygen saturation levels with music but also with music combined with NNS and with NNS alone [139]. Another crossover trial including 14 infants of 29–36 weeks PCA found a significant effect on heart rate, behavioral state, and pain scores only in infants over 31 weeks [175].

Auditory stimulation may be administered through different types of sounds, from music to direct or recorded maternal voice, or filtered voice and heart beat that would resemble the sound heard in the womb. Significant changes during the maturation process occurring in the last trimester of pregnancy with implication on the frequencies and levels of intensity that can be perceived by neonates of different GAs pose an important challenge when designing appropriate auditory interventions and methodologically sound studies.

Olfactory Stimulation

During their prenatal experience, human fetuses are exposed to the numerous compounds of the amniotic fluid, which play an active role in shaping the development of chemosensory sensitivity and preferences [176]. It has been demonstrated that newborns are able to discriminate odors and have head-orientation behavior toward their own amniotic fluid, showing their preference for a familiar versus non familiar odor [177]. In preterm infants, responses elicited by odorants are weak and irregular at 24 weeks PCA but reliable by week 28 [176]. Given the soothing effect of the smell of amniotic fluid in term neonates separated from their mothers following birth [177], the effect of olfactory stimulation for painful procedures has gained increasing interest.

To determine the soothing effect of familiar and unfamiliar odor in full-term infants undergoing a routine heel lance, 44 breast-fed newborns were randomized to 4 groups [178]: (1) infants naturally familiarized with their mother's milk odor (2), infants previously familiarized with vanilla odor

(3), infants not previously exposed to vanilla odor, and (4) infants who received no intervention. Results showed that the neonates in group 1 and 2 who received the odors during and after heel lance showed less distress during the recovery phase compared with the heel lance phase. Furthermore, the infants who were not exposed previously to the vanilla odor and those in the control group showed no difference in grimacing and cry during and after the heel lance. Babies who smelled their mother's milk exhibited significantly less motor agitation during the heel lance compared with the other groups. Whether familiarization to the odor was obtained through the mother or without the mother did not make a difference as shown in a replication of the previous study, in which the calming effects of familiar odor were visible during the heel-lance phase [179]. In healthy preterm newborns, a familiar odor compared to unfamiliar or no odor also reduced crying and grimacing [180]. A comparison between mother's milk, non-mother's milk, and formula milk given to healthy full-term neonates showed that crying, grimacing, and motor activity during heel lance were decreased only by exposure of the infant's own mother's milk [180].

Olfactory stimulation has been used in full-term and preterm infants during heel lance as a component of SS, an intervention that combines visual stimulation (looking the baby in the face to attract his attention), auditory stimulation (speaking to the infant gently but firmly), tactile stimulation (massaging the infant's face and back), and gustatory stimulation (glucose with pacifier) [137, 138, 181]. Within the original concept of SS, olfactory stimulation was provided by letting the infant smell the fragrance of baby oil on the therapist's hands [138], but a modified version without perfume has also been shown to be effective in reducing pain scores of full-term healthy neonates [181]. Moreover, the modified intervention was shown to be more effective on a cry scale [182] than 1 ml of 30 % glucose with pacifier, raising questions regarding the importance of the olfactory component of SS.

The mechanism underlying the comforting effect of intrauterine, maternal, and familiarized smell remains unclear but it has been postulated that it is an opioid-mediated system. This hypothesis derives, on one hand, from knowledge that the taste system and the olfactory system are linked and that the antinociceptive effect of sweet taste is opioid mediated [183]. Conversely, animal studies indicated that the opioid system modulates olfactory learning and odor preferences [184].

Maternal Proximity

Breast Milk and Breastfeeding

The mother–infant dyad has an innate mutual bond that is key to survival. Infants actively mediate this bond by eliciting distress cues when separated from their mother that in turn heightens a mothers' instinctive need to protect and comfort their young. Therefore, it is not surprising that researchers returned to this basic human premise to investigate whether maternal presence could diminish the effects of repeated procedural pain exposure during prolonged hospitalization. The first studies followed the oro-gustatory research and focused on the use of breast milk or breastfeeding to attenuate the pain associated with common newborn procedures such as heel lance, venipuncture, and intramuscular injection. In a systematic review of eleven clinical trials, six examining the effectiveness of supplemental breast milk and five examining breastfeeding, breast milk giving orally by syringe was no different than water and significantly less beneficial than sweet taste in both full-term and preterm infants undergoing routine procedural pain from heel lance and venipuncture [185]. In contrast, breastfeeding when compared to placebo was shown to provide analgesia. In addition, when comparing to sweet taste, breastfeeding has been shown to be equivocal [186] and may even be superior [187]. Healthy term neonates (37–42 weeks of gestation at least 60 h old) undergoing heel lance for metabolic screening had lower median PIPP scores in the breastfeeding group (3.0) than those infants receiving 1 ml sucrose solution (8.5). The benefits of glucose and breastfeeding may be cumulative when provided simultaneously [188]. The efficacy of breastfeeding to diminish the painful effects of immunization appears to continue to at least 1 year of age. Consistent findings have been reported in three studies. Breast-fed infants when compared to controls experienced significantly shorter duration of crying, 35.85 vs. 76.24 s, $P = 0.001$ [189] and 20.0 s (0–120) vs. 150.0 (0–180), $P = 0.001$ [190] and 125.33 vs. 148.66 [191]. NIPS scores were also significantly reduced when infants were breast-feed, B 3.0 (0–6) vs. 6.0 (0–7), $P = 0.001$ [190].

Maternal contact is likely to be the mediating factor why breastfeeding when compared to supplemental breast milk alone is effective. During heel lance, infants being held by mother and breast-fed or being held by mother with pacifier cried significantly less (33 and 45 %) compared to being held by non-mother with pacifier (66 %, $P < 0.01$ and $P = 0.03$) [192].

SCC Contact

SSC between an infant and mother is also referred to as kangaroo mother care (KMC) due to its similarity to marsupial maternal care [193]. During KMC, a diaper-clad infant is held upright, at an angle of approximately 60°, between the mother's breasts, providing maximal skin-to-skin contact between baby and parent. Full skin contact and maternal presence have been shown to be beneficial for both term and preterm infants. Advantages for the infant are numerous: stable heart and respiratory rates, balanced thermoregulation, decreased apnea and periodic breathing, improved weight gain, accelerated maturation of the autonomic and circadian

systems, and analgesia to painful therapeutic procedures [194–197]. KMC was originally implemented as an alternative to the incubator to maintain preterm infants' body temperature and increase survival rate in South America where incubators were in short supply [193]. During this time, it was serendipitously noted that infants spent more time in quiet sleep state [197, 199]. Since quiet state is associated with decreased pain response [31, 200], the idea developed to use KMC for procedural pain. In addition, it appeared that holding with skin-to-skin contact provided more comfort than holding with clothed body-to-skin contact [201]. The difference in skin-to-skin contact comfort may be related to inborn tactile receptor response and regulation of opiates, oxytocin, beta endorphins, and vagal tone [202, 203].

Initially studied in full-term neonates, 10–15 min of KMC prior to heel lance reduced crying by 82 %, grimacing by 65 %, and elevation in heart rate (8–10 vs. 36–38) compared to infants who stayed in a cot [204]. Later in the first study to examine the effects of KMC in preterm neonates, pain scores (PIPP) [32, 38], as well as the individual components of decreased facial action, heart rate acceleration, and increased arterial oxygen saturation changes, were reported as lower for the neonates who received KMC compared to those remaining in an incubator during heel lance [196]. Following these studies, numerous trials followed.

In a Cochrane review on skin-to-skin contact for procedural pain in infants, 13 studies that meet the inclusion criteria all show positive results [205]. KMC during heel lance significantly reduced pain scores in full- and in preterm neonates as young as 28 weeks GA [196, 206–210], as well as venipuncture [206] and intramuscular injection [211, 212]. KMC during heel lance has also been associated with a shortened duration of crying [213, 214], more robust heart rate variability [215], and better regulated neurobehavioral response assessed by the Newborn Individualized Developmental Care and Assessment Program (NIDCAP) [216]. Of interest, two of those studies [210, 211] showed that KMC was more effective than sweet taste.

Summary

Pain in neonates is an important issue in particular as neonates are a vulnerable population due both to their helplessness, their inability to report verbally, and their highly developing nervous system. Although they cannot self-report, there are validated ways to measure their pain, and new techniques hold promise for further specificity. There is a need to search for safe analgesics for this population. Such searches should begin with infants and not extrapolate down from other populations. Endogenous mechanisms show somewhat surprising effectiveness for procedural pain. Being inexpensive and easily implemented, the use of these strategies should be implemented [116].

References

1. McGraw MB. Neural maturation as exemplified in the changing reactions of the infant to pin prick. Child Dev. 1941;12:31–42.
2. Owens ME. Pain in infancy: conceptual and methodological issues. Pain (Amsterdam). 1984;20:213–30.
3. Owens ME. Assessment of infant pain in clinical settings. J Pain Symptom Manag. 1986;1:29–31.
4. Johnston CC, Strada ME. Acute pain responses in infants: a multidimensional description. Pain (Amsterdam). 1986;24:373–82.
5. Anand KJ, Sippell WG, Aynsley-Green A. Randomised trial of fentanyl anaesthesia in preterm babies undergoing surgery: effects on the stress response. Lancet. 1987;1(8524):62–6.
6. Anand KJS, Craig KD. New perspectives on the definition of pain. Pain (Amsterdam). 1996;67:3–6.
7. Anand KJ, Hickey PR. Halothane-morphine compared with high-dose sufentanil for anesthesia and postoperative analgesia in neonatal cardiac surgery. N Engl J Med. 1992;326(1):1–9.
8. Anand KJS, Aynsley-Green A. Measuring severity of surgical stress in newborn infants. J Pediatr Surg. 1988;23:297–305.
9. Carbajal R, Rousset A, Danan C, et al. Epidemiology and treatment of painful procedures in neonates in intensive care units. JAMA. 2008;300(1):60–70.
10. Johnston CC, Barrington K, Taddio A, Carbajal R, Filion F. Pain in Canadian NICU's: have we improved over the past 12 years? Clin J Pain. 2010;27(3):225–32.
11. American Academy of P, Committee on F, Newborn, Canadian Paediatric S, Fetus, Newborn C. Prevention and management of pain in the neonate. [An update reprint of Pediatrics. 2006;118(5):2231–41; PMID: 17079598]. Adv Neonatal Care. 2007;7(3):151–160.
12. Simons SH, van Dijk M, Anand KS, Roofthooft D, van Lingen RA, Tibboel D. Do we still hurt newborn babies? A prospective study of procedural pain and analgesia in neonates. Arch Pediatr Adolesc Med. 2003;157(11):1058–64.
13. Stevens B, McGrath P, Gibbins S, et al. Procedural pain in newborns at risk for neurologic impairment. Pain (Amsterdam). 2003;105(1–2):27–35.
14. Fitzgerald M, Beggs S. The neurobiology of pain: developmental aspects. [Review] [120 refs]. Neuroscientist. 2001;7(3):246–57.
15. Fitzgerald M, Walker SM. Infant pain management: a developmental neurobiological approach. Nat Clin Pract Neurol. 2009;5(1):35–50.
16. Grunau RE, Thanh Tu M. Long-term consequences of pain in human neonates. Anand KJS, Stevens BJ, McGrath PJ (ed.), 3rd editions, Pain Neonates and Infants: Elsevier 2007;3.
17. Fitzgerald M, Millard C, McIntosh N. Cutaneous hypersensitivity following peripheral tissue damage in newborn infants and its reversal with topical anaesthesia. Pain (Amsterdam). 1989;39:31–6.
18. Johnston CC, Stevens BJ. Experience in a neonatal intensive care unit affects pain response. Pediatrics (Evanston IL). 1996;98(5):925–30.
19. Grunau RE, Oberlander TF, Whitfield MF, Fitzgerald C, Lee SK. Demographic and therapeutic determinants of pain reactivity in very low birth weight neonates at 32 weeks' postconceptional age. Pediatrics (Evanston IL). 2001;107(1):105–12.
20. Grunau RE, Haley DW, Whitfield MF, Weinberg J, Yu W, Thiessen P. Altered basal cortisol levels at 3, 6, 8 and 18 months in infants born at extremely low gestational age. J Pediatr. 2007;150(2):151–6.
21. Walker SM, Franck LS, Fitzgerald M, Myles J, Stocks J, Marlow N. Long-term impact of neonatal intensive care and surgery on somatosensory perception in children born extremely preterm. Pain. 2009;141(1–2):79–87.
22. Hermann C, Hohmeister J, Demirakca S, Zohsel K, Flor H. Long-term alteration of pain sensitivity in school-aged children with early pain experiences. Pain (Amsterdam). 2006;125(3):278–85.
23. Hohmeister J, Demirakca S, Zohsel K, Flor H, Hermann C. Responses to pain in school-aged children with experience in a neonatal intensive care unit: cognitive aspects and maternal influences. Eur J Pain. 2009;13(1):94–101.
24. Goffaux P, Lafrenaye S, Morin M, Patural H, Demers G, Marchand S. Preterm births: can neonatal pain alter the development of endogenous gating systems? Eur J Pain. 2008;12(7):945–51.
25. Anand KJS, Hickey PR. Pain and its effects in the human neonate and fetus. N Engl J Med. 1987;19:1321–9.
26. Ranger M, Johnston CC, Anand KJ. Current controversies regarding pain assessment in neonates. Semin Perinatol. 2007;31(5):283–8.
27. Slater R, Cantarella A, Franck L, Meek J, Fitzgerald M. How well do clinical pain assessment tools reflect pain in neonates? PLoS Med. 2008;5(6e129):0928–33.
28. Slater R, Cantarella A, Yoxen J, et al. Latency to facial expression change following noxious stimulation in infants is dependent on postmenstrual age. Pain. 2009;146(1–2):177–82.
29. Stevens B, Franck L, Gibbins S, et al. Determining the structure of acute pain responses in vulnerable neonates. Can J Nurs Res. 2007;39(2):32–47.
30. Craig KD, Whitfield MF, Grunau RV, Linton J, Hadjistavropoulos HD. Pain in the preterm neonate: behavioural and physiological indices. Pain (Amsterdam). 1993;52:287–99.
31. Grunau RVE, Craig KD. Pain expression in neonates: facial action and cry. Pain (Amsterdam). 1987;28:395–410.
32. Stevens B, Johnston C, Gibbins S, Taddio A, Yamada J. The premature infant pain profile (PIPP): evaluation 13 years after development. Clin J Pain. 2010;26(9):813–30.
33. Als H. Towards a synactive theory of development: promise for the assessment of infant individuality. Infant Ment Health J. 1982; 3:229–43.
34. Gibbins S, Stevens B, Beyene J, Chan PC, Bagg M, Asztalos E. Pain behaviours in extremely low gestational age infants. Early Hum Dev. 2008;84(7):451–8.
35. Slater R, Cantarella A, Gallella S, et al. Cortical pain responses in human infants. J Neurosci. 2006;26(14):3662–6.
36. Slater R, Fabrizi L, Worley A, Meek J, Boyd S, Fitzgerald M. Premature infants display increased noxious-evoked neuronal activity in the brain compared to healthy age-matched term-born infants. Neuroimage. 2010;52(2):583–9.
37. Anand KJ. Pain assessment in preterm neonates. Pediatrics (Evanston IL). 2007;119(3):605–7.
38. Stevens B, Johnston C, Petryshen P, Taddio A. Premature infant pain profile: development and initial validation. Clin J Pain. 1996;12(1):13–22.
39. Johnston CC, Stevens B, Craig KD, Grunau RV. Developmental changes in pain expression in premature, full-term, two- and four-month-old infants. Pain. 1993;52(2):201–8.
40. Stevens BJ, Johnston CC, Horton L. Factors that influence the behavioral pain responses of premature infants. Pain (Amsterdam). 1994;59(1):101–9.
41. Hummel P, Puchalski M, Creech SD, Weiss MG. Clinical reliability and validity of the N-PASS: neonatal pain, agitation and sedation scale with prolonged pain. J Perinatol. 2008;28(1):55–60.
42. Lawerence J, Alcock D, McGrath PJ, Kay J, MacMurray SB, Dulberg C. The development of a tool to assess neonatal pain. Neonatal Netw. 1993;12:59–66.
43. Krechel SW, Bildner J. CRIES: a new neonatal postoperative pain measurement score. Initial testing of validity and reliability. Paediatr Anaesth. 1995;5:53–61.
44. Carbajal R, Paupe A, Hoenn E, Lenclen R, Olivier M. APN: evaluation behavioral scale of acute pain in newborn infants. [French]. Arch Pediatr. 1997;4(7):623–8.

45. Blauer T, Gerstmann D. A simultaneous comparison of three neonatal pain scales during common NICU procedures. Clin J Pain. 1998;14(1):39–47.

46. Hudson-Barr D, Capper-Michel B, Lambert S, Palermo TM, Morbeto K, Lombardo S. Validation of the Pain Assessment in Neonates (PAIN) scale with the Neonatal Infant Pain Scale (NIPS). Neonatal Netw. 2002;21(6):15–21.

47. Holsti L, Grunau RE. Initial validation of the behavioral indicators of infant pain (BIIP). Pain (Amsterdam). 2007;132(3):264–72.

48. Sparshott M. The development of a clinical distress scale for ventilated newborn infants: identification of pain and distress based on validated behavioural scores. J Neonatal Nurs. 1996;2:5–11.

49. Debillon T, Zupan V, Ravault N, Magny JF, Dehan M. Development and initial validation of the EDIN scale, a new tool for assessing prolonged pain in preterm infants. Arch Dis Child Fetal Neonatal Ed. 2001;85(1):F36–41.

50. Stevens BJ, Pillai Riddell R, Oberlander TE, Gibbins S, Anand KJS, McGrath PJ. Assessment of pain in neonates and infants, Pain in neonates and infants, vol. 3. Toronto: Elsevier; 2007. p. 67–90.

51. Duhn LJ, Medves JM. A systematic integrative review of infant pain assessment tools. [Review] [71 refs]. Adv Neonatal Care. 2004;4(3):126–40.

52. Johnston CC, Stevens BJ, Yang F, Horton L. Differential response to pain by very premature neonates. Pain. 1995;61(3):471–9.

53. Sweet SD, McGrath PJ. Physiological measures of pain. In: Finley GA, McGrath PJ, editors. Measurement of pain in infants and children. Seattle: IASP Press; 1998. p. 59–81.

54. Grunau RE, Holsti L, Haley DW, et al. Neonatal procedural pain exposure predicts lower cortisol and behavioral reactivity in preterm infants in the NICU. Pain. 2005;113(3):293–300.

55. Harrison D, Boyce S, Loughnan P, Dargaville P, Storm H, Johnston L. Skin conductance as a measure of pain and stress in hospitalised infants. Early Hum Dev. 2006;82(9):603–8.

56. Hellerud BC, Storm H. Skin conductance and behaviour during sensory stimulation of preterm and term infants. Early Hum Dev. 2002;70(1–2):35–46.

57. Storm H. Development of emotional sweating in preterms measured by skin conductance changes. Early Hum Dev. 2001;62(2):149–58.

58. Eriksson M, Storm H, Fremming A, Schollin J. Skin conductance compared to a combined behavioural and physiological pain measure in newborn infants. Acta Paediatr. 2008;97(1):27–30.

59. Oberlander T, Saul JP. Methodological considerations for the use of heart rate variability as a measure of pain reactivity in vulnerable infants. Clin Perinatol. 2002;29(3):427–43.

60. Slater R, Worley A, Fabrizi L, et al. Evoked potentials generated by noxious stimulation in the human infant brain. Eur J Pain. 2009;14(3):321–6.

61. Slater R, Cornelissen L, Fabrizi L, et al. Oral sucrose as an analgesic drug for procedural pain in newborn infants: a randomised controlled trial. Lancet. 2010;376(9748):1225–32.

62. Lagercrantz H. The birth of consciousness. Early Hum Dev. 2009;85(10 Suppl):S57–8.

63. Slater R, Boyd S, Meek J, Fitzgerald M. Cortical pain responses in the infant brain. Pain. 2006;123(3):332–4.

64. Bartocci M, Bergqvist LL, Lagercrantz H, Anand KJ. Pain activates cortical areas in the preterm newborn brain. Pain (Amsterdam). 2006;122(1–2):109–17.

65. Limperopoulos C, Gauvreau K, O'Leary H, Bassan H, Eichenwald EC, Ringer S. Cerebral hemodynamic changes during intensive care of premature infants. Pediatrics (Evanston IL). 2008;122(5):e1006–13.

66. Soul JS, du Plessis AJ. New technologies in pediatric neurology. Near-infrared spectroscopy. [Review] [53 refs]. Semin Pediatr Neurol. 1999;6(2):101–10.

67. Wolfberg AJ, du Plessis AJ. Near-infrared spectroscopy in the fetus and neonate. [Review] [110 refs]. Clin Perinatol. 2006;33(3):707–28.

68. Hoshi Y. Functional near-infrared optical imaging: utility and limitations in human brain mapping. Psychophysiology. 2003;40(4):511–20.

69. Becerra L, Harris W, Joseph D, Huppert T, Boas DA, Borsook D. Diffuse optical tomography of pain and tactile stimulation: activation in cortical sensory and emotional systems. Neuroimage. 2008;41(2):252–9.

70. Hall RW, Shbarou RM. Drugs of choice for sedation and analgesia in the neonatal ICU. Clin Perinatol. 2009;36(1):15–26.

71. Taddio A, Ohlsson A, Einarson TR, Stevens B, Koren G. A systematic review of lidocaine-prilocaine cream (EMLA) in the treatment of acute pain in neonates. Pediatrics. 1998;101(2):E1.

72. Jain A, Rutter N. Local anaesthetic effect of topical amethocaine gel in neonates: randomised controlled trial. Arch Dis Child Fetal Neonatal Ed. 2000;82(1):F42–5.

73. Larsson BA, Jylli L, Lagercrantz H, Olsson GL. Does a local anaesthetic cream (EMLA) alleviate pain from heel-lancing in neonates? Acta Anaesthesiol Scand. 1995;39(8):1028–31.

74. Larsson BA, Norman M, Bjerring P, Egekvist H, Lagercrantz H, Olsson GL. Regional variations in skin perfusion and skin thickness may contribute to varying efficacy of topical, local anaesthetics in neonates. Paediatr Anaesth. 1996;6:107–10.

75. Taddio A, Lee C, Yip A, Parvez B, McNamara PJ, Shah V. Intravenous morphine and topical tetracaine for treatment of pain in [corrected] neonates undergoing central line placement. [Erratum appears in JAMA. 2006;295(13):1518]. J Am Med Assoc. 2006; 295(7):793–800.

76. Lemyre B, Hogan DL, Gaboury I, Sherlock R, Blanchard C, Moher D. How effective is tetracaine 4% gel, before a venipuncture, in reducing procedural pain in infants: a randomized double-blind placebo controlled trial. BMC Pediatr. 2007;7:7.

77. Ballantyne M, McNair C, Ung E, Gibbins S, Stevens B. A randomized controlled trial evaluating the efficacy of tetracaine gel for pain relief from peripherally inserted central catheters in infants. Adv Neonatal Care. 2003;3(6):297–307.

78. Lindh V, Wiklund U, Hakansson S. Assessment of the effect of EMLA during venipuncture in the newborn by analysis of heart rate variability. Pain. 2000;86(3):247–54.

79. Larsson BA, Tannfeldt G, Lagercrantz H, Olsson GL. Venipuncture is more effective and less painful than heel lancing for blood tests in neonates. Pediatrics (Evanston IL). 1998;101(5):882–6.

80. Jain A, Rutter N. Does topical amethocaine gel reduce the pain of venipuncture in newborn infants? A randomised double blind controlled trial. Arch Dis Child Fetal Neonatal Ed. 2000;83(3):F207–10.

81. Acharya AB, Bustani PC, Phillips JD, Taub NA, Beattie RM. Randomised controlled trial of eutectic mixture of local anaesthetics cream for venipuncture in healthy preterm infants. Arch Dis Child Fetal Neonatal Ed. 1998;78(2):F138–42.

82. Quinn M, Carraccio C, Sacchetti A. Pain, punctures, and pediatricians. Pediatr Emerg Care. 1993;9:12–4.

83. Pinheiro JM, Furdon S, Ochoa LF. Role of local anesthesia during lumbar puncture in neonates. Pediatrics. 1993;91(2):379–82.

84. Kaur G, Gupta P, Kumar A. A randomized trial of eutectic mixture of local anesthetics during lumbar puncture in newborns. Arch Pediatr Adolesc Med. 2003;157(11):1065–70.

85. Brady-Fryer B, Wiebe N, Lander JA. Pain relief for neonatal circumcision. [Review] [99 refs]. Cochrane Database Syst Rev. 2004;4:CD004217..

86. Benini F, Johnston CC, Faucher DJ, Aranda JV. Topical anesthesia during circumcision in newborn infants. J Am Med Assoc. 1993;270:850–3.

87. Taddio A, Stevens B, Craig K, et al. Efficacy and safety of lidocaine-prilocaine cream for pain during circumcision. N Engl J Med. 1997;336(17):1197–201.

88. Lehr VT, Taddio A. Topical anesthesia in neonates: clinical practices and practical considerations. Semin Perinatol. 2007;31(5):323–9.

89. Yamada J, Stinson J, Lamba J, Dickson A, McGrath PJ, Stevens B. A review of systematic reviews on pain interventions in hospitalized infants. Pain Res Manag. 2008;13(5):413–20.

90. Brady-Fryer B, Wiebe N, Lander JA. Pain relief for neonatal circumcision. Cochrane Database Syst Rev. 2008;1.

91. Anand KJ, Johnston CC, Oberlander TF, Taddio A, Lehr VT, Walco GA. Analgesia and local anesthesia during invasive procedures in the neonate. Clin Ther. 2005;27(6):844–76.

92. Shah V, Taddio A, Ohlsson A. Randomised controlled trial of paracetamol for heel prick pain in neonates. Arch Dis Child Fetal Neonatal Ed. 1998;79(3):F209–11.

93. Macke JK. Analgesia for circumcision: effects on newborn behavior and mother/infant interaction. J Obstet Gynecol Neonatal Nurs. 2001;30(5):507–14.

94. Howard CR, Howard FM, Weitzman ML. Acetaminophen analgesia in neonatal circumcision: the effect on pain. Pediatrics (Evanston IL). 1994;4:641–6.

95. Taddio A, Manley J, Potash L, Ipp M, Sgro M, Shah V. Routine immunization practices: use of topical anesthetics and oral analgesics. Pediatrics (Evanston IL). 2007;120(3):e637–43.

96. Badiee Z, Torcan N. Effects of high dose orally administered paracetamol for heel prick pain in premature infants. Saudi Med J. 2009;30(11):1450–3.

97. Manley J, Taddio A. Acetaminophen and ibuprofen for prevention of adverse reactions associated with childhood immunization. [Review] [16 refs]. Ann Pharmacother. 2007;41(7):1227–32.

98. Prymula R, Siegrist CA, Chlibek R, et al. Effect of prophylactic paracetamol administration at time of vaccination on febrile reactions and antibody responses in children: two open-label, randomised controlled trials. Lancet. 2009;374(9698):1339–50.

99. Agrawal S, Fitzsimons JJ, Horn V, Petros A. Intravenous paracetamol for postoperative analgesia in a 4-day-old term neonate. Paediatr Anaesth. 2007;17(1):70–1.

100. Prins SA, Van Dijk M, Van Leeuwen P, et al. Pharmacokinetics and analgesic effects of intravenous propacetamol vs rectal paracetamol in children after major craniofacial surgery. Paediatr Anaesth. 2008;18(7):582–92.

101. Wilson-Smith EM, Morton NS. Survey of i.v. paracetamol (acetaminophen) use in neonates and infants under 1 year of age by UK anesthetists. Paediatr Anaesth. 2009;19(4):329–37.

102. Nandi R, Beacham D, Middleton J, Koltzenburg M, Howard RF, Fitzgerald M. The functional expression of mu opioid receptors on sensory neurons is developmentally regulated; morphine analgesia is less selective in the neonate. Pain. 2004;111(1–2):38–50.

103. Nandi R, Fitzgerald M. Opioid analgesia in the newborn. Euro J Pain: EJP. 2005;9(2):105–8.

104. Allegaert K, Simons SH, Vanhole C, Tibboel D. Developmental pharmacokinetics of opioids in neonates. [Review] [31 refs]. J Opioid Manag. 2007;3(1):59–64.

105. Bouwmeester NJ, Anderson BJ, Tibboel D, Holford NH. Developmental pharmacokinetics of morphine and its metabolites in neonates, infants and young children. Br J Anaesth. 2004;92(2): 208–17.

106. Lynn AM, Slattery JT. Morphine pharmacokinetics in early infancy. Anaesthesia. 1987;66:136–9.

107. Zuppa AF, Mondick JT, Davis L, Cohen D. Population pharmacokinetics of ketorolac in neonates and young infants. Am J Ther. 2009;16(2):143–6.

108. Koren G. Postoperative morphine infusion in newborn infants: assessment of disposition. J Pediatr. 1985;107:963–7.

109. Simons SH, van Dijk M, van Lingen RA, et al. Routine morphine infusion in preterm newborns who received ventilatory support: a randomized controlled trial. JAMA. 2003;290(18):2419–27.

110. Carbajal R, Lenclen R, Jugie M, Paupe A, Barton BA, Anand KJ. Morphine does not provide adequate analgesia for acute procedural pain among preterm neonates. Pediatrics. 2005;115(6):1494–500.

111. Anand KJ, Barton BA, McIntosh N, et al. Analgesia and sedation in preterm neonates who require ventilatory support: results from the NOPAIN trial. Neonatal Outcome and Prolonged Analgesia in Neonates [Published erratum appears in Arch Pediatr Adolesc Med. 1999;153(8):895]. Arch Pediatr Adolesc Med. 1999;153(4): 331–338.

112. Anand KJ, Hall RW, Desai N, et al. Effects of morphine analgesia in ventilated preterm neonates: primary outcomes from the NEOPAIN randomised trial. Lancet. 2004;363(9422):1673–82.

113. Bellu R, de Waal KA, Zanini R. Opioids for neonates receiving mechanical ventilation. Cochrane Database Syst Rev. 2005;1: CD004212.

114. Lago P, Tiozzo C, Boccuzzo G, Allegro A, Zacchello F. Remifentanil for percutaneous intravenous central catheter placement in preterm infant: a randomized controlled trial. Paediatr Anaesth. 2008;18(8):736–44.

115. Lago P, Garetti E, Merazzi D, et al. Guidelines for procedural pain in the newborn. Acta Paediatr. 2009;98(6):932–9.

116. American Academy of Pediatrics Committee on F, Newborn, American Academy of Pediatrics Section on S, et al. Prevention and management of pain in the neonate: an update. Pediatrics (Evanston IL). 2006;118(5):2231–41.

117. Shah V, Ohlsson A. The effectiveness of premedication for endotracheal intubation in mechanically ventilated neonates. A systematic review. Clinics Perinatol. 2002;29(3):535–54.

118. Kumar P, Denson SE, Mancuso TJ. Premedication for nonemergency endotracheal intubation in the neonate. Pediatrics. 2010; 125(3):608–15.

119. Lemyre B, Doucette J, Kalyn A, Gray S, Marrin ML. Morphine for elective endotracheal intubation in neonates: a randomized trial [ISRCTN43546373]. BMC Pediatr. 2004;4(1):20.

120. Choong K, AlFaleh K, Doucette J, et al. Remifentanil for endotracheal intubation in neonates: a randomised controlled trial. Arch Dis Child Fetal Neonatal Ed. 2010;95(2):F80–4.

121. Pereira e Silva Y, Gomez RS, Marcatto Jde O, Maximo TA, Barbosa RF, Silva AC Simoes e. Morphine versus remifentanil for intubating preterm neonates. Arch Dis Child Fetal Neonatal Ed. 2007;92(4):F293–4.

122. Melzack R, Wall P. Pain mechanisms: new theory. Science (Washington DC). 1965;150:971–9.

123. Benedetti F. Placebo and endogenous mechanisms of analgesia. Handb Exp Pharmacol. 2007;177:393–413.

124. Fitzgerald M, Millard C, MacIntosh N. Hyperalgesia in premature infants. Lancet (London). 1988;1(8580):292.

125. de Vries JIP, Visser GH, Prechtl HF. The emergence of fetal behaviour. I. Qualitative aspects. Early Hum Dev. 1982;7(4):301–22.

126. Pinelli J, Symington A. Non-nutritive sucking for promoting physiologic stability and nutrition in preterm infants [Systematic Review]. Cochrane Database Syst Rev 2007;1.

127. Corbo MG, Mansi G, Stagni A, et al. Nonnutritive sucking during heelstick procedures decreases behavioral distress in the newborn infant. Biol Neonate. 2000;77(3):162–7.

128. Campos RG. Rocking and pacifiers: two comforting interventions for heelstick pain. Res Nurs Health. 1994;17(5):321–31.

129. Elserafy FA, Alsaedi SA, Louwrens J, Mersal AY, Bin Sadiq B. Oral sucrose and a pacifier for pain relief during simple procedures in preterm infants: a randomized controlled trial. Ann Saudi Med. 2009;29(3):184–8.

130. Curtis SJ, Jou H, Ali S, Vandermeer B, Klassen T. A randomized controlled trial of sucrose and/or pacifier as analgesia for infants receiving venipuncture in a pediatric emergency department. BMC Pediatr. 2007;7:27.

131. Akman I, Ozek E, Bilgen H, Ozdogan T, Cebeci D. Sweet solutions and pacifiers for pain relief in newborn infants. J Pain. 2002;3(3):199–202.

132. Field T, Goldson E. Pacifying effects of nonnutritive sucking on term and preterm neonates during heelstick procedures. Pediatrics (Evanston IL). 1984;74:1012–5.

133. Miller HD, Anderson GC. Nonnutritive sucking: effects on crying and heart rate in intubated infants requiring assisted mechanical ventilation. Neonatal Intensive Care. 1994;46–48.

134. Stevens B, Johnston C, Franck L, Petryshen P, Jack A, Foster G. The efficacy of developmentally sensitive interventions and sucrose for relieving procedural pain in very low birth weight neonates. Nurs Res. 1999;48(1):35–43.

135. Boyle EM, Freer Y, Khan-Orakzai Z, et al. Sucrose and nonnutritive sucking for the relief of pain in screening for retinopathy of prematurity: a randomised controlled trial. Arch Dis Child Fetal Neonatal Ed. 2006;91(3):F166–8.

136. Carbajal R, Chauvet X, Couderc S, Olivier-Martin M. Randomised trial of analgesic effects of sucrose, glucose, and pacifiers in term neonates [see comments]. Br Med J. 1999;319(7222):1393–7.

137. Bellieni CV, Bagnoli F, Perrone S, et al. Effect of multisensory stimulation on analgesia in term neonates: a randomized controlled trial. Pediatr Res. 2002;51(4):460–3.

138. Bellieni CV, Buonocore G, Nenci A, Franci N, Cordelli DM, Bagnoli F. Sensorial saturation: an effective analgesic tool for heel-prick in preterm infants: a prospective randomized trial. Biol Neonate. 2001;80(1):15–8.

139. Bo LK, Callaghan P. Soothing pain-elicited distress in Chinese neonates. Pediatrics (Evanston IL). 2000;105(4):E49.

140. Campos RG. Soothing pain elicited distress in infants with swaddling and pacifiers. Child Dev. 1989;60:781–92.

141. Graillon A, Barr RG, Young SN, Wright JH, Hendricks LA. Differential response to intraoral sucrose, quinine and corn oil in crying human newborns. Physiol Behav. 1997;62(2):317–25.

142. Blass EM, Ciaramitaro V. A new look at some old mechanisms in human newborns: taste and tactile determinants of state, affect, and action. Monogr Soc Res Child Dev. 1994;59:1–80.

143. Stevens B, Yamada J, Ohlsson A. Sucrose for analgesia in newborn infants undergoing painful procedures. Cochrane Database Syst Rev. 2010;1:CD001069.

144. Gaspardo CM, Miyase CI, Chimello JT, Martinez FE, Martins Linhares MB. Is pain relief equally efficacious and free of side effects with repeated doses of oral sucrose in preterm neonates? Pain. 2008;137(1):16–25.

145. Harrison D, Loughnan P, Manias E, Gordon I, Johnston L. Repeated doses of sucrose in infants continue to reduce procedural pain during prolonged hospitalizations. Nurs Res. 2009;58(6):427–34.

146. Johnston CC, Filion F, Snider L, et al. Routine sucrose analgesia during the first week of life in neonates younger than 31 weeks' postconceptional age. Pediatrics. 2002;110(3):523–8.

147. Johnston CC, Filion F, Snider L, et al. How much sucrose is too much sucrose? Pediatrics (Evanston IL). 2007;119(1):226.

148. Stevens B, Yamada J, Beyene J, et al. Consistent management of repeated procedural pain with sucrose in preterm neonates: is it effective and safe for repeated use over time? Clin J Pain. 2005;21(6):543–8.

149. Akcam M, Ormeci AR. Oral hypertonic glucose spray: a practical alternative for analgesia in the newborn. Acta Paediatr. 2004;93(10):1330–3.

150. Eriksson M, Gradin M, Schollin J. Oral glucose and venipuncture reduce blood sampling pain in newborns. Early Hum Dev. 1999;55(3):211–8.

151. Deshmukh LS, Udani RH. Analgesic effect of oral glucose in preterm infants during venipuncture–a double-blind, randomized, controlled trial. J Trop Pediatr. 2002;48(3):138–41.

152. Carbajal R, Lenclen R, Gajdos V, Jugie M, Paupe A. Crossover trial of analgesic efficacy of glucose and pacifier in very preterm neonates during subcutaneous injections. Pediatrics. 2002;110(2 Pt 1):389–93.

153. Okan F, Coban A, Ince Z, Yapici Z, Can G. Analgesia in preterm newborns: the comparative effects of sucrose and glucose. Eur J Pediatr. 2007;166(10):1017–24.

154. Guala A. Glucose or sucrose as an analgesic for newborns: a randomised controlled blind trial. Minerva Pediatr. 2001;53(4):271–4.

155. Isik U. Comparison of oral glucose and sucrose solutions on pain response in neonates. J Pain. 2000;1(4):275–8.

156. Abad F, Diaz-Gomez NM, Domenech E, Gonzalez D, Robayna M, Feria M. Oral sucrose compares favourably with lidocaine-prilocaine cream for pain relief during venipuncture in neonates. Acta Paediatr. 2001;90(2):160–5.

157. Gradin M, Eriksson M, Holmqvist G, Holstein A, Schollin J. Pain reduction at venipuncture in newborns: oral glucose compared with local anesthetic cream. Pediatrics. 2002;110(6):1053–7.

158. van Sleuwen BE, Engelberts AC, Boere-Boonekamp MM, Kuis W, Schulpen TW, L'Hoir MP. Swaddling: a systematic review. [Review] [82 refs]. Pediatrics (Evanston IL). 2007;120(4):e1097–106.

159. Prasopkittikun T, Tilokskulchai F. Management of pain from heel stick in neonates: an analysis of research conducted in Thailand. J Perinat Neonatal Nurs. 2003;17(4):304–12.

160. Huang CM, Tung WS, Kuo LL, Ying-Ju C. Comparison of pain responses of premature infants to the heelstick between containment and swaddling. J Nurs Res. 2004;12(1):31–40.

161. Corff KE, Seideman R, Venkataraman PS, Lutes L, Yates B. Facilitated tucking: a nonpharmacologic comfort measure for pain in preterm neonates. J Obstet Gynecol Neonatal Nurs. 1995;24(2):143–7.

162. Ward-Larson C, Horn RA, Gosnell F. The efficacy of facilitated tucking for relieving procedural pain of endotracheal suctioning in very low birthweight infants. MCN Am J Matern Child Nurs. 2004;29(3):151–6. quiz 157–158.

163. Axelin A, Salantera S, Lehtonen L. 'Facilitated tucking by parents' in pain management of preterm infants-a randomized cross-over trial. Early Hum Dev. 2006;82(4):241–7.

164. Axelin A, Salantera S, Kirjavainen J, Lehtonen L. Oral glucose and parental holding preferable to opioid in pain management in preterm infants. Clin J Pain. 2009;25(2):138–45.

165. Mathai S, Natrajan N, Rajalakshmi NR. A comparative study of nonpharmacological methods to reduce pain in neonates. Indian Pediatr. 2006;43(12):1070–5.

166. Johnston CC, Stremler RL, Stevens BJ, Horton LJ. Effectiveness of oral sucrose and simulated rocking on pain response in preterm neonates. Pain. 1997;72(1–2):193–9.

167. Hepper PG, Shahidullah BS. Development of fetal hearing. Arch Dis Child. 1994;71(2):F81–7.

168. Hepper PG. Fetal memory: does it exist? What does it do? [Review] [59 refs]. Acta Paediatr Suppl. 1996;416:16–20.

169. DeCasper AJ, Fifer WP. Of human bonding: newborns prefer their mothers voices. Science (Washington DC). 1980;208:1174–6.

170. Standley JM, Moore RS. Therapeutic effects of music and mother's voice on premature infants. Pediatr Nurs. 1995;21(6):509–12. 574.

171. Kurihara H, Chiba H, Shimizu Y, et al. Behavioral and adrenocortical responses to stress in neonates and the stabilizing effects of maternal heartbeat on them. Early Hum Dev. 1996;46(1–2):117–27.

172. Johnston CC, Filion F, Nuyt AM. Recorded maternal voice for preterm neonates undergoing heel lance. Adv Neonatal Care. 2007;7(5):258–66.

173. Hartling L, Shaik MS, Tjosvold L, Leicht R, Liang Y, Kumar M. Music for medical indications in the neonatal period: a systematic review of randomised controlled trials. Arch Dis Child Fetal Neonatal Ed. 2009;94(5):F349–54.

174. Joyce BA, Keck JF, Gerkensmeyer J. Evaluation of pain management interventions for neonatal circumcision pain. J Pediatr Health Care. 2001;15(3):105–14.

175. Butt ML, Kisilevsky BS. Music modulates behaviour of premature infants following heel lance. Can J Nurs Res. 2000;31(4): 17–39.

176. Schaal B, Marlier L, Soussignan R. Olfactory function in the human fetus: evidence from selective neonatal responsiveness to

the odor of amniotic fluid. Behav Neurosci. 1998;112(6): 1438–49.

177. Varendi H, Christensson K, Porter RH, Winberg J. Soothing effect of amniotic fluid smell in newborn infants. Early Hum Dev. 1998;51(1):47–55.

178. Rattaz C, Goubet N, Bullinger A. The calming effect of a familiar odor on full-term newborns. J Dev Behav Pediatr. 2005;26(2): 86–92.

179. Goubet N, Strasbaugh K, Chesney J. Familiarity breeds content? Soothing effect of a familiar odor on full-term newborns. J Dev Behav Pediatr. 2007;28(3):189–94.

180. Goubet N, Rattaz C, Pierrat V, Bullinger A, Lequien P. Olfactory experience mediates response to pain in preterm newborns. Dev Psychobiol. 2003;42(2):171–80.

181. Bellieni CV, Cordelli DM, Marchi S, et al. Sensorial saturation for neonatal analgesia. Clin J Pain. 2007;23(3):219–21.

182. Bellieni C, Maffei M, Ancora G, et al. Is the ABC pain scale reliable for premature babies? Acta Paediatr. 2007;96(7):1008–10.

183. Gibbins S, Stevens B. Mechanisms of sucrose and non-nutritive sucking in procedural pain management in infants. Pain Res Manag. 2001;6(1):21–8.

184. Jahangeer AC, Mellier D, Caston J. Influence of olfactory stimulation on nociceptive behavior in mice. Physiol Behav. 1997;62(2): 359–66.

185. Shah PS, Aliwalas LL, Shah V. Breastfeeding or breast milk for procedural pain in neonates. Cochrane Database Syst Rev. 2008;1.

186. Carbajal R, Veerapen S, Couderc S. Breastfeeding as an analgesic for term newborns during venipunctures. Proc Acad Pediatr Soc. 2002;2105

187. Codipietro L, Ceccarelli M, Ponzone A. Breastfeeding or oral sucrose solution in term neonates receiving heel lance: a randomized, controlled trial. Pediatrics (Evanston IL). 2008;122(3): e716–21.

188. Gradin M, Finnstrom O, Schollin J. Feeding and oral glucose–additive effects on pain reduction in newborns. Early Hum Dev. 2004;77(1–2):57–65.

189. Efe E, Ozer ZC. The use of breast-feeding for pain relief during neonatal immunization injections. Appl Nurs Res. 2007;20(1): 10–6.

190. Dilli DK, Küçük IG, Dallar Y. Interventions to reduce pain during vaccination in infancy. J Pediatr. 2009;154(3):385–90.

191. Abdel Razek A, Az El-Dein N. Effect of breast-feeding on pain relief during infant immunization injections. Int J Nurs Pract. 2009;15(2):99–104.

192. Phillips RM, Chantry CJ, Gallagher MP. Analgesic effects of breast-feeding or pacifier use with maternal holding in term infants. Ambul Pediatr. 2005;5(6):359–64.

193. Charpak N, Ruiz-Pelaez JG, Charpak Y. Rey-Martinez kangaroo mother program: an alternative way of caring for low birth weight infants? One year mortality in a two cohort study. Pediatrics (Evanston IL). 1994;94(6:Pt 1):t-10.

194. Conde-Agudelo A, Diaz-Rossello JL, Belizan JM. Kangaroo mother care to reduce morbidity and mortality in low birthweight infants. [update of Cochrane Database Syst Rev. 2000;(4): CD002771; PMID: 11034759]. [Review] [21 refs]. Cochrane Database of Syst Rev. 2003(2):CD002771.

195. Engler AJ, Ludington-Hoe SM, Cusson RM, et al. Kangaroo care: national survey of practice, knowledge, barriers, and perceptions. MCN, Am J Matern Child Nurs. 2002;27(3):146–53.

196. Feldman R, Eidelman AI. Skin-to-skin contact (Kangaroo Care) accelerates autonomic and neurobehavioural maturation in preterm infants. Dev Med Child Neurol. 2003;45(4):274–81.

197. Johnston CC, Stevens B, Pinelli J, et al. Kangaroo care is effective in diminishing pain response in preterm neonates. Arch Pediatr Adolesc Med. 2003;157(11):1084–8.

198. Moore ER, Anderson GC, Bergman N. Early skin-to-skin contact for mothers and their healthy newborn infants. Cochrane Database Syst Rev. 2007;4.

199. Acolet D, Sleath K, Whitelaw A. Oxygenation, heart rate, and temperature in very low birthweight infants during skin-to-skin contact with their mothers. Acta Paediatr Scand. 1989;78: 189–93.

200. Bohnhorst B, Heyne T, Peter CS, Poets CF. Skin-to-skin (kangaroo) care, respiratory control, and thermoregulation. J Pediatr. 2001;138(2):193–7.

201. Stevens BJ, Johnston C, Petryshen P, Taddio A. Premature infant pain profile: development and initial validation. Clin J Pain. 1996;12(1):13–22.

202. Arditi H, Feldman R, Eidelman AI. Effects of human contact and vagal regulation on pain reactivity and visual attention in newborns. Dev Psychobiol. 2006;48(7):561–73.

203. Mooncey S, Giannakoulopoulos X, Glover V, Acolet D, Modi N. The effect of mother-infant skin-to-skin contact on plasma cortisol and beta-endorphin concentrations in preterm newborns. Infant Behav Dev. 1997;20(4):553–7.

204. Michelsson K, Christensson K, Rothganger H, Winberg J. Crying in separated and non-separated newborns: sound spectrographic analysis. Acta Paediatr. 1996;85(4):471–5.

205. Gray L, Watt L, Blass EM. Skin-to-skin contact is analgesic in healthy newborns. Pediatrics (Evanston IL). 2000;105(1):e14.

206. Johnston C, Campbell-Yeo M, Fernandes A, Inglis D, Streiner D, Zee R. Skin-to-skin care for procedural pain in neonates (Protocol). Cochrane Database Syst Rev. 2010;(3):Art. No.: CD008435. DOI: 008410.001002/14651858.CD14008435.

207. Akcan E, Yigit R, Atici A. The effect of kangaroo care on pain in premature infants during invasive procedures. Turk J Pediatr. 2009;51(1):14–8.

208. Johnston CC, Filion F, Campbell-Yeo M, et al. Enhanced kangaroo mother care for heel lance in preterm neonates: a crossover trial. J Perinatol. 2009;29(1):51–6.

209. Johnston CC, Filion F, Campbell-Yeo M, et al. Kangaroo mother care diminishes pain from heel lance in very preterm neonates: a crossover trial. BMC Pediatr. 2008;8:13.

210. Castral TC, Warnock F, Leite AM, Haas VJ, Scochi CG. The effects of skin-to-skin contact during acute pain in preterm newborns. Euro J Pain: EJP. 2008;12(4):464–71.

211. de Sousa Freire NjB, Santos Garcia JoB, Carvalho Lamy Z. Evaluation of analgesic effect of skin-to-skin contact compared to oral glucose in preterm neonates. Pain (Amsterdam). 2008;139(1): 28–33.

212. Chermont AG, Falcao LF, de Souza Silva EH, de Cassia Xavier Balda R, Guinsburg R. Skin-to-skin contact and/or oral 25% dextrose for procedural pain relief for term newborn infants. Pediatrics. 2009;124(6):e1101–7.

213. Kashaninia Z, Sajedi F, Rahgozar M, Noghabi FA. The effect of kangaroo care on behavioral responses to pain of an intramuscular injection in neonates. J Spec Pediatr Nurs. 2008;13(4):275–80.

214. Kostandy RR, Ludington-Hoe SM, Cong X, et al. Kangaroo care (skin contact) reduces crying response to pain in preterm neonates: pilot results. Pain Manag Nurs. 2008;9(2):55–65.

215. Ludington-Hoe SM, Hosseini R, Torowizc DL. Skin-to-skin contact (kangaroo care) analgesia for preterm infant heelstick. AACN Clin Issues. 2005;16(3):373–87.

216. Cong X, Ludington-Hoe SM, McCain G, Fu P. Kangaroo care modifies preterm infant heart rate variability in response to heel stick pain: pilot study. Early Hum Dev. 2009;85(9):561–7.

217. Ferber SG, Makhoul IR. The effect of skin-to-skin contact (kangaroo care) shortly after birth on the neurobehavioral responses of the term newborn: a randomized, controlled trial. Pediatrics (Evanston IL). 2004;113(4):858–65.

Assessing Disability in the Pain Patient

23

Steven D. Feinberg and Christopher R. Brigham

Key Points
- Assessing disability in the pain patient is often difficult due to both administrative and clinical issues, yet this assessment is essential.
- Clinically, quantifying pain remains problematic as chronic pain is a subjective phenomenon, often associated with confounding behavioral, characterological, personality, and psychological issues.
- Typically, the physician does not define "disability"; rather, the physician defines clinical issues, functional deficits, and, when requested, impairment. Disability is most often an administrative determination.
- The assessment of disability associated with chronic pain is complex, and the evaluator must approach the clinical evaluation with recognition of the many factors associated with the experience of pain and disability.
- The treating physician who has a doctor–patient relationship with the claimant may have a different perspective than the "independent" disability evaluator.
- While an independent medical evaluation has some similarities to a comprehensive medical consultation, there are significant differences.

S.D. Feinberg, M.D. (✉)
Feinberg Medical Group, 825 El Camino Real, Palo Alto, CA 94301, USA

Stanford University School of Medicine, Stanford, CA USA

American Pain Solutions, San Diego, CA USA
e-mail: stevenfeinberg@hotmail.com

C.R. Brigham, M.D.
Brigham and Associates, Inc, N. Kalaheo Avenue, Suite C-312, Kailua, HI 96734, USA

American Medical Association, Chicago, IL, USA
e-mail: cbrigham@cbrigham.com

Introduction

Assessing disability in the pain patient is often difficult due to both administrative and clinical issues, yet this assessment is essential. Administratively, it is complicated by numerous states, federal, and private systems and policies with different definitions and benefit systems. Clinically, quantifying pain remains problematic as chronic pain is a subjective phenomenon, often associated with confounding behavioral, characterological, personality, and psychological issues. Additionally, the terms impairment and disability are often misunderstood. Furthermore, underlying personality structure and motivation are often determinates for disability. Chronic-pain complaints may be linked with significant disability [1]. Typically, the physician does not define "disability"; rather, the physician defines clinical issues, functional deficits, and, when requested, impairment. Disability is most often an administrative determination.

Pain is the most common cause of disability, with chronic low back pain alone accounting for more disability than any other condition [2]. Disability related to back pain has increased, although there is no significant change in back injuries or pain [3, 4]. Headache disorders are frequently associated with work loss [5]. Despite advances in physiologic understanding and interventions, challenges associated with chronic pain and disability increase.

The pain associated with specific recognized physical conditions needs to be distinguished from somatoform pain disorder. The essential feature of somatoform pain disorder in DSM-IV [6] is preoccupation with pain in the absence of physical findings that adequately account for the pain and its intensity, as well as the presence of psychological factors that are judged to have a major role. Somatization is defined as a person's conscious or unconscious use of the body or bodily symptoms for psychological purposes or psychological gain [7, 8]. Somatization is characterized by the propensity to experience and report somatic symptoms that have no pathophysiologic explanation, to misattribute them to disease, and to seek medical attention for them. Somatization can be acute or chronic and may be associated with medical comorbidity, an underlying psychiatric syndrome, a coexistent personality disorder, or a significant psychosocial stressor [9]. Somatoform disorders, factitious disorders, and malingering represent various degrees of illness behavior characterized by the process of somatization.

It is important to recognize that in chronic-pain states, physical and psychological factors typically are both present and overlap and that a quality physical examination is critical before dismissing the problem as being purely psychological.

The *biopsychosocial* approach is currently viewed as the most appropriate perspective to the understanding, assessment, and treatment of chronic-pain disorders and disability [2–4, 10, 11]. Chronic pain reflects a complex and dynamic interaction among biological, psychological, and social factors.

Pain, impairment, and disability may coexist, or be independent [5]. Pain is a subjective experience defined by the International Association for the Study of Pain as "an unpleasant sensory and emotional experience associated with actual or potential tissue damage or described in terms of such damage" [12]. Impairment is defined in the AMA *Guides to the Evaluation of Permanent Impairment* (AMA *Guides*) [13] as "a significant deviation, loss, or loss of use of any body system or function in an individual with a health condition, disorder, or disease." Typically, the AMA *Guides* determines impairment on the basis of specific objective findings, rather than on subjective complaints. The AMA *Guides* defines disability as "an umbrella term for activity limitations and/or participation restrictions in an individual with a health condition, disorder or disease." Waddell notes that pain is a symptom, not a clinical sign, or a diagnosis, or a disease, whereas disability is restricted activity [14]. Managing pain does not guarantee that the disability will lessen or resolve. There is not a direct relationship between pain and disability.

Although it is appealing to define disability on the basis of objective as opposed to subjective factors, this is not always the case. The Institute of Medicine Committee on Pain and Disability and Chronic Illness Behavior concluded that "the notion that all impairments should be verifiable by objective evidence is administratively necessary for an entitlement program. Yet this notion is fundamentally at odds with a realistic understanding of how disease and injury operate to incapacitate people. Except for a very few conditions, such as the loss of a limb, blindness, deafness, paralysis, or coma, most diseases and injuries do not prevent people from working by mechanical failure. Rather, people are incapacitated by a variety of unbearable sensations when they try to work" [15].

Assessing disability in the pain patient is thus a challenging endeavor. While some individuals present with a clear and direct connection between pathology and loss of function, it is problematic to measure loss of functional ability in the individual whose behavior and perception of disability and functional loss is significant, sometimes far exceeding that which would be expected from the physical pathology. Some people with chronic pain seek the designation of being "disabled" because of perceived incapacity associated with their portrayed pain and physical dysfunction. For some, seeking such designation is a logical extension of suffering a loss of capacity and utilizing an available benefit system. Others may portray being disability as a reflection of anger, dissatisfaction, or a sense of entitlement.

For some, the designation of being disabled is more complex and may involve seeking attention and/or other benefits that for some observers may seem excessive, unreasonable, and unnecessary. The request for assistance or insurance benefits may take various forms such as a disability parking permit, avoiding waiting lines, housing assistance, help with household chores, and benefits such as monetary payments or subsidies. The individual may claim incapacity (including from work) and request disability benefits under various private, state, or federal programs.

The physician performing a clinical evaluation that will be used to determine disability should perform a biopsychosocial assessment, recognizing the array of factors that relate to the experience of pain and disability. From a physical perspective, it is necessary to clarify the physical pathology. Some pathology cannot be directly measured (headache, neuropathic pain, etc.), and other pathology may have been missed (tumor, herniated disk, complex regional pain syndrome). Secondary to problems with chronic pain, there may be other problems, such as physical deconditioning and secondary psychological issues. Two individuals with similar injuries and resulting pathological changes may present with distinctly different experiences and perceptions. The first may have little or no complaints or perceived disability, while the second individual may present with significant pain behavior and dysfunction.

There may be other nonphysical (psychosocial, behavioral, and cultural) ramifications that may help explain the second individual's pain presentation and assertion of functional loss despite physical findings that do not support the reported disability. Assuming the individual is presenting in an honest and credible manner, the physician then must opine on impairment or functional issues considering physical and these other nonphysical factors. If requested, the physician may also opine on disability. Opining on disability requires an understanding of specific definitions of disability and often specific occupational functional requirements.

Symptom magnification, i.e., illness behavior, is common, particularly in the context of subjective experiences such as chronic pain or litigation. When the individual is not credible or there is purposeful misrepresentation, such as malingering, it may not be possible to accurately define any disability.

The assessment of disability associated with chronic pain is complex, and the evaluator must approach the clinical evaluation with recognition of the many factors associated with the experience of pain and disability.

Symptom Magnification and Malingering

Symptom magnification, inappropriate illness behavior, and embellishment are not uncommon (malingering is less common but occurs and should be considered), particularly in medicolegal circumstances and entitlement programs. Therefore, evaluators need to consider whether the presenting complaints are congruent with recognized conditions and known pathophysiology and have been consistent over time. The evaluator should also determine if there is inappropriate illness behavior.

Pain behaviors (i.e., facial grimacing, holding or supporting affected body part or area, limping or distorted gait, shifting, extremely slow movements, rigidity, moaning, or inappropriate use of a cane) may indicate symptom magnification.

Nonorganic findings, i.e., findings that are not explained by physical pathology, may also support a conclusion of symptom magnification. Nonorganic findings have been described dating back to the early part of the twentieth century [16]. Since that time, a number of nonorganic signs have been defined [17]. In an effort to maximize information from the evaluation, physicians routinely test for nonorganic physical signs. Gordon Waddell, M.D., described five signs to assist in determining the contribution of psychological factors to patients' low back pain [18]. He was specifically interested in developing screening tests to determine the likelihood a patient would have a good outcome from surgery. The physician must perform all five Waddell tests—evaluation for excessive tenderness, regional weakness, overreaction, distraction, and simulation. Isolated positive signs have no clinical or predictive value, and only a score of three or more positive signs is considered clinically significant. These tests were not designed to detect malingering.

Malingering is defined in the *Diagnostic and Statistical Manual for Mental Disorders, Fourth Edition-Text Revised (DSM-IV-TR)* [19] as the "intentional production of false or grossly exaggerated physical or psychological symptoms, motivated by external incentives such as avoiding military duty, avoiding work, obtaining financial compensation, evading criminal prosecution, or obtaining drugs." The DSM-IV-TR states:

Malingering should be suspected if any combination of the following is noted:

1. Medicolegal context of presentation (e.g., the person is referred by an attorney to the clinician for examination)
2. Marked discrepancy between the person's claimed stress or disability and the objective findings
3. Lack of cooperation during the diagnostic evaluation and in complying with the prescribed treatment regimen
4. The presence of antisocial personality disorder

Malingering occurs along a spectrum—from embellishment to symptom magnification to blatant misrepresentation. The possibility of obtaining disability benefits or financial rewards or being relieved from other responsibilities, such as work, increases the likelihood of malingering. Patients may unconsciously or consciously exaggerate their symptoms. With malingering, the intent is purposeful. Ill-defined complaints occur in a circumscribed group, perhaps in a setting of poor morale or conflict, also may be viewed with suspicion. If there are suggestions of significant illness behavior or malingering, a careful investigation including a multidisciplinary evaluation and psychological testing may be required [20, 21].

Treating Physician Versus Independent Medical Evaluation

The treating physician who has a doctor–patient relationship with the claimant may have a different perspective than the "independent" disability evaluator. The treating physician often takes a patient-advocate role and may have little desire or experience to comment on disability, nor will that physician be able to define disability in an independent manner [22].

Frequently, conflict and distrust develops between claimants and the independent evaluating physicians who evaluate them and the claims examiners handling their claim. Patients often report that their problem is being discounting, while physician disability evaluators and claims representatives may express doubt and skepticism about claimants' chronic-pain complaints and reported loss of functional capacity.

The physician has the predicament of viewing the subjective reports in relationship with the objective evidence of tissue damage or organ pathology to come up with some final assessment about the extent to which the patient really is disabled from functional activities. It is not difficult to see how the treating physician advocating for the patient will have a different perspective than the "independent" physician evaluating a claimant for disability.

The "independent" medical evaluator (IME) is also not without his or her biases, and in some jurisdictions, only plaintiff and defense IMEs are the norm. The true IME is used by both sides and in some settings is referred to as the "agreed" medical evaluator (AME).

When the physician provides treatment, the doctor–patient relationship is one of trust. The physician is acting as an agent for the patient. When performing a disability evaluation, the physician is acting as agent for the state or agency requesting the evaluation. In 1992, Sullivan and Loeser recommended that physicians refuse to do disability evaluation on patients they are treating [23].

The problem with this is that adverse consequences may ensue for the patient who may be cut off from benefits absent a signed disability form.

Disability Versus Impairment

The two main terms when discussing disability are impairment and disability. The following definitions are from the AMA *Guides,* the World Health Organization (WHO), and from various state and federal programs.

The AMA *Guides to the Evaluation of Permanent Impairment,* Sixth Edition (hereafter referred to as the *Guides*), defines disability as "an umbrella term for activity limitations and/or participation restrictions in an individual with a health condition, disorder or disease." The AMA *Guides* defines *impairment* as "a significant deviation, loss, or loss of use of any body system or function in an individual with a health condition, disorder, or disease." The sixth edition, published in December 2007, introduces new approaches to rating impairment. The leadership for this edition was provided by Robert Rondinelli, M.D., an experienced physical medicine and rehabilitation physician; therefore, this edition reflects principles of this specialty. An innovative methodology is used to enhance the relevancy of impairment ratings, improve internal consistency, promote greater precision, and simplify the rating process. The approach is based on a modification of the conceptual framework of the International Classification of Functioning, Disability, and Health (ICF), although the fundamental principles underlying the *Guides* remain unchanged.

The World Health Organization (WHO) defines impairment as "any loss or abnormality of psychological, physiological or anatomical structure or function." Problems in body function or structure involve a significant deviation or loss. Impairments of structure can involve an anomaly, defect, loss, or other significant deviation in body structures.

The *International Classification of Functioning, Disability, and Health* (ICF) [24] changes the emphasis from the word "disability" to *activity* and *activity limitation* (WHO 2000). ICF defines activity as "something a person does, ranging from very basic elementary or simple to complex." Activity limitation is "a difficulty in the performance, accomplishment, or completion of an activity. Difficulties in performing activities occur when there is a qualitative or quantitative alteration in the way in which activities are carried out. Difficulty encompasses all the ways in which the doing of the activity may be affected."

Federal and state agencies generally use a definition that is specific to a particular program or service. To be found disabled for purposes of Social Security disability benefits, individuals must have a severe disability (or combination of disabilities) that has lasted, or is expected to last, at least 12 months or result in death and which prevents working at a "substantial gainful activity" level (1). Impairment is described as an anatomical, physiological, or psychological abnormality that can be shown by medically acceptable clinical and laboratory diagnostic techniques.

The Americans with Disabilities Act (ADA) has a three-part definition of *disability.* Under ADA, an individual with a disability is a person who (1) has a physical or mental impairment that substantially limits one or more major life activities, or (2) has a record of such an impairment, or (3) is regarded as having such an impairment. A *physical impairment* is defined by ADA as "any physiological disorder or condition, cosmetic disfigurement, or anatomical loss affecting one or more of the following body systems: neurological, musculoskeletal, special sense organs, respiratory (including speech organs), cardiovascular, reproductive, digestive, genitourinary, hemic and lymphatic, skin, and endocrine."

Regardless of the system, the term impairment defines a measurable change (any loss or abnormality psychological, physiological, or anatomical structure or function) and is consistent and measurable across different systems and programs. On the other hand, disability is a social construct in that each program or system defines it differently and assigns different weights and benefits to those definitions. One can be "disabled" in one system of benefits and not in another despite the same impairment. Disability usually results from an impairment that results in a functional loss of ability to perform an activity.

It is imperative to distinguish the difference between impairment and disability. One individual can be impaired significantly and have no disability, while another individual can be quite disabled with only limited impairment.

For example, a person with a below-knee amputation may be working full time quite successfully as a pianist and, therefore, would not meet the Social Security Administration (SSA's) definition of being disabled. On the other hand, this same pianist might have a relatively minor injury to a digital nerve that severely limits his/her ability to perform basic work activities such as playing a difficult piano concerto. In some disability systems, a person in this situation might meet the definition of partial disabled, even though he/she can do other work.

Perhaps, another way to distinguish the terms disability and impairment is as follows: Some diseases cause a negative change at the molecular, cellular, or tissue level which leads to a structural or functional change at the organ level, a measurable impairment. At the level of the person, there is a deficit in daily activities and this is the disability.

Because of this difference between impairment and disability, and despite the fact that many disability systems are work-injury-loss related, the widely used AMA *Guides* has stated that impairment ratings are not intended for use as direct determinants of work disability. The impairment rating is rather based on universal factors present in all individuals, the level of impact of the condition on performance of activities of daily living, rather than on performance of work-related tasks. The sixth edition of the AMA *Guides* states on p. 6 that "the relationship between impairment and disability remains both complex and difficult, if not impossible, to predict."

While it is true that the AMA *Guides* is a widely used source (the vast majority of state workers' compensation systems require some use of the different editions of the AMA *Guides*) for assessing and rating an individual's permanent impairments, there are a number of states and the federal government's SSA disability program that do not recognize the AMA *Guides* for rating impairment. In addition, the Veterans Administration has its own unique set of disability rating criteria. There is clearly no consensus on a universal system to measure impairment.

Depending upon the system, impairment is necessary for disability, but other factors are considered. Different disability programs attempt to combine medical information and the associated impairment with nonmedical factors that bear on the individual's ability to compete in the open labor market. Other considerations include age, educational level, and past work experience. Physicians typically provide the data regarding the medical condition and impairment, while nonmedical issues are the purview of disability adjudicators.

The AMA Guides and Chronic Pain

The *Guides* provides a discussion of the assessment of pain in Chapter 3—Pain-Related Impairment. The AMA *Guides* states that subjective complaints are included in the provided impairment ratings, and up to 3% whole person permanent impairment may be provided in only unusual circumstances, including that there is no other basis to rate impairment.

Pain specialist physicians may feel that the AMA *Guides* method of impairment rating do not adequately address the "disability" and functional loss caused by some chronic-pain states. Since the *Guides* limits itself for the most part to describing measurable objective changes or impairment, chronic-pain states, despite causing significant functional losses, are not provided significant impairment ratings.

The American Academy of Pain Medicine has characterized pain with updated terminology, namely, *eudynia* for nociceptive pain and *maldynia* for neuropathic pain. Eudynia (nociceptive pain) is a normal physiologic response to noxious events and injury to somatic or visceral tissue. It can be beneficial and serves as an early warning mechanism. Eudynia often is acute, but can also be persistent (e.g., cancer pain). Eudynia usually is correlated directly with the resultant impairment. In this scenario, pain would appropriately be incorporated into the organ system impairment rating. Maldynia or neuropathic pain often results in significant dysfunction. Whatever pathology exists, it is not well measured

with our current testing abilities and the clinician often has difficulty correlating the pathology with the level of reported dysfunction.

The AMA Guides and Maximal Medical Improvement (MMI)

The AMA *Guides* states that an impairment rating can only be done when the individual has reached maximal medical improvement (MMI), i.e., "the point at which a condition has stabilized and is unlikely to change (improve or worsen) substantially in the next year, with or without treatment." It is necessary to determine that the patient is stable and that no further restoration of function is probable. If the examinee shows up and is in the middle of a flare-up or has had a new injury that interferes with the examination, it is premature to do an impairment rating. In other words, the examinee must be stabilized medically for the physician to fairly assess the impairment rating. If the condition is changing or likely to improve substantially with medical treatment, the impairment is not permanent and should not be rated.

The AMA Guides and Activities of Daily Living (ADL)

The AMA *Guides* reflects the severity of the medical condition and the degree to which the impairment decreases an individual's ability to perform common activities of daily living (ADL), *excluding* work.

Throughout the fifth edition of the AMA *Guides*, the examiner is given the opportunity to adjust the impairment rating based on the extent of any activities of daily living (ADL) deficits (5th Ed). The fifth edition of the AMA *Guides* describes typical ADLs as:

- Self-care and personal hygiene (urinating, defecating, brushing teeth, combing hair, bathing, dressing oneself, eating)
- Communication (writing, typing, seeing, hearing, speaking)
- Physical activity (standing, sitting, reclining, walking, climbing stairs)
- Sensory function (hearing, seeing, tactile feeling, tasting, smelling)
- Nonspecialized hand activities (grasping, lifting, tactile discrimination)
- Travel (riding, driving, flying)
- Sexual function (orgasm, ejaculation, lubrication, erection)
- Sleep (restful, nocturnal sleep pattern)

In the sixth edition, a distinction is made between ADLs, basic activities (such as feeding, bathing, hygiene), and instrumented ADLs, complex activities (such as financial management and medications). This edition also distinguishes between activity "execution of a task or action by an individual" and participation "involvement in a life situation" and between activity limitations "difficulties an individual may have in executing activities" and participation restrictions "problems an individual may experience in involvement in life situations."

AMA Guides Impairment Rating Percentages

A 0% whole person impairment (WPI) rating is assigned to an individual with an impairment if the impairment has no significant organ or body system functional consequences and does not limit the performance of the common activities of daily living. A 90–100% WP impairment indicates a very severe organ or body system impairment requiring the individual to be fully dependent on others for self-care, approaching death. The *Guides* impairment ratings reflect the severity and limitations of the organ/body system impairment and resulting functional limitations.

The AMA *Guides* provides weighted percentages for various body parts, but since the total impairment cannot exceed 100%, the Guides provides a combined values chart to enable the physician to account for the effects of multiple impairments with a summary value. Subjective concerns, including fatigue, difficulty in concentrating, and pain, when not accompanied by demonstrable clinical signs or other independent, measurable abnormalities, are generally not given separate impairment ratings. Impairment ratings in the Guides already have accounted for commonly associated pain, including that which may be experienced in areas distant to the specific site of pathology.

The Guides does not deny the existence or importance of these subjective complaints to the individual or their functional impact but notes that there has not yet identified an accepted method within the scientific literature to ascertain how these concerns consistently affect organ or body system functioning. The physician is encouraged to discuss these concerns and symptoms in the impairment evaluation.

The AMA Guides and Work Disability

Impairment assessment is provided by the *Guides*; however, the *Guides* does not define disability. An individual can have a disability in performing a specific work activity but not have a disability in any other social role. An impairment evaluation by a physician is only one aspect of disability determination. A disability determination also includes information about the individual's skills, education, job history, adaptability, age, and environment requirements and modifications. Assessing these factors can provide a more realistic picture of the effects of the impairment on the ability to perform complex work and social activities. If adaptations

can be made to the environment, the individual may not be disabled from performing that activity (in this scenario though, the impairment is still present).

The *Guides* is not intended to be used for direct estimates of loss of work capacity (disability). Impairment percentages derived according to the Guides criteria do not measure work disability. Therefore, it is inappropriate to use the *Guides'* criteria or ratings to make direct estimates of work disability.

Independent Medical Evaluation (IME)

While an independent medical evaluation has some similarities to a comprehensive medical consultation, there are significant differences. An independent medical evaluation involves an examination by a health care professional at the request of a third party in which no medical care is provided.

The terminology for these evaluations varies in different areas of the country and includes terms like independent medical evaluation or examination (IME), or in California, an agreed medical evaluation (AME) or qualified medical evaluation or examination (QME). The AME serves both sides of a dispute at the same time and, in a sense, serves as the "medical judge." These evaluations otherwise are typically at the request of one side or the other (defense or plaintiff/applicant).

Medicine and law have different approaches. The practice of law is based on the advocacy system and is contentious and argumentative in nature by design. It is a system that allows different and conflicting points of view to be heard with resolution achieved by way of a jury, judge, or through arbitration. The practice of medicine is focused on diagnosing and treating patients to the best of the physician's ability to help them regain and maintain good health.

Physicians providing either a one-time consultation or ongoing medical care are accustomed to having their advice sought and followed by a usually grateful patient. Whereas in the legal system, physicians can expect to have their opinions challenged vigorously and in detail by skilled attorneys. In some cases, physicians may have their credentials and ability to testify as an expert questioned in a harsh and demeaning manner. While the attack may seem personal, in fact, it is only a method used by attorneys to discredit physicians' testimony to either have it thrown out or its value minimized. A skilled attorney will ask questions that are often difficult to answer, and physicians may find that the opportunity for explanation may be limited.

Possible Versus Probable

The gold standard for a medical opinion is "beyond a reasonable degree of medical probability." Physicians do not have to be 100% certain, but they must form opinions that are medically probably or greater than a 50% chance of being correct. Anything less than this is termed "possible." Anything is possible, but to be accepted as medically reasonable, with a causal relationship, the term probable must be used. It is actually wise to keep away from using specific percentages, as this is hard to substantiate.

Evaluation Process

An independent medical evaluation involves an examination by a health care professional at the request of a third party in which no medical care is provided or suggested. The physician is not involved in the medical care of the examinee (there is no physician/patient relationship or privilege with some exceptions—please see liability issues below) and serves to provide a medical opinion to clarify issues associated with the case. The disability evaluation report is not necessarily to facilitate the well-being of the patient. Medical expertise is assumed for a disability evaluation, as is impartiality and objectivity, but such is not always the case. Unlike a medical consultation, the disability evaluation is not confidential and, further, should be easily read and understood by nonmedical personnel. Standards for independent medical evaluations have been published [25].

Referral Sources

Disability evaluations are an integral part of case management and are utilized widely by insurers and attorneys in a variety of arenas, including workers' compensation, personal injury, and long-term disability.

Workers' compensation systems are no fault, but litigation issues often center around causation, the extent and duration of medical care needs, the length of temporary disability, the extent and cost of permanent impairment and/or disability, and issues of apportionment to nonindustrial causation. An insurance carrier or third-party administrator typically handles claims. Some employers are partially or fully self-insured.

Personal injury litigation including malpractice cases involves primarily the cause and extent of injuries and the level of associated disability. Once a lawsuit is filed, the defendant is generally allowed one IME. In these cases, the defendant is counting on the IME to be unusually thorough as the case may hinge on the examination findings and report conclusions.

Long-term disability cases range from Social Security benefits for persons expected to be totally disabled for at least 12 months to individuals who have purchased or been provided by their employer private disability insurance policies.

Report Quality Issues

While the quality of the physician's testimony at a deposition, arbitration, or trial may be critical, the initial-typed report is typically most important. This report is relied upon in any settlement negotiation and often becomes part of the evidence. The disability evaluation report should be valid, defensible, and readable. A well-written report will assist the physician during cross-examination and may even discourage the opposing attorney from calling the physician to testify. The report itself may lead to early case settlement or resolution. Most often, the physician will be judged by the quality of the written report.

A quality evaluation report is responsive to the specific questions asked by the referral source. The report should be understandable by nonmedical individuals. Often, a verbal report is provided prior to submission of a written report, thus giving the referrer the opportunity to further direct specific questions or concerns or to even defer on receiving a written report. The physician should always maintain integrity but should remember that there is no traditional doctor–patient relationship and the payer is the client.

Report Writing Technique

Evaluation reports should be without spelling errors and should be grammatically correct. The report structure should include appropriate formatting with headings and categories. Bold lettering, italics, underlining, numbering, and bullet points can be used for clarity and emphasis. All material and records reviewed should be listed. Paragraphs should be kept relatively short, and separate ideas should be put in distinct categories. Unnecessary repetition should be avoided. It is of critical importance to use unambiguous language that can be easily understood by the referral source.

Pre-evaluation Issues

Prior to examining the claimant, the physician's office will receive a request for a disability evaluation by the referral source. A chart should be made up and all verbal and written correspondence noted in the record. It is important to provide documentation regarding charges, and usually a curriculum vita will be requested. Some physicians insist on a prepayment advance prior to reviewing records, providing an examination report, or attending a deposition, arbitration, or trial. Charges should include costs for late cancellations, records review, the actual examination, report writing, research, meeting time with the referral source, deposition, arbitration, and trial testimony time. It is important to identify who will be notifying the examinee of the appointment date and time. It is appropriate to review records in advance to assure that all historical items are reviewed with the examinee.

Interactions with the Examinee

If the evaluation is being accomplished at the request of the examinee's attorney or as an agreed medical examiner, there is an implied understanding that the physician is serving in that individual's best interest. When examining for the defense (the "other side"), it is not uncommon to find an examinee who is, at a minimum, suspicious and maybe even hostile.

Depending on the jurisdiction, the claimant's attorney or representative and sometimes even a court reporter may attend the evaluation. This may or not be permissible, dependent on the setting. Any other individual attending the appointment should remain silent and not provide information except for significant others. The claimant may request to tape record the examination; however, whether this is permissible is dependent on the jurisdiction.

It is important in any scenario to carefully explain your role including the fact that the disability evaluation is not meant to be a comprehensive medical evaluation covering all possible problems and that no doctor–patient relationship is implied. Risk is reduced by having the examinee signed an informed consent form. There is usually no confidentiality. Typically, the disability evaluation physician's opinions and any recommendations are not discussed with the examinee unless such is specifically requested by the referral source.

It is recommended that the examinee be told to not perform any maneuver that her or she feels will be harmful to them. Adequate gown coverage is important and a chaperone is recommended.

Evaluation Report Writing

Introduction

Physicians are well aware of the usual details covered in a standard history and physical examination. The disability evaluation report goes into much greater detail in certain areas as compared to a medical consultation since often other factors contribute to the issues of portrayed pain and disability.

The examinee's pre-injury status is carefully detailed. It is very important to determine if there was any disability predating the injury. The history of the injury, subsequent events, and medical care up to the present time are carefully ascertained.

Any inconsistency between the individual's report and information found in the medical record is noted. It is important to remember that individuals often have selective memories and, sometimes, what they remember is not accurate. The medical record is of critical importance; however, it is possible that the health care professional left something out or misunderstood the examinee. Therefore, just because something is not reported in the medical record does not mean that it did not happen as described by the examinee.

A quality disability evaluation report takes all of these factors into consideration. The disability evaluation physician is neither a magician nor fortune-teller, but must assess all the information available and provide a medically reasonable explanation. All the disability evaluation physician can do is to give a sincere and honest opinion and state what is medically probable.

Identifying Information

The report starts out with the identifying information consisting of the date of the report, the name of address of the referral source(s), the name of the examinee, the claim or other identifying numbers (like the date of injury), and the date of the exam if different than the report date. For workers' compensation cases, the employer's name is often listed as well.

Purpose of the Examination

The report should be addressed directly to the referral source. The first report paragraph typically notes the purpose of the exam and any other specific questions asked or reasons for the evaluation. You may add a paragraph noting that the report is based upon the personal interview and examination of the examinee, combined with review of available medical records and radiographs and other submitted information. A list of all records reviewed is either listed in the body of the report or attached as an addendum. You may choose to ask to see examinee picture identification such as a driver's license. You should identify if the examinee was accompanied by an interpreter or any other person (significant other, friend, relative, lawyer, nurse, etc.) and whether the examinee tape recorded the examination. Document that the examinee was informed the purposes of the examination and that there was no doctor–patient relationship and that the examinee should not perform any maneuvers that the individual would consider harmful or injurious.

Examinee Introduction

The next paragraph lists the examinee's age, handedness, and marital status. In the workers' compensation arena, the employer, years on the job, and current work status can be listed.

Pertinent History

For most evaluations, there is a point in time when problems surfaced either due to a specific injury or illness or on a cumulative trauma basis, and this should be identified. You may identify that prior to some identified point in time, the examinee described being in good health without ongoing disability, or that second, the examinee had a pre-injury (or illness) history of pertinence. You should describe any *relevant* prior history of injuries or illness (this might include auto accidents, illnesses, prior work or other injuries, surgeries, etc.) and document a history from the examinee regarding the injury/illness itself and subsequent symptoms and medical care (including medications prescribed and tests/procedures accomplished). You should assess whether the history is consistent with the records, recognizing that examinees do not always recollect their medical history correctly nor are medical records always correct.

Current Symptoms

The current symptoms are carefully documented. A pain diagram can be useful. The examinee is given the opportunity to detail all symptoms and complaints. Any loss of function (activities of daily living) or loss of pre-injury capacity is described. Body parts involved include location and radiation of symptoms and referral patterns along with spatial characteristics, duration periodicity, and intensity/severity.

Pain complaints associated with disability are often described with two components: the character of the pain (i.e., continuous, non-fluctuating; continuous fluctuating; episodic; paroxysmal, etc.) and the quality of the pain (e.g., burning; freezing; sharp; pins and needles; aching; dull; hot; cold; numbing; and electrical).

Additional descriptors should be listed (tingling, numbness, weakness, swelling, color change, temperature change, sweating, skin or hair growth changes, etc.). Provocative or aggravating factors that worsen the pain and palliative factors that alleviate the symptoms should be detailed. The current intensity of the pain is described on a 10-point scale, where "0" represents no pain and "10" represents the worst pain imaginable. Any bowel, bladder, sexual, or sleep dysfunction should be described.

The presence of any examinee-perceived emotional (anxiety, depression, etc.) or cognitive dysfunction should be noted. Additional relevant information may be obtained from significant others.

Assess

1. What is the *cause of the pain* (the examinee's perspective of what tissue abnormalities are causing the current problem)?

2. The *meaning of the pain* (what is and is not causing further tissue damage, and what is the meaning of the complaint is, i.e., whether there is progression, sinister illness, and/or concern present).
3. The *impact of the pain* on the examinee's life including interference in vocational, social, recreational activities, etc. We recommend a listing of an average day and daily activities.
4. Note the examinee's *perception of appropriate treatment*. An individual who is directed toward a passive treatment approach will have little interest in an active, functional restoration approach.
5. Note the examinee's *goals* to be achieved with further treatment.

Functional History

Obtain information regarding activities of daily living (ADLs—feeding, grooming, bathing, dressing, and toileting) and physical functional activities during an average day (exercise, outdoor activities, shopping, recreation, household chores, etc.). A description of the examinee's daily routine and changes from pre-injury status are documented.

Current and Past Medications

Obtain a list of past and current medications. We find it helpful to request that the examinee brings all current medications to the examination. The examiner should assess medication effectiveness, side effects, and any evidence of misuse or abuse.

Review of Systems

Consider constitutional, head and neck, cardiovascular, respiratory, genitourinary, gastrointestinal, neurological, psychiatric, and musculoskeletal symptoms in the review.

Past Medical and Surgical History

The examiner should especially note relevant injuries and illnesses including accidents (auto and other). There should be a review of all past significant or similar medical diagnoses, treatments, allergies, previous hospitalizations, and surgical procedures plus any history of psychiatric disorders/treatments/hospitalizations. Note potentially significant other medical problems like diabetes, cardiovascular or pulmonary disease, hypertension, arthritis, gout, etc.

Family History

The examinee should be questioned about relevant family history issues especially any alcoholism, substance abuse, major injuries, disability, pain, etc. Disability, illness, or death in the family may affect how the individual responds to his or her own medical problems. A family history of certain diseases may explain symptoms in the examinee that have not previously been well explained.

Personal History

Information in this section can be of critical importance, and areas of concern include the following:
• Childhood, i.e., was the examinee's childhood normal, dysfunctional, or abusive (sexual/verbal/physical)?
• Education, i.e., years of formal education, military service, and any legal history (litigation or incarceration).
• Marital status, i.e., has the examinee ever been married, how many times, and for how long? Was there any associated abuse history?
• Children, i.e., if there are children, what ages and how many? Is there a significant other and is that person working or disabled?
• Current living situation.
• Illicit substance use or abuse? If positive, provide previous and current usage level.
• Tobacco, caffeine, and alcohol usage.
• Current income source, if any (family members, workers' compensation, pension, long-term disability, state disability, Social Security, etc.).
• Work history: The occupational history should include not only the titles, types, and physical intensity of previous jobs but also continuity and length of previous positions. Attitudes about work (work "ethic") can be of considerable importance.

Physical Examination

The physical examination is similar for the disability evaluation as it is for a medical consultation, but it is important to document negative, positive, and nonorganic findings. If you are performing an impairment evaluation, perform the assessment according to specific examination requirements in the AMA *Guides*. When giving testimony, an opposing attorney can make the disability evaluating physician feel quite uncomfortable when parts of the examination are not documented.

The examination integrates information obtained from physical findings to support or refute diagnoses suggested during the history taking. The examination may uncover physical findings not readily apparent from the history or even known to the patient.

The physical examination is not limited to but is directed to the concerned body parts, and when a change or abnormality is identified, the appropriate regional examination is expanded.

The *general observation* of the examinee includes a behavioral examination including such issues as cooperation and attentiveness, along with any pain behaviors or unusual activities. The individual's sitting and standing tolerance is noted and all measurements recorded. Nonphysiologic findings are also noted.

Patient descriptors can include the patient as a good, poor, or fair historian and, when appropriate, can include such terms as pleasant and cooperative (vs. unpleasant and uncooperative), angry or hostile, and/or garrulous or loquacious.

Any *pain behavior* should be noted (verbal—sighing, moaning, groaning and nonverbal—grimacing, guarding, splinting, clutching, bizarre gait).

Constitutional findings refer to the examinee's general appearance (e.g., body habitus, deformities, development, nutrition, and attention to grooming) and vital signs (e.g., height, weight, temperature, blood pressure, pulse, respirations). Any adaptive aids such as braces/splints and walking aids/wheelchair are noted including whether such is appropriate or inappropriate.

Other physical examination findings, dependent on the context of the evaluation, may include:
• *Head, eyes, and ears*—General appearance, deformities, assistive devices (e.g., hearing aids, glasses), and visual/auditory acuity.
• *Mouth, throat, and nose*—General appearance, general dental condition, and patency of airway.
• *Neck*—General appearance, vascular distension, auscultation for bruits, active range of motion (AROM) and passive range of motion (PROM), and lymph nodes.
• *Cardiovascular*—Auscultation of the heart, examination of peripheral pulses, inspection of vascular refilling, varicosities, swelling, and edema.
• *Respiratory and chest*—General appearance of the chest, breasts for masses or tenderness, auscultation of lungs and upper airways, observation of breathing pattern, and examination for peripheral clubbing or cyanosis.
• *Gastrointestinal/genitourinary*—Inspection of abdomen and pelvis, auscultation of bowels, palpation of abdominal organs, and rectal examination.
• *Genitourinary*—Directed as appropriate.
• *Integumentary*—Inspection and palpation of skin and subcutaneous tissues for color, mottling, sweating, temperature changes, atrophy, tattoos, lesions, scars, rashes, ulcers, and surgical incisions.
• *Musculoskeletal*—Inspection, percussion, and palpation of joints, bones, and muscles/tendons noting any deformity, effusion, misalignment, laxity, crepitation, masses, or tenderness; assessment of AROM and PROM and stability of joints; inspection of muscle mass, spinal alignment, and symmetry; and assessment of muscle strength and tone.

- *Provocative tests*—Maneuvers for thoracic outlet syndrome, Phalen's and Tinel's for carpal tunnel, foraminal compression for cervical radiculopathy, straight leg raising for sciatica, etc.
- *Neurologic*—Assessment of level of consciousness (alert, lethargic, stuporous, comatose) and mental status (e.g., orientation, memory, attention and concentration, thought processes and content, speech and communication/language and naming, fund of knowledge, insights into current condition) and assessment of cranial nerves. The neurologic examination also includes assessment of (1) sensation to pinprick, two-point discrimination, sensibility, vibration, and proprioception; (2) assessment of sphincter tone and reflexes (e.g., bulbocavernosus); (3) assessment of deep tendon reflexes (DTR) in the upper and lower extremities, including pathologic reflexes (e.g., Babinski, Hoffman, palmomental, etc.); (4) assessment of coordination (e.g., finger/nose, heel/shin, rapid alternating movements) and tandem gait; and (5) functional mobility including gait and station.
- *Nonphysiologic behaviors*—assessed such as Waddell signs (e.g., superficial skin tenderness, stimulation of back pain by axial loading or trunk rotation, differences in straight leg raising response between supine and sitting positions, regional nonanatomic weakness or numbness, and overreaction/disproportionate pain responses).

Impression

List the diagnostic categories and/or the differential diagnoses.

Discussion

We recommend a succinct summary of the history and physical examination followed by opinions (when requested) on the specific issues requested by the client.

Causation and apportionment are often critical issues to be discussed along with prognosis. The evaluator must be able to determine whether the problem or disability was preexisting or caused by an event or occurrence, which is not a subject of the claim. If there is a basis for causation for the claim in question, is it fully or partially responsible?

The evaluator must be able to distinguish between an *aggravation and an exacerbation*. An aggravation results from a new event or injury causing a worsening, hastening, or deterioration of a preexisting condition. An exacerbation is a temporary increase in the symptomatology of a preexisting condition.

The issue of whether and when the examinee has reached *maximal medical improvement* (MMI) may also be addressed. The disability evaluator may also be asked to discuss the

prognosis and future medical care needs of the condition and other costs as part of a life-care plan.

Lastly, the *face-to-face time* spent with the examinee should be listed (some physicians also document records review, research, and report preparation time as well) followed with the examiner's name and signature. Copies of the report to the appropriate parties should be noted.

Functional Capacity Evaluation

The disability evaluator may be asked to address the examinee's functional ability or work capacity. The opinion is based on a review of medical records, the historical and physical examination, test results, and the examinee's functional capacity. The evaluation is made difficult when the individual demonstrates pain behaviors and a suboptimal effort on examination and testing.

The report should include the number of hours to be worked per day, sitting, standing, and walking tolerance, as well as lifting and carrying capabilities. For the upper extremities, the ability to perform forceful and repetitive activities should be discussed. Other factors to be considered are reaching, pushing, pulling, grasping or gripping, bending, crouching, squatting, climbing, balancing, working on uneven terrain, and working at heights. For difficult cases, a formal functional capacity evaluation (FCE) may be helpful.

A physical or functional capacity evaluation (FCE) is a systematic process of assessing an individual's physical capacities and functional abilities. Testing, lasting one-half day to several days, is usually carried out by a physical or occupational therapist with special training and expertise in this area.

The FCE matches human performance levels to the demands of a specific job or work activity or occupation. The FCE establishes the physical level of work an individual can perform. The FCE is useful in determining job placement, job accommodation, or return to work after injury or illness. An FCE can provide objective information regarding functional work ability in the determination of occupational disability status.

The FCE is a tool that can be used to make objective and reliable assessments of the individual's condition. Its precise data format provides information that can be used in various contexts. The FCE may be used (1) to determine the individual's ability to safely return to work full time or on modified duty; (2) to determine if work restrictions, job modifications, or reasonable accommodations are necessary to prevent further injury; (3) to determine the extent to which impairments exist, or the degree of physical disability for compensation purposes; and (4) to predict the potential ability to perform work following acute rehabilitation or a work-hardening/work-conditioning program.

A physical or functional capacity evaluation (FCE) provides additional information beyond what can be determined by the physician-directed disability evaluation, but the FCE does have its limitations as well. The functional capacity of the examinee who does not provide a full effort cannot be accurately assessed. Further, while providing a greater depth of testing than the physician physical examination, the FCE can only measure capacity in a controlled environment over a short period of time and does not necessarily equate with full-time, real-world, everyday life and job tasks.

Reason for the Opinion

The evaluation physician cannot base opinions solely on only the basis of "education, training, and experience." Rather, the disability evaluator must provide a clear description of why a conclusion has been reached. What are the facts in the case that cause you to formulate that opinion? It is important to discuss unusual or abnormal findings.

Post-evaluation Issues

Disability evaluation reports should be completed and sent with appropriate billing to the referral source. The examinee and the treating physician are not provided copies of the disability evaluation report unless requested by the referral source although this is uncommon. Depending upon the particular situation, the referral source should be contacted by phone so the disability evaluator can discuss any opinions or recommendations. In some cases, a written report may not be required or desired at that time. This is particularly true when the opinion generated is not deemed to be in the best interest of the referral source's case.

Testimony

The disability evaluator should be prepared to be deposed and to attend an arbitration hearing or trial. Depositions are usually requested by the opposing counsel to gauge the potential effectiveness of the physician as a witness. Should the case go forward to arbitration or trial, the effectiveness of the disability evaluation physician goes beyond medical knowledge, but also involves the individual's presentation and demeanor in front of a judge and/or jury.

Credibility is always increased through the observer's perception of the physician's honesty and integrity. It is always best to be honest and not appear to be trying to "help" the case of the referral source. Any potential negative information or opinions should have been discussed previously with the referring attorney or claims person as to how to deal with it in the least damaging manner. While honesty and integrity are essential, there is no need to volunteer information that might be damaging to your referral source. It is ultimately the job of the disability evaluation physician to be an expert witness, not to "make" the case for the referral source. It is never appropriate to demean or demonize the claimant or treating physicians.

Physician Disability Evaluation Liability Issues

The claimant may not be pleased with the disability evaluator's opinions. In recent years, medical malpractice lawsuits against physicians who conduct disability evaluations have become more common. Despite the absence of a traditional physician–patient relationship, physicians who conduct disability evaluations still have various legal duties to the examinee, although this issue is in flux and ever changing [26]. Examinees generally can successfully sue IME physicians for negligently causing physical injury during the examination, failing to take reasonable steps to disclose significant medical findings to the patient, and disclosing confidential medical information to third parties without authorization, but they *cannot* successfully sue for inaccurate or missed diagnoses.

Summary

The evaluation of pain and disability is complex and multifaceted. The evaluating physician must approach such an evaluation from a biopsychosocial perspective. Often, these evaluations are performed in the context of an independent medical evaluation, i.e., an examination by a health care professional at the request of a third party in which no medical care is provided. The evaluation results in a report that must reflect a thorough evaluation, answer the specific issues requested by the client, and be easily understandable by non-medical individuals. These evaluations are part of the legal or advocacy system that may be contentious and argumentative. The skilled independent medical examiner must always maintain impartiality and provide conclusions that are supportable. A thoughtful and thorough evaluation is of considerable value to all involved.

References

1. Aronoff GM. Chronic pain and the disability epidemic. Clin J Pain. 1991;7:330–8.
2. Gatchel RJ, Okifuji A. Evidence-based scientific data documenting the treatment- and cost-effectiveness of comprehensive pain programs for chronic nonmalignant pain. J Pain. 2006;7:779–93.

3. Turk DC, Gatchel RJ, editors. Psychological approaches to pain management: a practitioner's handbook. 2nd ed. New York: Guilford; 2002.
4. Turk DC, Monarch ES. Biopsychosocial perspective on chronic pain. In: Turk DC, Gatchel RJ, editors. Psychological approaches to pain management: a practitioner's handbook. 2nd ed. New York: Guilford; 2002.
5. Robinson JP, Turk DC, Loeser JD. Pain, impairment, and disability in the AMA guides. Guides newsletter. Nov/Dec 2004.
6. American Psychiatric Association. Committee on nomenclature and statistics. Diagnostic and statistical manual of mental disorders. Rev. 3rd ed. Washington, DC: American Psychiatric Association; 1987. Diagnostic and statistical manual of mental disorders. 4th ed. Washington, DC: American Psychiatric Association; 1994.
7. Ensalada LH, Brigham C. Somatization. Guides newsletter. July–Aug 2000.
8. Lipowski ZJ. Somatization: the concept and its clinical application. Am J Psychiatry. 1988;145:1358–68.
9. Lipowski ZJ. Somatization and depression. Psychosomatics. 1990;31:13–21.
10. Gatchel RJ. Comorbidity of chronic mental and physical health disorders: the biopsychosocial perspective. Am Psychol. 2004;59: 792–805.
11. Gatchel RJ. Clinical essentials of pain management. Washington, DC: American Psychological Association; 2005.
12. Merskey H, Bogduk N. Classification of chronic pain: descriptions of chronic pain syndromes and definitions of pain terms. 2nd ed. Seattle: IASP Press; 1994.
13. Rondinelli R, editor. AMA guides to the evaluation of permanent impairment. 6th ed. Chicago: AMA Press; 2007.
14. Waddell G. The back pain revolution. 2nd ed. Edinburgh: Churchill Livingstone; 2004.
15. Institute of Medicine Committee on Pain, Disability, and Chronic Illness Behavior (Osterweis M, Kleinman A, Mechanic D, eds.). Pain and disability: clinical, behavioral, and public policy perspectives. Washington, DC: National Research Council; 1987. p. 28.
16. Collie J. Malingering and feigned sickness. London: Edward Arnold Ltd; 1913.
17. Brigham C, Ensalada LH. Nonorganic findings. Guides newsletter, Sept–Oct 2005.
18. Waddell G, McCulloch JA, Kummel E, Venner R. Nonorganic physical signs in low-back pain. Spine. 1980;5:117–25.
19. American Psychiatric Association. Diagnostic and statistical manual of mental disorders. Text revision. 4th ed. Washington, DC: American Psychiatric Association; 2000.
20. Rogers R, editor. Clinical assessment of malingering and deception. 2nd ed. New York: Guilford Publications; 1997.
21. Meyerson A. Malingering. In: Kaplan H, Sadock B, editors. Textbook of psychiatry. 7th ed. New York: Williams & Wilkins; 2000.
22. Barth RJ, Brigham CR. Who is in the better position to evaluate, the treating physician or an independent examiner? Guides newsletter, 8, Sept–Oct 2005.
23. Sullivan MD, Loeser JD. The diagnosis of disability. Arch Intern Med. 1992;152:1829–35.
24. WHO. International classification of functioning, disability and health: ICF. Geneva: World Health Organization; 2001.
25. Nierenberg C, Brigham C, Direnfeld LK, Burket C. Standards for independent medical examinations. Guides newsletter. Nov/Dec 2005
26. Baum K. Independent medical examinations: an expanding source of physician liability, offer insights and suggestions for limiting physician liability in these situations. Ann Intern Med. 2005;142: 974–8.

The Double Effect: In Theory and in Practice

24

Lynn R. Webster

Key Points

- The principle of double effect has roots in the Hippocratic Oath and moral teachings of the Catholic Church as outlined by Thomas Aquinas.
- The double effect allows serious harm to a person as a secondary effect resulting from a primary action that is good. To satisfy double effect, only the primary good action must be intended, the good outcome must not be produced by means of the bad effect, and the good must outweigh the harm caused.
- The principle has clinical relevance whenever an intervention performed to benefit a patient has the potential or certitude of also causing harm, such as when opioids are administered during end-of-life care.
- Everyday clinical decisions raise questions that involve the difficulty of determining clinician intent, disagreements regarding the limits of patient autonomy, the tension between proponents of compassionate pragmatism vs. moral absolutism, and interpreting the laws that govern the ending of human life.
- Opioids given as therapy for chronic, nonmalignant pain can also cause detriment as well as benefit to individuals and to society and may be considered in light of double effect.
- The question of whether double effect continues as a valuable clinical guide given recent technological advances and the current state of medical ethics remains unresolved.

Introduction

It is not always possible to perform clinical interventions that benefit a patient without also triggering some degree of harm. The double effect (DE) is both a moral and pragmatic principle to determine whether the good outcome resulting from an action outweighs any detrimental secondary effects. The principle's underpinnings are lodged in medieval, theological thought, and the continuing clinical significance of DE to a diverse, technological society is the subject of much debate among scientists and philosophers. In the scientific literature, DE is most often invoked to address questions of what is moral and ethical inend-of-life care.

The following discussion will trace the principle's beginnings, its usual clinical applications, and the areas where DE is most subject to differing interpretations. Reaching beyond the end-of-life debate, the analysis will turn to decisions that must be made while caring for patients who suffer chronic, nonmalignant pain. The question remains open as to whether the arguments raised serve to nullify, modify, or only reinforce the strictures of DE principle, in part or in whole.

The History and Specifics of Double Effect (DE)

The DE has been described variously as a rule, a principle, and a doctrine. The word "doctrine" connotes religious observance in keeping with DE's beginnings in the moral teachings of the Catholic Church as outlined by Thomas Aquinas [1]. In the *Summa Theologica* (II-II, Qu. 64, Art.7), Aquinas reasons, "Nothing hinders one act from having two effects, only one of which is intended, while the other is beside the intention" [2]. Reaching back further still, DE's emphasis on the physician's responsibility to safeguard the total life and well-being of a patient can be traced to the ancient Greek principle of non-maleficence encoded in the Hippocratic Oath.

L.R. Webster, M.D. (✉)
Lifetree Clinical Research and Pain Clinic,
3838 South 700 East, Suite 200, Salt Lake City,
UT 84106, USA
e-mail: lynnw@lifetreepain.com

T.R. Deer et al. (eds.), *Treatment of Chronic Pain by Integrative Approaches: the AMERICAN ACADEMY of PAIN MEDICINE Textbook on Patient Management*, DOI 10.1007/978-1-4939-1821-8_24,
© American Academy of Pain Medicine 2015

As interpreted today, DE principle allows bad effects to occur as the result of good action as long as four essential components are satisfied:

1. The primary act in itself must be morally good or at least indifferent.
2. Only the good effect must be intended and not the bad effect.
3. The good effect must not be produced by means of the bad effect.
4. The good achieved must sufficiently outweigh in proportion the harm caused.

The most typical clinical application cited to illustrate DE is the giving of opioids to ease end-of-life pain even when doing so may hasten death. Direct killing through the administration of a lethal drug such as KCl is forbidden. The giving of high-dose opioids, however, has pain relief as its aim and is permissible under DE.

A look at each DE criterion will show how this judgment follows:

- The No. 1 component, which says the primary action must not be morally wrong, appears to be satisfied here: Opioids are not in themselves evil agents, despite their somewhat checkered reputation among laypeople and even some physicians.
- The second component is met because the primary aim is pain control, while death is a potential but unintended secondary evil.
- The third requirement also appears to be met as death is a possible side effect but not the primary means of pain control.
- Most clinicians who treat terminally ill patients, the patients themselves, and their families assign a degree of benefit to a peaceful, pain-free death. They would agree that the fourth component of proportionality is satisfied when a patient who is already close to death and who would otherwise suffer excruciating, escalating pain is relieved of that suffering – even if to do so hastens the inevitable.

The reasoning behind this classic end-of-life scenario appears unimpeachable but is, in fact, anything but controversy free. The biggest areas of contention concern the difficulty of determining clinician intent, the arguments for and against limitations on patient autonomy, and the sometimes unshared view that the ultimate good lies in prolonging life. Furthermore, end-of-life care is only one area in which clinical interventions invoke DE; indeed, anytime an action is performed that raises the possibility of harm to the patient, DE questions are raised.

Intended or Only Foreseen Outcomes

An important distinction occurs between secondary bad outcomes that are "foreseen" and those that are "intended." Many are the examples where an outcome can be reasonably predicted considering the clinical action taken, yet the outcome is not intended (and may even be dreaded) by the physician. For instance, a clinician gives a needed medication that is likely to cause the side effect of nausea. The nausea is certainly not intended, although it is foreseen; thus, steps are taken to minimize the patient's discomfort.

Yet, intention may be difficult to discern. Some critics argue that it is no different to foresee an outcome when one reasonably expects it will occur than to intend that outcome. Take, for example, the clinician who administers a dose of opioids that reasonably could be expected to hasten a death. The question is whether the person performing that action intends a quicker death as a means of ending suffering. This would violate DE, which states that a harm that would be acceptable as a side effect must not occur as a primary means.

Others contend these are very different matters indeed. Sulmasy argues that a clinician who expects, desires, and even prays for a gravely ill patient's death still does not intend the death as a primary aim [3]. This type of reasoning comes from supporters of DE's clinical relevance, who argue that the ambiguities of intent need not render DE impracticable.

Some ethicists make a further distinction between outcomes that *may* occur as opposed to those that certainly will. The question is, for example, whether palliative care involving large doses of opioids is permitted when death is certain or when it is only possible.

Proportionality: How Much Harm Is Too Much?

The fourth rule of proportionality is very important in applying DE principle. It is not enough that bad effects merely be unintended and not the primary action – they must also fail to outweigh the good achieved.

One can see a continuum of proportional harm where the harm rendered is most grave at either end. At one end of the continuum, physicians, perhaps fearing regulatory or other sanctions, administer doses of opioids too weak to relieve pain. At the other end, physicians administer doses larger than needed for pain control that prove lethal. One can see that the proportionality of harm applies not just to doses that may hasten death but to the harm of allowing patients to suffer pain needlessly. In between the two poles lies the therapeutic window.

Applications of Good and "Evil"

In Catholic doctrine, DE differentiates between casts of evil from a religious point of view. No good outcomes must be achieved through evil acts performed with intent. Today, although most Americans are religious, dissent arises as to what constitutes "evil," raising the possibility that words like "detriment" and "harm," which are less fraught with theological judgment, could serve as pragmatic alternatives. Even commonly used terms like "compassion" and "morality" are open to interpretation. Analysts are obliged to wrestle with universal applications of this type of terminology and also with whether the intent behind a given action matters more than its result.

Moral Absolutism Versus Pragmatism

Moral absolutists take the view that the killing of innocents as a primary aim is never justified. A vivid example is that of the pregnant woman who must be rid of a fetus in order to live. The particulars could include eclampsia or malignant hypertension that would kill both the woman and the fetus unless action is taken. To the absolutist, to abort a fetus to save the life of the mother violates DE by perpetrating a primary evil; however, no violation occurs when one performs an operation to remove the uterus (a primary good), though the fetus dies as a result (a secondary evil). Although the operation goes against the argument of some ethicists who would insist that death should be only a possibility – never a certainty – in general, the action is permissible even by the precepts of moral absolutism as represented by Catholic theology: Removal of the uterus whereby the fetus *will* die is (morally) lawful; abortion is not.

Proponents of a viewpoint that could be termed *compassionate pragmatism* reject this solution as being tainted by circular logic and ask, "Why subject the mother to a needless operation?" They argue against the capacity of DE to resolve questions raised by euthanasia and abortion [3]. Why, for example, subject a woman with an ectopic pregnancy to an unnecessary operation – removal of the fallopian tube – to satisfy the requirement that a fetus death must be a side effect, not a means of treatment? Instead, pragmatists argue, why not administer an intramuscular injection of methotrexate to kill the fetus? could be administered. Again, in this example, the fetus will die anyway, and the woman, under the strictest DE interpretation, must undergo an operation to remove organs, thus enduring an unnecessary harm, the pragmatic argument goes [3].

The pragmatist is particularly concerned with apparent inconsistencies in the limits placed on patient autonomy by DE principle. For instance, Shaw points out that killing a person directly is forbidden, although sex changes – which would be seen as horrific mutilation under different circumstances – are allowed. The question raised is why patient autonomy reigns supreme in one instance but not the other:

> The prohibition of euthanasia must derive from a belief that direct killing of the innocent is supremely and always wrong in a way that dreadful mutilations are not. That belief may or may not be true. The patient should decide for himself. [4]

Despite the pragmatist's rejection of moral absolutism, questions of patient autonomy and clinician intent can complicate pragmatic decisions. For example, palliative care advocates who argue passionately for a dying patient's right to pain control often see physician-assisted suicide as an unacceptable overextension of the concept of patient autonomy, a contradiction of a physician's role as healer and an invitation to abuse the practice.

Reconciling the Terminology

Ethics and *morals* are two terms that describe the individual's responsibility to do right and not wrong in relation to one's fellow man. The two somewhat synonymous terms carry different connotations for many people. *Ethics*, with roots in the teachings of Aristotle, describes universal standards of upright character, while *morals* (from the Latin "mores") are more often invoked relative to the standards of a particular social group.

Yet ethics are created in an ongoing fashion and are often defined as the situation dictates. Such *situational ethics* are frequent in DE examples utilizing warfare where many types of gain to the aggressor are deemed "good" sufficient to outweigh the proportion of evil suffered by adversaries.

Cultural relativity also plays a role in what constitutes unallowable harm to a patient. Eastern cultures, for example, may not stress individual autonomy. In addition, some other modern societies do not share equally the United States' uneasiness with physician-assisted suicide; in the Netherlands, for example, acceptance of the practice is far broader [5], though some point to the Dutch as evidence of a "slippery slope" toward involuntary euthanasia.

One could also ask what is meant by "compassion" today. Physicians are expected to do more than present choices and informed consent to patients. They must also listen and empathize, understand the cultural and social significance of certain decisions to the patient, and help patients cope with stress, anxiety, and physical pain [6].

Whenever we apply relative terminology to medical practice, we are responsible for achieving results that are not only theoretically satisfying but also clinically beneficial. One must take special care not to utilize the concept of pragmatism to describe that which is merely convenient to the clinician. When ethics become too situational, the fourth DE component of proportionality may be given too much weight. This occurs when an achieved benefit such as mere clinical expediency is deemed sufficient to outweigh deleterious effects.

Fresh Thinking and Revised Criteria

Western society places great value on individual autonomy. To safeguard this principle, Quill, Dresser, and Brock have offered revised criteria that they believe mesh better with today's medical realities and that help mitigate some of the ethical ambiguities unforeseen by crafters of DE absolutism. They suggest medical decision making be guided by:

- The patient's informed consent
- The patient's degree of suffering
- The absence of less harmful treatment alternatives [7]

In this view, the patient's autonomy and the rule of proportionality are weighted more heavily than the inexact science of ascertaining a clinician's intent or the absolute prohibition against purposefully causing death.

Traditional Clinical Applications (Mostly End of Life)

The impact of DE on medicine is most clearly seen in cases of terminal illness. The application of DE to end-of-life care is contained in the following summation given by the *International Consensus Conference in Critical Care*:

> The patient must be given sufficient analgesia to alleviate pain and distress; if such analgesia hastens death, this "double effect" should not detract from the primary aim to ensure comfort. [8]

DE says death is not a medical treatment and cannot be utilized as a primary aim. Prohibitions would include physician-assisted suicide, euthanasia (voluntary or involuntary) and – in the strictest interpretation – even the withholding of life-sustaining treatment in some instances.

One can see physician actions as a descending ladder organized from the greatest to the least degree of intervention (Fig. 24.1).

Before addressing the different categories of physician action using medical ethics or personal conscience, it is first advisable to understand what the law says about DE.

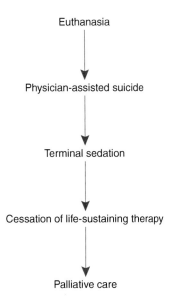

Euthanasia

Physician-assisted suicide

Terminal sedation

Cessation of life-sustaining therapy

Palliative care

Fig. 24.1 Descending ladder of physician action in end-of-life care

Double Effect and the Law

The fear that DE opens the door to legalized euthanasia is a prime motivator behind the precepts that get codified into law. The principle has in the past come into conflict with laws forbidding acts or omissions that hasten death. Australian law, for example, clarifies that acting to kill or allowing a person to kill oneself is unacceptable. Palliative care must be "reasonable" and "in good faith" and is never to be confused with euthanasia [9].

In the United States, recent federal focus has been on forbidding clinicians to help people die. The Pain Relief Promotion Act (PRPA) (H.R.2260), which would have imposed stiff penalties on clinicians for assisting the suicide of a patient, was passed by the House of Representatives in 2000 only to stall in committee, never becoming law. The proposal was alternately praised and damned by physicians. The American Medical Association (AMA) hailed the act for acknowledging that death may be hastened by appropriate, aggressive palliative care. But critics decried the attempt to override state law, putting federal authorities in charge of medical determinations such as how high a dose indicates "intent" to assist suicide rather than to relieve pain [10].

The failure of the PRPA was followed by a challenge from the US Attorney General to Oregon's physician-assisted suicide law attempting to outlaw the prescribing of medications to assist with a suicide on the grounds that to do so does not serve "a legitimate medical purpose" under the federal Controlled Substances Act. In the end, the US Supreme Court refuted the challenge, specifying that Congress has not granted medical decision-making power to the attorney general, though it is possible such power could still be granted in the future [11, 12].

The Supreme Court has affirmed that patients have a right to palliative care and also upholds states' rights to pass their own laws regarding physician-assisted suicide; a majority of states have passed laws forbidding the assisting of suicide [13, 14].

US criminal law forbids causing death but protects posing a risk to life if the risk is justified by expected benefits. US law also says a physician is to stop treatment when a competent patient requests, even with the foreknowledge of death. When palliative care does not bring adequate relief, "there is a growing consensus [in the United States] that sedation to the point of comfortable sleep is permissible" [15]. Thus, the law and common medical practice stand against DE, which says the cause of death cannot be intentional. In general, US law recognizes the right to discontinue life-sustaining therapy but stops short of endowing a patient with the right to die. Some supporters of a patient's right to die find the distinction counterintuitive, asking why the refusal of life-supporting therapy is protected, but the choice to ask a physician for assistance in ending one's life is not [16].

The argument for the patient's right to die is offset by the belief that laws allowing assisted suicide are based on a "cynical argument ... that killing pain and deliberately killing patients are essentially similar, that neither laws nor doctors can effectively distinguish them, that therefore we must allow *both* if we allow either" [17]. So the argument continues unabated.

Is the DE Argument Based on a "Myth?"

Opioids confer enormous benefits for the dying, including the relief of pain and dyspnea. Their side effects include:

- Sedation
- Respiratory depression
- Hypotension
- Vomiting
- Myoclonus
- Delirium
- Anxiety
- Agitation

Do they also hasten death? Some experts in pain and palliative care say no and would render moot DE's relevance to questions of high-dose opioids administered to the dying. Several researchers argue that little evidence supports the precipitation of death so often associated with the giving of opioids at the end of life [18, 19]. Fohr performed an exhaustive literature review, concluding that the belief that opioids hasten death via respiratory depression is "more myth than fact" and further posits that a false belief in DE leads to the undertreatment of pain because physicians fear to hasten death [19]. The American Academy of Pain Medicine (AAPM) and the American Pain Society (APS) uphold the principle that patients on opioid therapy develop tolerance quickly to the risk of respiratory depression and that pain itself antagonizes the effect, further reducing the risk [20].

It is argued that opioids given to dying patients may appear to hasten a death that is instead the result of the disease process and also that benzodiazepines and barbiturates are more likely to induce a sedation that could lead to death than are opioids. However, other literature supports the potential of opioids for hastening death – particularly in patients with sleep apnea – [21–23] and warns against counting on tolerance to confer complete protection to respiratory depression. Research has found that development of tolerance to respiratory depression is highly variable and may lag behind tolerance to other effects, never becoming complete even for long-term opioid users [24, 25].

Categories of Clinician Action

Clinical actions in the treatment of terminal patients throw into sharp relief society's views on patient autonomy and clinician intent. Many commentators take pains to differentiate the DE-supported use of opioids that may hasten death from the practice of euthanasia. Though some argue for euthanasia or physician-assisted suicide as humane practices, the prohibitions of law and of many individual consciences would disagree. Therefore, the largest gray areas in DE application exist in the categories of terminal sedation and the cessation of life-sustaining therapy, both of which do occur commonly in medical practice.

"Foreseen" and "intended" consequences can be in the eye of the beholder, depending on whether one believes the action achieved is good in proportion to the bad. Research does support the assertion that clinicians, particularly non-specialists, fear to hasten death [26]. The danger exists that, hamstrung by ambiguities, clinicians may refuse to give adequate pain control.

Euthanasia

Euthanasia is the intentional administering of medication or other interventions to cause a patient's death. This can be either voluntary at the request of a competent patient who has received informed consent or involuntary, lacking the request of a competent patient. In DE terms, the intention (to relieve pain) may be laudable, but the primary action (voluntary killing) is impermissible.

The following experience, the memory of a then 26-year-old intern illustrates the daily experiences of clinicians who work with dying patients:

> I will never forget this patient because the experience was terribly painful. He was over 90 and in the VA hospital waiting to die. He did not have a terminal illness – he was just old. He could walk only with tremendous pain. He could perform no other meaningful activities. He was half blind, had partial hearing, couldn't sleep, and was tormented with bowel and bladder problems. He hurt all over, and he had no family. This man did not want to live. Every time I passed his bed, he would grab at me, cry and plead for me to help him die. He suffered physically and emotionally as much as anyone can suffer. His only hope was to escape. I was obliged to observe him being tortured by his own existence. I had nightmares of hearing him scream. Obviously I couldn't comply with his request. My own personal conscience tells me I couldn't have done it then, and I couldn't do it now. But that doesn't mean I don't believe someone could.

The intern who chronicled that memory is the first author of this chapter, now many years removed. The question at stake is whether the preservation of life is always the ultimate value. DE forbids causing a grave harm as an end in itself, but could the law of proportionality sometimes support the belief that allowing a person to suffer excruciating pain with no hope of relief is itself an unjustifiable harm?

Those who argue that active euthanasia – not just acts of omission and "letting die" – can be a compassionate, clinical act are buoyed by the belief that consequences, such as a pain-free death, matter as much or more than absolute prohibitions against deliberate killing [27].

The absolutist would disagree sharply, lobbying for limitations on patient autonomy and the need to scrutinize the clinician's intent as opposed to the clinical outcome. One worry is that a clinician, endowed with too much decision-making power, could succumb to skewed intentions and – overfocused on ending pain – begin euthanizing without consent. Some experts argue it is relatively easy to prove intent by reviewing the medical record of drugs given and actions taken; but this supposition depends mightily on the qualifications of the person doing the looking.

Physician-Assisted Suicide

Physician-assisted suicide refers to the providing of medications or other interventions to a patient who intends to use them to end his or her life [7]. In general, it is assumed that the physician knows what the patient intends. The value assigned to patient autonomy is thus brought directly into conflict with the DE prohibition against intending a patient's death.

Distinctions of intention may be unclear: How, for example, can a physician know for certain what a patient will do with medications sufficient to either relieve pain or to cause death (if taken in high enough quantities)? Is it sufficient to violate DE if a physician knows a death will result from his action, even if it is the patient's own final action that brings the death about?

In addition to the prohibitions enforced by law, a fair number of medical professionals and associations oppose physician-assisted suicide, believing it reflects a failure to provide adequate palliative care and psychological support to the dying. The American Medical Association (AMA) has announced its firm opposition to physician-assisted suicide as a contradiction of the physician's role as healer. The familiar arguments that pit the right to a pain-free death and patient autonomy against the need to safeguard life and guard against a "slippery slope" of suspect clinician intent also apply here.

Terminal Sedation

Terminal sedation refers to the administration of a dose larger than is needed for analgesia with the goal of sedating the patient to the point of unconsciousness to relieve untreatable pain. This action often occurs in tandem with the cessation of life-sustaining therapies. The intentionality of causing death is incompatible with DE, although many physicians perform this action, which is supported by current medical ethical standards and allowed by law. The practice is not meant to provide mere clinical expediency and should be driven only by the patient's symptoms. It requires informed consent from the patient or the permission of a surrogate. Critics complain that terminal sedation is comparable to slow euthanasia and could be easily abused by clinicians.

Cessation of Life-Sustaining Therapy

Cessation of life-sustaining therapy involves the withholding or withdrawing of life-sustaining medical treatments from the patient to let him or her die. This is where DE conflicts most strongly with commonly accepted medical ethics and clinical reality. A survey showed that 39 % of physicians who had sedated patients while stopping life-sustaining treatment had not just foreseen but had intended to hasten the death of the patient [7].

Fear of violating the absolute prohibition against intentionally causing death may lead some physicians to refuse to withdraw nonbeneficial, life-sustaining treatment, even when such a refusal clearly violates the wishes of the patient and the patient's family. The nitty-gritty of the debate is summarized thus "Many persons and groups reject the position that death should never be intentionally hastened when unrelievable suffering is extreme and death is desired by the patient" [7]. Here, pragmatic compassion butts heads with moral absolutism.

Palliative Care

Palliative care concentrates on improving quality of life for terminal patients. It involves the administering of opioids or other medications to relieve pain with the potential incidental consequence of causing respiratory depression sufficient to result in the patient's death. Courts have upheld a patient's right to palliative care as long as the primary purpose is to relieve pain, not to hasten death.

For some commentators and clinicians in the field, it is sometimes difficult to distinguish between the dose of medication that relieves suffering and the dose of medication that ends a life in order to bring about the same aim: the relief of suffering. In particular, it may be difficult to distinguish between euthanasia and palliative care when death is not just a potential but a known outcome of interventions.

Some clarification can be found in the knowledge that morphine and other opioids are pain-relieving aids, not mere agents of death as would be carbon monoxide. Some also insist that a lag is needed between pain relief and death, meaning doses that instantly kill a patient constitute euthanasia rather than palliative care [9].

In some cases, the confusion causes needless suffering. It has been estimated that greater than 90 % of pain associated with severe illness is relievable if established guidelines are followed [15]. Yet the literature contains examples of physicians and nurses refusing to administer "as needed" doses of opioids – even to patients who are close to death and suffering excruciating pain from advanced malignancies – for fear of "causing" a patient's death [15].

In the matter of palliative care, the line between the dose that kills and the dose that relieves pain grows narrower as the patient reaches the end. In practice, healthcare providers in hospice and palliative care accept hastened death as the price of giving optimal treatment to patients who are dying. Some admit they have hastened a death to end unendurable pain, then ponder whether they have crossed a line where their "intent" was to administer death rather than symptom relief.

The fact remains that if the disease process were not present, the need to end suffering would not be either. Yet neither is the DE component of proportionality to be forgotten:

> After all, physicians are not permitted to relieve the pain of kidney stones with potentially lethal doses of opiates simply because they foresee but do not intend the hastening of death! A variety of substantive medical and ethical judgments provide the justificatory context: the patient is terminally ill, there is an urgent need to relieve pain and suffering, death is imminent, and the patient or the patient's proxy consents. [28]

Impact of the Technology on DE Debate

Current techniques sometimes provide alternatives that manage pain without hastening death. In this way, advances in technology change the DE conversation. Many proponents of palliative care who campaign strenuously for better pain control for the dying believe that those who plead for allowing patients to die may be motivated by an unwillingness or inability to provide adequate interventions. A call to increase the skills and training of those who care for the dying appeared in the letters column of the *New England Journal of Medicine*: "It is sad that our care of the dying has lagged behind other forms of medical care, justifying the fear of many persons that they will not be able to die with dignity and comfort" [29].

A patient's comfort as he or she nears death may well depend as heavily on the absence of psychological and emotional agony as it does on the relief of physical pain. In general, using sedation to relieve a patient's psychic symptoms courts greater controversy than using the same dose to address physical symptoms.

Technology is important to this distinction. The advent of spinal opioid treatment, which delivers opioid analgesia without triggering psychic effects, is one advance in pain treatment that reframes the question of what constitutes adequate relief of suffering at the end of life. The following cases presented at the 2002 *American Pain Society* meeting illustrate the point:

> Two of three patients, all of whom suffered advanced malignancies, intractable pain, and unacceptable side effects such as mental clouding, were implanted with an intrathecal pump to deliver analgesia. Both patients attained greater than 50 percent pain relief and increased cognitive function. However, this latter benefit came at a price: an increase in anxiety, depression, and difficult issues that presented conflicts with family members [30].

When pain can be relieved at the end of life without significant psychic side effects, who is there to help patients deal with the extraordinary psychological burden presented by their situation? Palliative care *must* seek to answer this question.

DE Applications to a Nonterminal, Chronic-Pain Population

The precepts of DE apply outside the realm of terminal illness, encompassing any clinical intervention that measures harm against benefit. Physicians and other clinicians who specialize in the care of patients suffering from chronic, non-malignant pain are accustomed to weighing the benefit against the harm, from clinical and regulatory standpoints, even if they have never thought of the process in terms of DE. One can see DE applications in microcosm and macro-cosm, pertaining to the individual and the relative good of society as a whole.

The giving of opioids to manage chronic, nonmalignant pain can be considered a primary good, thus satisfying the first component of DE. However, what if opioids are being given knowingly to someone who is not gaining adequate pain relief from opioids and who suffers from an active addiction? The intent might be to help that person forestall the agony of withdrawal symptoms, so ostensibly the goal is to ease suffering. However, the clinician should consider that any benefit gained is likely to be short term and that to continue to provide opioids to people with addiction may tip the balance.

On a macro level, overdose deaths involving pain medications are increasing [31]. Based on historical data, a small percentage of patients with chronic, nonmalignant pain who are prescribed opioids could die, either by intentional or unintentional overdose. Some may also die from suicide if pain is not treated. The secondary evil occurs as a result of the good intent and primary action: the giving of opioids to relieve pain and improve physical function and quality of life for the majority of patients. Thus, the fourth component of proportionality is important in determining how much good is achieved at the risk of ill effect.

Assume a few patients in a pain practice may inject, distribute, or otherwise misuse opioids prescribed for pain. The intended good effect is pain relief, and the detrimental effect is drug abuse or addiction from overdose. Opioid prescribing for chronic pain is based on the belief that the large numbers of patients who use their medications as directed derive substantial benefit, outweighing the harm caused by a smaller number of patients who misuse them. However, if a clinician's prescribing becomes careless, resulting in a larger number of patients harmed than helped by opioids, at that point, the prescribing clinician's action would not meet the rule of proportionality.

Summary

DE has been described as a means of explaining exceptions to the absolute prohibition to purposefully ending human life [28]. Supporters maintain its value as a moral compass and clinical aid. However, DE principle is frequently challenged as containing too much ambiguity to serve as a truly useful clinical guide, and modifications through compassionate pragmatism are intended to bring DE in line with current medical ethics.

Whatever a clinician's personal convictions, it is imperative to clarify the wishes of patients or their surrogates and to give whatever treatments provide the greatest comfort and cause the least harm. While supporting patient autonomy, one should try to ensure that a patient's expressed desire to die does not stem from inadequate, though available, pain control or lack of psychological support. DE is one guide for a clinician to consult, along with relevant laws and accepted medical practices, when in the view of the patient, the benefit of living no longer outweighs the pain endured in meeting the inevitable end.

Acknowledgment Beth Dove of Dove Medical Communications, Salt Lake City, Utah, contributed technical writing and manuscript review. (Note: Please note the spelling of Dove – not Dover – Medical Communications).

References

1. Mangan J. An historical analysis of the principle of double effect. Theol Stud. 1949;10:41–61.
2. Aquinas T. (13th c). Summa Theologica II-II, Q. 64, art. 7, "Of Killing". In: Baumgarth WP, Richard J, Regan SJ, editors. On law, morality, and politics. Indianapolis/Cambridge: Hackett Publishing Co; 1988. p. 226–7.
3. Sulmasy DP. Killing and allowing to die: another look. J Law Med Ethics. 1998;26(1):55–64.
4. Shaw AB. Two challenges to the double effect doctrine: euthanasia and abortion. J Med Ethics. 2002;28(2):102–4.
5. Purdy L. Ending life [book review]. JAMA. 2006;295(7):830–1.
6. Tauber AI. Patient autonomy and the ethics of responsibility. Cambridge: MIT Press; 2005.
7. Quill TE, Dresser R, Brock DW. The rule of double effect – a critique of its role in end-of-life decision making. N Engl J Med. 1997;337(24):1768–71.
8. Carlet J, Thijs LG, Antonelli M, et al. Challenges in end-of-life care in the ICU. Statement of the 5th International Consensus Conference in Critical Care: Brussels, Belgium, April 2003. Intensive Care Med. 2004;30(5):770–84. Epub 2004 Apr 20.
9. McGee A. Double effect in the criminal code 1899 (QLD): a critical appraisal. QUT Law Just J. 2004;4(1):46–57.
10. Orentlicher D, Caplan A. The pain relief promotion Act of 1999: a serious threat to palliative care. JAMA. 2000;283(2):255–8.
11. Annas GJ. Congress, controlled substances, and physician-assisted suicide – elephants in mouseholes. N Engl J Med. 2006;354(10):1079–84.
12. Kapp MB. The U.S. Supreme court decision on assisted suicide and the prescription of pain medication: limit the celebration. J Opioid Manag. 2006;2(2):73–4.
13. Vacco v. Quill, 117 S.Ct. 2293. 1997.
14. Washington v. Glucksberg, 117 S.Ct. 2258. 1997.
15. Quill TE, Meier DE. The big chill – inserting the DEA into end-of-life care. N Engl J Med. 2006;354(1):1–3.
16. Canick SM. Constitutional aspects of physician-assisted suicide after Lee v. Oregon. Am J Law Med. 1997;23(1):69–96.
17. Reality check on the pain relief promotion act. Secretariat for Pro-Life Activities, United States Conference of Catholic Bishops, 3211 4th Street, N.E., Washington, DC 20017–1194 (202) 541–3070. http://www.nccbuscc.org/prolife/issues/euthanas/reality2. htm. Accessed 17 Aug 2006.
18. Sykes N, Thorns A. The use of opioids and sedatives at the end of life. Lancet Oncol. 2003;4(5):312–8.
19. Fohr SA. The double effect of pain medication: separating myth from reality. J Palliat Med. 1998;1(4):315–28.
20. The use of opioids for the treatment of chronic pain: a consensus statement from American Academy of Pain Medicine and American Pain Society. Approved by the AAPM Board of Directors on 29 June 1996. Approved by the APS Executive Committee on 20 Aug 1996. http://www.ampainsoc.org/advocacy/opioids.htm. Accessed 19 July 2005. Under review.
21. Farney RJ, Walker JM, Cloward TV, Rhondeau S. Sleep-disordered breathing associated with long-term opioid therapy. Chest. 2003;123(2):632–9.
22. Wang D, Teichtahl H, Drummer O, Goodman C, Cherry G, Cunnington D, Kronborg I. Central sleep apnea in stable methadone maintenance treatment patients. Chest. 2005;128(3):1348–56.
23. Webster LR, Grant BJB, Choi Y. Sleep apnea associated with methadone and benzodiazepine therapy [abstract]. Poster presented at the 22nd annual meeting of the American Academy of Pain Medicine (AAPM), San Diego, 2006.
24. White JM, Irvine RJ. Mechanisms of fatal opioid overdose. Addiction. 1999;94(7):961–72.
25. Santiago TV, Pugliese AC, Edelman NH. Control of breathing during methadone addiction. Am J Med. 1977;62(3):347–54.
26. Schwartz JK. The rule of double effect and its role in facilitating good end-of-life palliative care: a help or a hindrance? J Hosp Palliat Nurs. 2004;6(2):125–33.
27. Snelling PC. Consequences count: against absolutism at the end of life. J Adv Nurs. 2004;46(4):350–7.
28. McIntyre A. Doctrine of double effect. In: Edward NZ, editors. The stanford encyclopedia of philosophy. Summer 2006 ed. 2006. http://plato.stanford.edu/archives/sum2006/entries/double-effect/. Accessed August 20, 2012.
29. Patterson JR, Hodges MO. The rule of double effect [letter]. N Engl J Med. 1998;338(19):1389.
30. Cahana A. Is optimal pain relief always optimal? Bioethical considerations of interventional pain management at the end of life. Am Pain Soc Bull. 2002;12(3):1–4.
31. Webster LR. Methadone-related deaths. J Opioid Manag. 2005;1(4):211–7.

Failure to Treat Pain

Kenneth L. Kirsh, Steven D. Passik, and Ben A. Rich

Key Points

- Despite issues of misuse and abuse with opioid analgesics, pain continues to be undertreated and many barriers exist to proper access to pain care.
- In place of a pure disease model, there is a need to get back to incorporating issues of palliation into medicine in order to live up to the calling to reduce suffering.
- While there has been a trend towards under-prescribing controlled medications for pain out of fear of regulatory sanction, several cases have shown that undertreatment of pain can also be a cause for civil liability.
- The failure to treat pain is fundamentally a failure of empathy and prescribers need to acknowledge their own strengths and weaknesses in this area in an open and honest fashion.
- In addition to issues of empathy, prescribers need to be aware of social psychological phenomenon such as observer-subject bias and the psychoanalytic notion of projective identification when assessing and treating patients with chronic pain issues.

K.L. Kirsh, Ph.D. (✉)
Department of Behavioral Medicine, The Pain Treatment Center of the Bluegrass, 2416 Regency Rd, Lexington, KY 40503, USA
e-mail: doctorken@windstream.net

S.D. Passik, Ph.D.
Department of Psychology and Behavioral Sciences,
Memorial Sloan-Kettering Cancer Center, 641 Lexington Avenue,
7th Floor, New York, NY 10022, USA
e-mail: passiks@mskcc.org

B.A. Rich, JD, Ph.D.
School of Medicine Alumni Association Endowed Chair of Bioethics,
University of California, Davis School of Medicine, 4150 V Street,
Suite 2500, Sacramento, CA 95817, USA
e-mail: barich@ucdavis.edu

Introduction

Simply stated, there is an epidemic of undertreated pain, and it has been recognized as a major public health problem [1]. The question that begs to be answered, candidly and definitively, is how such a state of affairs could have developed at the very time when advances in medical science and technology offer a wide variety of pharmacological and non-pharmacological measures for the management of pain. The problem of undertreated pain is complex, and therefore, so too must be any plausible explanation of it.

Barriers to Effective Pain Management

The barriers to pain management are so well recognized by now that they might, somewhat pejoratively, be characterized as "the usual suspects" (see Table 25.1). With the advent of managed care, a barrier that has increased in significance is the lack of adequate reimbursement by third party payers for pain management [2]. There are also patient-centered barriers that, to a significant degree, mirror the clinician-related problems of ignorance and fear concerning the use of opioids in pain management [3]. Until recently, one might reasonably anticipate that patients would share such knowledge deficits since what they did know about pain management would be largely dependent upon what their clinicians could impart to them. However, with the rise of the internet, many patients now have access to a wealth of information on pain management that may or may not be within the working knowledge of the clinicians whom they encounter.

An elucidation of these barriers actually raises more questions than it answers. During a time when the ethical and legal debate over physician-assisted suicide came to a head in the 1990s, national health-care organizations (representing physicians, nurses, and other types of health-care professionals) insisted that the role of their professions was to treat

Table 25.1 Barriers to effective pain management

Inadequate clinical and continuing education on the assessment and management of pain
Insufficient understanding of the adverse clinical and psychological impact of undertreated pain on patients and their families, and consequently, a failure to make pain relief a priority in patient care
The virtual absence of monitoring of pain management by clinicians or accountability for demonstrable deficiencies in clinician knowledge, skills, and attitudes with regard to the assessment and management of pain
A regulatory environment that has historically been, and to a significant extent continues to be, hostile to appropriately aggressive pain management practices

Table 25.2 Comparison of the curative versus palliative model

Curative model	Palliative model
Analytic and rational	Humanistic and personal
Clinical puzzle solving	Patient as person
Mind-body dualism	Mind-body unity
Disvalues subjectivity	Privileges subjectivity
Biomedical model	Biocultural model
Discounts idiosyncrasy	Privileges idiosyncrasy
Death = failure	Unnecessary suffering = failure

disease and relieve suffering, not cause or hasten a patient's death [4]. Yet, just as the health professions were reaffirming their clinical priority and professional responsibility to relieve suffering, the clinical literature was documenting their manifest failure to do so [5]. This failure was not merely a phenomenon of rural, outpatient settings where a lack of state-of-the-art pain management strategies might be anticipated but in the citadels of the most prestigious academic medical centers [6]. Clearly, a major disconnect between the goals and aspirations of the health professions on the one hand, and the real life experience of patients on the other had been revealed. If, as the opponents of physician-assisted suicide maintained, virtually all pain can be safely and effectively managed, and doing so is one of the primary professional responsibilities of clinicians, then how could the previously identified barriers to effective pain management have produced this epidemic of undertreated pain?

The Culture of Medicine and the Culture of Pain

One response is that the prescriber's purported duty to relieve pain and suffering is much more rhetoric than a reflection of a genuinely felt sense of professional responsibility [7]. Twenty-five years ago, in a seminal article on the subject, Cassell wrote that the major goal of medicine is to reduce or relieve suffering [8]. Nearly 10 years later, he elaborated on this issue, stating that modern medicine largely fails to relieve suffering adequately [9].

A major issue involves the biomedical model of disease and the curative model of medical practice, which causes the prescriber to focus on the pathophysiology of disease rather than the patient's experience of illness. Unless and until clinicians can focus on the patient as person, rather than the body as the locus of a disease process, they cannot begin to address pain and suffering. The major problem posed by the curative model of medical practice is that its essential features stand in stark contrast, indeed, diametric opposition to those of the palliative model (see Table 25.2) [10].

In the curative paradigm, pain is a symptom of an underlying medical condition. Patient reports of pain constitute information that facilitates the diagnosis of the underlying condition and the formulation of a treatment plan. From this perspective, measures intended to reduce or possibly even eliminate the pain would be counterproductive, as they would (theoretically) deprive the clinician of potentially important information. This propensity to categorize pain as a clinical datum to be processed rather than a personal experience calling for a compassionate response by the clinician can itself exacerbate the problem by causing the patient to feel abandoned.

The Cultivation of Ignorance

The barrier of knowledge deficits on the part of clinicians in the assessment and management of pain has been documented in the clinical literature for decades [11]. These deficits can be directly linked to the virtual absence of pain management in the medical school curriculum [12]. This curricular void has produced not just knowledge deficits that clinicians themselves recognize but also myths and misinformation about the risks (especially addiction to opioid analgesics) and potential side effects of opioids that are perpetuated in the informal medical curriculum from one generation of physicians to another [13]. A clinician in the full grip of these pervasive myths and misinformation could, and commonly did, invoke the ancient medical maxim of primum non nocere as the moral basis for withholding opioid analgesics from patients who required them for pain relief.

The Proliferation of Fear

Surveys of physicians consistently reveal a high level of anxiety concerning regulatory oversight of their prescribing of opioid analgesics [14]. The primary fear factor has been a well-established pattern and practice of state medical boards of charging physicians with "overprescribing" pain medications, particularly opioid analgesics for patients with chronic nonmalignant pain [15]. More recently, physicians who treat large numbers of chronic nonmalignant pain patients have been increasingly made the targets of DEA (Drug Enforcement Administration) investigations and federal criminal prosecutions for "drug trafficking" [16]. In a host of guidelines and policy statements, physicians are admonished to balance a patient's need for opioid analgesics with their purported responsibility as prescribers to prevent drug abuse, diversion, and trafficking [17]. The combination of these factors perpetuated what one commentator has characterized as an "ethic of underprescribing" in the medical community [18]. Such an ethic, of course, runs counter to the ancient and core value of the medical profession concerning the relief of suffering.

The fear factor was significantly complicated when a few health-care institutions and professionals were held liable for substantial damages in civil actions alleging a failure to manage pain. The first such case was brought against a skilled nursing facility in North Carolina. The crux of the complaint was that a nursing administrator had discontinued a pain management regimen for an elderly patient with metastatic prostate cancer because she considered it to be excessive. A jury found the facility that employed her guilty of gross negligence and assessed compensatory and punitive damages in the amount of $15 million [19]. Ten years later, a California jury awarded damages of $1.5 million to the family of an elderly patient who died of lung cancer. The basis for the award was that the patient's pain had been ineffectively managed by the physician who had been responsible for his care during a 5-day hospitalization prior to his death [20]. This case achieved substantial national notoriety for a number of important reasons. First, because tort reform legislation in California precluded the recovery of damages in a medical malpractice suit for pain and suffering following the death of the patient, the civil action against the physician and hospital was brought under the state elder abuse statute, which allowed such a postmortem award. Second, prior to the litigation, the Medical Board of California had investigated a complaint against the physician by the patient's family. Its reviewing expert had found the physician's pain management to be inadequate, yet the board declined to take any disciplinary action. The stark contrast between how the board saw the case and how the jury saw the case seemed to epitomize the disparity noted much earlier by Cassell.

Such cases established what was, but should not have been, an entirely new precedent (i.e., liability of health-care institutions and professionals for undertreating pain). The underlying premise of these civil actions was quite straightforward – pain management is like any other aspect of patient care in that if it is done negligently or otherwise inappropriately; it can give rise to professional liability and the award of substantial monetary damages [21]. Such jury verdicts indicate that lay jurors take the clinician's responsibility to relieve pain and suffering very seriously. Similarly, state medical boards began to recognize that failure to properly manage a patient's pain might constitute unprofessional practice and thereby justify disciplinary action against a prescriber who had, in effect, subjected a patient to unnecessary pain or suffering. In 1999, Oregon became the first state to impose sanctions on a physician solely and exclusively for failure to properly manage the pain of several of his patients who were gravely ill or dying [22]. Subsequently, in 2003, the Medical Board of California pursued disciplinary action against a physician for failing to demonstrate in his care of an elderly patient dying of mesothelioma that he understood the nature and properties of some of the analgesics he prescribed for the patient [23]. Given the failure of the California Board to take any action in the case just 2 years earlier, this suggests a remarkable shift in attitude and approach to allegations of substandard pain management practice.

The Emerging Paradigm

Failure to appropriately assess and treat pain is now generally recognized as a form of substandard care and unprofessional practice. Many state medical board policies, and the model policy of the Federation of State Medical Licensing Boards, admonish physicians that effective pain management is an essential feature of quality patient care. Failure to provide such care, or to refer a patient to a clinician who can provide it, can constitute the basis for disciplinary action and/or malpractice liability. Organizations such as the American Academy of Pain Medicine and the American Pain Society, among others, have promulgated clinical practice guidelines to assist clinicians in fulfilling their responsibilities to all patients with pain. However, it would be presumptuous and overly simplistic to conclude that simply promulgating guidelines and promoting continuing professional education will magically remove the barriers to pain relief [24]. There are attitudes and ways of thinking in the culture of medicine and the health professions that contribute significantly to the problem of undertreated pain.

The Role of Empathy

The failure to treat pain is fundamentally a failure of empathy. From a clinical and psychological perspective, there are multiple pragmatic and psychological factors that argue against the ability of the health-care provider and the patient to relate to one another. If they could, it is hard to argue that the problem of undertreated pain would be of the magnitude that it has been, even when we take the previously mentioned barriers into account. Perhaps those involved in patient care will ultimately be better served if they simply learn to accept the fact that they are unable to rely solely on their empathy. While they may be, at their core, good caring people, this is not sufficient to make them competent or effective in the treatment of pain. Ultimately, the use of rating scales and aids that facilitate the objective measure of pain, and thereby communication about it, are the only hope in allowing for better, more empathic pain care. Ultimately, the souring of the regulatory and legal climates surrounding pain management creates fear, and fear widens the gulf between doctor and patient [25].

When students begin health-care training, it is easy to elicit from them expressions that their primary motivation for doing so is the desire to help people. What aspect of intervening in the care of another human being meets this criterion more readily than treating pain? When young medical trainees first enter their clinical rotations, they are psychologically very close to patients. A study of the content of the nightmares experienced by trainees revealed that residents at the beginning of training often find themselves in the patient role in a nightmare, such as being operated on without anesthesia [26]. It is important to make a marked distinction between this early form of sympathy, wherein a trainee over-identifies with the patient and the more appropriate level and skill of empathy, which entails putting oneself objectively in the viewpoint of another without taking on their emotional investment in the situation. Medical education provides the necessary distance to allow for empathy and perspective taking, as opposed to actually feeling the pain of the patient. This distance is probably necessary to allow physicians to do what they must do to other human beings in situations where, if there were too much emotional investment, perhaps it would be impossible to perform painful procedures. Thus, distance begins to develop, and by the end of training, residents' nightmares more commonly put them in the physician role. But is this distance good or bad thing when they are called upon to treat pain?

When we hear that older, non-white females have the highest likelihood of being undertreated for their cancer pain or that Hispanics are half as likely to receive pain medications in emergency rooms when they have the same long bone fractures as whites, are we to believe that medicine is ageist, racist, and sexist [27–29]? Or that in AIDS patients, being uneducated is a risk factor for poor pain care (along with a history of a substance abuse)? [30] Or is it possible – that in fields historically dominated by younger, educated, white men – that being different from your physician works against you somehow and drives the likelihood of their ability to empathize with your suffering even further underground?

These issues have perhaps been best studied in cancer. That the undertreatment of pain is a problem in oncology only reinforces the fact that the problem of undertreatment is even more profound in nonmalignant pain. In cancer clinics, studies have been done to examine how well oncologists and oncology nurses can intuit their patients' suffering. In studies of the agreement of patients' self report with reports given by

their professional caregivers about their estimations of the patients' pain, depression, and overall quality of life, agreement tends to occur for the lowest intensity of the symptom [31–34]. Thus, as long as the patients say that they are not in a lot of pain or are not too depressed or that there are no major problems in quality of life, their physicians and nurses agree with them. But when problems become more intense, the agreement falls off dramatically, leading to a marked tendency to underestimate the suffering of patients in many different facets.

Pragmatic Factors

There are many pragmatic considerations that detract from the experience of empathy for people in pain. They can be roughly categorized into system-related, patient-related, and professional-related barriers. The first, system-related barriers, includes time pressures created by the very brief time in which the physician and patient are in the room together and reimbursement issues that fail to adequately compensate the physician for treating pain and thereby lower attention to and interest in pain management [25, 35–38]. Second, patient-related barriers include the multiple fears patients harbor that inhibit them from aggressively and accurately reporting pain and suffering to their physicians – from the fear of addiction to fears of being a bad patient and fears of distracting the physician from the treatment of their primary disease to not wanting to acknowledge pain for fear that it may represent progression of disease [39]. These barriers lead to inhibited communication about pain, which in turn fails to provide the physician with the building blocks for empathy and concern. Beliefs such as "no news is good news" and "don't ask, don't tell" are quite common among patients. Finally, there are physician-related barriers, such as the failure to acquire adequate knowledge of pain assessment and management and the fear of regulatory oversight.

Unconscious Processes: The Mechanics of (Unempathic) Judgment

Cognitive and social psychologists have described numerous unconscious aspects of how humans make judgments that are out of awareness and have referred to these as the "mechanics of judgment" [40–44]. For example, when four items are randomly placed in four different positions, the item in the third position is preferred and chosen an inordinate number of times. This is not something people are generally aware of, yet it colors the perceptions of quality and preference. This use of subtle preferences and prototypes goes on out of conscious awareness. To what extent do physicians' judgments of pain and suffering in their patient, so important to the ability to empathize, fall victim to such mechanical aspects of the way humans think and make judgments? Are patients thought to be in pain or not, to require attention or not, because of processes that go on out of awareness for the person making the assessment? When one hears that there is a consistent inability to match the patient's assessment of their pain, depression, or quality of life, one might come to believe that the physician might be using a prototype of "what an outpatient with cancer feels" than what the individual patient sitting in front of them actually feels. This would be a fruitful avenue for further research.

Social psychologists have identified one such unconscious process that would seem most relevant to this discussion, namely, the observer-subject bias [45]. When one person looks at another's behavior and is asked to make a judgment about why that person is acting the way that they are, the observer is likely to posit a *characterological* explanation for the behavior (often termed the fundamental attribution error). On the other hand, when one is asked why they themselves are behaving in the way that they are, they tend to posit *situational* explanations (often termed the self-serving bias).

Unconscious Content

Is there unconscious sadism and hostility towards people in pain harbored by practitioners of medical and related disciplines that impede pain management? In classic papers on the undertreatment of pain, the insightful and brutally honest Sam Perry believed this to be the case [46, 47]. Are the pain patients who are nonresponsive to our ministrations actually thwarting our desires to help? Does this lead to engendering anger and sadistic impulses? Are patients who are seen to be "bringing their problems onto themselves," such as addicts and obese people, deserving of our scorn? If not, how do we explain the callous treatment they sometimes receive (i.e., carrying out painful procedures without the provision of adequate analgesia)? In a classic paper "Hate in the Counter-Transference," Winnicott [48] examines how patients who are depressed and self-destructive (like so many people in chronic pain) engender unconscious hate in their caregivers that can drive the patient into despair. Do people who have been the victims of abuse and neglect (like so many people in chronic pain) manage to unconsciously and unwittingly engage us in faulty caregiver scenarios that perpetuate more of the same? This process has been called projective identification by the psychoanalysts and is as germane to the care of people with pain as they are to psychoanalytic treatments of non-pain patients [49–51]. Yet psychoanalysts continually involve themselves in introspection and their own psychotherapy and supervision to examine themselves for such tendencies. Would all of us who treat patients benefit from doing the same?

Summary

The problem of undertreated pain can be solved. To do so, we need to address the medical and legal climates and the realities of a clinical situation that detract from empathic care. These realms are intricately tied to one another. In the end, professionals will need to accept the fact that, while they are caring people, there are too many barriers to the treatment of pain and the provision of empathic care that they simply cannot be overcome flying by the seats of our collective pants. We will have to accept our limitations and then work to overcome them with technologic and educational initiatives that promote communication and empathy such as screening tools and other aids.

References

1. Brenna SF, editor. Chronic pain: America's hidden epidemic. New York: Atheneum/SMI; 1978.
2. Hoffman DE. Pain management and palliative care in the era of managed care: issues for health insurers. J Law Med Ethics. 1998;26:267–89.
3. Bostrom M. Summary of the mayday fund survey: public attitudes about pain and analgesics. J Pain Symptom Manage. 1997;13: 166–8.
4. Quill TE, Lo B, Brock DW. Palliative options of last resort. JAMA. 1997;278:2099–104.
5. Cleeland CS, Gonin R, Hatfield AK, et al. Pain and it's treatment in outpatients with metastatic cancer. N Engl J Med. 1994;330: 592–6.
6. The SUPPORT Principal Investigators. A controlled trial to improve care for seriously ill hospitalized patients. JAMA. 1995;274:1591–8.
7. Foley KM. Pain relief into practice: rhetoric or reform? J Clin Oncol. 1995;13:2149–51.
8. Cassell EJ. The nature of suffering and the goals of medicine. N Engl J Med. 1982;306:639–45.
9. Cassell EJ. The nature of suffering and the goals of medicine. New York: Oxford University Press; 1991.
10. Fox E. Prominence of the curative model care, a residual problem. JAMA. 1997;278:761–3.
11. Von Roenn JH, et al. Physician attitudes and practice in cancer pain management. Ann Intern Med. 1993;119(2):121–6.
12. Weiner RS. An interview with John J. Boncia, M.D. Pain Pract. 1989;1:2.
13. Hill CS. When will adequate pain treatment be the norm? JAMA. 1995;274:1881–2.
14. Skelly FJ. Fear of sanctions limits prescribing pain drugs. Am Med News. 1994;15:19.
15. Hoover v. Agency for Health Care Administration, 676 So. 2d 1380 (Fla. Dist. Ct. App. 1996).
16. Brushwood DB. The chilling effect is no myth. Available at http://www.doctordeluca.com/Library/WOD/ChillingEffectNoMyth04.htm. Accessed on 13th July 2012.
17. Suthers JW. Professional Standards Committee of the Colorado Prescription Drug Abuse Task Force. Colorado Guidelines of Professional Practice for Controlled Substances. Denver, CO: Colorado Prescription Drug Abuse Task Force; 3rd ed. 1999.
18. Martino AM. In search of a new ethic for treating patients with chronic pain: what can medical boards do? J Law Med Ethics. 1998;26:332–49.

19. Estate of Henry James v. Hillhaven Corp., 89 CVS 64 (Super. Ct. Hertford Co., N.C. 1991).

20. Bergman v. Chin, M.D. No. H205732-1 (Cal. App. Dept. Super. Ct. Feb. 16, 1999).

21. Rich BA. A prescription for the pain: the emerging standard of care for pain management. William Mitchell Law Rev. 2000;26:1–91.

22. In the Matter of Paul A. Bilder, M.D. Stipulated Order. Oregon Board of Medical Examiners; 1999. Available at: http://www.drug-policy.org/docUploads/Bilder_v_Oregon_Stipulated_Order.pdf. Accessed on 13th July 2012.

23. Accusation of Eugene Whitney, M.D. Medical Board of California. Case No. 12-2002-133376. 2003.

24. Max MB. Improving outcomes of analgesic treatment: is education enough? Ann Intern Med. 1990;113(11):885–9.

25. Passik SD, Kirsh KL. Fear and loathing in the pain clinic. Pain Med. 2006;7(4):363–4.

26. Marcus ER. Medical student dreams about medical school: the unconscious developmental process of becoming a physician. Int J Psychoanal. 2003;84(Pt 2):367–86.

27. Cleeland CS. Undertreatment of cancer pain in elderly patients. JAMA. 1998;279(23):1914–5.

28. Cleeland CS, Gonin R, Baez L, Loehrer P, Pandya KJ. Pain and treatment of pain in minority patients with cancer. The Eastern Cooperative Oncology Group Minority Outpatient Pain Study. Ann Intern Med. 1997;127(9):813–6.

29. Todd KH, Samaroo N, Hoffman JR. Ethnicity as a risk factor for inadequate emergency department analgesia. JAMA. 1993;269(12):1537–9.

30. Breitbart W, Passik S, McDonald MV, Rosenfeld B, Smith M, Kaim M, Funesti-Esch J. Patient-related barriers to pain management in ambulatory AIDS patients. Pain. 1998;76(1–2):9–16.

31. Grossman SA, Sheidler VR, Swedeen K, Mucenski J, Piantadosi S. Correlation of patient and caregiver ratings of cancer pain. J Pain Symptom Manage. 1991;6(2):53–7.

32. Passik SD, McDonald M, Dugan W, Theobald D. Oncologists' recognition of depression in their patients with cancer. J Clin Oncol. 1998;16(4):1594–600.

33. McDonald M, Passik SD, Dugan W, Rosenfeld B, Theobald D, Edgerton S. Nurses' recognition of depression in their patients with cancer. Oncol Nurs Forum. 1999;26(3):593–9.

34. Fisch MJ, Titzer ML, Kristeller JL, Shen J, Loehrer PJ, Jung SH, Passik SD, Einhorn LH. Assessment of quality of life in outpatients with advanced cancer: the accuracy of clinician estimations and the relevance of spiritual well-being – a Hoosier Oncology Group Study. J Clin Oncol. 2003;21(14):2754–9.

35. Mechanic D, McAlpine DD, Rosenthal M. Are patients' office visits with physicians getting shorter? N Engl J Med. 2001;344(3):198–204.

36. Ohtaki S, Ohtaki T, Fetters MD. Doctor-patient communication: a comparison of the USA and Japan. Fam Pract. 2003;20(3):276–82.

37. Balkrishnan R, Hall MA, Mehrabi D, Chen GJ, Feldman SR, Fleischer Jr AB. Capitation payment, length of visit, and preventive services: evidence from a national sample of outpatient physicians. Am J Manag Care. 2002;8(4):332–40.

38. Joranson DE. Are health-care reimbursement policies a barrier to acute and cancer pain management? J Pain Symptom Manage. 1994;9(4):244–53.

39. Ward SE, Goldberg N, Miller-McCauley V, Mueller C, Nolan A, Pawlik-Plank D, Robbins A, Stormoen D, Weissman DE. Patient-related barriers to management of cancer pain. Pain. 1993;52(3):319–24.

40. Gati I, Tversky A. Weighting common and distinctive features in perceptual and conceptual judgments. Cognit Psychol. 1984;16(3):341–70.

41. Kahneman D. A perspective on judgment and choice: mapping bounded rationality. Am Psychol. 2003;58(9):697–720.

42. Kahneman D, Tversky A. On the reality of cognitive illusions. Psychol Rev. 1996;103(3):582–91; discussion 592–6.

43. Johnson-Laird PN, Girotto V, Legrenzi P. Reasoning from inconsistency to consistency. Psychol Rev. 2004;111(3):640–61.

44. Redelmeier DA, Koehler DJ, Liberman V, Tversky A. Probability judgement in medicine: discounting unspecified possibilities. Med Decis Making. 1995;15(3):227–30.

45. Haro JM, Kontodimas S, Negrin MA, Ratcliffe M, Suarez D, Windmeijer F. Methodological aspects in the assessment of treatment effects in observational health outcomes studies. Appl Health Econ Health Policy. 2006;5(1):11–25.

46. Perry SW. Irrational attitudes toward addicts and narcotics. Bull N Y Acad Med. 1985;61(8):706–27.

47. Perry SW. Undermedication for pain on a burn unit. Gen Hosp Psychiatry. 1984;6(4):308–16.

48. Winnicott DW. Counter-transference. III. Br J Med Psychol. 1960;33:17–21.

49. Rizq R. Ripley's Game: projective identification, emotional engagement, and the counselling psychologist. Psychol Psychother. 2005;78(Pt 4):449–64.

50. Waska R. Addictions and the quest to control the object. Am J Psychoanal. 2006;66(1):43–62.

51. Yahav R, Oz S. The relevance of psychodynamic psychotherapy to understanding therapist-patient sexual abuse and treatment of survivors. J Am Acad Psychoanal Dyn Psychiatry. 2006;34(2):303–31.

Index

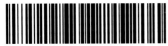

35261827R00195